Perioperative Safety

Perioperative Safety

Donna S. Watson, RN, MSN, CNOR, ARNP-BC
Senior Clinical Educator
Covidien Energy-Based Devices
Boulder, Colorado

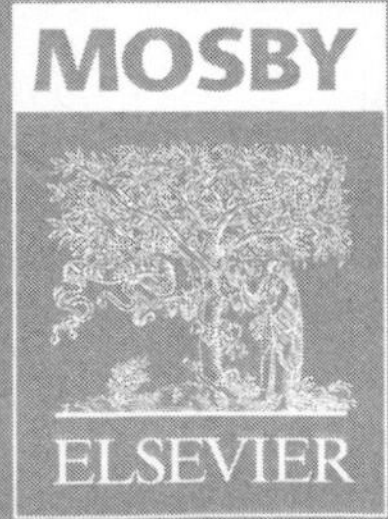

MOSBY
ELSEVIER

3251 Riverport Lane
St. Louis, Missouri 63043

PERIOPERATIVE SAFETY

ISBN: 978-0-323-06985-4

Notices

Knowledge and best practice in this field are constantly changing. As new research and experience broaden our understanding, changes in research methods, professional practices, or medical treatment may become necessary.

Practitioners and researchers must always rely on their own experience and knowledge in evaluating and using any information, methods, compounds, or experiments described herein. In using such information or methods, they should be mindful of their own safety and the safety of others, including parties for whom they have a professional responsibility.

With respect to any drug or pharmaceutical products identified, readers are advised to check the most current information provided (i) on procedures featured or (ii) by the manufacturer of each product to be administered to verify the recommended dose or formula, the method and duration of administration, and contraindications. It is the responsibility of practitioners, relying on their own experience and knowledge of their patients, to make diagnoses, to determine dosages and the best treatment for each individual patient, and to take all appropriate safety precautions.

To the fullest extent of the law, neither the Publisher nor the authors, contributors, or editors, assume any liability for any injury and/or damage to persons or property as a matter of products liability, negligence or otherwise, or from any use or operation of any methods, products, instructions, or ideas contained in the material herein.

Library of Congress Cataloging-in-Publication Data
Perioperative safety / [edited by] Donna S. Watson.
p. ; cm.
Includes bibliographical references and index.
ISBN 978-0-323-06985-4 (pbk. : alk. paper)
1. Surgical nursing—Safety measures. 2. Surgery—Safety measures. 3. Hospital patients—Safety measures. I. Watson, Donna, MSN.
[DNLM: 1. Perioperative Nursing—methods—United States. 2. Medical Errors—prevention & control—United States. 3. Perioperative Care—methods—United States. 4. Safety Management—methods—United States. WY 161 P4457 2011]
RD99.P47 2011
617'.02310289—dc22

2009052945

Acquisitions Editor: Tamara Myers
Associate Developmental Editor: Tina Kaemmerer
Publishing Services Manager: Anne Altepeter
Senior Project Manager: Doug Turner
Book Designer: Charlie Seibel

Printed in the United States of America

Last digit is the print number: 9 8 7 6 5 4 3 2 1

To my mother,

Linda S. Settle

Thank you for your sacrifices,
the support with the many life challenges,
my zest for life, and the goal to always succeed!

CONTRIBUTORS

Kelly H. Austin, MS
Certified Health Physicist
Dade Moeller & Associates
Gaithersburg, Maryland

Kay A. Ball, PhD, RN, CNOR, FAAN
Perioperative Consultant/Educator
K&D Medical Inc.
Lewis Center, Ohio

Jennifer S. Barnett, MSN, ARNP, FNP-BC, NP-C
Advanced Registered Nurse Practitioner
Cascade Vascular Associates
Tacoma, Washington

Sandra C. Garmon Bibb, DNSc, RN
Associate Professor and Chair
Department of Health, Risk, and Contingency Management
Department of Defense
Uniformed Services University of the Health Sciences
Bethesda, Maryland

Linda Brazen, MSN, BSN, RN, CNOR
Clinical Nurse Specialist/Educator
University of Colorado Hospital
Aurora, Colorado

Sandy L. Brown, RN
Registered Nurse
Franciscan Health System
Tacoma, Washington

Peggy Camp, MSN, BSN, RN
Division Clinical Resource Director
Hospital Corporation of America Supply Chain
Denver, Colorado

Lisa M. Cole, MSN, RN, CNOR
Perioperative Clinical Nurse Specialist
United States Air Force
Galveston, Texas

Alecia D. Cooper, MBA, RN, BS, CNOR
Senior Vice President of Clinical Services
Medline Industries
Mundelein, Illinois

Linda J. DeCarlo, MBA, MSN, RN, RNFA, CNOR, FNP-BC
Advanced Registered Nurse Practitioner
Northwest Vein Center
Gig Harbor, Washington

Reuben J. DeKastle, MSHA, BN, RN, CNOR
Clinical Educator
St. Luke's Health System
Boise, Idaho

Vangie Dennis, RN, CNOR, CMLSO
Clinical Manager
Gwinnett Medical Center
Duluth, Georgia

Laura D. DeSnoo, LTC Nurse Corps USA, MSN, RN, CNOR
Chief, Central Sterile Processing
Walter Reed Army Medical Center
Washington, District of Columbia

Deborah Dlugose, RN, CCRN, CRNA
President
Wright Professional Associates, Inc.
Oldsmar, Florida

Claire R. Everson, RN, CNOR, CCAP
Perioperative Clinical Educator
Banner Desert Medical Center
Mesa, Arizona

Debra L. Fawcett, PhD, RN
Manager
Infection Prevention & Control
Wishard Health Services
Indianapolis, Indiana

Jarrell Fox
Manager
Transfusion-Free Medicine and Surgery
Franciscan Health System
Tacoma, Washington

Allan Frankel, MD
Safety Faculty
Institute for Healthcare Improvement;
Principal and Clinical Co-Lead
Pascal Metrics
Washington, District of Columbia

Jill M. Garrett, RN, CPHQ
Perioperative Care Manager
Memorial Health System
Colorado Springs, Colorado

BradLee Goeckner, MSN, RN, LCDR, CNOR
Lieutenant Commander
Clinical Coordinator, Perioperative Clinical Specialist
United States Navy
Naval Medical Center
San Diego, California

Peter B. Graves, BSN, RN, CNOR
Senior Clinical Nurse
Molnlycke Health Care US, LLC
Norcross, Georgia

Rodney W. Hicks, PhD, RN, FNP-BC, FAANP, FAAN
Professor
UMC Health System Endowed Chair for Patient Safety
Texas Tech University Health Sciences Center
Lubbock, Texas

Aileen Killen, PhD, RN
Director
Patient Safety Program
Memorial Sloan-Kettering Cancer Center
New York, New York

Cecil King, MS, RN, CNOR, APRN
Clinical Educator
Perioperative Services
Cape Cod Hospital
Hyannis, Massachusetts

Beverly A. Kirchner, BSN, RN, CNOR, CASC
President
Genesee Associates, Inc.
Southlake, Texas

Michael W. Leonard, MD
Physician Leader for Patient Safety
Kaiser Permanente
Evergreen, Colorado

Sharon A. McNamara, MS, RN, CNOR
Director
Surgical Services
Wakemed Health and Hospitals
Raleigh, North Carolina

Elbridge A. Merritt, BSN, CNOR, CRCST, CHL
Chief, Central Material Supply
Landstuhl Regional Medical Center
Landstuhl, Germany

Jan Odom-Forren, PhD, MS, RN, CPAN, FAAN
Perianesthesia Consultant
Louisville, Kentucky;
Assistant Professor
College of Nursing
University of Kentucky
Lexington, Kentucky

Vivian M. Sersen, MSN, RN, CNOR, PCNS, CDR, NC, USN
Commander
Nurse Corps
United States Navy
National Naval Medical Center
Bethesda, Maryland

Anita Shoup, MSN, RN, CNOR
Perioperative Clinical Nurse Specialist
Swedish Medical Center;
Clinical Faculty
University of Washington
School of Nursing
Seattle, Washington

Brenda C. Ulmer, MN, RN, CNOR
Global Manager
Professional Education
Covidien Energy-Based Devices
Boulder, Colorado

Rebecca Vigil, RN
Registered Nurse
Franciscan Health System
Tacoma, Washington

V. Doreen Wagner, PhD, RN, CNOR
Assistant Professor
Kennesaw State University
Kennesaw, Georgia

Chasity Burrows Walters, MSN, RN
Patient Safety Facilitator
Memorial Sloan-Kettering Cancer Center
New York, New York

Linda J. Wanzer, MSN, RN, CNOR
Director
Perioperative Clinical Nurse Specialist Program
Department of Defense
Uniformed Services University of the Health Sciences
Bethesda, Maryland

REVIEWERS

Sheila L. Allen, RN, BSN, CNOR, CRNFA(E)
Clinical Educator/Consultant
Meeker, Colorado

Joy Don Baker, PhD, RN-BC, CNE, CNOR, NEA-BC
Associate Clinical Professor and Director
Distance Education
School of Nursing
University of Texas at Arlington
Arlington, Texas

Kay A. Ball, PhD, RN, CNOR, FAAN
Perioperative Consultant/Educator
K&D Medical Inc.
Lewis Center, Ohio

Barbara Bowen, MSN, RN, CRNP, CRNFA
President
Perioperative Consulting and Surgical Services, LLC
Collegeville, Pennsylvania

Larry Gene Burke, Jr., AAS, CST
Director of Surgical Technology
Augusta Technical College
Augusta, Georgia

Sharon M. Burns, EdD, CRNA
Associate Director/Associate Professor
Nurse Anesthesia Program
Midwestern University
Glendale, Arizona

Sheila L. Davis, AAS, CST
Surgical Technology Instructor
Temple College
Temple, Texas

Kathleen A. Gross, MSN, RN, BC, CRN
Registered Nurse
Owings Mills, Maryland

Charlotte L. Guglielmi, MA, BSN, RN, CNOR
Perioperative Nurse Specialist
Beth Israel Deaconess Medical Center
Boston, Massachusetts

Rachel Hottel, MSN, RN, CNOR
Advanced Practice Nurse
University of Iowa Hospitals and Clinics
Iowa City, Iowa

Julia Jackson, MEd, CST, FAST
Infection Control Practitioner
University of Michigan Health System
Ann Arbor, Michigan

Sherry M. Lawrence, MSN, RN, CNOR, ONC
Instructor
College of Nursing
University of South Alabama
Mobile, Alabama

Leigh W. Moore, MSN, RN, CNOR, CNE
Associate Professor
Nursing
Southside Virginia Community College
Alberta, Virginia

Janice A. Neil, PhD, RN
Associate Professor
East Carolina University
Greenville, North Carolina

Dorothy L. Nichols, BBA, RN, CNOR
Surgical Technology Program Director
Southern Union State Community College
Opelika, Alabama

Tera Pape, PhD, RN, CNOR
Associate Professor
Texas Woman's University
College of Nursing—Denton Campus
Denton, Texas

Patricia A. Pavlikowski, MA, BSE, RN, CST, CNOR
Program Director for Surgical Technology
Conemaugh Valley Memorial Hospital;
Adjunct Instructor
University of Pittsburgh at Johnstown
Johnstown, Pennsylvania

Leigh Ann Peteani-DiFusco, MSN, RN, CNOR
Clinical Nurse Specialist
Perioperative Complex
The Children's Hospital of Philadelphia
Philadelphia, Pennsylvania

Sarah Reidunn Pool, RN, MS
Resource Nurse Manager
Mayo Clinic
Rochester, Minnesota

Barbara Putrycus, MSN, RN
Director of Quality, Infection Control, and Regulatory Compliance
Surgical Services
Oakwood Hospital and Medical Center
Dearborn, Michigan

Catherine Napoli Rice, EdD, RN
Professor of Nursing
Western Connecticut State University
Danbury, Connecticut

Bernadette T. Higgins Roche, EdD, APN, CRNA
Administrative Director
Northshore University Health System
School of Nursing Anesthesia
Chicago, Illinois

Jacqueline Ross, MSN, RN, CPAN
Patient Safety Analyst
The Doctors Company
Napa, California

Paul St. Jacques, MD
Director of Perioperative Informatics
School of Medicine
Vanderbilt University
Nashville, Tennessee

Victoria Steelman, PhD, RN, CNOR, FAAN
Advanced Practice Nurse
University of Iowa Hospitals and Clinics
Iowa City, Iowa

Candace N. Taylor, BSN, RN, CPAN
Supervisor
Post Anesthesia Care Unit
Cedar Oaks Surgery Center
Warrensburg, Missouri

Denise Witt, MA, RN, CNOR, CST
Professor
Allied Health Science
Nassau Community College
Garden City, New York

PREFACE

The concept of health care safety and practice is not unique to any one discipline. Instead, it is the focus on safety that drives practice and unifies the various disciplines to work toward the common goal of personal, professional, and patient safety.

Throughout my career, I have collaborated with leaders in nursing and medicine who value their patients, the issue of safety, and individual contributions. These leaders all share defining characteristics that include the willingness to take risks to benefit the patient, to ask difficult questions that most would rather avoid, and to promote change toward a culture of patient safety that benefits the patient and the profession.

In 2002 and 2003, as the national president for the Association of periOperative Registered Nurses (AORN), I had the unique opportunity to work with many exceptional perioperative leaders and focus on a common goal for the AORN with the Patient Safety First initiative. Many leaders influenced this project as it evolved. However, I would like to recognize the initial thought leaders, who include then–AORN executive director, Tom Cooper; AORN president-elect, Betty Shultz; AORN vice president, Michelle Burke; AORN secretary, Sharon McNamara; AORN treasurer, William Duffy; AORN board members Lorraine Butler, Debra Fawcett, Paula Graling, Charlotte Guglielmi, Anita Jo Shoup, Debora Tanner, and Nathalie Walker; and sponsor of the Patient Safety First Initiative, Dan Sandel of Sandel Medical Industries.

My passion for and commitment to safety continues with this publication, *Perioperative Safety*. This book is written for the practicing perioperative registered nurse; however, it also has practical implications for nursing students, medical students, residents, interns, and industry health care representatives. *Perioperative Safety* includes concepts, principles, recommendations, and best practices that focus on patient and health care–worker safety. Each chapter is written by respected leaders in perioperative practice whose efforts continuously challenge the status quo to promote safety.

Unit I, "Overview of Perioperative Safety," reviews essential components of patient safety that focus on why systems continue to fail achieving the true attainment of a safe culture. Solutions focus on leadership engagement, team training, competency issues, and ideas that promote a just culture. National and local strategies that are proving to be effective in improving patient safety are also discussed.

Unit II, "Patient Safety," addresses by chapter some of the leading issues specific to patient safety; these include medication error, prevention of surgical fires, bloodless surgery and patient safety issues, moderate sedation, deep venous thrombosis prevention, foreign body mishaps and prevention, surgical site infections, positioning injuries, hypothermia, and electrosurgery. Each of these chapters provides an in-depth analysis of the issue, evidence-based research, and the recommendations for best practices to promote a safe environment. Each chapter also presents the most current information to assist with changing practices, updating policy and procedure, and increasing awareness to improve safety.

No publication on safety is complete without addressing the safety of the health care worker. Unit III, "Workplace Safety," provides an update on the most current information, with national and government recommendation on issues for health care–worker safety. Chapter topics include current workplace safety issues and trends, hazards from chronic exposure to surgical smoke, sharps injuries, laser risk, lumbar injuries, latex allergies, radiation exposure, infectious disease exposure, and dealing with abusive and disruptive behaviors. Each chapter reviews current recommendations and provides practical suggestions for implementation.

Unit IV, "Looking Ahead," discusses the challenges that are unique to the operating room with respect to technology and patient safety. Examples of policies and procedures developed in response to new technologies are presented. The final chapter is dedicated to suggestions on how to successfully implement and establish a culture of safety.

Perioperative Safety is written by leading experts in the field of perioperative practice, with the focus on safety of the patient and the health care worker. As such, this book is a must-have resource for any facility that is focusing on improving or enhancing a culture of safety with real solutions to actual safety problems and issues. It is my hope that this publication will be an impetus for every facility to renew its commitment to a solid culture of safety. A safe environment in which to work and to be treated will indeed positively affect the patient, the health care worker, and the community.

Special Thank You

Thank you to Tamara Myers (acquisitions editor) for believing in this project, and to Tina Kaemmerer (developmental editor) and Doug Turner (senior project manager) for maintaining the vision and focus of the book.

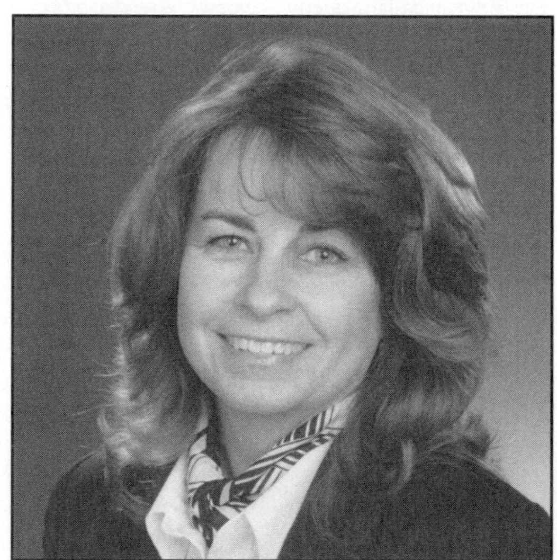

Donna S. Watson

CONTENTS

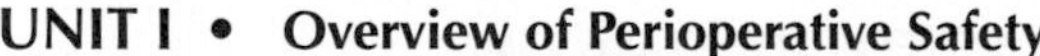

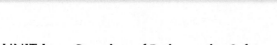

UNIT I • Overview of Perioperative Safety

ESSENTIAL COMPONENTS FOR A PATIENT SAFETY STRATEGY

Chapter 1

Allan Frankel, MD • Michael W. Leonard, MD

The safety of operating rooms depends largely on the professional and regulatory requirements that mandate skill levels, documentation standards, appropriate monitoring, and well-maintained equipment. Prescriptive and detailed protocols exist for almost every procedure performed, and although variation based on surgical and anesthesia preference is allowed, overall there is excellent management of the technical aspects. Experienced operating room physicians, nurses, and technicians come to rely on these operating room characteristics to support the delivery of safe care. Most practitioners, however, at some time have had the experience of working in suboptimal operating room conditions. This may be attributed to the level of procedural complexity in even the simplest of operative procedures when the level of complexity is not matched by the necessary team coordination, leadership engagement, or departmental perspective that encompasses all the prerequisites for reliable delivery of care. There are many causes for this current state, which include, depending on the country, the mechanisms for reimbursement that impede alignment of interests between physicians and hospitals (Ginsburg et al, 2007); the limited interdisciplinary training of the various disciplines (i.e., surgery, anesthesia, nursing, and technician), which promotes a hierarchical structure and undervalues core team characteristics; and the historical perceptions about the roles of physicians, nurses, and ancillary personnel, which have not kept pace with the changing nature of current health care delivery (Baker et al, 2005).

As far back as 1909, Ernest Avery Codman, a Boston orthopedic surgeon, openly challenged the then-current orthodoxy and proposed that Boston hospitals and physicians publicly share their clinical outcomes, complications, and harm. Wisely, he resigned his hospital position shortly before going public with this request, so he could not be thrown off the staff. Despite that, criticisms of him and his ideas were severe. Today his wishes are being realized across the United States at a rapidly accelerating pace (Mallon, 2000). The 1991 Harvard Practice Study, which evaluated errors in 30 hospitals in New York State, ultimately led to the now highly quoted number of 98,000 unnecessary deaths per year attributed to health care error. The Harvard Practice Study forced the health care industry to reflect on problems in patient care resulting in patient harm (Brennan et al, 1991; Leape et al, 1991). From these reflections a science of comprehensive patient safety has developed from disciplines such as engineering, cognitive psychology, and sociology. Combined with the increasing pace of electronic health record deployment, the movement toward demonstrable quality and value in medical care is advancing quickly.

THE CASE FOR SAFE AND RELIABLE HEALTH CARE

The 1991 Harvard Practice Study was the seminal article leading to the 1999 Institute of Medicine (IOM) report, *To Err Is Human* (Kohn et al, 2000), and that report has led to great public and business awareness of quality and safety problems in the health care industry. The media have fueled the public's interest, and businesses have formed advocacy groups, such as Leapfrog (Delbanco, 2004), to focus attention on this critical topic. The U.S. government program Medicare, with approximately $600 billion in annual spending, recently announced it would not pay for care resulting from medical errors (Centers for Medicare & Medicaid Services [CMS], 2008). Large private insurers are quickly following suit. Aetna just announced it will not pay for care related to the 28 "never events" defined by the National Quality Forum (Aetna Won't Pay, 2008).

Rapidly developing transparency in the market about safety and quality will be a major driver in health care change. Beth Israel Deaconess Hospital in Boston posts its quality measures on its Web site, including its recent Joint Commission accreditation survey (Beth Israel Deaconess Medical Center, 2008). New York Health and Hospitals, the largest public care system in the United States, has committed to following this example. The State of Minnesota publicly posts on the Internet all its hospitals' reported never events, such as wrong site surgeries and retained foreign objects during surgery (MDH Division of Health Policy, 2008). Several other states are quickly emulating this practice. Geisinger Clinic in Pennsylvania now offers a warranty on heart surgery (Ableson, 2007), in which specified complications are cared for without charge. Given the impressive care processes they have developed, this is a logical way to communicate their superior care and compete in the market. The successful hospitals and health systems in this new rapidly transparent market will be the ones that apply systematic solutions to enhance patient safety. Other bright spots in the systematic approaches taken by large care systems include Kaiser Permanente and Ascension in the areas of surgical and obstetric safety and through Institute for Healthcare Improvement (IHI) initiatives, such as the 100,000 Lives Campaign and the 5 Million Lives Campaign (IHI, 2008).

There has been a great deal of activity to improve the safety and quality of care since the IOM report. Currently there are pockets of excellence, but broadly there is much more work to do, and there are fundamental gaps in the quality and safety of health care. Well-intentioned projects and efforts to improve patient safety have met with variable results. Overall, however, in the absence of systematic, solutions-based approaches, health care organizations are unlikely to achieve sustained excellence in clinical safety and quality. This chapter describes the necessary elements for a comprehensive program to help ensure safe and reliable care for every patient every day. The surgical environment is an obvious one to which these programs should be applied, and perioperative nursing will play a significant role in shaping the efforts for patient safety and safe nursing practice.

THE OPERATING ROOM AS A SYSTEM

To begin, think of safety from an engineering perspective, which considers how safe a system is based on how reliably it produces its product or based on the frequency of its defects. Engineers think about the following:

- The reliability of achieving the desired outcome not just once but repeatedly
- Evaluating the processes leading to the desired outcome
- Analyzing in detail the indivisible steps that make up the process

In operating rooms the process has dozens and in some cases hundreds of sequential steps. The reliability of each of the steps (i.e., whether or not each step occurs as it should) determines whether or not the desired outcome will be achieved.

Ultimately, system safety and reliability are determined by the rate of defects in each step. When defect rates are multiplied, it becomes increasingly likely that they will lead to an undesired outcome. The result could, but will not always, be of clinical harm to patients. Patients may be fine, but the process nevertheless may have significant flaws that predispose patients to a greater-than-reasonable risk for harm. This is an indication that, although a current patient did not suffer an adverse event, the next patient might not be so lucky.

If the clinical perspective is combined with the engineer's viewpoint, a reliable operative procedure will see patients safely through because all of the steps in the processes have reliably small and known defect rates.

PROCESS STEPS

Consider that each step in the process is an individual and indivisible action. For example, the circulating nurse obtains the patient's chart before the procedure. The simple act of holding the chart in one's hands or reviewing the computerized patient record is a step in the process of evaluating a patient before beginning a surgical procedure.

Once a chart is available, there is a series of other steps that include identifying and confirming patient identification, review of current history and physical, confirmation of correct surgical consent, and other essential laboratory and clinical data as determined by the facility. These steps depend on several processes of their own, such as a secretary or assistant placing the chart in a convenient location and checking that the correct information is in the correct place. In the case of an electronic record, that may include steps such as making certain that the person collecting the data appropriately enters the information. Each of the process steps undertaken has its own failure rate and determines whether or not the information is present in the chart when it reaches the nurse.

Viewed from this perspective, any operative procedure performed in any location is made up of dozens to hundreds or thousands of steps. Each step taken has an intrinsic defect rate; some might be single steps, but many also will have associated processes that determine their defect rate. To the degree that each step's defect rate can be quantified, the safety of a system is measurable. The measure is not only whether the outcome is achieved, but also whether the processes may be replicated over and over again. To a large extent, safety is a system property determined by a system's reliability.

ACHIEVING RELIABILITY IN SYSTEMS

Operating rooms have done a remarkably good job of making themselves reliable and safe, albeit in a health care industry that has been slow to incorporate many key features of reliable systems (Cooper and Gaba, 2002). The Harvard anesthesia practice standards (Eichhorn et al, 1988), generated in the 1980s and adopted across the United States, are a shining example of standardization of anesthesia care that has helped improve the safety of the specialty. These standards identified minimum monitoring expectations now commonly used in every surgical procedure. They affect all of perioperative nursing and influenced the broad adoption of pulse oximetry and capnography.

Another rich source of reliability in operating rooms in the past has been promoting the interoperability of its practitioners. Although one anesthesia provider or nurse may begin a procedure, it has been likely that many other members in a department would be capable of replacing that person and might be called on to do so. This continues to be likely in many departments in which transfers of care occur daily. However, the limitations in interoperability are growing as equipment and surgical specialties become more specialized and require increasingly sophisticated knowledge of technique and machinery. The implications of increased specialization and technical complexity inevitably will influence decisions about caseload and case type regarding timing of cases, after-hours procedures, and, in all likelihood, credentialing of all operating room practitioners.

Reliability is feasible only when six interdependent factors are effectively integrated (Leonard et al, 2004a):

- An environment of continuous learning
- A just and fair culture (Marx 2001; Marx, 2003)
- An environment of enthusiasm for teamwork
- Leaders who are engaged in safety and reliability through the use of data (Frankel et al, 2003; Frankel et al, 2005)
- Effective flow of information
- Intelligent engagement of patients in their own care

Integration occurs only through concerted effort at multiple levels, starting with a goal, which takes precedence over all others, to achieve reliability. Organizations and departments that pursue greater reliability find that the end result positively influences patient care and employee satisfaction (Yates et al, 2004); it is obvious even to outside observers. To some extent this applies to all operating room practitioners as they arrive in a location to participate in a procedure. The initial reaction, that gut feeling about the quality of relationships and the safety of the environment, should be taken seriously, for it is likely to be a good barometer of the risk inherent in the environment (CMS, 2008).

AN ENVIRONMENT OF CONTINUOUS LEARNING

One example of a paradigm for a learning environment is Toyota Industries. It leads the auto industry in size and sales, and the enthusiasm of its car owners is well known. Toyota employees make suggestions for improving the work they do an average of 46 times per year and do so with the knowledge that a significant number of their suggestions will be tested and, if found worthy, adopted and spread. This process of applying the insights of the frontline workers to change and improvement applies not only to the production of Toyota's cars but also to the fundamental work of improvement itself (Spear, 2004). If a change in a procedure takes 1 month today, Toyota would be seeking ideas so that a year from now it could perform that change in 3 weeks. If Toyota receives 10 useful suggestions daily from a department, then 1 year from now its goal would be to receive 12 or 15. Toyota's perspective is that improvement is always feasible and there is always waste to be removed from its processes. The fact that in a prior quarter wasted effort and materials decreased as a result of focused improvement efforts is immaterial. There is, unrelentingly, always more to be achieved (Liker, 2004; Liker and Hoseus, 2008).

For decades, physicians and hospitals have had a guild relationship in which single physicians plied their trade within the walls of a hospital but with singularly insular perspectives. In the past 20 years a different health care industry has begun to emerge, built on a flood of hard evidence from randomized controlled clinical trials. Groups of clinicians are now providing service-line delivery across the spectrum of care-associated specific diseases (Ableson, 2007).

An environment of continuous learning in health care requires the presence of certain structural elements and the ability to execute ideas. The most basic structural element is the meeting of the clinical, unit-based leadership to consider information about unreliable events and decide on actions to remedy them (Mohr and Batalden, 2002). Surgical procedures will take place safely only in those clinical units whose leaders are able to orchestrate this process. Nursing must be an integral part of the leadership discussions in that unit. Multidisciplinary staff should meet on a regular basis to examine the straightforward operational issues in units, from items as specific as getting drugs to the right places in each room to the flow of patients through the entire suite.

The information collected at such meetings should be collated and evaluated so that remedies to any problems, potential problems, or concerns may be pursued. As in other industries with reputations for high reliability (Freiberg and Freiberg, 1998), listening to the front line and acting on their concerns is key to ensuring a safe process. This requires an environment or culture that makes it easy to bring problems to light and a teamwork structure that supports this process.

A JUST AND FAIR CULTURE

A just and fair culture in health care is one in which individuals fully appreciate that, although they are accountable for their actions, they will not be held accountable for system flaws (Reason, 1997; Marx, 2001). This culture provides a framework for looking at errors and adverse events to quickly and consistently determine if an individual nurse or physician involved in the event has behavioral or technical skill problems, whether or not he or she was set to fail by system flaw. This means evaluating the culpability of an individual after an error, accident, or adverse event by using a simple algorithm (Figure 1-1) that asks the following (Reason, 1997):

- Did the individual mean to cause harm?
- Did the individual come to work impaired (by drugs, alcohol, and so forth)?
- Did the individual follow reasonable rules that others who have similar knowledge and skills would have followed?
- Did the individual have a history of participating in or causing unsafe acts?

If the answers are, respectively, no, no, yes, and no, then no personal blame accrued. In this culture the organization believes that a reasonable mechanism exists to evaluate untoward events, regardless of the outcome of the event, and the organization acts accordingly. Implicit in this, and an extension of it, is that actions are evaluated based on what is best for patients and not on who is advocating the actions. Hierarchy, formal or informal, is not material in discussions of this sort.

When medication errors are being evaluated, the majority of the time the algorithm identifies capable conscientious individuals who are working in an unsafe system and on whom no blame should be placed. James Reason, who first articulated the algorithm described previously, is clear when describing his model that blaming individuals for events beyond their control does not fix a problem or make a system safer, although it might satisfy the patient's concerns or the legal issues about accountability. This model allows quickly separating individual issues from system ones. What is critical is creating a safe environment that

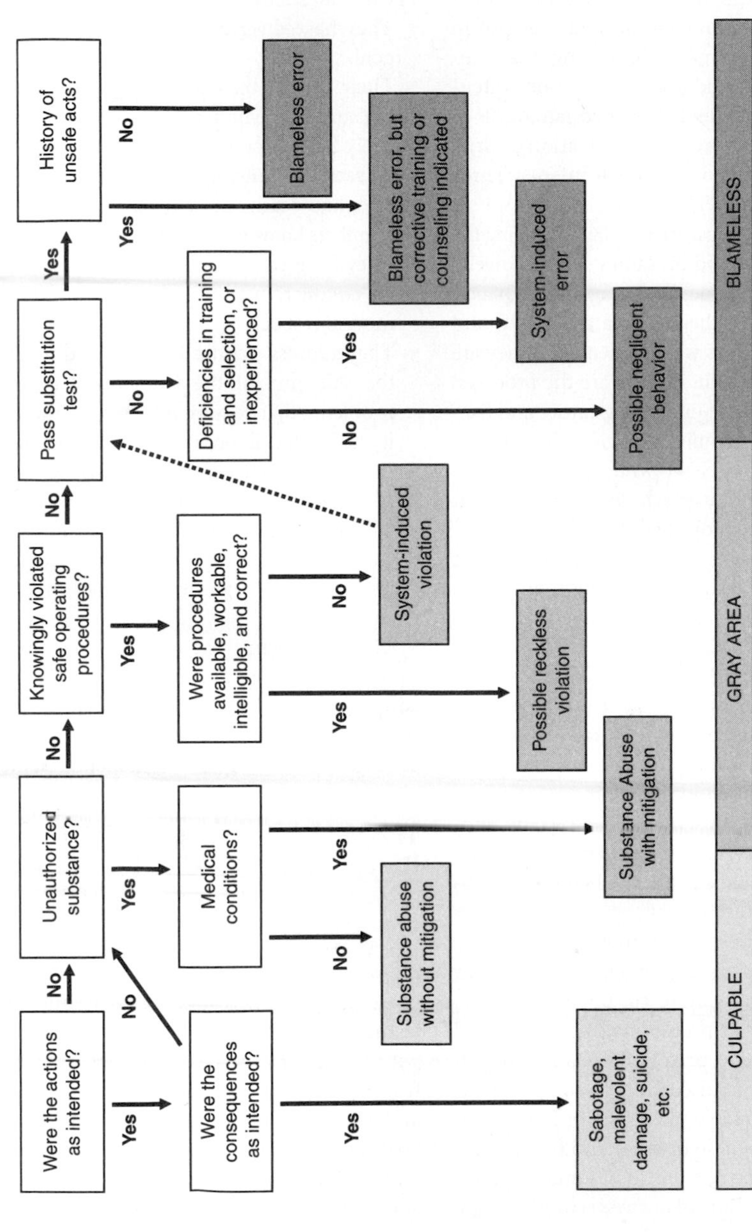

Figure 1-1 Reason's Simple Algorithm. (From Reason JT: *Managing the risks of organizational accidents*, Aldershot, Hampshire, England, and Brookfield, Vt, 1997, Ashgate.)

allows good nurses, physicians, and others to tell us when they make mistakes or have near misses.

Tragic examples highlight the need for this objective and clear evaluation mechanism, such as the overdoses in Indianapolis in 2006 of the blood thinner heparin. After the wrong concentration of heparin, 100 times too concentrated, was put in the automated pharmacy dispensing machine, nine very skilled individuals—six newborn intensive care unit nurses and three neonatologists—mistakenly took the wrong concentration of drug and administered it to very small infants. Three fatalities resulted (WRTV, 2008).

A similar episode occurred in 2007 involving the actor Dennis Quaid and his family in Los Angeles (Fox News, 2008). The media coverage of the Quaids' cases has highlighted their trauma as patients and the outrage that occurs when patients feel they are not being told the truth. Missing are the processes required to identify the underlying causes and fixes of these errors. They require an engineering and systematic approach that begins with an objective view of the events and from which flow insights about systematic flaws and individual culpability.

Thought leaders on both sides of the Atlantic have developed schema to address this topic. James Reason in the 1990s described his incident analysis tree (Reason, 1997). In the past decade David Marx developed his Just Culture Algorithm for evaluating the choices made by frontline providers, which incorporates and expands on Reason's work. In both cases the goal is to ensure appropriate accountability and an environment where every decision made by senior leadership and middle management is based on integrity and ethics.

In some serious patient injuries, there are contributing factors that are universally agreed upon. Other individual actions or events require careful analysis, teasing away bias or misconception, to arrive at a fair and just conclusion regarding culpability.

The advantage of promoting, nurturing, and supporting a climate perceived as fair is that it opens the door for discussion about problems and makes it acceptable to explore opportunities for improvement and to disagree and find resolution through testing and the quest for continuous improvement. A culture of fairness is fundamental to the implementation of a safe system. Every time a patient is brought into an operating room, the degree to which a fair and just culture is present in part determines the degree to which the environment supports the safety of the procedure.

THE GOOD HEALTH CARE TEAM

What is a good health care team? A good team is a group of interdependent individuals who have the following characteristics (Hackman, 1990; Pryor et al, 2006):

- They have diverse skills and share a common goal.
- Their output through synergy is greater than the sum of the individuals within the group.
- They have an appreciation of the roles played by each team member, including the leaders.
- They know each other's expertise so well that team members know where to turn to solve a problem.
- They have each agreed individually on norms of conduct, one of which is nonnegotiable mutual respect.
- They address technical problems directly using the skill mix of the team but face complex problems that require adaptation and flexibility through collaboration and open discussion.
- Individuals may express concerns without fear of retribution and know that their concerns will engender only two possible responses: their concerns will be acted on, or knowledge will be respectfully brought to light that mitigates the concern.

Excellent teams have team leaders who clarify the expected norms of conduct each time the team comes together. In addition to having agreed-on norms of conduct, outstanding teams have the added support of organizational endorsement.

TEAM LEADERS: THE CRITICAL ROLE OF LEADERSHIP

The active and committed engagement of executive and clinical leaders in systematically improving safety and quality is essential. One of the greatest challenges is aligning the frequently large number of strategic priorities in an organization with a simple, focused message that resonates with frontline clinicians caring for patients. Alignment and clarity of an organization's patient safety goals and work is critical. Senior leaders need to clearly communicate the priority of safe and reliable care and model these behaviors on a daily basis. Effective leaders continually reinforce the values and "this is the way we provide care within our organization." Excellent examples of how to do this well come from (1) the communication at Ascension Healthcare to everyone working in

of conduct, a series of predetermined steps should be followed that ultimately, and only if necessary, lead to the removal of that team member. For leaders to be effective this is essential.

Worthy of mention is Amy Edmondson's observations of operating room teams implementing what at the time was an innovative and new procedure—minimally invasive cardiac surgery (Edmondson and Wooley, 2003; Edmondson, 2004). The most effective groups were those for whom debriefing was a natural component of the ongoing minute-by-minute team function. This highlights the need for an environment that promotes continuous learning. It also serves to highlight the value of infrastructure that captures concerns and insights and takes action to ameliorate problems and concerns.

Determining how to make debriefings a natural part of clinical environments is not part of most clinicians' thinking. Most clinical environments are not configured to undertake debriefings primarily because there is insufficient appreciation of their value, a lack of understanding about how to do them efficiently, and incomplete knowledge of what to do with the information. Productivity-centered units and departments leave little to no time for even the briefest reflection. In fact, if time is taken to debrief, it usually is in the aftermath of a severe adverse event, and even then the debriefing is conducted in a manner not likely to generate the best results.

Evaluations of severe adverse events should be conducted as close as possible to the time of the event. After 24 hours, the minds of participants begin to fill in memory's blank or gray areas, reshaping the events to meet personal predispositions, to help protect oneself, or to explain away the uncomfortable (Schacter, 2001). Effective debriefing occurs at the most critical times only if it is practiced in the most mundane times, as in the debriefings that occur after a day's normal and successful activities. Daily, routine debriefings provide the opportunity to highlight the good work done by a team and nearly always create the opportunity to learn something about how to improve.

Operating rooms in the United Kingdom, United States, and Canada are experimenting with debriefing as part of team training efforts and through collaboratives run by the Institute for Healthcare Improvement (2008). Almost every site is struggling with aspects of the debriefing, beginning with the question of when to do them. Most of those who have been successful have settled on a debriefing process that occurs during general anesthesia, between the start of skin closure and patient emergence. There is no ideal time for debriefing to occur; however, during this time, all the operating room participants tend to be together, and usually there is a moment of stability and calm before the patient emerges. Remember that the debriefing discussion, if done well, can be as brief as 2 minutes. If well coordinated and if each member of the team understands its purpose, the debriefing can yield an extraordinary amount of information.

In a culture in which debriefing is fully developed and routinely practiced, members of the team might in real time notice aspects of the procedure that are worthy of mention and tuck them away until the debriefing takes place. The result is a rapid debriefing discussion about things that went exceptionally well and should be repeated, those that were problematic and need to be fixed, and insights that might be fodder for future improvement tests. In such a setting, because the team members are accustomed to the debriefing drill, they know who should speak first (usually the most junior member or the individual who has the least authority), and they know how to express the issues and in what order. There also is a person assigned the responsibility of collecting the same information on a form, which in a well-developed scenario is readily and easily accessible, and that individual—surgeon, nurse, technician, or anesthesia practitioner—knows where to deposit the form (Figure 1-2).

Team members also know that the form serves a useful purpose, that the comments noted on the form are evaluated by departmental leaders, and that the comments are taken seriously. They know this because they see changes take place as a result of the comments and because they receive direct feedback when a specific comment they have made is acted on. For that feedback to occur, the well-designed collection instrument has a place for individual names so that leaders know where the comments originate, which procedures are being commented on, and what time of day the comments are made. This does not mean that every form must have all of this information; if a provider decides to pick up a form and insert an anonymous comment, that is acceptable, too. The culture is one of fairness so that providers are not hesitant about adding their names to the concerns expressed by others.

Patient Label ____________________

Date ____________________

What did we do well?

- ☐
- ☐
- ☐

What could we have done better?

- ☐
- ☐
- ☐

Did we learn anything that we should take into account for the next procedure?

- ☐
- ☐
- ☐

Comments

Signature (Optional) ____________________

FIGURE 1-2 Sample debriefing form.

COMMUNICATION TECHNIQUES

Simple communication techniques increase the likelihood that transmission and reception of information occur accurately and in a timely fashion (Leonard et al, 2004b; Gandhi et al, 2005).

Closing the Loop

Closing the loop, also known as readback or hearback, is the simple technique of repeating back verbally what is requested or described in a manner that ensures accurate comprehension (Brown, 2004). It is one of the most fundamental communication safety techniques. In technical conversations, the process is simple. "I need furosemide 10 mg, please" receives a response of "furosemide 10 mg." Note that the hearback in this case does not have to include a "thank you" or any other reflexive social response. The agreed-on norm of conduct is a succinct repeat back devoid of extraneous words. Closing the loop in this way requires other agreed-on norms. For example, requests by a surgeon to a surgical technician for a particular instrument may require no verbal response if the placement of the instrument in the appropriate place is obvious (e.g., surgeon's hand). It is likely, however, that unusual requests always should have a closing of the loop to ensure mutual understanding.

Closing the loop is equally important in complex descriptions, such as the history of a patient during a handoff or when a surgeon is describing a patient and procedure to an anesthesiologist, anesthesia provider, nurse, or technician. Closing the loop in communication entails a brief readback of the information imparted to ensure the receiving practitioner understands what has been described.

Acronyms

A second communication form that promotes critical thinking and frames actions to be taken is the use of acronyms.

SBAR

One common acronym is SBAR (situation, background, assessment, recommendation) (AORN, 2009). In departments where SBAR is used extensively, individuals can frame the conversation by actually saying, "I'm going to give you an SBAR," thereby telegraphing to the recipient the order of the information about to be imparted. Table 1-1 gives some examples of the many ways to use an SBAR.

The ***s***ituation is equivalent to the headline in a newspaper. It should be brief, succinct, and capture the attention of the recipient. "The situation is that we've lost 300 mL of blood in the last few minutes" is an example of a clear and concerning situation statement.

Background follows in which slightly more expansive information is given to explain the situation. "The blood loss increased when the abdomen was open, after the retractor was tucked further under the liver, and you started to suction deep in the abdomen."

Assessment is the evaluation or critical thinking part and is one of SBAR's strengths in that it promotes the analysis of contributing and causative factors that may help all team members focus on the problem at hand. "This bleeding seems excessive. I don't know the problem, but I'm concerned." In and of itself the concern is

TABLE 1-1 Situation, Background, Assessment, Recommendation: Examples of SBARs

		EXAMPLES		
	Description	**Anesthesia Provider to Surgeon**	**Father to Teenage Daughter**	**Young RN to MD**
Situation	The 3-second "headline" to capture the intended recipient's attention	"The blood pressure dropped precipitously to 80/palpable when you moved the mesentery."	"You may not take the car this weekend."	"I'd like to give you an SBAR. Mrs. Jones seems confused today for the first time since I've worked with her."
Background	Descriptive information, the known facts and events	"The blood pressure was stable up to that point."	"Last weekend you came home an hour after we agreed was your curfew."	"I've cared for her all week, and she's always been pleasant and oriented. Her labs and vital signs are all normal."
Assessment	The transmitter's critical thinking, conclusion, or reason for concern	"I think the traction you're putting on the mesentery is causing a parasympathetic response and causing the BP to drop."	"You are not showing the kind of adult level of responsibility that I'd expect from someone who drives a car on weekend evenings."	"Something's happened to her. I don't know what it is, but I'm concerned."
Recommendation	Actions that appear reasonable to the transmitter in response to the situation and based on his or her assessment	"Please release the traction, and let's see what happens."	"If you can show greater responsibility this week, we can start again next week."	"Please, could you evaluate her? When will you be able to come, and what can I do until you arrive?"

BP, Blood pressure; *RN*, registered nurse.

enough to warrant the discussion and is a reasonable assessment if a team member's gut feeling is the only precipitant for the SBAR.

The ***r***ecommendation further drives critical thinking: "Are you looking for the source of bleeding, and should I call for blood to the OR?" The surgeon may know or see something that the nurse or anesthesia provider does not and at this point may add to or alter the suggested actions. Regardless, the SBAR format clarifies for all a structured process of thinking and information sharing. When done well, it also promotes learning.

I PASS the BATON

"I PASS the BATON" was created by the Department of Defense Patient Safety Program as part of *Healthcare Communications Toolkit to Improve Transitions in Care* (TeamSTEPPS, 2006). The mnemonic is intended to help practitioners remember important details in a handoff. ***I*** is the introduction, when a transmitter of information introduces himself or herself. ***P*** is the name of the patient, including other identifiers such as age, sex, and location. ***A*** is the assessment, identifying the procedure or the patient's problem, or how far the practitioner is in the process of caring for the patient. ***S*** is the situation, the current status of circumstances, areas of uncertainty, or recent changes. ***S*** stands for safety concerns, such as critical laboratory values or other critical reports, threats, or pitfalls. ***B*** stands for the background and includes comorbidities, previous episodes—whether hospitalizations or illnesses—current medications, and family history. ***A*** refers to the actions to be taken and a brief rationale for them. ***T*** stands for timing and might include the level of urgency, the explicit timing necessary, or a prioritization of action. ***O*** stands for ownership and identifies who is responsible, including individuals, a team, and also the patient and family members. ***N*** stands for next and includes anticipated changes or contingencies.

Mnemonics like I PASS the BATON may be useful in formalized handoffs, especially if visual cues are placed in the areas where handoffs occur. The challenge is teaching individuals to expect that communication will occur in this formalized fashion, so that the transmitter is comfortable framing the information in this way and the recipient expects to hear the information in a specific order.

The 5 P's

Standardizing handoff information using simple checklists ensures that important facts are routinely transmitted and lessens the likelihood of misunderstanding or errors of omission. The "5 P's," similar to I PASS the BATON, categorizes handoff information discretely to help the oncoming care providers know the key aspects of care. ***P***atient demographics are followed by an explanation of the ***p***lan of care. The ***p***urpose explains why the plan of care has been put into place and promotes critical thinking by the providers. Lastly, ***p***roblems and ***p***recautions identify the hurdles the care practitioner may encounter in achieving the plan. One organization, Sentara Health, reported significantly improved quality of handoffs by using this technique (Yates, 2004). However, as with I PASS the BATON, the categories' simplicity and elegance does not mean that the checklist is easy to implement. Concerted effort by departments is required to change practice patterns, and checklists like the 5 P's must be marketed by leadership as important and then tested and implemented by the frontline providers who will use them. Leadership engagement makes it clear that these efforts are strategic, and frontline engagement is critical to promoting a sense of ownership and control by involved caretakers. As with many aspects of team practice, the concepts are simple but can often be hard to implement.

Critical Language

The third communication technique is critical language, an agreed-on phrase that stops acti-vity, described in other industries as "stopping the line." When a team member perceives a risk and believes that there is limited time to address it, a critical phrase is a useful and powerful mechanism to gain attention of all team members and momentarily stop all activity. Agreeing on a term may help a junior team member overcome the hesitancy to speak up or the common problem of speaking up indirectly and possibly delaying needed quick action. Many obstetric units now use the term, "I need clarity," as the critical statement known to all team members; its use stops activity so that a group evaluation may be made of the perceived risk. In the obstetrics setting, when every patient is alert and aware and families are often in attendance, the term also is neutral so as to not cause unnecessary alarm.

The test of effective teams and leaders occurs not only when a concern is real, because then action is obvious and the team member who picked up the problem is congratulated, but also when a concern is inaccurate—this is when the real test of teamwork and leadership occurs. The response by other team members in the latter case determines the health of the team and whether the environment in the future will be a learning, supportive, and reliable one. Intolerance of team members when they speak up and are wrong is a sure mechanism to decrease the likelihood they will speak up in the future.

This should not be misconstrued as a requirement to tolerate mediocrity. If individuals repeatedly misunderstand or misrepresent a situation, then it is entirely possible that they need remediation or are in the wrong position. Well-functioning teams are cognizant of the difference between excellent evaluation of concerns that sometimes are wrong and incompetent evaluations that slow the team from doing its work. As long as the actions taken are appropriate, discussed openly, and pass a general test of reasonableness by team members, the environment for outstanding team practice will remain viable.

SITUATION AWARENESS AND CONFLICT RESOLUTION

Conflict is an intrinsic part of teamwork (Hackman, 1990). A team's synergy derives from the inputs of each team member and the ineffable combining of perspectives and efforts to produce a sum greater than the individual parts. The strength of a team comes from the ability to evaluate, reconcile, combine, and mesh these perspectives into a viewpoint that uses the best of all. Along the way, it is likely that team members occasionally will feel strongly—and differently—and find themselves in conflict about the team's plan. Much of the time these differences are grist for great relationships, and team members likely will appreciate the reconciliation process because it often is educational. Occasionally differences of opinion flare into disagreement, and the glue of the team membership is tested. At these times, hierarchy or strength of personality may determine the course of action rather than what is in the best interest of the patient. Formalized practices to manage conflict can help ensure that the best course of action prevails. An adage that is helpful is "The sun never sets on a disagreement between two team members." Departments should have a codified mechanism for conflict resolution, committed to by all team members, to sit down with those they argue with to resolve the issues as a regular and required course of daily action. This is a true test of leadership because many of the serious discussions in this setting are unlikely to be successful if left solely to the two team members who disagree. A moderator often is necessary, a leader who has the formal authority and the informal respect to facilitate a discussion that leads to resolution or clearing the air.

Norms of conduct about challenging team members can help in this regard, and rules of engagement can be agreed on as a departmental or organizational expectation. Members of the department must agree to abide by these constructs, and department leaders must be willing to censure those who do not follow them. An important part of making these conduct norms real is gaining open commitment by all department members that they will abide by them. This may entail public commitment in departmental meetings and the signing of a document in which the norms of conduct are described.

One challenge rule that has shown promise as a mechanism to resolve disagreements is a set of escalating challenges that, if they do not resolve the differences, lead to collaboration with others. One set is to use the words *curious, concerned, challenge,* and *collaborate.* If a team member is troubled by a course of action taken by another team member, he or she might say, "I'm curious why you've chosen this particular course of action." In departments where the challenge rules are understood, the recipient might realize that the team member addressing him or her has started a challenge process. If the response does not satisfy the team member's curiosity, he or she might next say, "I'm concerned about the course of action we're taking." This increases the challenge, and the recipient should now clearly appreciate that a negotiation needs to occur if a further challenge is to be avoided. If the response does not alleviate the concern, the team member may move up to the third level of challenge and say, "I'm not comfortable with this course of action, and I feel I have to challenge it." If circumstances permit, this challenge should lead to a set of prescribed actions, the primary one being involvement of a third party who has the expertise or objectivity to help resolve the difference of opinion. It may be necessary to identify who these arbiters are, although in some groups it may be adequate to call on any other member of the team to help.

The department would have to agree on a mechanism to help the two team members resolve their differences should an arbiter be unavailable. In some situations a decision needs to be made rapidly or no third person is available, for example, during middle-of-the-night emergency procedures. In that case, hierarchy or accountability for the patient may have to be the deciding factor, although departments might experiment with other, better solutions (a senior person is assigned responsibility for clinical and challenge situations, with the clear understanding that the threshold for calling is to be set at a very low level).

No solution takes into account every situation, but a formal and clear set of conduct norms pertaining to conflict resolution is essential to ensure that the inevitable deviation of behavior from norms is managed effectively.

LEADERS ENGAGED IN SAFETY AND RELIABILITY THROUGH THE USE OF DATA

The components of reliability and team practice that support safe care require leadership engagement before implementation. All leaders must understand the concepts well enough to explain them to others and must believe that they are important.

If there is agreement to move forward, education and practice are necessary for safety to flourish. Without ongoing practice, measurement, and continuous learning, the procedures described in this article are likely to be discontinued, even in departments that find them valuable. They consume some time and require a different paradigm than is current in health care today and a kind of reflection that many individuals avoid. Team excellence requires organizational and individual concentration.

If used wisely, a powerful tool that leaders will find essential is the measurement of safety culture within an operating room, hospital, or health care system. Evaluation of provider attitudes toward safety, teamwork, management, and improvement offers a valuable perspective on the strengths and weaknesses of specific clinical care areas and the relationships between care providers. Further, if they cannot be measured, how can they be managed? The Safety Attitudes Questionnaire (Sexton et al, 2006) is one validated instrument that has been used in more than 2000 hospitals. Hospitals can measure safety culture at a clinical unit level and then map these units and compare them with specific high-risk clinical areas: obstetrics, surgery, critical care, emergency medicine, oncology, and areas identified by claims and injury within the hospital from its own data. Interventions in each clinical unit then can be chosen to strengthen specific weaknesses, and safety culture can be tracked over time, in combination with other operational or outcome measures, to follow improvement. Between safety culture and direct observation—another measurement tool becoming increasingly well understood—organizations now have powerful tools to engage clinical teams in constructive dialogue about their strengths in and barriers to delivering optimal care. Feeding back this information is a powerful driver to help improve team cultures over time. The development of Web-based platforms to allow easy safety culture data entry, analysis, and report generation is an active area of interest and research. In the coming years, health care and health care culture, like every other sector, will become ever more illuminated by metrics.

HEALTH LITERACY

Health literacy is the ability of patients and their families to understand the process and goals of their medical care. Awareness of and consistent approaches to this issue can have a huge impact on the quality and safety of clinical care. There are five levels of health literacy. Virtually all the readers of this chapter are level 5—quite literate. Approximately 20% of the U.S. population is level 1, which means they have a difficult time reading the headlines of a newspaper. Many others are level 2, which means they have difficulty reading a bar graph, interpreting a bus schedule, or understanding a pie chart on the front page of *USA Today*. In major metropolitan U.S. markets, 40% to 70% of the population is literacy level 2 or below. They are seriously at risk for having lower health status and increased costs.

Some simple, effective tools are available through the American Medical Association (NIFL, 2002). The first technique is Ask Me 3 (Mika et al, 2007), which means that every patient and his or her family members should leave a medical encounter with knowledge of three key aspects of the patient's care:

1. What is my basic medical or surgical problem?
2. Why is it important I know this?
3. What needs to happen for me to get better?

The second technique is called a teach-back. Instead of asking patients, "Do you know what we talked about?" and having them politely nod their heads whether they understand or not (and often they do not), we now ask, "You've heard us talk about this; please take a moment and tell me how you'll explain this to your family." This closed-loop technique greatly increases the chances that patients and their families actually do understand the process and goals of their medical care. This technique is easily implemented. Individuals at the Iowa Healthcare Collaborative (2009) have developed one of the most comprehensive implementation programs on health literacy. The program includes systematic training for all clinical staff, during which patients who have had literacy issues share their stories with clinical staff.

DISCLOSING UNANTICIPATED ADVERSE EVENTS AND JUST CULTURE

An ethical environment that is considered just and fair also must include the ability to have honest, open conversations with patients and their families in the aftermath of an adverse event. Most physicians, nurses, and hospital leaders traditionally have had little or no formal training in having these difficult conversations during major life experiences for vulnerable patients. There is an increasing body of evidence that having skilled individuals facilitate open, honest discussions after an adverse event not only provides much better care but also greatly reduces the risk for lawsuits (Gallagher and Levinson, 2005; Browning et al, 2007; Gallagher et al, 2007).

COPIC, the largest malpractice carrier in Colorado, has had an early intervention program for the past several years through which premium reductions are the incentive for physicians to report within 24 hours any adverse event or negative patient interaction. COPIC then uses skilled personnel to reach out directly to patients and their families to see how they can help support and, when feasible, resolve the situation. These personnel are trained to be supportive, to ensure that the patients believe they have a straightforward ally to work with and that they will not be abandoned by their health care provider as a result of the disagreement or mishap. If patients want an attorney, they have to drop out of the program. COPIC has resolved more than 3000 cases, writing a check to one in four patients for an average of approximately $5000. Only seven patients have dropped out and retained lawyers; two have filed lawsuits (Berlinger, 2005).

Kaiser Permanente has a national ombudsman mediator program adopted from the National Naval Medical Center in Bethesda, Maryland. There are trained ombudsman mediators in almost all Kaiser hospitals whose job is to take care of clinicians, patients, and their family members following an adverse outcome. These individuals report directly to the chief executive officer in each hospital and centrally to Kaiser Risk Management to ensure clarity of reporting and to minimize the likelihood that their actions will be influenced by the priorities of hospital departments. Their goal is to be an impartial advocate so that those involved can engage in a productive dialogue that helps resolve the issues. This program has been well received by all participants, and early indications are that it probably helps reduce claims.

CONCLUSION

For many reasons, health care overall has been slow to adopt the reliability engineering well known for decades to other industries. National health care systems have their own reasons, and in each there are confounding factors that blind leadership, physicians, and nurses to many of the concepts listed. In the United States the primary problem is in the methods of reimbursement because payment has been unrelated to quality or safety (Lee et al, 1990).

Although prescient and leading-edge health systems are moving forward, significant parts of the U.S. health system have not begun this process. However, the general trend is likely to favor those who adapt to the new paradigm. Because outcomes are now measurable, benchmarking increasingly is associated with pay or performance, and increasingly well-coordinated consumers favors well-organized and forward-thinking groups.

Comprehensive patient safety and quality solutions share fundamental principles. They tend to require a holistic framework that is part of a core strategy, a carefully constructed structural framework that matches the strategic goals, and execution at a variety of levels.

First, changing the culture of patient safety through leadership engagement and team training ensures that people across hospitals and health care systems are more likely to achieve the goals required for safe and reliable care. The success of technology implementation is equally dependent on effective leadership engagement and teamwork, and, if well implemented, these efforts go further than improving safety and technology; they mitigate clinical, operational, and financial risk by improving organizational ability to make all types of needed changes.

Second, healthy patient safety solutions should be measurable, unit specific, dynamic, and risk adjusted. Cultural assessment, measures obtained through direct observation, and actions tracked as a component of learning-to-action cycles all aid in assessing the patient safety milieu.

Third, all our work is for patients and should be patient focused. Patients must be considered team members and, to ensure comprehension of their clinical problems, health literacy concepts must be applied. At the same time, they are our patients—which requires effective disclosure policies to support them and clinicians when care goes wrong.

Fourth, the ideal approach in managing cost-effective safety programs is to deliver the best in clinical practice and scientific rigor in a manner that adjusts across large organizations and networks. The only way to ensure ongoing improvement is knowing how to spread change in a standardized manner where providers, through cycles of learning, can speak up about their insights and concerns and see actions generated as a result. A just culture increases the likelihood that individuals will speak up.

And, fifth, because changing culture demands judgment and takes time, programs that draw on leading clinical expertise and sustainable operational modeling are likely to deliver safe and reliable care, especially when flourishing under the disciplines of ongoing assessment, action, and accountability.

Increasingly, precise invasive treatments performed as part of prescriptive protocols achieve, when performed well, targeted and reliable results. This trend ensures increasing operating room complexity. A culture of reliability is not optional, it is essential, and today we have the knowledge to achieve it.

REFERENCES

Ableson R: In bid for better care, surgery with a warranty, *New York Times*, 2007, available at http://www.nytimes.com/2007/05/17/business/17quality.html. Accessed July 23, 2008.

Aetna won't pay for never events: *Wall Street Journal*, 2008, available at http://online.wsj.com/article/SB120035439914089727.html. Accessed January 15, 2008.

Association of periOperative Registered Nurses: "Hand-off" tool kit to improve transitions in care within the perioperative environment, available at http://www.aorn.org/docs_assets/55B250E0-9779-5C0D-1DDC8177C9B4C8EB/44F40E88-17A4-49A8-86B64CAA80F91765/HandOff_Executive.pdf. Accessed August 2, 2009.

Baker DP, et al: The role of teamwork in the professional education of physicians: current status and assessment recommendations, *Jt Comm J Qual Patient Saf* 31:185–202, 2005.

Berlinger N: *After harm: medical error and the ethics of forgiveness*, Baltimore, 2005, Johns Hopkins University Press.

Beth Israel Deaconess Medical Center: *Our awards & recognition: Beth Israel Deaconess Medical Center—Boston, hospital, quality, awards, recognition, best hospital, safety*, 2008, available at http://www.bidmc.harvard.edu/display.asp?node_id=8345. Accessed July 23, 2008.

Bohmer RM, Edmondson AC: Organizational learning in health care, *Health Forum J* 44:32–35, 2001.

Brennan TA, et al: Incidence of adverse events and negligence in hospitalized patients: results of the Harvard Medical Practice Study I, *N Engl J Med* 324:370–376, 1991.

Brown JP: Closing the communication loop: using readback/hearback to support patient safety, *Jt Comm J Qual Saf* 30(8):460–464, 2004.

Browning DM, et al: Difficult conversations in health care: cultivating relational learning to address the hidden curriculum, *Acad Med* 82:905–913, 2007.

Centers for Medicare & Medicaid Services: *Eliminating serious, preventable, and costly medical errors—never events*, available at http://www.cms.hhs.gov/apps/media/press/factsheet.asp?Counter=1863&;;intNumPerPage=10&checkDate=&checkKey=&srchType=1&numDays=3500&srchOpt=0&srchData=&keywordType=All&chkNewsType=6&intPage=&showAll=&pYear=&year=&desc=false&cboOrder=date. Accessed July 23, 2008.

Collins J: *Good to great: why some companies make the leap—and others don't*, London, 2001, Random House Business Books.

Cooper JB, Gaba D: No myth: anesthesia is a model for addressing patient safety, *Anesthesiology* 97:1335 1337, 2002.

Davidson JH: *The committed enterprise*, Oxford, 2002, Butterworth-Heinemann.

Delbanco SF, Suzanne: Delbanco on the Leapfrog Group and employer purchasing power, interview by Pamela K. Scarrow, *J Healthc Qual* 26:18–21, 2004.

Edmondson AC: Learning from failure in health care: frequent opportunities, pervasive barriers, *Qual Saf Health Care* 13(Suppl 2):ii3–ii9, 2004.

Edmondson AC, Wooley AW: Understanding outcomes of organizational learning interventions. In Easterby-Smith M, Lyles MA, editors: *The Blackwell handbook of organizational learning and knowledge management*, Blackwell handbooks in management, Weinheim, Germany, 2003, Wiley-Blackwell.

Eichhorn JH, et al: Anesthesia practice standards at Harvard: a review, *J Clin Anesth* 1:55–65, 1988.

Ericsson KA: *The Cambridge handbook of expertise and expert performance*, Cambridge, England, 2006, Cambridge University Press.

Fox News: *Dennis Quaid's twins among three newborns given drug overdose*, available at http://www.foxnews.com/story/0,2933,312357,00.html. Accessed July 23, 2008.

Frankel A, et al: Patient safety leadership walkrounds, *Jt Comm J Qual Saf* 29:16–26, 2003.

Frankel A, et al: Patient safety leadership walkrounds at Partners Healthcare: learning from implementation, *Jt Comm J Qual Patient Saf* 31:423–437, 2005.

Freiberg K, Freiberg J: *Nuts! Southwest airlines' crazy recipe for business and personal success*, New York, 1998, Broadway Books.

Gallagher TH, Levinson W: Disclosing harmful medical errors to patients: a time for professional action, *Arch Intern Med* 165:1819–1824, 2005.

Gallagher TH, et al: Disclosing harmful medical errors to patients, *N Engl J Med* 356:2713–2719, 2007.

Gandhi TK, et al: Closing the loop: follow-up and feedback in a patient safety program, *Jt Comm J Qual Patient Saf* 31:614–621, 2005.

Ginsburg PB, et al: Distorted payment system undermines business case for health quality and efficiency gains, *Issue Brief Cent Stud Health Syst Change* 112:1–4, 2007.

Hackman JR: *Groups that work (and those that don't): creating conditions for effective teamwork*, San Francisco, 1990, Jossey-Bass.

Heifetz RA: *Leadership without easy answers*, Cambridge, Mass, 1994, Belknap Press of Harvard University Press.

Helmreich RL, et al: The evolution of crew resource management training in commercial aviation, *Int J Aviat Psychol* 9:19–32, 1999.

Institute for Healthcare Improvement (website): http://www.ihi.org/ihi. Accessed July 23, 2008.

Iowa Healthcare Collaborative: *Health literacy*, available at http://www.ihconline.org/toolkits/healthliteracy.cfm. Accessed August 3, 2009.

Kohn LT, et al: *To err is human: building a safer health system*, Washington, DC, 2000, National Academy Press.

Leape LL, et al: The nature of adverse events in hospitalized patients: results of the Harvard Medical Practice Study II, *N Engl J Med* 324:377–384, 1991.

Lee PR, et al: Physician payment reform: an idea whose time has come, *Med Care Rev* 47:137–163, 1990.

Leonard M, et al: *Achieving safe and reliable healthcare: strategies and solutions (management series)*, Chicago, 2004a, Health Administration Press.

Leonard M, et al: The human factor: the critical importance of effective teamwork and communication in providing safe care, *Qual Saf Health Care* 13(Suppl 1):i85–i90, 2004b.

Liker JK: *The Toyota way: 14 management principles from the world's greatest manufacturer*, New York, 2004, McGraw-Hill.

Liker JK, Hoseus M, Center for Quality People and Organizations: *Toyota culture: the heart and soul of the Toyota way*, New York, 2008, McGraw-Hill.

Mallon B: *Ernest Amory Codman: the end result of a life in medicine*, Philadelphia, 2000, Saunders.

Marks MA, et al: Performance implications of leader briefings and team-interaction training for team adaptation to novel environments, *J Appl Psychol* 85:971–986, 2000.

Marx D: *Patient safety and the "just culture": a primer for health care executives*, New York, 2001, Columbia University Copyright 2008 by the Trustees of Columbia University in the City of New York.

Marx D: How building a "just culture" helps an organization learn from errors, *OR Manager* 19(1):14–15, 2003.

MDH Division of Health Policy: *Adverse health events reporting law: Minnesota's 28 reportable events—Minnesota Dept. of Health*, 2008, available at http://www.health.state.mn.us/patientsafety/ae/adverse27events.html. Accessed July 23, 2008.

Mika VS, et al: Ask me 3: improving communication in a Hispanic pediatric outpatient practice, *Am J Health Behav* 31(Suppl 1):S115–S121, 2007.

Mohr JJ, Batalden PB: Improving safety on the front lines: the role of clinical microsystems, *Qual Saf Health Care* 11:45–50, 2002.

NIFL-HEALTH 2002: *[NIFL-HEALTH:3700] re: AMA's health literacy*, 2002, available at http://www.nifl.gov/nifl-health/2002/0197.html. Accessed July 23, 2008.

Pryor DB, et al: The clinical transformation of Ascension Health: eliminating all preventable injuries and deaths, *Jt Comm J Qual Patient Saf* 32:299–308, 2006.

Reason JT: *Managing the risks of organizational accidents*, Aldershot, Hampshire, England, and Brookfield, Vt, 1997, Ashgate.

Roberto MA, et al: Facing ambiguous threats, *Harv Bus Rev* 84:106–113, 2006.

Schacter DL: *The seven sins of memory: how the mind forgets and remembers*, Boston, 2001, Houghton Mifflin.

Sexton JB, et al: The safety attitudes questionnaire: psychometric properties, benchmarking data, and emerging research, *BMC Health Serv Res* 6:44, 2006.

Spear SJ: Learning to lead at Toyota, *Harv Bus Rev* 82:78–86, 2004.

TeamSTEPPS multimedia resource kit [TeamSTEPPS: Team strategies and tool to enhance performance and patient safety, developed by the Department of Defense and published by the Agency for Healthcare Research and Quality], AHRQ Publication No. 06-0020-3, Rockville, Md, 2006, Agency for Healthcare Research and Quality, available at http://teamstepps.ahrq.gov/index.htm. Accessed August 2, 2009.

The Joint Commission: *Universal protocol for preventing wrong site, wrong procedure, and wrong person surgery*, Oakbrook Terrace, IL, 2003, The Joint Commission, available at http://www.jointcommission.org/NR/rdonlyres/E3C600EB-043B-4E86-B04E-CA4A89AD5433/0/universal_protocol.pdf. Accessed October 2, 2009.

WRTV, Indianapolis: *Family wants medicine label changed after preemie deaths—staying healthy news story*, 2008, available at http://www.theindychannel.com/health/9903031/detail.html. Accessed July 23, 2008.

Yates G: *Sentara Healthcare*. In Panel 1—Promising quality improvement initiatives: reports from the field, AHRQ summit—Improving health care quality for all Americans: celebrating success, measuring progress, moving forward, Washington, DC, 2004.

Yates GR, et al: Sentara Norfolk General Hospital: accelerating improvement by focusing on building a culture of safety, *Jt Comm J Qual Saf* 30:534–542, 2004.

INITIATIVES TO IMPROVE PATIENT SAFETY

Alecia Cooper, MBA, RN, BS, CNOR

The United States faces a paradoxical health care situation. On the one hand, the level of care available, at least at certain facilities, is among the best in the world, and many major medical breakthroughs and innovations occur in the United States. On the other hand, the U.S. health care system is dysfunctional to the point that justifiable concerns are being raised about patient safety. Approximately 15 million incidents of medical harm occur each year, averaging 40,000 such events a day (Institute for Healthcare Improvement, 2009b). In a large study (n = 44,000) of operations performed between 1977 and 1990, it was found that 5.4% of all surgical patients suffered complications, nearly half of which were attributable to error (Kohn et al, 2000). It has been found that 40% to 60% of surgical site infections are preventable and that antibiotics are overused, underused, misused, or used at the wrong time in 25% to 50% of all operations. The result is that as many as 13,027 perioperative deaths and 271,055 surgical complications could have been prevented (Kanter, 2007). A 2007 study found that hospital-acquired infections were associated with 99,000 deaths (Klevens, 2007). A well-known 1999 report stated that medical errors cost the U.S. health care system between $17 billion and $29 billion (Kohn et al, 2000). The full extent of the problem is so vast that it has not yet been rigorously quantified.

DEFINING HEALTH CARE

One of the first challenges in addressing safety in U.S. health care is that there may not be a uniform way to define "U.S. health care." The *Dartmouth Atlas*, published by the Dartmouth Institute for Health Policy and Clinical Practice, found U.S. health care is "remarkably uneven," with wide variations in the frequency of primary care, visits to medical specialists, hospitalization rates, and other characteristics (Wennenberg et al, 2008). These variations challenge popular assumptions about health care. At first glance, one is tempted to make a lot of assumptions that the *Dartmouth Atlas* subsequently refutes. For instance, facilities that spend more on care do not necessarily deliver better care. Conversely, some of the best care in the United States is provided by lower-cost providers. It might seem reasonable to assume that different severities of illness are reflected in different spending levels, but that is also not the case. Therein lies the heart of the issue: high costs are more indicative of quality and safety issues than higher levels of care (Wennenberg et al, 2008).

HEALTH CARE COSTS

In discussing why care costs much more at certain institutions, the *Dartmouth Atlas* attributes such variations to supply-sensitive care, in which the supply of a specific resource (such as number of specialists or hospital beds per capita) influences use rates. Although supply sensitivity influences health care spending, it does not necessarily deliver better care. Whether viewed from the patient's perspective (outcomes, technical quality, satisfaction with care provided) or the physician's viewpoint (quality of communication among physicians, continuity of care), higher spending is not associated with better care either for Medicare beneficiaries (in isolation) or for all patients who have serious illnesses cared for at major U.S. academic medical centers.

The relationship between cost and safety in U.S. health care is complex. Medical errors carry a huge price tag for institutions, payers, and patients and their families. Yet the current U.S. health care system is not set up for payers to exercise much control over the quality of care delivered.

CURRENT HEALTH CARE SYSTEMS

Congress has called for fundamental reforms of the Centers for Medicare & Medicaid Services (CMS), moving it to a more proactive role from its previous role as "passive payer" that provides incentives for health care consumption with no links back to quality or appropriateness. The original Medicare program was designed to pay for care, as ordered, and to treat as inconsequential the quality of care. Medicare had no incentives (or even passive penalties) for such commonsense tactics as preventive medicine, withholding excessive care, or thorough patient education (Valuck, 2009). Under the Deficit Reduction Act of 2005, Section 5001(b), CMS was authorized to develop a pay-for-performance or value-based purchasing (VBP) program for hospitals that would tie reimbursement to achievement of certain benchmarks or goals in quality and efficiency. VBP is considered a major paradigm shift in U.S. health care. Although financial reform is no doubt needed, it is perhaps even more important to consider the role VBP could play in improving patient safety.

GOVERNMENT INITIATIVES

The hospital VBP plan, launched in 2009, uses measures, data infrastructure and validation steps, incentive structure, and public reporting. In setting up this program, CMS identified that care ought to be safe, effective, efficient, patient centered, timely, and equitable. The goal is first to quantify where hospitals are and then establish ways to measure improvement. Hospitals will be awarded a Total Performance Score, an aggregate of scores based on attaining certain benchmark levels and based on their own improvement over the preceding year. This Total Performance Score translates into an incentive payment plan. The hospital VBP plan has elevated patient safety to a key element of the Total Performance Score. Although safety is now tied to financial incentives, it may be of even more value that hospitals have been given ways to measure their levels of safety, to report safety data, to compare their data against established benchmarks, and to use safety scores as a way to identify specific areas for improvement. Of course, tying financial incentives to performance in a field fraught with uncontrollable variables can be a difficult leap of faith for hospital administration. Every health care provider knows that there are times when a clinical team can do everything right and still get a poor outcome.

The American Hospital Association (AHA) supports VBP but advocates moving forward carefully and with deliberation to avoid the creation of convoluted or counterproductive incentive-based payment plans. The AHA has set forth guidelines to create a workable incentive program that includes focusing on improving quality (rather than cutting costs), incremental implementation, and using measures that are evidence based, tested, feasible, and statistically sound and that recognize differences in patient populations (AHA, 2009b). VBP initiatives are some of the most fundamental changes in American health care in recent times, but other initiatives already have been used successfully to help address the safety issues in U.S. hospitals.

In 1996 the Institute of Medicine (IOM) of the National Academies in the United States launched a phased, multiyear initiative aimed at the large but important goal of improving the quality of health care in the United States. The first phase (1996-1999) reviewed medical literature to capture the scope of the problem, which can be summed up as the overuse, underuse, and misuse of available health care resources. In the second phase (1999-2001), the Committee on Quality of Health Care in America formulated metrics and a road map to help "cross the quality chasm" from what medical consensus determines to be sound health care practice versus what U.S. patients actually receive. Now in its third phase, this initiative seeks to put its vision into practice by creating a "more patient-responsive health system" (IOM, 2009).

Initiatives to improve patient safety may seem fairly straightforward on the surface, but crafting them can be complicated. Such measures, both public and private, have been successful in accomplishing the goals they set for themselves and finding resonance with the clinical community. The result has been a wave of initiatives that has created its own confusion. In 2006 the AHA launched the AHA Quality Center to help hospital leaders keep abreast of the many new and effective measures to improve quality and patient safety (AHA, 2009a).

An effective initiative must involve two distinct entities—health care services and health care systems—and help restructure their interaction (Clancy, 2007). The Agency for Healthcare Research and Quality (AHRQ) of the U.S. Department of Health and Human Services formulated *Ten Patient Safety Tips for Hospitals.* The tips may be grouped into setting up quality programs at the hospital (continuous improvement, reporting systems, proper decision-making tools), creating an efficient working environment for clinicians (teamwork, limiting shifts, using appropriate-level staff, minimizing interruptions), and fundamental medical safety tips (such as infection prevention and proper use of chest tubes and urinary catheters) (AHRQ, 2009).

Part of AHRQ's role is to provide data necessary to formulate initiatives and assess quality levels. One such successful effort is the creation of the Consumer Assessment of Healthcare Providers and Systems (CAHPS), a program that develops patient surveys to evaluate the patient's perception of his or her care. Data pose a unique problem in patient safety initiatives. As the U.S. health care market increasingly asks consumers to make important decisions about their own health care, the need for comprehensible patient safety data becomes urgent. Hospitals now follow no uniform national standards regarding what data they collect, how they collect data, and how these data are transmitted. Apples-to-apples comparisons can be impossible across systems. Variations in which data are collected and how they are collected can occur even among hospitals in the same system. For this reason the National Voluntary Hospital Reporting Initiative, a public-private collaborative, launched a three-state pilot program in 2003 to standardize hospital data across all systems. The goal is to collect similar data in similar ways so that meaningful comparisons can be made across the continuum of care and among facilities (American Health Quality Association, 2003).

Even today, the degree to which health care in the United States is consistent with basic quality standards is largely unknown, in part because quality studies tend to be highly focused and not indicative of overall care received by the average consumer (McGlynn and Brook, 2001). Thus it may be possible to obtain safety statistics for a specific procedure done in a specific time period at certain hospitals, but not broad safety statistics. This paucity of information contributes to the persistent belief in the United States that quality is not a serious national health care issue. In a comprehensive study, phone interviews with a random sampling of adults (n = 6712) in 12 U.S. metropolitan areas evaluated performance on 439 indicators of quality of care for 30 acute and chronic conditions and for preventive care. Aggregate scores found that only about half (54.9%) of patients received recommended care (McGlynn et al, 2003). What remains unknown is the real price tag for those patients who did not receive recommended care—in financial terms and in human suffering and even loss of life.

Institute for Healthcare Improvement Initiatives

The Institute for Healthcare Improvement (IHI) (2009b) launched a groundbreaking initiative in 2004 with its aptly named 100,000 Lives Campaign, aimed at reducing deaths attributable to preventable medical errors. More than 3000 hospitals came together for an initial program credited with saving 122,000 lives in its first 18 months. Encouraged by national and grassroots-level resonance, IHI launched its 5 Million Lives Campaign in 2006, aimed at preventing 5 million cases of medical harm over a 2-year period (IHI, 2009b). More than 3800 facilities enrolled in 5 Million Lives, including more than 1500 rural hospitals (which have a special rural affinity group to address their unique needs). Building on the first six proven interventions of the 100,000 Lives Campaign, the 5 Million Lives Campaign added six more (Box 2-1).

Participating hospitals picked at least one of the interventions to address and were encouraged to implement several. The 100,000 Lives and 5 Million Lives initiatives demonstrate the role that a single hospital, acting independently, can play in improving patient safety. Although sweeping national programs are important, this sort of well-promoted initiative of individual facilities also has been effective.

The eighth intervention of the 5 Million Lives campaign refers to the Surgical Care Improvement Project (SCIP), a well-known program for surgical safety. SCIP's genesis was in 2002, when CMS and the Centers for Disease Control and Prevention (CDC) launched the Surgical Infection Prevention Project. Findings from this project on preventable surgical site infections and inappropriate use of antibiotics resulted in the creation of SCIP, a suite of national initiatives to improve the care of Medicare patients receiving surgery. The original goal of SCIP was to reduce preventable surgical morbidity and mortality by 25% by 2010. Using outcome, process, and test measures, SCIP periodically identifies measurable outcomes of preventable complications specific to the surgical setting (Table 2-1).

At the beginning of 2009 IHI launched a new campaign called the IHI Improvement Map, which retains the 12 patient safety interventions from

BOX 2-1 IHI Proven Interventions

The 5 Million Lives Campaign challenges U.S. hospitals to adopt 12 changes in care that save lives and reduce patient injuries:

THE SIX INTERVENTIONS FROM THE 100,000 LIVES CAMPAIGN

- **Deploy Rapid Response Teams**... at the first sign of patient decline
- **Deliver Reliable, Evidence-Based Care for Acute Myocardial Infarction**... to prevent deaths from heart attack
- **Prevent Adverse Drug Events (ADEs)**... by implementing medication reconciliation
- **Prevent Central Line Infections**... by implementing a series of interdependent, scientifically grounded steps
- **Prevent Surgical Site Infections**... by reliably delivering the correct perioperative antibiotics at the proper time
- **Prevent Ventilator-Associated Pneumonia**... by implementing a series of interdependent, scientifically grounded steps

NEW INTERVENTIONS TARGETED AT HARM

- **Prevent Harm From High-Alert Medications**... starting with a focus on anticoagulants, sedatives, narcotics, and insulin
- **Reduce Surgical Complications**... by reliably implementing all of the changes recommended by SCIP, the Surgical Care Improvement Project (www.medqic.org /scip)
- **Prevent Pressure Ulcers**... by reliably using science-based guidelines for their prevention
- Reduce Methicillin-Resistant ***Staphylococcus aureus*** (MRSA) infection... by reliably implementing scientifically proven infection control practices
- **Deliver Reliable, Evidence-Based Care for Congestive Heart Failure**... to avoid readmissions
- **Get Boards on Board**... by defining and spreading the best known leveraged processes for hospital boards of directors, so that they can become far more effective in accelerating organizational progress toward safe care

IHI, Institute for Healthcare Improvement.
From Institute for Healthcare Improvement: *Protecting 5 million lives from harm,* available at http://www.ihi.org/NR/rdonlyres/EB78B6DB-0955-4C9C-A9B8-599E1E53DF6D/0/5MillionLivesCampaignBrochure0207.pdf. Accessed on August 18, 2009.

the 5 Million Lives campaign and adds 3 more: (1) the World Health Organization (WHO) Surgical Safety Checklist, (2) prevention of catheter-associated urinary tract infections, and (3) ability to link quality and financial management—engage the chief financial officer and provide value for patients (IHI, 2009a). The WHO Surgical Safety Checklist (Figure 2-1) gained recognition following a study describing how its use significantly reduced patient morbidity and complications (Haynes et al, 2009). In hospitals where the checklist was used, postoperative complication rates fell by 36% on average, and death rates fell by a similar amount (Haynes et al, 2009).

Although such national-level initiatives seem lofty and academic, they are practical solutions to issues related to patient safety and care. For example, evidence-based guidelines have shown that delivering antibiotics to a surgical patient within 1 hour before the first incision can significantly reduce surgical site infections. The National Nosocomial Infections Surveillance system of the CDC has found that rigorous implementation of this guideline alone reduced surgical site infections up to 44%, with other organizations reporting similar results (Bratzler et al, 2005). Simple and low-cost preventive measures often result in documentable quality improvements.

SCIENCE OF SAFETY

About 2 million adverse events involving drugs occur each year, caused by prescribing error, improper product selection or use, known side effects, or some yet-to-be-identified problem. These adverse drug events account for approximately 100,000 deaths a year (Lazarou et al, 1998). From this knowledge the science of safety has emerged, helping us to grapple with the dilemma of modern health care—the trade-off between access and safety. For example, assume that several adverse events prompt the U.S. Food and

TABLE 2-1 Surgical Care Improvement Project National Hospital Inpatient Quality Measures

Set Measure ID #	Measure Short Name
INFECTION	
SCIP Inf-1	Prophylactic antibiotic received within one hour prior to surgical incision.
SCIP Inf-2	Appropriate antibiotic received.
SCIP Inf-3	Prophylactic antibiotic discontinued within 24 hours after surgery end (48 hours for cardiac surgery).
SCIP Inf-4	Cardiac surgery patients with controlled 6 am postoperative blood glucose.
SCIP inf-6	Appropriate hair removal for surgery patients.
SCIP Inf-9	Urinary catheter removed on postoperative (POD) Day 1 or POD Day 2
SCIP Inf-10	Surgery patients with perioperative temperature management.
VENOUS THROMBOEMBOLISM	
SCIP VTE-1	Recommended VTE prophylaxis ordered.
SCIP VTE-2	Appropriate VTE prophylaxis received within 24 hours prior to surgery to 24 hours after surgery.
CARDIAC	
SCIP Card-2	Surgery patients on beta-blocker therapy prior to arrival who receive a beta-blocker during perioperative period.

Modified from Centers for Medicare and Medicaid Services (CMS), The Joint Commission (TJC): *Specifications manual for national hospital inpatient quality measures (specifications manual)*, version 3.0c, 2009, available at: http://www.qualitynet.org/dcs/ContentServer?c=Page&pagename=QnetPublic%2Fpage%2FQnetTier4&cid=1228695698425. Accessed December 14, 2009.
The *Specifications Manual for National Hospital Inpatient Quality Measures* (Version 3.0c, November 06, 2009) is the collaborative work of the Centers for Medicare & Medicaid Services and The Joint Commission. The *Specifications Manual* is periodically updated by the Centers for Medicare & Medicaid Services and The Joint Commission.

Drug Administration (FDA) to remove a drug from the market. What about the many patients who could have benefited from that drug? Taking the drug off the market will prevent some adverse events (safety), but at what cost to the patients who benefit from the drug and tolerate it well.

In the United States, the FDA determines in a premarket phase whether a drug's benefits outweigh its associated risks for the labeled use in the intended population. Despite being one of the most rigorous approval processes in the world, the FDA system simply cannot uncover every possible safety problem. In most cases, early clinical trials are not large enough, diverse enough, or long enough to uncover all of the potential issues. Future studies and ongoing use often turn up rare, serious adverse events that may occur only with long-term use or in specific population subgroups or in combination with other treatments. New information about drug safety is often obtained after a drug has been on the market for a period of time.

The FDA handles this through so-called postmarket surveillance programs, which study adverse events reported for commercially available drugs. Postmarket surveillance relies on voluntary reporting from clinicians, facilities, and hospitals to manufacturers, who in turn are required by law to report adverse events to the FDA. Although manufacturers are generally compliant in the process, the system is inherently reactive in that it relies on voluntary reports from many people who may be unaware of the vital importance of reporting postmarket adverse events. Postmarket surveillance thus provides the FDA with, at best, sketchy information on how products actually perform in real-world clinical situations.

In 2007 the Sentinel Initiative was created as part of the FDA Amendments Act. It allows the use of Medicare data from CMS in the postmarket surveillance process. Relying on public-private partnerships, the Sentinel Initiative uses current electronic data to determine how prescription drugs are affecting patients. The Sentinel Initiative

SURGICAL SAFETY CHECKLIST (FIRST EDITION)

Before induction of anaesthesia ▸▸▸▸▸▸▸▸▸▸ Before skin incision ▸▸▸▸▸▸▸▸▸▸▸▸▸▸▸▸ Before patient leaves operating room

SIGN IN

☐ **PATIENT HAS CONFIRMED**
- IDENTITY
- SITE
- PROCEDURE
- CONSENT

☐ **SITE MARKED/NOT APPLICABLE**

☐ **ANAESTHESIA SAFETY CHECK COMPLETED**

☐ **PULSE OXIMETER ON PATIENT AND FUNCTIONING**

DOES PATIENT HAVE A:

KNOWN ALLERGY?
☐ NO
☐ YES

DIFFICULT AIRWAY/ASPIRATION RISK?
☐ NO
☐ YES, AND EQUIPMENT/ASSISTANCE AVAILABLE

RISK OF >500ML BLOOD LOSS (7ML/KG IN CHILDREN)?
☐ NO
☐ YES, AND ADEQUATE INTRAVENOUS ACCESS AND FLUIDS PLANNED

TIME OUT

☐ **CONFIRM ALL TEAM MEMBERS HAVE INTRODUCED THEMSELVES BY NAME AND ROLE**

☐ **SURGEON, ANAESTHESIA PROFESSIONAL, AND NURSE VERBALLY CONFIRM**
- PATIENT
- SITE
- PROCEDURE

ANTICIPATED CRITICAL EVENTS

☐ **SURGEON REVIEWS:** WHAT ARE THE CRITICAL OR UNEXPECTED STEPS, OPERATIVE DURATION, ANTICIPATED BLOOD LOSS?

☐ **ANAESTHESIA TEAM REVIEWS:** ARE THERE ANY PATIENT-SPECIFIC CONCERNS?

☐ **NURSING TEAM REVIEWS:** HAS STERILITY (INCLUDING INDICATOR RESULTS) BEEN CONFIRMED? ARE THERE EQUIPMENT ISSUES OR ANY CONCERNS?

HAS ANTIBIOTIC PROPHYLAXIS BEEN GIVEN WITHIN THE LAST 60 MINUTES?
☐ YES
☐ NOT APPLICABLE

IS ESSENTIAL IMAGING DISPLAYED?
☐ YES
☐ NOT APPLICABLE

SIGN OUT

NURSE VERBALLY CONFIRMS WITH THE TEAM:

☐ **THE NAME OF THE PROCEDURE RECORDED**

☐ **THAT INSTRUMENT, SPONGE, AND NEEDLE COUNTS ARE CORRECT** (OR NOT APPLICABLE)

☐ **HOW THE SPECIMENT IS LABELLED** (INCLUDING PATIENT NAME)

☐ **WHETHER THERE ARE ANY EQUIPMENT PROBLEMS TO BE ADDRESSED**

☐ **SURGEON, ANAESTHESIA PROFESSIONAL, AND NURSE REVIEW THE KEY CONCERNS FOR RECOVERY AND MANAGEMENT OF THIS PATIENT**

THIS CHECKLIST IS NOT INTENDED TO BE COMPREHENSIVE. ADDITIONS AND MODIFICATIONS TO FIT LOCAL PRACTICE ARE ENCOURAGED.

FIGURE 2-1 WHO Surgical Safety Checklist. (Modified from World Health Organization: *Surgical safety checklist,* available at http://www.who.int/patientsafety/safesurgery/ss_checklist/en/index.html.)

will develop a new electronic system to enable the FDA to query a broad array of information to identify postmarket adverse events (Association for the Advancement of Medical Instrumentation, 2009).

The Association for the Advancement of Medical Instrumentation (AAMI) final regulation makes it possible for federal agencies, states, and academic researchers to use claims data from the Medicare prescription drug program (Part D) for public health and safety research, quality initiatives, care coordination, and other research and analysis. The objective of the Sentinel Initiative is to launch the Sentinel System, a national, integrated electronic system for monitoring medical procedure safety. This effort is a phased long-term initiative with pilot programs now under way. Its goal is to allow data mining and research activities across multiple data systems while protecting patient privacy (AAMI, 2009).

Other FDA initiatives for patient safety include MedSun, the Medical Product Safety Network, launched in 2002 by the Center for Devices and Radiological Health to help identify, understand, and solve similar problems with medical devices. More than 350 health care facilities, primarily hospitals, participate, and there are subnetworks, such as KidNet (for pediatric and neonatal intensive care units) and HeartNet (for electrophysiology laboratories), to capture specific data (FDA, 2009).

Like many recent quality initiatives, the Sentinel System relies on electronic health care data. As president, George W. Bush set forth a goal that most Americans should have an interoperable electronic health record by the year 2014. Related technologies, such as e-prescribing and electronic decision support tools, will help improve risk management systems, better protect the public, and potentially reduce health care costs (AAMI, 2009). Previous postmarket surveillance systems relied on paper data, which meant that it could take years for patterns of adverse events to emerge from reports. It is hoped that electronic surveillance will allow problems to percolate to agency and clinical awareness rapidly.

The Sentinel System seeks to build on existing electronic infrastructure rather than build new systems from scratch, so as much as possible data sources will be managed and maintained by their owners. Working with the Nationwide Health Information Network, the Sentinel System will integrate systems to allow for queries of multiple data sources. Part of the Sentinel Initiative involves standardizing data, creating user-friendly interfaces to input and access data, and formulating standard terminology for use in electronic records. One of its several goals is transparency, in that protocols, data, and results should be made available to consumers.

The goal of allowing consumers better insight into hospital safety and performance is not a new one. With many Americans charged by their health care insurance, employers, and even health care providers to make more of their own decisions about health care, the U.S. public rightly demands—and requires—more information, yet few hospitals offer the degree of data transparency consumers need. In 2002 the AHA launched the Hospital Quality Alliance (HQA) to promote such transparency and to make reliable, credible, useful information on hospital quality available to the public. Joined by various prestigious national organizations (e.g., the American Association of Retired Persons, the AFL-CIO, Blue Cross Blue Shield Association [BCBSA]), the originally voluntary alliance sought to make safety data available to consumers. Congress soon linked submission of HQA-requested data to receipt of the full Medicare market-basket update for hospital inpatient payment. Data are available for public access (U.S. Department of Health and Human Services, 2009). The success of the HQA initiative is clearly evident in its year-over-year growth. The role of standardized, transparent, coherent data cannot be overemphasized.

Data Collection

The burden of record keeping falls on the hospitals, however, who often must add staff (or take staff away from patient care) to manage the time-consuming tasks of data collection and reporting. At present, hospitals face multiple requests for data (often similar versions of the same data) from insurers, employer groups, accreditation organizations, and government agencies. For that reason, the HQA strongly advocates that data on quality be reported once to the HQA in one format, which will save time, streamline reporting, help standardize data, and bolster the value of HQA's transparency initiative. Meanwhile, the HQA continues to identify key areas of quality that can be measured and reported. On the docket are infection prevention, surgical care, pediatric care, and care for patients who have chronic conditions. Efficiency data will also be collected. These data may become the foundation on which CMS bases future pay-for-performance programs, an action supported by the AHA (2009b).

After October 1, 2007, Inpatient Prospective Payment System (IPPS) hospitals were required to submit data on claims for payment indicating whether diagnoses were present on admission (POA). After October 1, 2008, CMS cannot assign a case to a higher DRG based on the occurrence of one of the selected conditions if that condition was acquired during hospitalization. Box 2-2 lists all of the conditions for which guidelines and interventions exist and that are deemed to be reasonably preventable.

In addition, effective January 15, 2009, CMS no longer provides Medicare coverage for surgery if it is the wrong procedure or if it is performed on the wrong patient or the wrong body part. The decision applies to all procedures described in the surgery section of the Current Procedural Terminology, as well as other invasive procedures, such as percutaneous transluminal angioplasty and cardiac catheterization. Minimally invasive procedures involving biopsies or placement of probes or catheters requiring entry into a body cavity through a needle or trocar are also included (CMS, 2009a, 2009b, 2009c).

Conditions (which must be high cost, high volume, or both) under consideration for future lists include ventilator-associated pneumonia and *Staphylococcus aureus* septicemia (CMS, 2009d). The POA criterion has caused some concern at the clinical level because it requires new procedures to be mapped out and implemented, but it represents an important shift in institutional thinking away from passive payment for health care consumption toward incentives for preventive care, a principle most clinicians heartily endorse.

BOX 2-2 Hospital-Acquired Conditions

The 10 categories of hospital-acquired conditions are:

1. Foreign Object Retained After Surgery
2. Air Embolism
3. Blood Incompatibility
4. Stage III and IV Pressure Ulcers
5. Falls and Trauma
   - Fractures
   - Dislocations
   - Intracranial Injuries
   - Crushing Injuries
   - Burns
   - Electric Shock
6. Manifestations of Poor Glycemic Control
   - Diabetic Ketoacidosis
   - Nonketotic Hyperosmolar Coma
   - Hypoglycemic Coma
   - Secondary Diabetes With Ketoacidosis
   - Secondary Diabetes With Hyperosmolarity
7. Catheter-Associated Urinary Tract Infection (UTI)
8. Vascular Catheter-Associated Infection
9. Surgical Site Infection Following:
   - Coronary Artery Bypass Graft (CABG)—Mediastinitis
   - Bariatric Surgery
     - Laparoscopic Gastric Bypass
     - Gastroenterostomy
     - Laparoscopic Gastric Restrictive Surgery
   - Orthopedic Procedures
     - Spine
     - Neck
     - Shoulder
     - Elbow
10. Deep Vein Thrombosis (DVT)/Pulmonary Embolism (PE)
    - Total Knee Replacement
    - Hip Replacement

From Centers for Medicare & Medicaid Services: *Hospital-acquired conditions*, available at http://www.cms.hhs.gov/HospitalAcqCond/06_Hospital-Acquired_Conditions.asp. Accessed August 20, 2009.

Never Events

The National Quality Federation (NQF) set forth a list of Serious Reportable Adverse Events in 2002. These events have since been nicknamed "never events" because not only are these errors preventable, they should never occur. Never events are unambiguous, indicative of a problem in the facility's safety system, and important for public accountability. Of the 28 never events, those involving surgery include surgery on the wrong body part, surgery on the wrong patient, wrong surgery on the patient, foreign object left in the patient, postoperative death in a normal-health patient, and implantation of the wrong egg. Recent proposals suggest that payers may opt not to pay for never events. A few states have started requirements that never events be reported. One such state, Minnesota, averages about 100 such event reports a year (Leapfrog Group, 2009b). Statistics on never events are lacking because reporting for most facilities is discretionary and usually not done. Based on Minnesota statistics, however, it is reasonable to assume that never events do occur, probably more frequently than most consumers realize. Initiatives to combat never events have been set forth, and the NQF advocates that a root cause analysis be performed when a never event does occur.

PRIVATE INITIATIVES

Although many safety initiatives come from the government, medical organizations, and health care providers, some patient safety initiatives have been launched by payers. The BCBSA worked with the Harvard Medical School's Department of Health Care Policy and formulated seven initiatives under the banner "collaborating with providers" in 2007. Among these initiatives are Hospital Patient Safety (Anthem Blue Cross and Blue Shield in Virginia) and Quality-In-Sights Hospital Incentive Program (Q-HIP) (Blue Cross and Blue Shield, 2007). Data from network hospitals are collected and interpreted to provide feedback on key quality and safety metrics. Launched in 2003 in 16 network hospitals, the program has since expanded to more than 60 facilities.

Quality Physician Performance Program (Q-P3) was a spinoff of Q-HIP in the same participating facilities. It uses outcomes, processes, and quality measures to reward evidence-based medicine and best practices. Results showed that complication rates in 2004 for angioplasty and cardiac catheterization procedures decreased by 50% and 29%, respectively, over the preceding year.

Blue Cross Blue Shield of North Dakota launched a pilot collaborative initiative for diabetes management in 2005. Patients receive a suite of services, including medication comprehension and self-management education. Compared with nonstudy patients, pilot study patients had lower costs for care, fewer emergency department visits, and fewer inpatient admissions.

Blue Cross Blue Shield of Massachusetts and CareFirst Blue Cross Blue Shield partnered in an initiative to move from paper to electronic prescriptions. This initiative involved a series of interventions across multiple stakeholders. One of the largest such initiatives in the nation, the program offered free e-prescribing devices, services, and software to up to 2500 providers. In its first 4 years, more than 10 million electronic prescriptions were generated through the collaborative. In 2006, e-prescriptions resulted in 15,000 drug interaction warnings and 7400 drug allergy warnings being generated by the system and delivered to the prescribing physician as an alert message.

Blue Cross Blue Shield of South Carolina launched the Web Precert initiative to shape hospital precertification into a streamlined online procedure. The organization reports that 46% of all precertification requests and inquiries are now managed online, saving time and reducing long-distance phone calls.

Premier has set up Perspective, a national clinical database of 500 of its network hospitals for benchmarking and quality improvement activities (Premier, 2009a). Hospitals submit data to Perspective for analysis; in particular, outcome data are compared and areas for improvement identified (Premier, 2008). Related tools include Premier's Safety Surveillor, a Web-based tool aimed at optimizing antimicrobial use to improve outcomes (Premier, 2009b). It helps to manage a facility's infection control surveillance and combat hospital-acquired infections. Other tools for analyzing and measuring quality metrics are also available (Premier, 2009a).

The Joint Commission, which offers accreditation programs for hospitals, formulates National Patient Safety Goals (NPSGs) by highlighting problematic areas in health care, reviewing the medical evidence, and then consulting with safety and medical experts to determine specific solutions. Insofar as possible, solutions are formulated to be both specific and systemwide. In June 2007 The Joint Commission's Board of Commissioners approved the 2008 National Patient Safety Goals. The system allowed a 1-year phase-in period that included defined expectations for planning, development, and testing (by milestones) at 3, 6, and 9 months in 2008. Full implementation commenced in January 2009. The NPSGs are as follows (The Joint Commission, 2009b):

- Improve the accuracy of patient identification.
- Improve the effectiveness of communication among caregivers.
- Improve the safety of using medications.
- Reduce the risk of health care–associated infections.
- Accurately and completely reconcile medications across the continuum of care.
- Reduce the risk of patient harm resulting from falls.
- Encourage patients' active involvement in their own care as a patient safety strategy.
- The organization identifies safety risks inherent in its patient population.

- Improve recognition and response to changes in a patient's condition.

During 2009 The Joint Commission undertook an extensive review of the current NPSGs and the process for their development. As a result, there will be no new NPSGs developed for 2010. The review was undertaken in response to concerns about the challenge some goals represent and the need for additional information about effective approaches to addressing these challenges (The Joint Commission, 2009a).

The Association of Professionals in Infection Control and Epidemiology set forth its Vision 2012 to establish itself as the recognized leader in infection prevention and control by health care practitioners, policy makers, health care executives, and consumers. Among its many related initiatives are development of public reporting standards, playing a leadership role in emergency preparedness, and promoting zero tolerance for health care–associated infections (Association for Professionals in Infection Control and Epidemiology, 2009). Likewise, the Association of PeriOperative Registered Nurses (AORN) has formulated several initiatives specifically to guide nursing professionals in the surgical suite. Tool kits available to AORN members and nonmembers for deployment at the local level include prevention and response to surgical fires, correct-site surgery, safe medication administration, "just culture" (for reporting and analyzing medical errors with the goal of improving patient safety, not hiding wrongdoing), communication in patient handoff, and human factors in health care.

One of the most original groups in initiatives for patient safety is the Leapfrog Group. In 1998 several employers with large health care expenditures came together, finding themselves in the untenable position of spending vast sums for health care with no way to assess quality or compare providers. In 1999 the IOM issued a report suggesting that large employers should take steps for market reinforcement of patient safety standards. Calling its initiatives "leaps," the Leapfrog Group officially started in 2000.

Working with the NQF, the Leapfrog Group formulated 30 Safe Practices for Better Healthcare, which offer initiatives in four areas and tie back to never events. The Leapfrog Group has an unusual initiative with regard to never events. Although such preventable errors should ideally never occur, if and when they do, the Leapfrog Group offers special recognition to those hospitals that report them and take other appropriate steps, such as apologizing to the patient and family, performing a root case analysis, and waiving related charges. The theory is that those facilities that take aggressive steps to learn from such preventable errors will more rapidly approach the goal of zero never events (Leapfrog Group, 2009b).

The Leapfrog Hospital Survey publishes reports on the efforts of more than 1300 hospitals to improve the efficiency of care and has set forth "purchasing principles" by which Leapfrog members (employers who provide health care coverage) are expected to abide. Chief among these principles are educating and informing enrollees about the safety, quality, and affordability of health care, educating consumers about care comparisons, and rewarding providers for advances in safety, quality, and affordability. In 2006 the Leapfrog Group launched its inaugural reward program for hospitals, based on five measures of quality and efficiency. Measures are scored by participating hospitals and their data vendors. Hospitals rated "excellent" or "show improvement" along both dimensions qualify for rewards. This initial program is likely to be expanded with other steps. The Leapfrog Group is currently assessing ongoing pay-for-performance projects by other organizations to help in formulation of its own incentives (Leapfrog Group, 2009a).

Perioperative care contributes significantly to patient outcomes and overall quality of surgical care. With about 50 million operations annually in the United States, it is a vast field with vast potential (NQF, 2009). The National Voluntary Consensus Standards for Surgery and Anesthesia launched a perioperative care initiative endorsed by the NQF, funded by CMS, and encompassing 28 measures at the hospital level, 10 measures for ambulatory surgery, and 12 measures for clinicians.

The Hospital Quality Incentive Demonstration (HQID), a joint project between CMS and Premier, was the first national project designed to determine if economic incentives to hospitals would be effective in improving the quality of care to inpatients. Initially set up for 2 years, the project was extended 3 more years. Premier collected a set of more than 30 evidence-based clinical quality measures from more than 250 of its hospitals around the country. The quality measures were determined by HQID, which tracks process and outcome measures in five clinical areas: acute myocardial infarction, heart failure, coronary artery bypass graft (CABG), pneumonia, and hip and knee replacements. Using CABG surgery as an example, the initiative reviews such measures as the following (Premier, 2009a):

- Aspirin prescribed at discharge for CABG
- Prophylactic antibiotic received within 1 hour of surgical incision
- Prophylactic antibiotic selection for surgery patients
- Prophylactic antibiotic discontinued within 24 hours after surgery
- Inpatient mortality rate
- Postoperative hemorrhage or hematoma
- Postoperative physiologic and metabolic derangement

The HQID project was a test of one VBP model and serves as a guideline for the current CMS proposal before Congress, which ties payment to quality of care or specified outcomes.

The advantage of this program is that it should help determine standard, meaningful measures for health care quality. Financial incentives are intended to help focus hospitals on benchmarking and measurement tools that, in turn, identify those areas needing improvement. This program represents an important milestone in the U.S. health care system because this is the first time on a national level that participating hospitals could qualify for additional Medicare payments based on performance in clearly defined clinical areas. More than 250 hospitals joined this program at its inception, agreeing to have their Medicare reimbursements tied directly to the quality of care they provide. Although this may seem like a small step, it indicates the fundamental change in thinking going on in many U.S. hospitals. Clearly, patient safety, clinical outcomes, and reimbursement are being considered as interrelated items in ways that benefit not only payers and patients, but also potentially hospitals and other health care providers.

Fundamental financial questions remain, however. What do quality and safety initiatives actually cost the health care system? For CMS the HQID program is cost neutral in that incentive payments are offset by the reduction in cost of care. To be specific, in the third year of HQID more than a million patients were treated in one of the five clinical areas of the initiative; participating hospitals improved overall quality by an average of 15.8%, more than 2500 lives were saved, and CMS ended up paying about $24 million in incentive payments. Other initiatives are hoped to be cost-saving programs. It is sometimes hard to define specific costs that such programs save, however. For example, if an initiative prevents a patient from developing a surgical site infection, what expense does that truly save the system? At best, cost savings can be captured as statistical extrapolations. Just as we may not truly appreciate the full scope of the problem of patient safety in our hospitals, we may not (at least in the short term) fully appreciate how much money these initiatives actually do save the system (Premier, 2008a).

CONCLUSION

Although there is increasing political awareness and a lively public discussion about America's "broken" health care system, the main focus has always been universal health insurance or other equitable solutions to extending health care benefits to the entire population. Without diminishing the importance of this laudable goal, it is unrelated to the problems discussed here in variation in patient care, misuse of health care resources, and patient safety issues. Patient safety must rise to public and political awareness as an important and independent goal in and of itself in improving U.S. health care. Patient safety initiatives at the national and local level, launched by public and private stakeholders and embracing large goals or small steps, have proved to be remarkably effective in improving patient safety, reducing medical errors, and saving money. Such initiatives may begin with sweeping concerns, but they ultimately boil down to a list of tactics. Many of these tactical steps are simple, inexpensive, and not particularly difficult to implement. It is highly encouraging that the solutions to many knotty and seemingly overwhelming health care problems can be found in a series of small, specific steps crafted in the form of specific health care initiatives. Even more encouraging, these initiatives seem to find that reducing error, improving patient safety, and upgrading care across the nation are actually associated with lower health care costs.

REFERENCES

Agency for Healthcare Research and Quality: *Ten patient safety tips for hospitals,* available at http://www.ahrq.gov/qual/10tips.htm. Accessed June 8, 2009.

American Health Quality Association: *Supporting the National Voluntary Hospital Reporting Initiative,* press release, October 9, 2003, available at http://www.ahqa.org/pub/media/159_678_4585.cfm. Accessed June 8, 2009.

American Hospital Association: *The American Hospital Association quality care center,* http://www.hospitalconnect.com/hospitalconnect_app/search/ahaqualitycenter_results.jsp?q=reference&site=AHAQUALITYCENTER&client=AHAQUALITYCENTER_FRONTEND&proxystylesheet=AHAQUALITYCENTER_FRONTEND&filter=1&output=xml_no_dtd&oe=ISO-8859-1. Accessed August 13, 2009a.

American Hospital Association: *Improving quality and patient safety,* available at http://www.aha.org/aha/letter/2007/070124-cl-vbp-p4p.pdf. Accessed June 4, 2009b.

Association for the Advancement of Medical Instrumentation: *Sentinel initiative launched to improve patient safety and quality of care,* press release, available at http://www.aami.org/news/2008/052708.fdacms.html. Accessed June 5, 2009.

Association for Professionals in Infection Control and Epidemiology: *Vision 2012,* available at http://www.apic.org/AM/Template.cfm?Section=About_APIC&;Template=/CM/ContentDisplay.cfm&ContentFileID=4688. Accessed June 5, 2009.

Blue Cross and Blue Shield initiatives recognized for increasing patient safety and efficiency: press release, September 10, 2007, available at http://www.bcbs.com/news/bcbsa/collaborating-with-providers-2007.html. Accessed June 5, 2009.

Bratzler DW, et al: Use of antimicrobial prophylaxis for major surgery: an advisory statement from the National Surgical Infection Prevention Project, *Arch Surg* 140:174–182, 2005.

Centers for Medicare & Medicaid Services: *Decision memo for surgery on the wrong body part (CAG-00402N),* available at http://www.cms.hhs.gov/mcd/viewdecisionmemo.asp?id=222. Accessed May 5, 2009a.

Centers for Medicare & Medicaid Services: *Decision memo for surgery on the wrong patient (CAG-00403N),* available at http://www.cms.hhs.gov/mcd/viewdecisionmemo.asp?id=221. Accessed May 5, 2009b.

Centers for Medicare & Medicaid Services: *Decision memo for wrong surgery performed on a patient (CAG-00401N),* available at http://www.cms.hhs.gov/mcd/viewdecisionmemo.asp?id=223. Accessed May 5, 2009c.

Centers for Medicare & Medicaid Services: *Hospital-acquired conditions,* available at http://www.cms.hhs.gov/HospitalAcqCond/06_Hospital-Acquired_Conditions.asp. Accessed June 4, 2009d.

Clancy CM: *Testimony on health care quality initiatives: before the Subcommittee on Health of the House Committee on Ways and Means,* Rockville, Md, May 18, 2007, Agency for Healthcare Research and Quality, available at http://www.ahrq.gov/news/qtest319.htm. Accessed June 4, 2009.

Haynes AB, et al: A surgical safety checklist to reduce morbidity and mortality in a global population, *N Engl J Med* 360: 491–499, 2009.

Institute for Healthcare Improvement: *IHI improvement map,* available at http://www.ihi.org/IHI/Programs/ImprovementMap. Accessed May 5, 2009a.

Institute for Healthcare Improvement: *IHI's 5 million lives campaign* (website) http://www.ihi.org/IHI/Programs/IHIOpenSchool/IHICampaignWebsite.htm. Accessed June 5, 2009b.

Institute of Medicine: *Crossing the quality chasm: the IOM Health Care Quality Initiative,* available at http://www.iom.edu/CMS/8089.aspx. Accessed June 3, 2009.

Kanter G: *SCIP: preventing surgical site infections,* PowerPoint presentation, 2007, available at http://www.mass.gov/Eeohhs2/docs/dph/patient_safety/07conference_kanter.ppt. Accessed June 5, 2009.

Klevens RM, et al: Estimating health care associated infections and deaths in U.S. hospitals, 2002, *Public Health Rep* 122:160–166, 2007.

Kohn LT, et al editors: *To err is human,* Washington, DC, 2000, National Academy Press.

Lazarou J, et al: Incidence of adverse drug reactions in hospitalized patients: a meta-analysis of prospective studies, *JAMA* 79:1200–1205, 1998.

Leapfrog Group: *Hospital rewards program,* available at http://www.leapfroggroup.org/for_hospitals/fh-incentives_and_rewards/hosp_rewards_prog. Accessed June 8, 2009a.

Leapfrog Group: *Leapfrog Group position statement on never events,* available at http://www.leapfroggroup.org/for_hospitals/leapfrog_hospital_quality_and_safety_survey_copy/never_events. Accessed June 5, 2009b.

McGlynn EA, Brook RH: Keeping quality on the policy agenda, *Health Aff* 20:82–90, 2001.

McGlynn EA, et al: The quality of health care delivered to adults in the United States, *N Engl J Med* 348:2635–2645, 2003.

National Quality Forum: *National voluntary consensus standards for surgery and anesthesia: additional performance measures,* available at http://www.qualityforum.org/projects/ongoing/surgicalfacilities/index.asp. Accessed June 8, 2009.

Premier, Inc.: *Patient lives saved as performance continues to improve in CMS, Premier healthcare alliance pay-for-performance project,* press release, June 17, 2008, available at http://www.premierinc.com/about/news/june08/p4pProject061708.jsp. Accessed June 8, 2009.

Premier, Inc.: *CMS/Premier Hospital Quality Incentive Demonstration (HQID),* available at http://www.premierinc.com/quality-safety/tools-services/p4p/hqi/index.jsp. Accessed June 8, 2009a.

Premier, Inc.: *Premier Safety Surveillor™—infection control,* available at http://www.premierinc.com/about/downloads/ss-infection-control-66.pdf. Accessed June 5, 2009b.

The Joint Commission: *National Patient Safety Goals,* available at http://www.jointcommission.org/PatientSafety/NationalPatientSafetyGoals. Accessed May 5, 2009a.

The Joint Commission: *2008 National Patient Safety Goals,* available at http://www.jcrinc.com/common/PDFs/fpdfs/pubs/pdfs/JCReqs/JCP-07-07-S1.pdf. Accessed June 5, 2009b.

U.S. Department of Health and Human Services: *Hospital Compare—a quality tool provided by Medicare,* available at http://toolbar.yahoo.com/config/slv4_done?.act=3&.dflt=1&.intl=us&.region=us&.partner=none&.guest=none&.cpdl=upghp&.mf1=&.cxurl=http://new.toolbar.yahoo.com. Accessed August 13, 2009.

U.S. Food and Drug Administration: *About MedSun,* available at http://www.fda.gov/MedicalDevices/Safety/MedSunMedicalProductSafetyNetwork/ucm112683.htm. Accessed June 8, 2009.

Valuck TB: *CMS' progress toward implementing value-based purchasing,* PowerPoint presentation, available at http://www.rheumatology.org/practice/qmc/CMS-Perspective-TValuck.asp. Accessed June 4, 2009.

Wennberg JE, et al: *Tracking the care of patients with severe chronic illness: the Dartmouth Atlas of Health Care 2008,* available at http://www.dartmouthatlas.org. Accessed June 5, 2009.

USE OF MEDMARX DATA FOR THE SUPPORT AND DEVELOPMENT OF PERIOPERATIVE MEDICATION POLICY

Vivian M. Sersen, MSN, RN, CNOR, PCNS, CDR, NC, USN •
Sandra C. Garmon Bibb, DNSc, RN

Perioperative evidence-based practice depends on synthesis of data from internal and external benchmarking (Titler, 2006). Development of perioperative medication policy should be guided by synthesis of these data and by recommendations from perioperative professional organizations and regulatory agencies. However, limited evidence of this synthesis exists in the literature to guide policy development for safe medication practices for this critical specialty (Beyea et al, 2003). Responding to this gap in knowledge, the United States Pharmacopeia (USP) and the Uniformed Services of the Health Sciences Graduate School of Nursing collaborated in a partnership to analyze perioperative medication error reports from the MEDMARX database. The Association of periOperative Registered Nurses (AORN), the American Society of PeriAnesthesia Nurses (ASPAN), and other volunteer experts served as the USP Council of Experts, which reviewed and provided input for the final report, *MEDMARX Data Report: A Chartbook of Medication Error Findings From the Perioperative Settings From 1998-2005* (Hicks et al, 2006).

The MEDMARX database contains a unique classification system for medication errors that supports coding of all records of medication errors according to the extent of harm, including potential errors causing no harm. These invaluable data have the capability to guide the development of medication policy in the high-risk perioperative environment through identification of causative factors and trends. Yet, there is minimal descriptive summary in the literature on how MEDMARX data are currently being used to support the development of perioperative medication policy. The purpose of this chapter is to review results of an initial research study that describes how MEDMARX data are being used to support the development and revision of a population health medication policy across the perioperative continuum. This will allow individuals responsible for the development and updating of perioperative medication policies to apply and use evidence-based practice to determine and set policy. Chapter 5 provides further details related to MEDMARX data with specifics of medication error prevention.

REVIEW OF LITERATURE

Population health focuses on improving health outcomes, eliminating health disparities, and reducing health care costs for a particular group of people (Bibb, 2002; Department of Defense, 2005a; Department of Defense, 2005b; Bibb et al, 2006). Central to improving the outcome for surgical patient populations is the reduction of patient safety risk factors. The U.S. epidemic of patient safety problems was documented in the Institute of Medicine's (IOM's) report in 1998 (Institute of Medicine, 1998). This landmark report indicated that 98,000 deaths occurred each year as a result of medical errors. More recently, the IOM report from November 2003 titled *Patient Safety: Achieving a New Standard for Care* calls for a unified national health information infrastructure as a requirement to make patient safety a standard of care (Institute of Medicine, 2003).

Patient Safety Risk

With medical mistakes ranking sixth among the leading causes of death in U.S. hospitals today, it is urgent to identify probable causative factors (Nosek et al, 2005). According to recent USP data, a large portion of medical mistakes in the hospital setting are medication errors, with 235,000 errors reported in the 2003 MEDMARX annual summary report (Hicks et al, 2004b) and 950,000 adverse drug events reported in MEDMARX as of January 2006 (USP, 2006).

In an immediate effort to decrease patient safety risk in hospitals across the United States, the U.S. Congress approved a billion-dollar patient safety initiative (National Patient Safety Foundation, 2005). Shortly after Congress endorsed these measures for all health care facilities, many literary and Web-based resources emerged. Some of these initiatives assessed and evaluated practices at both the unit and hospital level, with increased analyses of systems within health care facilities.

The MEDMARX Database

In 1998 USP created a central depository for anonymous medication error reporting through a subscription service, the MEDMARX database. Since then, annual reports have been published identifying common trends and causative factors among like facilities and similar groups of patients. By analyzing the trends and factors contributing to medication mistakes in various facilities, a clearer picture of the problem areas has emerged. Once identified, these causative factors can be reduced or eliminated through evidence-based interventions to maximize the effectiveness of safe medication practices.

USP owns another older and less-used database for voluntary reporting of errors, the Medication Error Reporting (MER) database. This database contains roughly one-tenth the data sets reported to MEDMARX. Although it is a free, anonymous service, MER lacks the number of data sets needed to generate reports of trends from its users. Although the number of medication errors should not be the sole criterion for determining a useful database, it does afford the analysis of causative factor trends (Department of Defense, 2005a). Therefore the MEDMARX database is preferred over the MER database for secondary analysis. As stated in the USP e-newsroom, "This third annual report, *Summary of Information Submitted to MEDMARX in the Year 2001: A Human Factors Approach to Medication Errors,* is the most comprehensive compilation of medication error data submitted by hospitals and health systems nationwide" (Borden and Gifford, 2006).

Unsafe Perioperative Practices

The operating room and postanesthesia care unit share unsafe medication administration practices, including nonspecific policies for unit stock medications, communication of verbal orders, and written case card preference sheets. MEDMARX data has identified these specific unsafe practices in all phases of the perioperative continuum throughout the literature. Once the cause is known, systems involved in the unsafe process can be evaluated and gaps identified to further develop or modify existing medication policy (Beyea et al, 2003; Hicks et al, 2004a).

In 2002 The Joint Commission (TJC) announced plans to establish its first set of National Patient Safety Goals (NPSGs) (TJC, 2008a). In 2005 The Joint Commission NPSGs added reconciliation of medications across the continuum of care as their eighth specific goal (TJC, 2006). The 2009 NPSG Goal 8 requires accredited institutions to "accurately and completely reconcile medications across the continuum of care" (TJC, 2008b). This goal provides elements of performance on how to achieve the NPSGs, requiring that all patients have a complete list of medications that they are currently taking on their chart at all times. This information is communicated throughout each phase of their care. In addition, a process allowing for comparison of ordered medication to medications on the patient's current list is required (TJC, 2008b). NPSG.08.01.01 requires that medications at all times must be accurate. Elements of Performance for NPSG.08.01.01 require that upon admission the patient must have a current list of medications that includes the medication, dose, route, and frequency. The patient and members of the family may participate in creating an accurate list. Any discrepancies should be addressed to prevent the potential for a medication error. NPSG.08.02.01 requires communication of the reconciled medication list to the provider of the next level of service. When the list is reconciled, the process should be documented. NPSG.08.03.01 involves patient education at the time of discharge. The patient and/or family should receive education and a current list of reconciled medications. The patient should be instructed to discard any old medication list he or she may have and replace it with the current version. NPSG.08.04.01 states that facilities may use a modified medication reconciliation process in areas such as the emergency department, convenient care, office-based surgery, outpatient radiology, ambulatory care, and behavioral care (TJC, 2008b). The importance of medication reconciliation is essential to patient safety.

Professional organizations such as AORN and ASPAN have also assisted perioperative nurses and perioperative practitioners with identification of gaps within their practice environment and have provided valuable tools to improve patient safety in risk-prone areas. AORN has multiple resources for the perioperative nurse in practice and as guides for updating current medication policy, such as *AORN Safe Medication Administration Took Kit* (AORN, 2005), *Safe Medication Practices in the Perioperative Setting* (AORN, 2009), *Managing the Patient Receiving Moderate Sedation/Analgesia* (AORN, 2009), and *Managing the Patient Receiving Local Anesthesia* (2009). These are valuable resources for the perioperative nurse for the development of medication competencies and increasing awareness of safe medication administration by the perioperative team. In addition, ASPAN's *Position Statement on Safe Medication Administration* (ASPAN, 2005) provides guiding principles and guidelines for the safe administration of medications. The nurse should be knowledgeable about these valuable resources and use them in the process of policy development or revision of existing medication administration policies.

An Underutilized Asset

MEDMARX data are being used for performance improvement projects in the surgical population, revealing the database as a user-friendly tool (Beyea et al, 2003; Hicks et al, 2007). Perioperative nurses and practitioners could benefit from a comprehensive list of studies using the MEDMARX database for a quick review of existing trends in medication errors. From this list, perioperative nurses could envision the body of evidence-based research studies available and integrate this knowledge into future medication policy and best medication practices (Hamric and Hanson, 2003). In addition, medication error trends that have not been explored, and thus require further study, will be easily identified as gaps in the current body of knowledge. It is only through the exploration of these gaps that nurses and practitioners can achieve a healthy, safe outcome for the surgical patient population.

Significant gaps relating to medication error causes have been identified over the past 6 years, yet there exists no collection of interventions that have been taken to correct these causative factors, as identified in medication policy documents in the literature (Cousins, 1998; Cowley et al, 2001; Beyea et al, 2003, Santell et al, 2003; Beyea et al, 2004; Hicks et al, 2004a, Hicks et al, 2004b, Jones et al, 2004; Niccolai et al, 2004; Nosek et al, 2005). Practitioners such as advanced practice nurses (APNs) are an excellent resource and are often consulted to update policy based on the latest standards, while incorporating evidence-based findings in the defense of modified policy (Heitkemper and Bond, 2006). A list of studies using secondary analysis of the MEDMARX database to support perioperative medication policy, and assist in the identification of future research needed, would be an invaluable asset for the perioperative nurse, the APN, or anyone involved with policy development (Zuzelo, 2003; Nicoll and Beyea, 1999).

The study described in this chapter was conducted using the methodologic approach and data collection tools piloted in a study conducted by Bibb et al (2006) to identify and describe clinical databases and data sets used to support development of population health programs and population health policy (Figure 3-1). The study described focused specifically on the use of MEDMARX data in the support and development of medication policy in the perioperative setting.

Conceptual Definition—Perioperative Medication Safety Policy

The definition of perioperative medication policy includes standards set by regulatory agencies—The Joint Commission, the U.S. Food and Drug Administration, the Department of Defense, and the Department of Health and Human Services—in conjunction with recommendations from professional organizations (AORN and ASPAN), state requirements, and facility instructions, which guide the development of evidence-based medication practices in the perioperative environment (Department of Defense, 2005a; Titler, 2006; AORN, 2009).

Operational Definition—Perioperative Medication Safety Policy

Unit-based adjuncts, such as instructions, protocols, explanations, and checklists, are used to implement a facility's perioperative medication policy. Specific examples of such adjuncts are laminated medication safety cards with preapproved

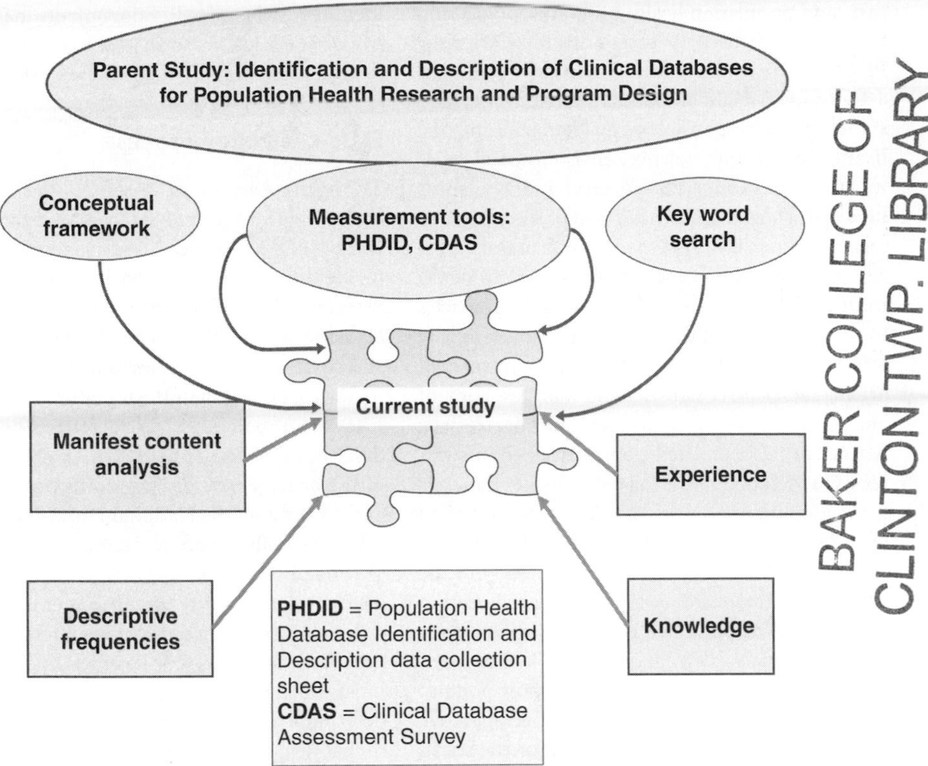

FIGURE 3-1 Conceptual framework for MEDMARX policy document study. (From Devine V, Bibb S: Use of MEDMARX data for the support and development of perioperative medication policy, *Perioper nurs clin* 3[4]:323, 2008.)

calculations listed, preapproved surgeon's preference cards with desired "formulary" medications specific for the patient and case listed, and point-of-care pharmacist access.

Specific Aims

The specific aims of this study were as follows:

- To describe the use of the MEDMARX database in the development and revision of population health medication policy across the perioperative continuum
- To identify a list of population health medication policies that have been developed or revised as a result of secondary data analysis of the MEDMARX database
- To create a list of population health medication policies that could be developed and supported using the MEDMARX database
- To generate a list of population health medication research topics that could be addressed for future study by perioperative nurses

METHODS

The research design for this study was descriptive. The methodologic approach was adopted from a study by Bibb et al (2006), in which a systematic search of the literature using the Cumulative Index to Nursing and Allied Health Literature (CINAHL) and the National Library of Medicine's search service (PubMed) bibliographic databases, covering the years 2003 and 2004, was performed to locate completed population health studies conducted by means of secondary analysis of existing clinical or administrative data. Key words associated with theoretic definitions of clinical database, secondary analysis, military health care, federal health care, and population health programs, policy, and research were used to locate abstracts. Healthy People 2010 leading health indicators (physical activity, overweight and obesity, tobacco use, substance abuse, responsible sexual behavior, mental health, injury and violence, environmental quality, immunization, access to care) and key words *safety* and *deployment health* were also used to locate abstracts. A systematic confirmatory process and exclusion algorithm were used to determine which abstracts and corresponding articles to include in the study. A data collection template was used to guide extraction of data from each article. Descriptive statistics and manifest content analysis were used to analyze and summarize data. A total of 52 completed population health studies were included in the analysis. Twenty data sets were identified. One of the data sets identified was the MEDMARX database. Identification of the MEDMARX data set was associated with the key words *secondary analysis* and *safety.* Location and analysis of published studies associated with secondary analysis of data from the MEDMARX data set and used in the development of population health medication policy for the perioperative setting was the focus of the analysis for the study. After the MEDMARX data set was identified as the data set for the focus of this study, a new systematic search of the literature was conducted to identify articles or policy documents that used the MEDMARX database in research, programs, or development of policy or policy-like documents.

Data Collection Process

Thirty-five key words, based on the conceptual definitions for the study, in combination with the word *MEDMARX*, were used in a search algorithm to identify articles and documents (Table 3-1). A systematic confirmatory process and exclusion algorithm were used to determine which abstracts and corresponding articles to include in the study. A systematic search of the literature from January 1, 1998, through July 31, 2005, retrieved 37 articles describing the use of MEDMARX data. Nineteen of the articles were discovered through CINAHL and 18 through the National Library of Medicine (PubMed) bibliographic databases.

The abstracts or summaries of these articles were printed to verify that they met the inclusion criteria. However, because of insufficient information in the summaries or abstracts to complete the inclusion algorithm, full articles were retrieved to determine which abstracts met inclusion criteria.

Six articles were excluded from the study because they did not meet the inclusion criteria. The remaining 10 articles were included in this study and were analyzed for content (Box 3-1).

TABLE 3-1 Summation of Key Words Used for Bibliographic Searches

Number of Hits	Number of Abstracts Saved	Key Words
5	3	"MEDMARX" and "secondary analysis"
0	0	"MEDMARX" and "military health policy"
1	1	"MEDMARX" and "policy"
5	3	"MEDMARX" and "safety"
5	0	"MEDMARX" and "patient safety"
19	9	"MEDMARX" and "medication errors"
1	0	"MEDMARX" and "adverse drug reactions"
1	0	"MEDMARX" and "perioperative patient safety"
0	0	"MEDMARX" and "perioperative medication policy"
0	0	"MEDMARX" and "operating room policy"
0	0	"MEDMARX" and "intraoperative medication policy"
37	**16**	**Total articles 16, minus 6 exclusions = 10 articles in study**

Description of Data Analysis

A data collection template was used to guide extraction of qualitative and quantitative data from each article. Quantitative data were coded and entered into SPSS version 12.0 for statistical analysis. Descriptive statistics were used to describe and summarize quantitative data. Manifest content analysis was used to analyze qualitative data and to identify themes related to use of MEDMARX data to support policy development.

RESULTS

Presentation of Results

The first aim of this study was to describe the use of the MEDMARX database in the development and revision of population health medication policy across the perioperative continuum. None of the 10 articles included in the study contained evidence that MEDMARX data were being used to create or revise medication policy.

The second aim of this study was to identify a list of population health medication policies that have been developed or revised as a result of secondary data analysis of the MEDMARX database. Again, none of the 10 articles included in the study contained evidence that MEDMARX data were being used to create or revise medication policy.

A summary table of all articles used in the study, with main content summarized, illustrates the gap of written evidence to support policy creation and modification based on MEDMARX findings (Table 3-2).

The third aim was to create a list of population health medication policies that could be developed and supported using the MEDMARX database. To create this list, themes were extracted from all of the articles using manifest content analysis, using phrases that depicted specific medication policies throughout the articles (Bibb, 2002; Bibb et al, 2006) (Box 3-2).

Population health medication research topics that could be addressed in future study by perioperative nurses and practitioners are identified in Table 3-3. To create this table, themes were extracted from all of the articles using manifest content analysis, using phrases that conveyed the need for further research throughout the articles.

DISCUSSION

Discussion of Major Findings

The major gap in the literature regarding policy change or modification supports this study's

BOX 3-1 Articles Used in Study

1. Beyea SC et al: Medical errors in the OR—a secondary analysis of MEDMARX, *AORN J* 77(1):122, 125-129, 132-134, 2003.
2. Beyea SC et al: Medication errors in the LDRP: identifying common errors through MEDMARX reporting, *AWHONN Lifelines* 8(2):130-140, 2004.
3. Cousins DD: Developing a uniform reporting system for preventable adverse drug events, *Clin Ther* 20(Suppl C):C45-58, 1998.
4. Cowley E: Medication errors in children: a descriptive summary of medication error reports submitted to the United States Pharmacopeia, *Curr Ther Res* 62(9): 627-640, 2001.
5. Hicks RW et al: Medication errors in the PACU: a secondary analysis of MEDMARX findings, *J PeriAnesth Nurs* 19(1):18-28, 2004.
6. Hicks RW et al: Selected medication-error data from USP's MEDMARX program for 2002, *Am J Health Syst Pharm* 61(10):993-1000, 2004.
7. Jones KJ et al: Translating research into practice: voluntary reporting of medication errors in critical access hospitals, *J Rural Health* 20:335-343, 2004.
8. Niccolai CS et al: Unfractionated heparin: focus on a high-alert drug, *Pharmacotherapy* 24(8 Pt 2):146S-155S, 2004.
9. Nosek RA et al: Standardizing medication error event reporting using MEDMARX. *Legal Medicine*, 2002, available at http://www.operationgivingback.facs.org/stuff/contentmgr/files/afdc13485baf0179425b669e4e4e8a4a/miscdocs/rules_of_engagement.pdf. Accessed December 1, 2009.
10. Santell JP et al: Medication errors: experience of the United States Pharmacopeia (USP) MEDMARX reporting system, *J Clin Pharmacol* 43(7):760-767, 2003.

TABLE 3-2 Recommendations From the Literature for Medication Policies That Could Be Developed Using the MEDMARX Database

Literary Recommendations for Future Perioperative Medication Policy Development	No. of Supporting Articles From Box 3-1
High-alert medication protocol (second verifier)	1, 2, 4–6, 8, 10
Competency evaluation of staff regarding medication policy	1–4, 7, 8, 10
Automated medication delivery system (decreasing reliance on floor-stocked medications)	1, 2, 6, 7, 10
Technological system–based improvements (bar coding, built-in safety alert software, computerized prescriber order entry [CPOE], medication error reporting)	3, 6, 7, 9, 10
Use point-of-care pharmacist model	1, 2, 4, 5, 7
Standardized acronyms, abbreviations, and medication doses	1, 2, 4, 6
Preprinted standard order forms with approved dosing nomograms	2, 5, 8
Telephone order/verbal order verification protocol with procedural steps listed	1, 8
Medication labeling policy of all medications (including sterile field)	1
Increased communication during transfer of patient (medication reconciliation)	1

BOX 3-2 Policies That Could Be Developed Using MEDMARX Data

STANDARDIZED MEDICATION ORDERING SYSTEM
- Computerized surgeon's preference cards with an automatic pharmacy order placed upon ordering case cart (surgical supplies)
- Built-in safety alerts

STANDARDIZED MEDICATION DELIVERY SYSTEM
- Automated dispensing system to decrease floor stock for operating room and bar coding all medication

STANDARDIZED MEDICATION ADMINISTRATION SYSTEM
- Second verifier required for all pediatric and high-alert medications: label all medications
- Surgeon preference cards as physician order for all perioperative medication

PHARMACY INTEGRATION IN ALL PERIOPERATIVE PRACTICES
- Preapproval of all unit formularies for floor stock
- Pharmacy involvement needed to mix medications and prepare high-alert medications
- A point-of-care pharmacist is available

argument for an increased use of the MEDMARX database to influence medication safety policy in the perioperative setting. This evidence-based change should be a priority for all perioperative nurses and practitioners to immediately decrease the patient safety risk through policy development. Some of the recommended policy themes are simple and can be integrated into existing policy immediately, with the more complex recommendations of system change requiring interdisciplinary resource planning.

Research topics that were identified from the literature are areas within the perioperative nursing specialty that require further study (see Table 3-3). Without this additional research, perioperative medication policy cannot be modified to best reflect safe medication practices for the surgical patient. Future research is essential for development of policies in the perioperative setting that are based on evidence-based findings.

Increased research is needed to identify specific causes of near misses to proactively change systems at risk to prevent medication errors from occurring. With 95% of all of the medication error reports in the MEDMARX database being "nonharm" categories, this database is the only one that should be used in the identification of preventable medication errors (Hicks et al, 2004b).

TABLE 3-3 Research Topics That Could Be Developed Using MEDMARX Data

Research Topic	Themes	Specifics Regarding Necessity of Research
Perioperative specialty units could benefit from research.	Causative data for medication errors and near misses in specialty areas are needed.	Identifies trends for harmful or near-miss medication errors, and practices changes following implementation of policy (i.e., same-day surgery, operating room holding area, and gastrointestinal/endoscopy units)
Operating rooms could benefit from research.	Operating rooms are high-risk medication safety areas.	Focuses on quality assurance monitors regarding perioperative policy statements, with observation and documentation data to support that the policy is being practiced
Participating MEDMARX subscribers could benefit from research.	Benchmark facilities	Compares and contrasts medication errors in similar health care facilities to identify causes and examine medication policies

Identification of Limitations

Limitations of this study included researcher subjectivity and bias, because there was only one researcher. In addition, there was a small sample size of 10 articles.

Implications for Nursing

Perioperative nurses and practitioners are equipped with the skills required to analyze secondary data from nationally recognized databases for medication errors. They are also educated in recognizing areas of further research that is needed to expand the evidence-based knowledge in their nursing specialty (Heitkemper and Bond, 2006; AORN, 2009). The MEDMARX database is a rich source of data for someone who recognizes its immense potential to improve medication administration safety and prevent medication errors for the surgical patients of tomorrow.

CONCLUSION

Future research on the effect of an electronic database such as MEDMARX on safe medication practices in the perioperative milieu would support revisions of perioperative medication policy as a risk-reduction strategy to increase safe patient care. Through the tracking of medication errors in clearly defined categories, linked with specific degrees of harm or no harm, an accurate assessment of a facility's medication delivery process could then be made. These identified risks should be incorporated into a comprehensive plan of action, targeting specific areas of the medication delivery process in the surgical environment and therefore supporting the development of new medication policy. Only through further research in perioperative medication policy and risk-reduction strategies identified from medication error electronic databases can we begin to evaluate effective evidence-based practice in the quest for a medication error–free perioperative environment.

REFERENCES

Association of PeriAnesthesia Nurses: *Position statement on safe medication administration*, 2005, available at http://www.aspan.org/ClinicalPractice/PositionStatements/SafeMedicationAdministration/tabid/3281/Default.aspx. Accessed August 16, 2009.

Association of periOperative Registered Nurses: *Perioperative standards and recommended practices*, Denver, 2009, The Association.

Association of periOperative Registered Nurses: *AORN safe medication administration tool kit*, Denver, 2005, available at http://www.aorn.org/PracticeResources/ToolKits/SafeMedicationAdministrationToolKit/. Accessed October, 21, 2009.

Beyea SC, et al: Medication errors in the LDRP: identifying common errors through MEDMARX reporting, *AWHONN Lifelines* 8(2):130–140, 2004.

Bibb SC: Healthy People 2000 and population health improvement in the Department of Defense military health system, *Mil Med* 167:552–555, 2002.

Bibb SC, et al: *Identification and description of existing datasets available for use in population health research and program design in the Department of Defense*, Karen A. Rieder Nursing Research Poster Session, San Antonio, Texas, November 2006.

Borden S, Gifford E: *USP identifies leading medication errors in hospital emergency department*, available at http://vocuspr.vocus.com/vocuspr30/xsl/uspharm/Profile.asp?Entity=PRAsset&. Accessed May 5, 2006.

Cousins DD: Developing a uniform reporting system for preventable adverse drug events, *Clin Ther* 20(Suppl C): C45–C58, 1998.

Cowley E, et al: Medication errors in children: a descriptive summary of medication error reports submitted to the United States Pharmacopeia, *Curr Ther Res Clin Exp* 62(9):627–640, 2001.

Department of Defense: *Department of Defense directive: health promotion and disease/injury prevention,* available at http://www.dtic.mil/whs/directives/corres/html2/d101010x.htm. Accessed August 22, 2005a.

Department of Defense Tricare Management Activity: *Medical management guide,* available at http://www.mhsophsc.org?public/spd.cfm?spi=mmguide. Accessed August 22, 2005b.

Devine V, Bibb S: Use of MEDMARX data for the support and development of perioperative medication policy, *Perioper Nurs Clin* 3(4):323, 2008.

Hamric AB, Hanson CH: Educating advanced practice nurses for practice reality, *J Prof Nurs* 19(5):262–268, 2003.

Heitkemper MM, Bond EF: *Clinical nurse specialists: state of the profession and challenges ahead,* available at http://www.medscape.com/viewarticle/480355. Accessed March 6, 2006.

Hicks RW, et al: Medication errors in the PACU: a secondary analysis of MEDMARX findings, *J Perianesth Nurs* 19(1): 18–28, 2004a.

Hicks RW, et al: Selected medication-error data from USP's MEDMARX program for 2002, *Am J Health Syst Pharm* 61:993–1000, 2004b.

Hicks RW, et al: *MEDMARX data report: a chartbook of medication error findings from the perioperative settings from 1998–2005*, Rockville, Md, 2006, USP Center for the Advancement of Patient Safety.

Hicks RW, et al: Medication errors in the PACU, *J Perianesth Nurs* 22:413–419, 2007.

Institute of Medicine: *Institute of Medicine report*, 1998. available at http://www.iom.edu/?id=12735. Accessed March 28, 2006.

Institute of Medicine: *Patient safety: achieving a new standard for care*, 2003, available at http://www.iom.edu/Object.File/Master/27/174/PatientSafety-web.pdf. Accessed October 6, 2009.

Jones KJ, et al: Translating research into practice: voluntary reporting of medication errors in critical access hospitals, *J Rural Health* 20:335–343, 2004.

National Patient Safety Foundation (website): http://www.npsf.org. Accessed November 20, 2005.

Niccolai CS, et al: Unfractionated heparin: focus on a high-alert drug, *Pharmacotherapy* 24(8, Pt 2):146S–155S, 2004.

Nicoll LH, Beyea SC: Policy analysis as a strategy for clinical decision making, *AORN J* 70(2):310–312, 1999.

Nosek RA, et al: Standardizing medication error event reporting in the U.S. Department of Defense. In Henriksen K et al, editors: *Advances in patient safety: from research to implementation*, vol 4, pp 361–374. "Programs, tools, and products. Surveillance tools." AHRQ Pub. No. 05-0021-4. Rockville, Md, 2005, Agency for Healthcare Research and Quality.

Santell JP, et al: Medication errors: experience of the United States Pharmacopeia (USP) MEDMARX reporting system, *J Clin Pharmacol* 43(7):760–767, 2003.

The Joint Commission: *Sentinel Event Alert,* Issue 35, June 25, 2006, available at http://www.jointcommission.org/SentinelEvents/SentinelEventAlert/sea_35.htm. Accessed August 16, 2009.

The Joint Commission: *Facts about the national patient safety goals,* June 19, 2008a, available at http://www.jointcommission.org/PatientSafety/NationalPatientSafetyGoals/npsg_facts.htm. Accessed August 16, 2009.

The Joint Commission: *The Joint Commission accreditation program, hospital national patient safety goals,* 2008b, available at http://www.jointcommission.org/NR/rdonlyres/31666E86-E7F4-423E-9BE8-F05BD1CB0AA8/0/HAP_NPSG.pdf. Accessed August 16, 2009.

Titler PR: *Nursing research: methods and critical appraisal for evidence-based practice*, ed 6, St. Louis, 2006, Mosby.

United States Pharmacopeia: The MEDMARX database, available at http://www.usp.org. Accessed April 10, 2006.

Zuzelo PR: Clinical nurse specialist practice—spheres of influence, *AORN J* 77:361–369, 2003.

COMPETENCE, NURSING PRACTICE, AND SAFE PATIENT CARE

Linda Brazen, MSN, BSN, RN, CNOR

Competent, competence, competences, competency, competencies—all describe, but in no way define, the complex of knowledge, skill, and ability that is the hallmark of successful practice in any profession, including the nursing profession. Attempts to define competence as a concept, to create a model of competence, or to measure it have been made for almost 20 years in the nursing education, staff development, and practice literature.

Yet, although competence is relevant to all health care disciplines, consumers of health care, academic and clinical educators, student nurses, employers, and administrators, there is not even a common understanding or consensus of what competence is or is not (Tilley, 2008). Implicitly though, competence is essential.

THE COMPETENCE CONTINUUM

Nursing faculty struggle to create curricula that provide content and teaching strategies to best prepare students with entry-level competencies. Health care facilities with registered nurse (RN) employees struggle with entry-level competence. Nursing administrators and directors struggle with obtaining the finances to support competence development, especially as it relates to safe patient care issues. Unit-based managers struggle to keep staff competent in light of constantly increasing technologies. Clinical educators and staff-development specialists struggle to assess, validate, and maintain all the points along the continuum of competence: from the entry-level competences of graduate nurses, to the initial-competence of new hires, to the new- and ongoing-competence needs of staff. Distinguishing the intent and purpose of competence provides a consensus about the requisite knowledge, skill, and ability inherent in professional clinical nursing practice.

Academic nursing education curriculum is designed to provide students with a baseline of knowledge and a real-time skill base that ensures that they are generically "safe" clinicians upon graduation. Because of this intention, student nurses are prepared for success in earning a professional nursing license. There are issues in licensure that are beyond the scope of this chapter. Specific to competence, however, it may be argued that the licensure examination is a static test of knowledge for a dynamic practice; it does not and cannot provide an indication of accuracy in future performance. A more common idea is that an RN license provides a measurable criterion for schools and colleges of nursing and employers. The license is intended to ensure that graduates from various types of nursing education programs will be equally successful.

In the workplace, employers use the RN license as a baseline indicator of an ability to do a job, competence notwithstanding. However, nurses starting their career or those hired into a care setting that they have no experience in are not always prepared to do the job. Employers who recognize this liability but use the recruit-to-retain strategy to hire candidates who value competence as a process that continues after their licensure, rather than an end product, are most successful. The quality, not the quantity, of new hires should be considered because what RNs do with their basic education has become the indicator of success in this quantum age of nursing practice (Porter-O'Grady, 2008).

The gap between knowledge gained through nursing education and its application to nursing practice is a conundrum when considering competence. Similarly, the gap between knowledge gained in the work setting and its implementation in practice is another challenge. Patients, as the recipients of nursing care, need competent RNs, and RNs need career competence.

Competence is absolutely necessary, but is still without definition.

Continuing Competence

Competence is an issue in nursing education, for employers of nurses, and for nursing itself. There are regulatory agencies, professional organizations, accrediting bodies, and, in the clinical practice arena, a certification process that creates challenges and opportunities for attaining and measuring RN competence. All of these entities consider and influence issues of competence. Because nursing is primarily a clinical, practice-based profession, the influence of these organizations reaches far into health care settings, traditionally the largest employers of RNs. The Joint Commission (TJC), the accrediting organization for health care facilities, requires employers to have programs in place that assess, maintain, and provide their employees with an ongoing process to maintain and gain competence.

Performance evaluation is a separate requirement and process of The Joint Commission; it relates to issues of competence at the organizational and individual employee level. The Joint Commission added National Patient Safety Goals (NPSGs) to its standards that measure, in part, the organization's and its employees' competence and performance. The Joint Commission does not prescribe how to improve or to measure an organization's or an employee's performance. The expectation is that catastrophic errors and near-miss patient incidents in health care settings will never occur. The Joint Commission added a never event list to the NPSGs in 2006. It continues to review organizational performance, and update and create new standards as needed, to attain the goal of eliminating never events in patient care (Catalano, 2008).

The standards of practice set by specialty nursing organizations are used by health care facilities and RN employees to develop competencies. Most specialty nursing organizations publish evidence-based guidelines for practice and support evidence in ongoing research. The results are then shared in professional journals. An additional set of guidelines and recommended practices, published with the standards of practice, are available from the organizations. These are used to develop workplace policies that support RN patient care competence. The Association of periOperative Registered Nurses (2008) has published guidelines that support the NPSGs.

Other groups that also contribute to professional competence issues, literature, and practice settings are the credentialing bodies for each specialty practice. Research is lacking to demonstrate a link between certification examinations and improved patient outcomes (Wittaker, 2008). However, a number of credentialing organizations are exploring how to validate competence so that portability and reciprocity are options for certified RNs who change employers or move to another state. Continuing career competence, through certification by examination and by participation in competence and skills-based activities, would be profiled and transferable throughout the RN's career and from employer to employer.

Organizational Competence

The goal of accreditation for the performance of a health care facility is to decrease the competition to be all things to all consumers and to increase the ability to do what the organization does best. Historically the word *competent* was used in accreditation manuals to indicate the quality of the organization by employing quantitative measurements such as fewer undesirable patient outcomes compared with a neighboring organization. A patient could use these measurements to determine the safety of the health care organization. A health care organization was considered competent if fewer patient risks were associated with it. In addition, it was implied that employees of a competent organization were themselves competent. In the scheme of accreditation, the mechanistic term *capacity* was often associated with a quantitative organizational measure and a perception of quality employees. Competent and accredited facilities demonstrated two performance measures: successful patient outcomes and the capacity to employ staff to provide such outcomes. Relative to the concept of competence, entry-level knowledge and skill combined with the RN license were considered equivalent to the knowledge and skill of the career-level competent RN in assigning roles and responsibilities. A large amount of health care, nursing education, and nursing practice literature was published in this era about competency as it related to entry-into-practice issues, including the comprehensive work of Patricia Benner (2008).

In 1991 the word *competent* in The Joint Commission manual was changed to *competence.* This was a deliberate move on the part of The Joint Commission Agenda for Change. The administrative and accreditation changes were designed to be less prescriptive and more process oriented. In turn, health care facilities were expected to be more process oriented and to use competence as a criterion of performance. Instead of organizations attempting to provide all care to all consumers, each organization identified its competence according to what it did best; for example, organ transplant surgery, a birthing center, or a specialization such as oncology. Because employee competence was a critical component of an organization's competence, the design of competence programs for employees was an indication of organizational performance. Employee competence programs included organizational expectations and identification of observable and measurable actions indicating individual performance. An employee who successfully demonstrated the combined performance of knowledge and skill had achieved competence. Implicit in the achievement was the expectation of continuing competence, which will be addressed in a later section of this chapter.

The terms *competent, competence,* and *competency* are often used interchangeably. Relative to accreditation standards, it may important to note that in addition to changing the word, the competence standard was moved from its original place in the nursing care standards section (1987–1991) to the staff education standards, where it remained until 1994. Then it was moved into the human resources article, where it remains as of this writing.

NATIONAL PATIENT SAFETY GOALS

Accreditation has evolved over the years, but what has remained constant is that it is a process, not a standardized or terminal point, along a continuum of patient care. Regardless of changes in the process of accreditation, The Joint Commission sets the primary benchmark for the safety and quality of care provided to future and current consumers of health care. Patients, as the consummate consumers of services provided by health care organizations, have become actively engaged in determining the nature and quality of their own care and services. Through the years, The Joint Commission has fostered and nurtured progressive and prospective process improvement initiatives in accredited health care organizations. This has been supported by consumers declaring that catastrophic errors and near-miss patient safety incidents are not acceptable. A representative group was invited to work with The Joint Commission to explore and prioritize the elimination of untoward patient incidents. They reviewed current goals, suggested new goals, and recommended requirements, based on evidence and best practices, designed to prevent such incidents from occurring. These goals are presented in the NPSG section of the accreditation manual. Any organization, accredited or seeking accreditation, that offers health care, treatments, and services relevant to the NPSGs is responsible for implementing the applicable requirements or effective alternatives. A term used in reference to The Joint Commission Safe Patient Care Initiative is the *safety trilogy.* Components of the safety trilogy are (1) trends in sentinel events, (2) preventive patient safety programs related to near-miss incidents, catastrophic errors, and never events, and (3) the NPSGs.

ASSOCIATION OF PERIOPERATIVE REGISTERED NURSES

In general, the NPSGs are focused on systemwide solutions. As professional patient care providers, perioperative RNs, including those primarily in the intraoperative phase of patient care, are equally responsible for creating a culture of patient safety. Creating and maintaining a culture of patient safety is a measure of organizational and employee competence. The subsets of patient safety culture include, but are not limited to, the following:

- A reporting culture, in which practice errors and near misses allow staff in the organization to learn from the experience
- A learning culture, in which gaining knowledge (i.e., learning) from experience is superseded by a willingness to implement major changes geared toward preventing any untoward incidents in the future
- A wary culture, in which members of all patient care teams are continually alert for the unexpected
- A just culture, in which all members of a patient care team are acutely aware of the distinction

between acceptable and unacceptable behaviors, including appropriate and inappropriate behaviors.

Inherent in any patient safety culture is the mindset that all employees of the organization share its values, attitudes, and beliefs and that reporting without blaming is a strategy that supports and improves patient safety. To encourage employee commitment to this mindset, an organization may use differing strategies, and technologies may be introduced to promote safe patient cultures. Learning to learn from knowledge, experience, and skill is the core of employee competence. If an entry-level employee's competence requirements are to learn unfamiliar or new technologies, to learn about communication expectations, and to learn that changing practice often reduces errors, then maintaining a "learning" process as a competence during the employee's tenure with the organization is achievable.

AMERICAN NURSES CREDENTIALING CENTER

The gap between education and practice will always be a challenge because it is created by a difference in competence as an outcome-based activity, not a terminal event. In nursing education the outcome is to learn nursing. By achieving RN licensure, the graduate student nurse is generically "safe." In nursing practice, however, the outcomes are always and only patient oriented. Because the practice role of competency from an educational perspective identifies and measures learning outcomes (also known as entry-level competencies), the result is that the competency of entry-level RNs has had to be met by employers through externships, internships, residency programs, orientations, in-service training, and worksite continuing education programs.

Employers also had to meet the continuing, ongoing, and career competence of employed RNs. Often this was achieved through certifications, portfolios, and progressive skill building to bridge performance expectations in the workplace. Clinical-based RNs have concerns about the quality of care they provide and the safety of their patients, and they want to work with competent peers. Knowing that a practicing RN is ready and able to provide care at the highest level of ability is also important to patients, colleagues in other health care disciplines, legislators, and organizations (Pacini, 2005). Accountability to oneself to be a competent peer is tantamount to being a safe caregiving professional. Everyday nursing practice takes place in dynamic health care systems that are bursting with new knowledge and skills to learn and a multitude of decisions that must be made to keep patients safe.

It is a challenge for a practicing RN to maintain competence and to demonstrate competence if employment changes. In an attempt to facilitate competence portability and competence reciprocity, the American Nurses Credentialing Center (ANCC) created Nursing Skills Competency Accreditation (ANCC, 2009; Yoder-Wise, 2008). The program is designed as a voluntary process for health care facilities to provide educational or training activities that yield or validate a nursing skill or subset. The ANCC Commission on Accreditation validates that a provider meets established standards based on predetermined criteria. Unlike the ANCC program that accredits organizations for Magnet Status, accreditation is awarded to an individual educational activity that meets design criteria. The activity must have both a didactic and a skills-demonstration component and requires validation and reliability. The program is a tool for employers and individual nurses to use to identify educational programs that are appropriately designed to validate nursing skills and skill sets. Employers and health care consumers can have confidence that an RN who has completed an accredited activity has met competency requirements (Yoder-Wise, 2008).

COMPETENCY AND CREDENTIALING INSTITUTE

The quality of certification in nursing practice is indicated by the number of certified RNs. The value of a health care facility's employing certified RNs is that it receives the ANCC Magnet Status Accreditation. The Competency and Credentialing Institute (CCI) is the leader in credentialing the operating room (OR) nursing community and has supported and facilitated a number of competency credentialing education programs since 1979 (CCI, 2009). Credentialing entails achieving success on a national examination. Competence entails maintaining credentials through participation in specific educational activities, which include, but are not limited to, ANCC-approved continuing education. In 2007

CCI convened the national Think Tank to explore how those in nursing can collaborate to develop a framework for continuing competence. As definitions of competence were reviewed and themes emerged, action items were identified for the nursing profession to consider when developing or implementing continuing competence programs and activities (CCI, 2008). These themes included the following:

- Competence is evolutionary; it is a process and an outcome.
- Educational process needs reform; competency-driven learning and student self-awareness are critical.
- Information literacy needs to be developed. Knowledge is dynamic, evolutionary, and experiential; needing to know is not as important as needing to retain.
- Impact on policy issues must be considered. Social, public, health, and economic influences are dynamic factors in health care worker competence systems.
- Working and learning in multidisciplinary teams is an essential component for the delivery of safe patient care.
- Data management is crucial because the effective use of data can help determine what constitutes safe patient care and safe nursing practice.

COMPETENCE APPLICATIONS

Health care organizations can have the most competent RN staffs, but if the environment is not supportive of professional practice, safe practice for patients will fail. Infrastructure programs are important for entry- and career-level competence assessment, development, and maintenance. However, competence in relation to patient safety and patient outcomes may require innovative approaches such as developing the competence process after both patient safety and patient outcomes are established. Instead of using static policies as a guide for care practice, a competence in a specialty of nursing could be the catalyst for the RN to design, manage, and coordinate the patient's care according to the variables presented (Tilley, 2008). Alternatively, a Synergy Model could optimize the nurse-patient relationship by matching the needs of the patient with the competencies of the RN, ensuring a safe passage through the health care system for the patient (Kerfoot and Cox, 2005). Continuing a reverse mode of thought would mean that entry-level competence assessment, staff orientation, and all the other methods of staff education would also need to change. Fundamentally the premise of the model is that patient characteristics drive nurses' competences (Pacini, 2005).

Gaps in knowledge, skill, and ability to provide safety for patients through the phases of care may be narrowing. In 2005, using a Robert Wood Johnson Foundation Grant, respected leaders from nursing education programs embarked on the Quality and Safety Education for Nurses (QSEN) Project (2009). The project's long-range goal is to reshape professional identity formation in nursing to include commitment to quality and safety competencies. To date, six specific quality and safety competencies for nursing have been identified and developed, and targets for the knowledge, skills, and attitudes to be developed in nursing prelicensure programs have been proposed. The six core competences are (1) patient-centered care, (2) teamwork and collaboration, (3) evidence-based practice, (4) quality improvement, (5) safety, and (6) informatics. The second phase of QSEN includes partnering with representatives to discuss potential graduate education competencies and working with 15 pilot schools that voluntarily committed to change their curricula toward incorporating quality and safety competencies. The QSEN Project is an academic response that may bridge the knowledge, skill, and ability gaps in competence for nursing students when they are hired into their first professional clinical position. The project is a model that, perhaps in combination with the myriad of new-graduate programs created by health care facilities to address the gap, may solve the issue of entry-level competence.

The other end of the nursing competence continuum concerns the gaps in knowledge, skill, and ability of practicing nurses. Career competence includes achievement and maintenance of specific competencies associated with an RN's area of expertise and practice setting (Allen et al, 2008). As an RN, career core competence includes the abilities to think in action, to have confidence and clarity in decision making, and to retrieve information. In the depth and breadth of health care, education, and nursing literature over the years, multiple models, methods, and strategies have been used to control the competence continuum in workplace settings. Clinical nursing practice is desperate for a blueprint that ensures achievement and maintenance of competences that will improve clinical nursing and provide patients with safe journeys through their health care experiences. To date what is conclusive is that on the whole we have a very poor understanding of our own ability to change health care worker behaviors (Pyrek, 2008). Delivery of knowledge content has rarely embraced measuring the outcomes of learning (i.e., competences). As a result, health care employers face the dual struggle of evaluating competency and managing the regulatory and accrediting challenges of patient safety. Measuring competence annually by evaluating RN clinical bedside skills does not guarantee that an RN possesses the actual knowledge, skill, and ability to care for patients and to care for them in changing patient situations.

COMPETENCE, OPERATING ROOM NURSING PRACTICE, AND SAFE PATIENT CARE

Self-assessment is both a challenge and an opportunity when it comes to accountability. Society has conditioned people to believe that high self-esteem is more important than anything else. One unfortunate side effect is that people can come to view anything other than praise as a personal attack or a sign that they are not knowledgeable and talented. Self-assessment is a critical component of any professional's behavior, and competence is an ethical component. Self-assessment requires a person to examine and be accountable for his or her actions and competency. Ethically, if one's actions are parallel with expectations of society and regulatory, accrediting, and credentialing agencies, self-assessment is an opportunity to be accountable for one's own practice.

Safe patient care in OR care settings requires competence in OR nursing practice. At the core of that practice is the higher-level-practice concept of advocacy. An OR RN advocating for patients in need of operative procedures guards them against errors and provides them with competent practices when they are at their most vulnerable. Efforts toward the goals of self-assessment, accountability, and competence are in place through mutual collaborative initiatives such as the Council on Surgical and Perioperative Safety (Banschback, 2008) and the Joint Commission International Center for Patient Safety (2009).

Competence and accountability at a day-to-day level of practice are both a challenge and an opportunity. It has long been a challenge to assess intraoperative patient outcomes associated only with RN competence (Kleinbeck and McKennet, 2000). As indicators of what patients should expect from nursing care during surgical or other invasive procedures, the outcomes have never been intended to be only the result of a patient's time in the OR. Nonetheless, how the patient actually benefited as a result of an RN's advocacy has not been identified through the number of tasks and interventions performed and documented by the intraoperative RN during the patient's intraoperative experience.

The impact of emphasizing the RN's actions, rather than how the patient benefits from those actions, is unknown at this time. Instead of being fearful that unlicensed staff will encroach on an RN's practice, RNs in the OR setting can turn this perceived challenge and their tasks and interventions into an opportunity for a patient's safe journey. The opportunity at a day-to-day level is found not in asking who is responsible for the patient's safety, but in realigning the question into a framework that through competence and accountability makes all of us as professionals responsible.

Under pressure from insurers, federal agencies, and regulatory agencies, hospitals are starting to agree to not charge a patient who experiences a never event, because a never event should not have happened (Fulmer, 2008). The cost of treatment resulting from surgical objects left in a patient during surgery, patient falls, catheter-caused urinary tract infections, and pressure ulcers will no longer be reimbursed because these errors occurred during a hospital stay. The incentive for health care workers to be vigilant to competence, accountable for practice, and responsible for working in collaboration is clear. Building a culture of safety using high-reliability principles is key to the future success of health care facilities as employers of professional RNs. To support these efforts, standardized practice strategies have been designed (Joint Commission International Center for Patient Safety, 2009; World Health Organization, 2007). In the literature, evidence can be found that relates how systems and interactions between system components influence performance and patient safety (Christian et al, 2006).

CONCLUSION

There will always be health care consumers, and there will always be a need to help them have safe health care experiences. Patient outcomes that indicate achievement of safe patient care are needed for RNs. The RN's competence must be based on a reality of patient-focused phenomena and patient-focused outcomes. Traditional psychomotor approaches to skill acquisition and cognitive delivery methods for knowledge acquisition have not fostered changes in health care worker behaviors. Evidence-based entry-level and career competence strategies need to incorporate abilities including, but not limited to, attention to patient safety and cue recognition of emerging patient crisis. There is also a need for support from the organizational level for human and fiscal resources to design and develop relevant content (Rapala, 2005). Optimal patient care depends on the best match between a patient's needs, the nurse's advocacy practice, and nursing competence. When entry-level through career-level competence is finally defined, philosophical and operational changes in clinical staff education activities such as orientation, professional and staff development, in-service training, continuing education, and management development will need to occur.

REFERENCES

Allen, et al: Evaluating continuing competence: a challenge for nursing, *J Contin Educ Nurs* 39(2):81, 2008.

American Nurses Credentialing Center: *Overview of ANCC: Nursing skills competency program—a new kind of nursing accreditation*, available at http://www.nursecredentialing.org. Accessed June 23, 2009.

Association of periOperative Registered Nurses: *Perioperative standards and recommended practices*, Denver, 2008, The Association.

Banschback SK: Mutual accountability for the common goal of patient safety, *AORN J* 88(1):11–13, 2008.

Benner P: *From novice to expert: excellence and power in clinical nursing practice*, Menlo Park, Calif, 2008, Addison-Wesley.

Catalano K: *Joint Commission and National Patient Safety Goals: update for 2008.* Paper presented at the Association of periOperative Nurses 55th Congress, Anaheim, Calif, March 30-April 4, 2008.

Christian CK, et al: A prospective study of patient safety in the operating room, *Surgery* 139(2):159–173, 2006.

Competency and Credentialing Institute: *The CCI continued competence forum: from pieces to policy*, available at http://www.cc-institute.org/tt07, Accessed March 11, 2008.

Competency and Credentialing Institute (website): http://www.cc-institute.org/abus.aspx. Accessed June, 23, 2009.

Fulmer M: The basics: hospitals won't get to bill for errors, *MSN Money*, March 7, 2008. available at. http://www.articles.moneycentral.msn.com/Insurance/InsureYourHealth. Accessed June 23, 2009.

Joint Commission International Center for Patient Safety, n.d., available at: http://www.jcipatientsafety.org. Accessed June 23, 2009.

Kerfoot KM, Cox M: The synergy model: the ultimate mentoring model, *Crit Care Nurs Clin North Am* 17:109–112, 2005.

Kleinbeck SVM, McKennet M: Challenges of measuring intraoperative patient outcomes, *AORN J* 72(5):845–853, 2000.

Pacini CM: Synergy: a framework for leadership development and transformation, *Crit Care Nurs Clin North Am* 17: 113–119, 2005.

Porter-O'Grady T: A glimpse over the horizon: a new future for nursing practice. In *A continuing education program designed specifically for the University of Colorado in Denver, College of Nursing*, Denver, 2008, Office of Professional Development and Extended Studies.

Pyrek K: Zero tolerance for infections: a winning strategy, *Infection Control Today*, January 24, 2008, available at http://www.infectioncontroltoday.com. Accessed June 23, 2009.

Quality and Safety Education for Nurses: *Overview*, available at http://qsen.org/competencydomains. Accessed June 23, 2009.

Rapala K: Mentoring staff members as patient safety leaders: The Clarian Safe Passage Program, *Crit Care Nurs Clin North Am* 17(2):121–126, 2005.

Tilley D: Competency in nursing: a concept analysis, *J Contin Educ Nurs* 39(2):58–64, 2008.

Wittaker S, et al. Assuring continued competence: policy questions and approaches—how should a profession respond? *Online J Issues Nurs* 5(3):2000. available at http://www.nursingworld.org/MainMenuCategories/ANAMarketplace/ANAPeriodicals/OJIN/TableofContents/Volume52000/No3Sept00/ArticlePreviousTopic/ContinuedCompetence.aspx. Accessed June 23, 2009.

World Health Organization Collaborating Center for Patient Safety Solutions: Performance of correct procedure at correct body site: patient safety solutions, *Patient Safety Solutions*, vol 1, solution 4, May 2007, available at http://www.ccforpatientsafety.org/common/pdfs/fpdf/presskit/PS-Solution4.pdf. Accessed June 23, 2009.

Yoder-Wise: Continuing competence: one state's efforts, *J Contin Educ Nurs* 39(2):51–52, 2008.

PERIOPERATIVE SAFE MEDICATION USE

A Focused Review

Linda J. Wanzer, MSN, RN, CNOR • Rodney W. Hicks, PhD, RN, FNP-BC, FAANP, FAAN • BradLee Goeckner, MSN, RN, LCDR, CNOR • Lisa Cole, MSN, RN, CNOR

In 1859 Florence Nightingale (1970) wrote in *Notes on Nursing*, "It may seem a strange principle to enunciate as the first requirement in a hospital that it should do the sick no harm." This tenet had already been the basis for physicians, given the centuries-old standard of first and foremost, do no harm. Yet there remains public concern among patients who enter the health care system, and rightly so. Within the past decade the Institute of Medicine (IOM) brought renewed attention to this hallowed tenet through its seminal report, *To Err Is Human: Building a Safer Health System*, when it asserted that up to 98,000 deaths occurred annually as the result of medical errors (Kohn et al, 2000). Citing data that health care institutions had caused harm or death (Kohn et al, 2000), the IOM went further in describing the health care system of the twenty-first century. In the newer model of patient safety through the avoidance of iatrogenic injury, safety would be the new and minimally accepted standard of care (IOM, 2004). Because of these reports, patient safety has become a mantra for all within health care.

Safe medication use has always been just one important aspect of patient safety. Violations of safe medication principles, policies, and processes and the resultant medication errors now serve as the markers of evidence for warranted concern. Such markers gain worldwide attention through headline stories that reflect personal tragedies of countless victims. Although the full extent of medication errors is unknown, there are indicators that such system failures are pervasive, which reflects poorly on the world's most advanced health care system. The IOM claimed that up to 7000 deaths were directly attributable to medication errors (Kohn et al, 2000). Other investigators have estimated that errors can affect 20% of all routinely administered medication doses (Barker et al, 2002). Researchers from the U.S. Food and Drug Administration investigated the agency's medication error database, the Adverse Event Reporting System, and found that 10% of the reported errors over a 6-year period resulted in death (Phillips et al, 2001). Still other investigators have claimed that up to 9% of all hospital admissions result from medication errors (Winterstein et al, 2002). In fact, as of December 31, 2007, medication errors were the fourth leading reported sentinel event in hospitals across the United States according to the sentinel event statistics reported by The Joint Commission. Given that all medication errors are preventable (National Coordinating Council for Medication Error Reporting and Prevention, 2008), it is no wonder that safe medication use became a focal point in numerous initiatives aimed at reducing the burden of iatrogenic injuries.

Since the release of *To Err Is Human*, great strides have been made to better understand the complexity of the health care system and how that complexity affects patient safety (Rudman et al, 2002). In turn, this understanding has guided the development of or revisions to professional guidelines (Association of periOperative Registered Nurses [AORN], 2008), national and international campaign initiatives focused on safety (World Health Organization [WHO], 2006), and state and federal laws (Shojania et al, 2001). Many of these activities have influenced safe medication practices to help move the health care delivery system to one that ensures that patient safety is the standard of care (Leape, 2002).

The purpose of this chapter is to expand the perioperative team's knowledge about current safe medication practices by (1) building the knowledge base using definitions from a national taxonomy and a leading patient safety organization, (2) presenting findings from multiple sources that represent some of the known failure points that reflect the state of the science, and (3) proposing and identifying solutions to address the failure points. This discussion should allow perioperative clinicians to gain an appreciation of how the complex system within the perioperative environment predisposes otherwise competent practitioners to be involved in medication errors.

NATIONALLY AND INTERNATIONALLY RECOGNIZED CONCEPTS ASSOCIATED WITH ERRORS

The Value of Medication Error Reporting

Event reporting systems can be powerful tools to build knowledge when the findings are used to improve systems and educate providers (Wachter, 2004). The intent behind such systems is to collate and analyze the risks associated with related activities to propose remedial and preventive actions (Leape, 2002). A reporting system includes multiple components: empiric and theoretic models, a variety of tools built from domain content, and analysis by domain experts (Nyssen et al, 2004).

Even before *To Err Is Human* was published, the United States Pharmacopeia (USP) had suggested significant patient safety initiatives drawn from the evidence of two national medication error reporting programs: the USP Institute for Safe Medication Practices Medication Errors Reporting Program and MEDMARX. The Medication Errors Reporting Program is a voluntary program open to all clinicians in all settings. This database, which is operated in cooperation with the Institute for Safe Medication Practices, collects information and provides data to regulatory agencies, professional organizations, and the pharmaceutical industry in an effort to educate about preventing future adverse drug events. MEDMARX, launched in 1998, is an Internet-accessible, anonymous medication error database used by hospitals and health systems and is available through an annual subscription service. MEDMARX provides subscribers with an opportunity to track adverse medication events within the facility, review errors reported by other facilities in the database, conduct comparisons between facilities, and examine quality improvement initiatives that other facilities have implemented in response to medication errors (Hicks et al, 2004). Although the facilities that report to MEDMARX currently constitute less than 10% of all U.S. hospitals and health care systems, USP has amassed the largest repository of medication error data currently available in the world, with more than 1.25 million case reports from more than 770 facilities. It is important to note that the number of case reports represents only those that have been voluntarily reported to MEDMARX.

When discussing the concept of reporting, it is important to recognize that two aspects occur: (1) errors are reported, and (2) errors are not reported. Errors that are not reported can be further segmented into those intentionally not reported and those that are not detected. The Iceberg Model is an excellent representation of this phenomenon. Researchers studying the relationship between detected and reported errors have found wide variances between what is reported (the tip above the water) and what is undetected and remains unreported (the ice mass below the water) (Barker et al, 2002; Flynn et al, 2002; Shaw-Phillips, 2002). Furthermore, extending the analogy and comparing reporting with not reporting, the mass that remains "under water" represents lost opportunities to learn from mistakes that could be used to improve health care systems.

Leape (2002) identified seven characteristics of successful reporting systems based on published expert opinions: (1) nonpunitive (free of fear of retaliation), (2) confidential (deidentified patient, reporter, and institutional information), (3) independent (analysis is done by an organization without power to punish), (4) expert analysis (content experts), (5) timely (prompt), (6) responsive (dissemination of results), and (7) systems oriented (focused on changes in systems and processes rather than on individual performances). Applying these characteristics to perioperative conditions (including errors) yields richness within practice to advance the profession.

National Coordinating Council for Medication Error Reporting and Prevention

Before discussing medication errors, the common languages used to report, analyze, and discuss medication errors and the medication use process (MUP) must be understood. Our understanding today of medication errors can be attributed to several sources, including early work done by the National Coordinating Council for Medication Error Reporting and Prevention (NCC MERP). Formed in July 1995 from 22 different constituent-based organizations, NCC MERP (2008) and its members cooperatively addressed the multidisciplinary causes of medication errors to promote safe medication use. NCC MERP (2008) produced the nation's first comprehensive taxonomy for studying medication errors and established the nationally recognized definition of a medication error:

> *A medication error is any* **preventable** *event that may cause or lead to inappropriate medication use or patient harm while the medication is in the control of the health care professional, patient, or consumer. Such events may be related to professional practice, health care products, procedures, and systems, including prescribing; order communication; product labeling, packaging, and nomenclature; compounding; dispensing; distribution; administration; education; monitoring; and use.*

The value of any taxonomy lies in its usefulness for providing a standard approach to record, interpret, and track phenomena. The NCC MERP Taxonomy of Medication Errors is the most useful tool known to evaluate medication error studies, given that it encompasses all disciplines involved in safe medication use.

Medication Error Severity

NCC MERP also created the Index for Categorizing Medication Errors to determine the outcome or effect of the medication error on the patient. The index contained four major subscales: (1) potential for error (category A); (2) actual error that did not reach the patient (category B); (3) actual error that reached the patient but did not result in harm (category C or D); and (4) actual error that reached the patient and resulted in harm (category E, F, G, H, or I). The reliability of this scale ($\kappa = 0.60$) was established in 2007 by a group of researchers at the Ohio State University (Forrey et al, 2007).

Medication Use Process

The MUP is a systems approach that defines the typical manner in which medications move through an institution in terms of prescribing, dispensing, and administering to patients (Nadzam, 1998). According to USP, each step or point in the MUP is referred to as a node (Hicks et al, 2004). Each node represents domains of professional responsibilities, including the corresponding series of checks and balances and professional judgments that seek to ensure safe medication use. Table 5-1 lists the nodes of the MUP and the corresponding definitions.

Nursing school curricula and nursing practice have historically drawn heavily on one safe medication practice known as the "five rights," which was intended to ensure that the right patient received the right dose of the right drug at the right time and by the right route. Nurses have used this guiding practice extensively. Furthermore, it has served as the legal standard for safe practice, because satisfying each of the "rights" offered maximum protection against medication errors. However, this practice is not foolproof, given that the national medication error reporting program MEDMARX contains data suggesting that one-third of the reported medication errors that occurred between 2002 and 2006 took place during medication administration (Hicks et al, 2008).

The continued prevalence of medication errors during drug administration indicates that the practice of five rights alone is not adequate to keep patients safe from medication errors. The Illinois Court of Appeals found this when it rendered its decision that hospitals were responsible for the negligence of nurses performing physicians' orders by giving medications that were clearly contraindicated for the patient (Medication Ordered Is Contraindicated, 2007). In this case there was an underlying "assumption"

TABLE 5-1 The Medication Use Process

Node	Definition
Procuring	The formal action of how organizations obtain products
Prescribing	The action of a legitimate prescriber to issue a medication order
Transcribing	Anything that involves or is related to the act of transcribing an order by someone other than the prescriber for order processing
Dispensing	A phase that begins with a pharmacist's assessment of a medication order and continues to the point of releasing the product for use by another health care professional
Administering	A phase in the MUP in which the drug product and the patient interface
Monitoring	The phase that involves evaluating the patient's physical, emotional, or psychologic response to the medication and then recording such findings

From Hicks RW et al, editors: MEDMARX data report: a report on the relationship of drug names and medication errors in response to the Institute of Medicine's call for action, Rockville, Md, 2008, Center for the Advancement of Patient Safety, US Pharmacopeia.
MUP, Medication use process.

that there was correct execution of tasks in all of the preceding steps within the MUP that ultimately proved to be inaccurate. Directly resulting from this case, two additional rights (the right indication and the right documentation) have been added to the standard for using medications safely. Furthermore, this case set legal precedence that in effect raised the bar by indicating that the five rights should not be the sole "safety net" for medication administration. Rather, undertaking a review of all steps of the entire MUP before administering a medication should be required to protect the patient.

CASE STUDY

A surgeon unknowingly writes an order for regular insulin, 10 units, in the wrong patient's chart. The patient for whom the surgeon is writing the insulin order is not diabetic. A pharmacist fills the order and sends the medication to the operating room (OR). The pharmacist perpetuates the error by labeling the medication with the name of the patient on the order sheet. A perioperative nurse, with faulty information, confirms the five rights and administers the insulin, further perpetuating the original error, and this patient becomes a victim of a medication error.

The five rights failed as a safety net for the nurse and the patient in this case study. In addition, had this been a real case, based on the appellate court ruling from Illinois, the organization would have been liable in giving the patient the insulin because the patient was not diabetic. This case study demonstrates how the addition of the two new rights (the right indication and the right documentation) to the current five rights could add a new dimension to the safety net for medication administration and could assist nurses in understanding the potential for medication errors throughout the MUP.

STATE OF THE SCIENCE IN PERIOPERATIVE SAFE MEDICATION USE

The OR is a unique environment. What occurs behind the pneumatic doors of the OR takes a special skill set that is not required within many other specialties in health care. Few researchers have focused on specific problems associated with safe medication use in the OR (Beyea et al, 2003). Rather, studies have investigated other important clinical topics such as instrument and sponge counts, new technologies, and fire safety. Therefore the literature offers very limited guidance for practitioners to improve safe medication use in the OR. Some of the earliest literature comes from researchers reporting findings collected through the Australian Incident

Monitoring Study (Runciman et al, 1993) that support the conclusion that system failures contributed to human errors in the OR setting. In fact, most of the current knowledge about medication errors in the OR stems from studies led by anesthesiologists; thus national safety experts recognize anesthesiology as the founding discipline of patient safety.

Wanzer and Hicks (2006), using the NCC MERP taxonomy, recently conducted a review of 10 articles that examined medication errors in the OR (Table 5-2). This focused review provided one look within the unique environment of the OR regarding medication safety and improving clinical outcomes. The investigators concluded that the science involving perioperative safe medication use was in its early stages. They supported this claim by drawing on systematic reviews of the literature, descriptive studies, and secondary analyses because there were few randomized clinical evaluations to provide evidence. Support for their conclusion included the inconsistency of the methods used to identify errors, variations in measuring patient outcomes, and lack of consensus about what constituted an error.

Included in the review was a study done by Beyea et al (2003) on 731 medication errors reported to MEDMARX between August 1998 and March 2002. The investigators found that 10% of the errors resulted in patient harm, including one case in which the error was associated with a patient's death. This reported incidence of harm was nearly five times greater than the remaining cases in the MEDMARX database. Furthermore, given that the data originated from multiple institutions, it was evident that medication errors that originated in the OR were not isolated events.

MEDMARX Chartbook

The most comprehensive review to date of OR medication errors can be found in USP's 2006 MEDMARX chartbook of perioperative medication errors (Hicks et al, 2006), which examined 3773 errors in accordance with the variables of the NCC MERP taxonomy. In addition, multiple analyses detailed the variables by age of the patient, which resulted in a more comprehensive review. The report also contained several case illustrations that further described the errors.

Of the 3773 errors in the OR, the investigators concluded that 7.2% resulted in harm, which compares unfavorably with the entire database, in which harm was associated with 1.4% of all events. Further analyses by age of the patient suggested that pediatric patients (patients younger

TABLE 5-2 Studies Reporting Perioperative Errors

Author (Year)*	Setting	Design	Sample (n)
Abeysekera et al (2005)	Anesthesia	Descriptive	896
Beyea et al (2003)	Operating room	Descriptive	731
Currie et al (1993)	Anesthesia	Descriptive	144
Fasting and Glsvoid (2000)	Anesthesia	Prospective design with intervention	55,426
Jensen et al (2004)	Anesthesia	Review article	98
Khan and Hoda (2005)	Anesthesia	Descriptive	768
Liu and Koh (2003)	Anesthesia	Survey	116
Orser and Byrick (2004)	Anesthesia	Secondary analysis	232
Webster et al (2004)	Anesthesia	Randomized clinical evaluation	15
Wheeler and Wheeler (2005)	Anesthesia	Review article	221

From Wanzer LJ, Hicks RW: Medication safety within the perioperative environment, *Annu Rev Nurs Res* 24:127-155, 2006.
* Full citations for each of these articles can be found in the references section at the end of the chapter.

than 17 years) had higher incidences of harm (16.7%) than adults (11.3%) and geriatric patients (10.0%). Nearly half of the records reviewed did not include the patient's age, and harm was present in this cluster in 2.4% of events. The report suggested that risk for medication error was greater in pediatric patients than any other population.

Case Study From the Report

In one fatal case an adult male was undergoing operative repair for a nasal fracture and facial lacerations after a bicycle accident. Following the placement of pledgets soaked with cocaine, the area was injected with what was thought to be lidocaine with epinephrine; unfortunately, he was injected with epinephrine 1:1000, which contributed to his death.

Node of the Medication Use Process

The node of the MUP was examined in 3216 records, and slightly more than half (56.3%) of the records were associated with the administering phase. As with error severity, the data supported that slightly higher percentages were associated with pediatric patients (69.4%) than with adult (68.4%) or geriatric (68.7%) patients.

The report describes a low percentage of transcribing and dispensing errors, which reflects the clinical practice in the OR setting. Most medications used in the OR are a result of a verbal order or a standing order on the surgical preference card. Often it is not possible to interrupt the work flow and write down medication orders. Likewise, this specialty setting rarely transcribes medication orders to a Kardex or a physician's order form to process the order through the pharmacy department. Furthermore, few surgical environments have the luxury of a pharmacist dedicated to the OR. Rather, a common approach is to obtain the medications from an automated dispensing device or from open stock within the OR and then deliver the medication to the sterile field.

Case Study From the Report

A nurse was making a buffered solution to inject during an ophthalmic procedure. Instead of adding 1.6 mL of sodium bicarbonate to a 20-mL bottle of 2% lidocaine, 1.6 mL of sodium bicarbonate was added to 1.6 mL of 2% lidocaine and the medication was injected. The nurse discovered this error when preparing the same medication for the next case.

Type of Error

Pareto type of representations suggest that 80% of problems stem from 20% of the conditions (Curry, 2001). This principle was also evident in the MEDMARX data report—nearly 75% of the reported errors involved only 4 of the 14 types of error selections. The most commonly reported types of errors that occurred in the OR were omission errors, wrong drug errors, prescribing errors, and wrong amount errors.

Omissions of products (meaning the medication was never given) were often associated with antimicrobial products and were typically seen in the use of intravenous piggybacks, whereby the containers were never activated or were simply not infused. With regard to wrong drug administration, the leading cause of harm was related to the administration of the wrong pain medications.

Case Study From the Report

An older adult patient was undergoing a procedure in which a resectoscope was being used. Lactated Ringer's was inadvertently hung instead of sorbitol, resulting in bleeding and increased anesthesia time.

Further subanalyses of the MEDMARX report revealed that omission errors disproportionately affected the geriatric population and that wrong amount errors negatively affected pediatric patients. The report indicated that most of the errors resulted from breakdowns in communication among health care workers following handoffs. The report also cited the failure of adequate documentation leading to medication errors (Hicks et al, 2006).

Case Study From the Report

A provider thought that an unlabeled syringe was an antibiotic; instead, the syringe contained a muscle relaxant. Because of the error, the pediatric patient remained intubated, which prolonged the case.

Cause of Error

The leading cause of error was performance deficit (41.8%), followed by procedure/protocol not followed (27.2%), and communication (18.1%). These findings were in line with overall trends in medication errors; however, it is important to note that other causes of errors (contraindicated/ drug allergy, dispensing-device involved, packaging/ container design, and verbal orders) had higher percentages of occurrence in the OR environment than in the overall database of medication errors. The data further outlined the lack of proper labeling and storage and look-alike and sound-alike issues that were involved in the errors.

Case Study From the Report

A surgeon gave a verbal order for intravenous digoxin and misspoke the dose. The anesthesia provider did not catch that the order was a tenfold overdose and delivered the medication. An improper dose along with a verbal order contributed to the death of this infant.

Contributing Factors

Contributing factors are transient conditions (such as situational, organizational, or environmental) that alone do not lead to errors (Hicks et al, 2006). Rather, contributing factors affect the precise execution of the MUP and cause failures that result in errors. Because of their transient nature, contributing factors are difficult to anticipate, difficult to recognize, and difficult to manage.

In 40% of the medication errors reported, there was no contributing factor identified. Distractions were the highest contributing factor and accounted for 26% of the medication errors reported. This finding was not unexpected, given the dynamic nature of the work environment in the OR. Six of the identified contributing factors deal with the impact of staffing patterns on the error events. Nursing shortages have increased the use of temporary/agency staff and necessitated the need for float staff/cross coverage, resulting in the working staff being less familiar with the institution's policies and procedures. The report also identified that inexperienced staff members contributed to some of the errors.

Products Involved in Medication Errors

The MEDMARX report identified 343 different products involved in medication errors in the OR. Product classes included antimicrobials, analgesics, sedatives, and parenteral intravenous fluids. The report reviewed products in all of the populations examined and by errors that both did and did not result in harm. The five most frequently reported products involved in harmful errors were cefazolin, heparin, fentanyl, midazolam, and morphine. It is noteworthy that of the top five products involved in errors, four were classified as high-alert medications as defined by The Joint Commission. Of these products, cefazolin was one of the many antimicrobials involved in omission errors. With regard to central nervous system (CNS) products, errors typically involved the wrong amount being given. The most serious errors that have occurred as a result of the wrong product being administered include the following:

- Excessive dose (twentyfold extra) of heparin administered during a plastic case, leading to loss of soft tissues
- Intra-articular epinephrine (wrong route and wrong drug), leading to cardiac arrest
- Potassium chloride administered by way of infusion pump, leading to cardiac arrest
- Vecuronium given intravenously instead of cefazolin, resulting in paralysis
- Bupivacaine given intravenously instead of by infiltration, resulting in seizures
- Epinephrine (1:1000 instead of 1:10,000) injected instead of lidocaine, resulting in death
- Excessive dose (tenfold overdose) of digoxin administered to an infant, resulting in cardiac toxicity and death

Cross-Tabulation Analysis of Type of Error by Product/Class of Agent

A cross-tabulation analysis allows a deeper analysis of two variables. The MEDMARX report examined the leading types of errors and the products or classes of agents involved in the errors. The most common type of error was omission, and these errors predominantly involved antimicrobial agents. Wrong-drug errors most frequently involved CNS agents. Error in prescribing included antimicrobials, CNS agents, and nonsteroidal antiinflammatory drugs. Errors involving the wrong amounts involved CNS agents and anticoagulants. Finally, drugs prepared incorrectly included lidocaine, heparin, and midazolam. These findings point to where quality improvement efforts can start to eliminate the burden of such errors.

Level of Care Rendered Following an Error

In 58% of the cases reported, the medication errors required no additional care. The level of care given following a medication error can range from a simple task such as increasing vital signs monitoring to the highest level of care requiring life-sustaining measures through resuscitation. It should be understood, however, that any additional care means increased resource use, regardless of whether the resources are time, supplies, or equipment. Furthermore, in today's health care industry, the outward focus is on the cost in terms of dollars. The requirement for additional tests or treatment or an increase in length of stay further increases health care costs.

INITIATIVES FOR IMPROVING PERIOPERATIVE MEDICATION SAFETY

In addition to the microsystem fixes within various clinical settings, macrosystem changes are appearing at the local, national, and health care organizational levels. These changes are becoming noticeably apparent as increasing numbers of regulatory and professional organizations are collaborating and spearheading initiatives, policies, and recommendations that are aimed at transforming the health care system into a system of safety. The Joint Commission, the IOM, the Food and Drug Administration, the Institute for Safe Medication Practices, USP, the Association of periOperative Registered Nurses (AORN), the Agency for Healthcare Research and Quality (AHRQ), and the World Health Organization, along with numerous others, continue to engage in systems-level patient safety initiatives in an attempt to assist health care organizations with addressing medication errors. Although many of these organizations are responsible for the positive movement toward elimination of medication errors, this section focuses on the AHRQ (and its call for changing the culture of safety), The Joint Commission's initiatives, and the AORN recommended standards and practice guidelines because these three organizations have content that specifically addresses the issues of safe medication use within the perioperative environment.

Culture of Safety

Improving the outcomes of medication use requires changing the culture of the organization. The AHRQ conducted a recent patient safety culture survey that documented baseline culture from 519 hospitals. Based on 160,176 respondents, AHRQ identified that nonpunitive responses to errors was one area for significant improvement. Furthermore, the survey revealed that staff perception was that hospitals treated mistakes punitively, including filing copies of error reports in personnel files. This finding along with other data suggests that organizations are better at addressing the individual component of error on a regular basis (by notifying the individual, by implicating other staff members, and by providing education or training) than they are at addressing systems-level causes. This finding is not surprising, given that interventions directed at the practitioner are easier to implement. Improving the culture, however, requires removing blame from individuals and focusing attention on the root causes of the errors. In addition, the ideal culture of safety seeks out opportunities to learn from mistakes to avoid future recurrences.

The Joint Commission

The Joint Commission has assisted organizations with focusing directly on system changes through efforts such as the National Patient Safety Goals and the Medication Management Standards. The Joint Commission's most public foray into quality care was the release of the National Patient Safety Goals, which began in 2002. Since then The Joint Commission has annually published a list of evidence- or expert-based concerns for patient safety for inclusion in the accreditation process (JCAHO, 2005). Including the National Patient Safety Goals as part of the accrediting process elevated the importance of patients and their role in safety by directly linking the goals to the accreditation process (which is often required to receive reimbursement from the Medicare payment system). Although all patient safety goals are applicable to perioperative clinicians, goal 3 specifically calls on clinicians to label all medications and containers on and off the sterile field. This goal was developed following several serious events.

The Joint Commission's 2004 Medication Management Standards set the tone for greater emphasis on medication safety throughout an organization. The standards called for those practitioners involved in the medication management system to have readily accessible patient-specific information, such as allergy history, pertinent laboratory results, and a list of other current medications.

Another medication management standard addresses the storage requirement for medications. Organizations must also actively plan for storage of products that look alike or sound alike. An important element in this standard deals with handling of expired products. The pharmacy department must ensure removal of expired products from the clinical unit and segregate the product from other nonexpired products to ensure removal from use.

Another standard pertains to pharmacy oversight for all medication orders. Such oversight ensures appropriateness of product, dose, therapeutic indication, and a number of other safety elements. Although the 2004 standards are more prescriptive than previous standards and recognize the important role that pharmacists play in ensuring safe medication use (Rich, 2004), it is invaluable for all perioperative clinicians to be familiar with the depth and breadth of the current standards.

AORN Recommended Standards and Guidelines

The IOM report *To Err Is Human* stimulated much of the activity surrounding the advancement of patient safety seen across the nation, including actions by professional organizations. The AORN, the voice for the perioperative profession, has long been a proponent of patient safety and safer medication practices. The AORN reaffirmed the profession's commitment to patient safety in 2002 after the IOM report by orchestrating several task forces charged specifically with developing initiatives, standards, position statements, and recommended practice guidelines related to staff and patient safety. One of these task forces, the AORN Presidential Commission for Patient Safety, was instrumental in creating AORN's safety platform—Patient Safety First—which set the framework for improving the safety of patients in surgery across the nation. This commission had a direct impact on shaping medication management practices within the perioperative setting (Table 5-3). Throughout each of these accomplishments, strategies for practice improvement were outlined in an effort to focus on system solutions to encourage organizational change. In addition, the theme of creating a culture of medication safety is woven throughout each of the documents and tools in an effort to sustain the medication error prevention strategies implemented.

Additional Recommendations for Improved Medication Safety in Perioperative Practice

In addressing recommendations to improve practice, the sky is the limit. The health care provider is limited only by his or her own creative thinking. Table 5-4 outlines strategies to help enforce safe medication practices within the OR. These strategies are founded on the information obtained from the data reports specifically related to the OR that were accumulated during the analysis of the MEDMARX database.

TABLE 5-3 AORN "Patient Safety First" Accomplishments Related to Safety

Accomplishment	Relationship to Safety
AORN standards, recommended practices and guidelines	• Recommended practice guidelines for safe medication practices in perioperative practice settings across the life span • Guidance statement: do-not-use list of abbreviations • Creating a patient safety culture • Position statement on patient safety
AORN safety initiative	AORN Patient Safety First Event Reporting Program
AORN patient safety tool kits	• Medication Administration Tool Kit • Patient Handoff Tool Kit

AORN, Association of periOperative Registered Nurses.

TABLE 5-4 Recommendations for Safe Medication Practice

Interventions	Implementation Strategies/Rationale
Examine unit/facility policies related to medication use	Policies should do the following: Address the implementation of the read-back/repeat and verify process for verbal orders. Examine the potential of expanding the read-back process for all "standing order" medications in OR surgeon preference cards. Consider adding the element of a team review of medications to be used during the surgical procedure during the "time-out" process in relation to patient allergies and other contraindications.
Enforce a unit-based labeling policy	Ensure that all medications are labeled on and off the sterile field. Institute "leadership walk-arounds," whereby management performs spot checks to ensure the medication labeling policy is being followed.
Keep medication containers until end of surgical procedure	Ensure that staff keeps medication containers until end of procedure just in case there is an issue regarding medications delivered. Review all medication containers with staff during handoffs (breaks, lunch, or change of shift) as part of the medication reconciliation requirement.
Encourage pharmaceutical companies to expand involvement in product development specifically focused on the needs in the OR	To minimize errors in the labeling process, call on manufacturers to produce drug products in sterile ready-to-use packaging with duplicate sterile labels. To minimize errors seen in pediatric dose calculations, encourage the development of pediatric doses for commonly used products in the OR.
Technology purchases in the OR to improve medication safety	Obtain a commitment from leadership who can support the need for technology purchases in the OR to improve medication safety. Examine technology that prompts documentation focused on key elements supporting the transfer of patient information and that enables the process of medication reconciliation. Have the pharmacy develop standardized dose charts that can be placed in each OR suite and be readily available for staff use, or purchase personal digital assistants (PDAs) for all staff, with programs to support medication calculations and formulations. Create a process to continually update the surgeon preference cards through the use of PDAs. Nursing staff could download surgeon preference cards onto PDAs, allowing on-the-spot changes to occur in the OR, and dock them at the end of the day to update the system.
Patient handoff policy	Institute a patient handoff policy that improves team communication and incorporates medication reconciliation concurrently.
Review formulary for medications used in the OR	Review the facility formulary for high-alert medications. Standardize dosages, and reduce the number of products available.
Create charts or references for staff	Outline common allergies and the associated medications that are contraindicated for those allergies. Provide a corresponding list of medication substitutions to be used when contraindications are outlined. Identify common drug-drug contraindications that are typically seen in the OR. Download these charts/references onto staff PDAs for point-of-use availability of information.
Establish a "just culture"	Create a "just culture" supportive of safety. Monitor successes as improvements are made to create a culture of safety. Safety climate survey tools: http://www.qualityhealthcare.org http://www.Mers-tm.net/support.marx_primer.pdf http://www.psnet.ahrq.gov/resource.aspx?resourceID=1438 http://www.ihi.org/IHI/Topics/Patientsafety/SafetyGeneral/Tools/ChecklistForAssessingInstitutionalResilience.htm

Continued

TABLE 5-4 Recommendations for Safe Medication Practice—cont'd

Interventions	Implementation Strategies/Rationale
Implementation of The Joint Commission recommendations related to medication safety	The Joint Commission resources to guide safe medication use practices: Medication Management Standards National Patient Safety Goals Accreditation manual (standards) Workshops and publications
Implementation of AORN recommended practice guidelines and use of various patient safety tool kits	Practice guidelines focused on medication safety: Recommended practice guidelines for safe medication practices across the life span Do-not-use abbreviations Creating a patient safety culture Patient safety tool kits: Medication Administration Tool Kit Patient Handoff Tool Kit AORN Patient Safety First Event Reporting Program
Examine other sources for best practices in medication use	USP Web site: http://www.usp.org AHRQ Web site: http://www.ahrq.gov IOM Web site: http://www.iom.educ

AHRQ, Agency for Healthcare Research and Quality; *AORN,* Association of periOperative Registered Nurses; *IOM,* Institute of Medicine; *OR,* operating room; *USP,* United States Pharmacopeia.

CONCLUSION

Throughout this chapter, findings and associated recommendations for practice have been identified in an attempt to make a difference in safe medication administration within the OR. But dissemination of information is only half the battle. Lucian Leape (2002) described the phenomenon of an information graveyard, whereby information becomes buried in a data graveyard if not disseminated so that others can learn and make system changes to improve safety. Frontline practitioners must take the next step and use this critical information as supporting evidence to legitimize and make the changes needed to successfully translate these initiatives into safety practices at institutions nationwide. The health care system needs superheroes to fix the system, and leaders within the perioperative community need to become institutional champions to lead this effort for patient safety to ensure the safe delivery of medications to our patients.

REFERENCES

Abeysekera A, et al: Drug error in anaesthetic practice: a review of 896 reports from the Australian Incident Monitoring Study database, *Anaesthesia* 60(3):220–227, 2005.

Association of periOperative Registered Nurses: *Perioperative standards and recommended practices,* Denver, 2008, The Association.

Barker KN, et al: Medication errors observed in 36 health care facilities, *Arch Intern Med* 162(16):1897–1903, 2002.

Beyea SC, et al: Medication errors in the OR—a secondary analysis of MEDMARX, *AORN J* 77(1):122–134, 2003.

Currie M, et al: The Australian Incident Monitoring Study. The "wrong drug" problem in anaesthesia: an analysis of 2000 incident reports, *Anaesth Instensive Care* 21(5):596–601, 1993.

Curry D: The Pareto principle, *Field Notes* 10:3, 2001.

Fasting S, Glsvold SE: Adverse drug errors in anesthesia, and the impact of coloured syringe labels, *Can J Anaesth* 47(11):1060–1067, 2000.

Flynn EA, et al: Comparison of methods for detecting medication errors in 36 hospitals and skilled-nursing facilities, *Am J Health Syst Pharm* 59(5):436–446, 2002.

Forrey RA, et al: Interrater agreement with a standard scheme for classifying medication errors, *Am J Health Syst Pharm* 64(2):175–181, 2007.

Hicks RW, et al: *MEDMARX 5th anniversary data report: a chartbook of 2003 findings and trends 1999-2003,* Rockville, Md, 2004, Center for the Advancement of Patient Safety, US Pharmacopeia.

Hicks RW, et al: *MEDMARX data report: a chartbook of medication error findings from the perioperative settings from 1998-2005*, Rockville, Md, 2006, Center for the Advancement of Patient Safety, US Pharmacopeia.

Hicks RW, et al: *MEDMARX data report: a report on the relationship of drug names and medication errors in response to the Institute of Medicine's call for action*, Rockville, Md, 2008, Center for the Advancement of Patient Safety, US Pharmacopeia.

Institute of Medicine: *Patient safety: achieving a new standard for care*, Washington, 2004, National Academies Press.

Jensen LS, et al: Evidence-based strategies for preventing drug administration errors during anesthesia, *Anaesthesia* 59(5):493–504, 2004.

Joint Commission for the Accreditation of Healthcare Organizations: *Introduction to the National Patient Safety Goals*, 2005. available at http://www.jcaho.org/accreditediorganizations/patient+safety/05+npsg/index.htm. Accessed January 13, 2005.

Khan FA, Hoda MQ: Drug related critical incidents, *Anaesthesia* 60(1):48–52, 2005.

Kohn LT, et al: *To err is human: building a safer health system*, Washington, 2000, National Academies Press.

Leape L: Reporting of adverse events, *N Engl J Med* 347(20): 1633–1638, 2002.

Liu E, Koh K: A prospective audit of critical incidents in anaesthesia in a university teaching hospital, *Ann Acad Med Singapore* 32(6):814–820, 2003.

Medication ordered is contraindicated: court discusses nurse's legal responsibilities, *Legal Eagle Eye Newsletter* 15(1):1, 2007.

Nadzam DM: A systems approach to medication use. In Cousins DD, editor: *Medication use: a systems approach to reducing errors*, Oakbrook Terrace, Ill, 1998, Joint Commission on Accreditation of Healthcare Organizations.

National Coordinating Council for Medication Error Reporting and Prevention: *What is a medication error? 1998-2001*, available at http://www.nccmerp.org/. Accessed April 25, 2008.

Nightingale F: *Notes on nursing*, Princeton, NJ, 1970, Brandon/System Press.

Nyssen AS, et al: Reporting systems in healthcare from a case-by-case experience to a general framework: an example in anaesthesia, *Eur J Anaesthesiol* 21(10):757–765, 2004.

Orser BA, Byrick R: Anesthesia-related medication error: time to take action, *Can J Anaesth* 51(8):756–760, 2004.

Phillips J, et al: Retrospective analysis of mortalities associated with medication errors, *Am J Health Syst Pharm* 58(19): 1835–1841, 2001.

Rich DS: New JCAHO medication management standards for 2004, *Am J Health Syst Pharm* 61(13):1349–1358, 2004.

Rudman WJ, et al: The use of data mining tools in identifying medication error near misses and adverse drug events, *Top Health Inf Manage* 23(2):94–103, 2002.

Runciman WB, et al: The Australian Incident Monitoring Study: errors, incidents and accidents in anaesthetic practice, *Anaesth Intensive Care* 21(5):506–519, 1993.

Shaw-Phillips MA: Voluntary reporting of medication errors, *Am J Health Syst Pharm* 59(23):2326–2340, 2002.

Shojania KG, et al: *Making health care safer: a critical analysis of patient safety practices*, Evidence report/technology assessment No. 43, Rockville, Md, 2001, Agency for Healthcare Research and Quality .

Wachter RM: The end of the beginning: patient safety five years after "To err is human.", *Health Aff* W4:534–545, 2004.

Wanzer LJ, Hicks RW: Medication safety within the perioperative environment, *Annu Rev Nurs Res* 24:127–155, 2006.

Webster CS, et al: A prospective randomized clinical evaluation of a new safety-oriented injectable drug administration system in comparison with conventional methods, *Anaesthesia* 59:80–87, 2004.

Wheeler SJ, Wheeler DW: Medication errors in anaesthesia and critical care, *Anaesthesia* 60(3):257–273, 2005.

Winterstein AG, et al: Identifying clinically significant preventable adverse drug events through a hospital's database of adverse drug reaction reports, *Am J Health Syst Pharm* 59(18):1742–1749, 2002.

World Health Organization: *World alliance for patient safety*, Forward Programme 2006-2007, Geneva, 2006, World Health Organization.

FIRE PREVENTION IN THE PERIOPERATIVE SETTING

Perioperative Fires Can Occur Everywhere

Claire R. Everson, RN, CNOR, CCAP

Fire can start whenever heat, fuel, and oxygen converge together. During a surgical procedure, whether it is in a medical center, ambulatory surgery center, clinic, or physician's office, all three of these components are usually present. This potentially places every surgical patient at risk for a surgical fire. A surgical fire is defined as a fire that is located on or in the patient (ECRI, 2006).

A fire triangle is frequently described when discussing elements necessary for the occurrence of a fire. A triangle is a geometric figure formed of three sides and three angles. The angles do not need to be the same degree and the sides do not need to be equal; they just all need to be present for the triangle to exist. The same can be said of surgical fires. All three elements of the fire triangle must be present for a surgical fire to occur. These three elements are heat, fuel, and oxygen (Figure 6-1). The elements do not need to be equal; they just need to be present and in close proximity. It is essential for the perioperative nurse to be familiar with each component as it relates to prevention and patient safety.

The surgical fire is not a new problem or one specific to modern medicine and anesthesia. Woodbridge (1939) stated, "*Although statistically their importance is minute, they are of great emotional importance. The dramatic nature of the accident and of the death that may occur leads to publicity. The noise, the dramatic suddenness and the publicity all tend to produce a wave of fear and under the emotional tension of fear it is felt that something must be done, and done quickly.*" Turner (2000) provides a review of the history of surgical fires and explosions, including events from as early as 1745 to the introduction and acceptance of the first nonflammable anesthetic agent, halothane, in 1956. Many of these historical fires were caused by the fire triangle that involved an ignition/heat source of static electricity, inspired oxygen (or room air) mixed with a flammable anesthetic agent, and fuel. Of note was a 1930 statement by the American Medical Association Council on Physical Therapy, "A certain carelessness regarding this matter has developed" (William, 1930). Later that year, the American Medical Association Committee on Anesthesia Accidents stated, "care does not now completely forestall this hazard" and discussed the importance of "weighing the potential advantages and disadvantages of each anesthetic technique" (Henderson, 1930).

On June 24, 2003, The Joint Commission (2003) issued a *Sentinel Event Alert* titled "Preventing Surgical Fires." In the *Sentinel Event Alert* there is concern for underreporting of surgical fires. Estimates in 2003 from the U.S. Food and Drug Administration (FDA) and the ECRI Institute, a nonprofit health services research agency, suggested approximately 100 surgical fires. With the advent of mandatory state reporting of surgical fires, data are available that the ECRI Institute has used to better estimate occurrences of surgical fires in the United States. More than 50 million surgeries are now performed annually in the United States; the current estimate is that 550 to 650 surgical fires occur annually (ECRI, 2009).

Regulations require facility accountability. The American Association for Accreditation of Ambulatory Health Care Facilities, The Joint Commission, the Centers for Medicare & Medicaid Services, and other third-party payers are scrutinizing perioperative patient care for patient safety issues. The Joint Commission's National Patient Safety Goals, the Agency for Healthcare Research and Quality, and the National Quality Forum never events contribute recommendations for patient safety, including fire safety. Many of these recommendations are evidence based, sensible, and very similar among the various organizations. This makes it easier to apply recommendations

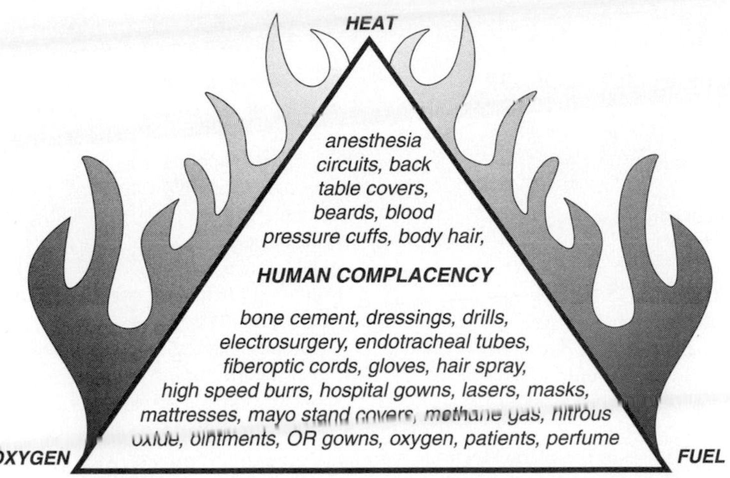

FIGURE 6-1 Fire triangle. (From Smith C: Surgical fires—learn not to burn, *AORN J* 80[1]:26, 2004.)

that are consistent, no matter which resource a facility chooses to use.

At the time of the 2003 Joint Commission *Sentinel Event Alert,* the ECRI Institute's analysis of case reports revealed that the most common ignition sources were electrosurgical equipment (68%) and lasers (13%); the most common fire locations were the airway (34%), head or face (28%), and elsewhere on or inside the patient (38%). An oxygen-enriched atmosphere was a contributing factor in 74% of all cases (ECRI, 2003). When these three elements of the triangle—an ignition source, an oxidizer, and a fuel source—come together in the wrong way at the wrong moment, a fire may occur (Box 6-1).

One important area of concern for the perioperative nurse is management of the fuel sources. Fuel sources include any material that may come in contact with the patient (e.g., drapes, gown, cap, towels, body hair, intestinal gases). The endotracheal tube in the airway, fine skin hair at the surgical site that may have been slicked back with petroleum jelly instead of a water-soluble jelly, surgical drapes, and even equipment are potential fire sources. There are similarities and differences in how each of these fuel sources may be prevented or suppressed.

The literature artificially discusses the issues as four topics. Although these topics are closely intertwined, they are divided for purposes of education and organization of thought as prevention, suppression, evacuation, and communication.

PREVENTION

Oxygen-Enriched Atmosphere

When the patient receives oxygen and anesthetic gases through a face mask or nasal cannula, there is a potential for the creation of an oxygen-enriched atmosphere as the oxygen and nitrous oxide vents into the atmosphere and accumulates under the surgical drapes. This accumulation is of particular concern for surgeries performed in the head and neck region. The proximity of the surgical site to the oxygen-enriched atmosphere increases the potential for a spark from the electrosurgery unit (ESU), electrocautery unit (ECU), or laser to ignite the surrounding oxygen-enriched atmosphere. Seventy-four percent of reported surgical fires occur in an oxygen-enriched atmosphere (ECRI, 2003). Therefore a patient's need for increased supplemental oxygen should always be communicated to the surgeon and the perioperative team members by the anesthesia provider or, in the case of procedure sedation, by the monitoring registered nurse (RN).

Heat Source

Keeping the active electrode of the ESU or ECU in a nonconductive holder when not in use is a simple step that can be taken to prevent surgical fires. Traditionally a "holster" is close to the scrub person, but a surgeon may prefer the active

BOX 6-1 The Fire Triangle (and the Affiliated Surgical Team Member)

HEAT SOURCES (SURGEON OR ASSISTANT)

Electrosurgical units
Electrocautery units
Lasers
Fiberoptic light sources and cables
Sparks from high-speed surgical drills and surgical burrs
Defibrillators
Glowing embers of charred tissue
Other electrical hemostatic devices
Ultrasonic hemostatic or cutting devices
Flexible endoscopes
Tourniquet cuffs
Needle electrodes versus flat-blade electrodes on an electrosurgery or electrocautery unit

FUEL SOURCES (SCRUB PERSON, CIRCULATING REGISTERED NURSE, SURGICAL TECHNOLOGIST)

Degreasers
Flammable prepping agents including tinctures (chlorhexidine gluconate [Hibitane], thimerosal [Merthiolate]), iodophor [DuraPrep])
Drapes
Towels
Gowns
Hoods
Masks
Surgical sponges
Dressings
Ointments, petrolatum (petroleum jelly)
Tincture of benzoin (74% to 80% alcohol)
Aerosols (e.g., Aeroplast)
Paraffin
White wax
Patient's hair (face, scalp, body)
Gastrointestinal tract gases (mostly methane)
Aerosol adhesives
Alcohol (also in suture packets)
Instrument and equipment drapes and covers
Egg-crate mattresses
Mattresses and pillows
Blankets
Adhesive tape (cloth, plastic, paper)
Ace bandages, stockinettes
Collodion (mixture of pyroxylin, ether, and alcohol)
Disposable packaging materials (paper, plastic, cardboard)
Smoke evacuator hoses
Some instrument boxes and cabinets

OXYGEN SOURCES (ANESTHESIA PROVIDER)

Oxygen-enriched atmosphere
Oxygen delivered through a nasal cannula
Oxygen delivered through a mask
Use of flammable endotracheal tube during airway procedures with laser
Nitrous oxide
Petroleum-based jelly on eyes
Flexible endoscopes
Anesthesia components (breathing circuits, masks, airways, tracheal tubes, suction catheters, pledgets)
Coverings of fiberoptic cables and wires (e.g., ESU leads, ECG leads)
Blood pressure cuffs
Stethoscope tubing

HUMAN FACTORS

Complacency
Distraction
Inattentiveness
Slow reaction
Improper firefighting techniques
Improper firefighting tools
Feeling rushed

ECG, Electrocardiogram; ESU, electrosurgery unit

electrode to be close at hand. Health care facilities should consider the availability of an additional holster to encourage safe practice. Providing a second holster could end the debate over using the holster versus keeping the active electrode conveniently close at hand. The risk of accidental activation by placing instrumentation or supplies (or by simply leaning) on it is also mitigated by using the holster. Mark Bruley from the ECRI Institute recommends that if the active electrode is not in immediate use (defined as 5 to 10 seconds), then it should be holstered or placed on the back table if it is a battery-operated device (Association of periOperative Registered Nurses [AORN], 2006).

When using a laser, the standby mode is also an important protective step to take. The communication between the surgeon and the laser operator is essential for patient safety, to prevent accidental activation. The laser operator should

<table>
<tr><th colspan="2">Fire Risk Assessment Score</th><th colspan="2">Circle appropriate option</th></tr>
<tr><td colspan="2">Alcohol-based prep solution had sufficient time for fumes to dissipate: ❑ Yes ❑ No ❑ N/A</td><td>Yes</td><td>No</td></tr>
<tr><td colspan="2">Surgical site or incisiion above the xiphoid</td><td>1</td><td>0</td></tr>
<tr><td colspan="2">Open oxygen source (patient receiving supplemental oxygen via any variety of face mask or nasal cannular)</td><td>1</td><td>0</td></tr>
<tr><td colspan="2">Available ignition source (e.g., electrosurgery unit, laser, fiberoptic light source)</td><td>1</td><td>0</td></tr>
<tr><td colspan="2">Score 3 = High risk; 2 = Low risk with potential to convert to high risk; 1 = Low risk;
0 = No risk/action required
Total Score:</td><td colspan="2">______</td></tr>
<tr><td>❑ FIRE RISK SCORE " 1 to 2 " precautions implemented
(mark all that apply)</td><td colspan="3">❑ FIRE RISK SCORE "3" precautions implemented
(mark all that apply)</td></tr>
<tr><td>❑ Observe prep drying times (minimum of 3 minutes)
❑ Protect heat sources (cautery pencil holster, etc.)
❑ Follow standard draping procedure

Fire Risk Score equal to 2, low risk with potential to convert to a level "3" risk (e.g., ET tube puncture, surgical intervention in thoracic cavity). Convert to high-risk precautions.</td><td colspan="3">❑ Titrate deliverable oxygen to 30% or below
❑ Observe prep drying times (minimum of 3 minutes)
❑ Follow appropriate draping protocol (i.e., incise drape)
❑ Use wet sponges
❑ Have basin of sterile saline available for suppression purposes only
❑ Have a 60-mL syringe full of saline for procedure within the oral cavity
❑ Protect heat sources (cautery pencil holster for electrosurgery, utilize standby mode or tum off heat source with fiberoptic light source when not in use)
❑ Minimize electrosurgery settings
❑ ECT (electroconvulsive therapy)—remove oxygen prior to treatment.</td></tr>
</table>

FIGURE 6-2 Fire risk assessment score. (From Christiana Care Health Services.)

have no other responsibilities that will take attention away from managing and monitoring the laser. This will necessitate an additional RN in the room to circulate the case, assist the anesthesia provider, obtain and provide supplies for the scrub person on the other side of the room, and assess the patient when the laser needs to be placed on standby. The operating surgeon should be the only person controlling the activation of the active electrode or laser delivery apparatus.

Communication is essential at all times during surgery. It is important to communicate when a member observes an aspect of care that places a patient at risk for injury. For example, if a member of the surgical team should observe a single spark or arc, this should be reported. The single event may not have been the only one and places the patient at risk for a surgical fire.

When the surgeon or assistant is applying the active electrode of an electrosurgery device or laser delivery device to the patient, a large portion of responsibility for the prevention of fire risk falls to the scrub person. This individual is in the field and must give constant attention to keeping the ESU electrode tip clean to prevent possible sparking and keeping the ESU handheld device safely holstered when inactive, yet have it ready for quick use should the need arise. Light cables and other hot equipment must be kept off drapes and other flammable fuel sources. A wet sponge must always be available when used near a heat source, and a full basin of saline or water must be kept at all times in case a small fire starts. While the surgeon is intent upon the surgical procedure, the scrub person must constantly monitor for and prevent fire triangle "opportunities."

Several facilities are including fire risk assessment as part of the universal protocol process. The most frequently applied fire risk tool was developed by the Christiana Care Health System (Mathias, 2006). The patient is assigned a fire risk score of 1 to 3. A score of 1 is low risk, a score of 2 is low risk with the potential to convert to high risk, and a score of 3 is high risk (see Figure 6-2). After verifying the patient's name and surgical site, marking the presence of instrumentation and implants needed, noting the location of the surgical site in proximity to the anesthesia gases, and the safe use of heat sources, the monitoring of supplies and fire risk assessment are discussed. This additional communication takes seconds but is a preventive strategy that should be encouraged.

Fuel Source

The surgical environment should be set up with fire prevention considerations. Perioperative staff must be educated in steps taken to prevent fires, both at the field and within the environment. This includes knowing the location of fire pull alarms, fire extinguishers, and evacuation routes.

When planning for the intervention, the circulator and the scrub person should discuss any anticipated risks. A full basin of sterile saline or sterile water should be kept on the field. The ESU handheld devices are to be placed into a nonconductive holster when not in use. Music, conversation, and other ambient room noise should be at a level to ensure that equipment alarms are audible for all team members. If the audio from the ESU generator or laser is difficult to hear over the room noise, then its volume should be raised to allow for awareness of any potential inadvertent activation of the active electrode.

Operating room (OR) staff at any role level should be encouraged to speak up if they believe that adequate surgical fire prevention strategies are not being taken. Management and leadership staff need to support this team concept with consistent and timely involvement in order for it to become an integral and accepted component of practice. In reports of surgical fires, staff have stated that they were aware of potential problems but that they were ignored or ridiculed. Occasionally the assumption is made that leadership would not enforce prevention strategies, but leadership is often unaware of the problems. The staff performing the procedure cannot assume that leadership knows that prevention strategies are not being followed if they do not inform leadership personnel.

The circulating nurse is in charge of the surgical skin preparation, even if it is delegated to a different individual. Regardless of the skin preparation agent used, the flammability hazard is decreased if the agent is allowed to dry completely and manufacturer's instructions for use are followed. The registered nurse, as a patient advocate, observes and assesses for dripping or pooling of the prepping agent and monitors appropriate drying time before draping. With the increased use of waterless gels for the surgical hand scrub, the surgeon and assistant may enter the room more quickly and stand waiting, perhaps impatiently, for the prepping agent to adequately dry. The circulator and perioperative team play an essential role by confirming the dryness of the prepping agent before draping. In some institutions the dryness of the preparation is part of a patient safety checklist that is documented.

The scrub person, as patient advocate, can delay draping until adequate drying time is allowed. This requires support from the leadership team. The surgical drapes may burn or melt in an oxygen-enriched atmosphere when heat is applied. Even if the drapes do not flame, melting can ignite the flammable materials below, such as towels, warming blankets, or the patient's gown (OR surgical fire training, 2005). When possible, the drapes should be arranged to facilitate flow of anesthetic gases to the floor. ORs require adequate ventilation and scavenger systems, and these systems are also valuable in fire prevention strategies. The use of incise drapes has many purposes, one of which is to decrease or prevent venting of the oxygen-enriched atmosphere to the surgical site. For it to function as a prevention strategy, the seal between the incise drape and the skin needs to be monitored during the procedure.

The edges of chuck or cloth towels used to "square off" the incision site need to be kept well away from the incision site. Surgical sponges should be moistened in saline close to the time of anticipated use so they do not dry out on the sterile back table or Mayo stand. They may also need to be moistened periodically while in use to avoid becoming a fuel source.

SUPPRESSION

In the event of a fire outbreak, the fire triangle must be disrupted by diminishing or removing one or all of its sides (Table 6-1). When a fire occurs—flames, smoke, or fumes—the literature states that the surgical team has about 2 to 3 seconds to react and to call for help. In 30 seconds or so, a small fire can progress to a life-threatening, large fire. The RACE acronym (rescue, alarm, contain, evacuate) can be used as part of the required annual education and training to enable staff to respond immediately in the proper fashion without hesitation. If the environment is the fire source (e.g., ceiling tiles, overhead surgical lights, or smoke coming through the ventilation system), do not waste time—evacuate the patient and the team.

Rescue

In an airway fire, the anesthesia provider must immediately shut off the anesthetic gases and disconnect the circuit if the endotracheal tube is the source of the fire. If these steps are not taken, the

TABLE 6-1 Suppression Adjusted by the Type of Fire

Endotracheal Tube Fire	Oral Cavity Fire	Surgical Site Fire	Drape Fire	Equipment Fire
Communicate with team.	Communicate with team.	Communicate with team.	Communicate with team.	Communicate with team.
Shut off medical gases.	Shut off medical gases.	Shut off medical gases.	Shut off medical gases.	Shut off medical gases.
Disconnect circuit.	Disconnect circuit.			Protect self and patient first; evacuate if needed.
Extubate, removing the melting ET tube before it adheres too much to surrounding tissue.	Irrigate mouth with sterile saline to put out fire.	Dump sterile saline on the drapes, sponges, or fuel for the fire.	Pull the drapes off the patient to the ground. Roll them if possible to try to smother fire.	If you can get to the electrical outlet safely, you are not in danger, and no sparks from the outlet, then pull the plug.
Place ET tube in saline or water to extinguish fire.	Treat patient.	Move drapes, and look under them for fire.	Drapes are fluid resistant, so be accurate when pouring fluid on them.	If the correct, clean agent, fire extinguisher is available and you and the patient are safe, use the fire extinguisher.
Control patent airway.		Look under patient.	Look all around and under the patient.	
Treat patient.		Assess patient for injury.	Assess patient for injury.	
		Treat patient if needed.	Treat patient if needed.	

Data from Association of periOperative Registered Nurses: *Fire safety tool kit: be prepared to prevent and respond*, DVD, Denver, 2006, The Association.

possibility of pulling a blowtorch of flames through the trachea and oral airway is very real. Once retrieved from the patient, the endotracheal tube should be placed in fluid to help extinguish the fire. After the source of an airway fire is removed, immediate action must be taken to ensure that a patent airway is provided for the patient and that the extent of airway damage is assessed to determine an appropriate treatment plan by the surgeon.

When the drapes are ignited, patting the flames is ineffective—it only moves the flames in many directions. If the prepping solution dripped or pooled under the patient, the fire may be present there, too. There are different steps for different-size drape fires (Box 6-2).

Alarm

Even if a fire is small and easily extinguished and the surgery proceeds, leadership must be notified immediately. What may have been considered a superficial drape fire may be smoldering underneath. Additional help may be required to gather needed supplies or medications, document the occurrence, or monitor and assist with ongoing interventions. Leadership staff can help play a critical role in the timely and efficient management of the patient's treatment by providing an additional support person or stepping in to assist their team themselves.

Policy should drive when to call the internal disaster number, when to pull the fire alarm, and when to call the fire department. It should also address who should respond to an internal department alarm and when facilities should be notified. If the facility is a freestanding ambulatory surgery center or a physician's office, the fire department should always be notified.

BOX 6-2 Containing the Flames of a Surgical Fire

SMALL FLAMES OR A SMALL AREA

Communicate to the team.

Pour normal saline slowly so the fire does not spread.

Use a towel or sponge, and with your arm between the patient's head and the fire, lay it over the flame and sweep toward the patient's feet.

Lift the material used to smother the flame to vent heat.

Assess for any further flames, smoke, or fumes.

Assess the patient for any injuries, and treat.

LARGE FLAMES OR A LARGE AREA

Communicate to the team.

Remove the drape to the ground, rolling it on itself to smother the fire.

Do not move the drape into what may need to be your evacuation route from the room.

Assess the surgical field for a secondary fire of the underlying drapes or towels.

Assess the patient for injury, and treat.

Circulator ensures that the flames are extinguished, which may include the use of a fire extinguisher.

Data from Association of periOperative Registered Nurses: *Fire safety tool kit: be prepared to prevent and respond*, DVD, Denver, 2006, The Association.

Contain

Doors should always be kept closed. This helps to eliminate the risk of a fire spreading. Additional containment steps are listed in Box 6-2. Do not put the endotracheal tube or removed drape(s) in the trash; they may still be hot and become a source of a secondary fire, even if the flames are extinguished.

When discussing suppressing or working to suppress a real fire, it is important to understand that there will be by-products from the fire. Because of the materials in procedural areas, it will never simply be a fire that converts the fuel into water, carbon dioxide (CO_2), and other oxides. Incomplete combustion of materials in procedural areas may produce toxic carbon monoxide, acidic free hydrogen, soot, ash, and debris. Plastics—hydrocarbons with other elements to create properties such as flexibility—produce the most toxic combustion products. These products include hydrogen chloride, hydrogen fluoride, cyanide, mustard gas, phenol, and aldehydes. Victims of these fires, including the surgical team, would asphyxiate before burning to death (ECRI, 1992).

EVACUATION

Evacuation is the last part of the acronym RACE. Horizontal evacuation of the patient and the team should be considered when the drape fire still burns on the floor, when there is a fire in the overhead lights, or in the presence of smoke and fumes. Communication needs to occur so that the plan is known to all, including the rest of the department. The evacuation may be as simple as moving to a different OR or to a separate fire compartment, or be as complex as a department evacuation. When the decision to evacuate is made, communication will also contain the risk of the fire spreading externally from the room (Table 6-2).

Understanding the evacuation plan may be more complex than was anticipated during the annual review. It is not just knowing the route, but knowing what to do if the route is blocked—where to take the patient and how to move the patient if he or she is on a fracture table or during a robotic procedure. The complexities of the environment are individual to each department, so they need to be discussed. The AORN *Fire Safety Tool Kit: Be Prepared to Prevent and Respond* (2006) includes tools that can be used when preparing facility evacuation plans in detail.

It must be recognized that a fire may occur in which the fire involving the patient is too huge or the smoke is too dense or the fumes are too overpowering to save the patient. If this happens, it is senseless to add to the victim count. The staff members will need support as they face and work through this tragedy for many months.

COMMUNICATION

Communication of the fire plan needs to be constant and is important in the prevention and suppression of fires and in the safe evacuation of the entire team. Because surgical fires are rare occurrences, simulation training and annual drills with debriefing sessions are critical.

The time to communicate during a fire is limited and valuable. Although it is human to ask, "What do we do?" in this rare event, the communication time needs to be better spent. Rather than asking the question, each team member should communicate what he or she is actively doing.

Communication used as a preventive step is much easier than trying to communicate during a fire. The perioperative team should learn to provide verbal confirmation consistently throughout the surgical procedure about anything that can become a fire risk. Examples of important communication related to fire risk include the following: the skin preparation is dry before draping, the laser is placed on standby, the light source or other heat sources are on standby, the ESU device is holstered, and supplemental oxygen to the patient has been increased.

Another critical, although uncomfortable, communication component needs to be addressed. Whenever a fire is occurring, the families of patients need to be kept informed about the interventions that are being performed as this mishap is taking place and the steps that will be taken afterward to evaluate and prevent it from occurring again.

TABLE 6-2 Complementary Evacuation Steps for Personnel

Surgeon	Scrub Person	Anesthesia Provider	Circulator
Stabilize the surgical site.	Protect the surgical site.	Shut off anesthesia machine and gases.	Communicate the need to evacuate that room to the department.
Prepare site for transport, pack with sponges, cover with towels.	Gather necessary instruments and sponges.	Break down monitors, leads; prepare airway and IV lines for move.	Assist with preparing the patient to move.
Give final directions to circulator.	Assist in moving the OR table.	Stabilize patient; gather needed medications.	Help move the OR table.
Assist in moving the OR table.		Coordinate move of the OR table after unlocking it.	

IV, Intravenous; *OR,* operating room.
Data from *OR surgical fire training: how to prevent and respond to surgical fires,* DVD, 2005, HCPro.

As patient and family advocates, we need to be aware of the impact that a surgical fire will have on the patient and his or her family and friends. This critical component needs to be part of the plan, and a representative from the facility should be assigned to communicate with them. The options include administration and risk management personnel; however, perioperative leadership may be better able to answer technical questions. What families share by way of interviews and blogs is the frustration they experience when no one seems to know what is happening or when the families feel they are being ignored because facilities fear legal action. Families could benefit from knowing that their health care team is also frustrated, because surgical fire occurrences are rare and there may not be a preexisting care plan beyond RACE. This frustration led one family to develop the Web site http://www.surgicalfire.org in fulfillment of the mother's wishes.

EDUCATION AND COMPETENCY ASSESSMENT

There are multiple issues that need to be included in fire safety, including the many topics that do not occur in the 2- to 3-second reaction time allowed in the event of a perioperative fire. Education and training of staff is mandated by every regulatory agency. It is important to note, however, that this education and training is needed by not only registered nurses and surgical technologists but also the surgeons, anesthesia providers, anesthesia technicians, technologists, orderlies, nursing assistants, environmental staff, and unit clerks. In addition, health care industry representatives, radiology technologists, and students should be included in annual education and drills. Key points to include are fire risk, risk reduction, prevention, suppression strategies, and the development of policies, procedures, and evacuation plans.

The content of orientation and continuing education is strongly suggested in many regulatory manuals. The AORN (2008) guidance statement "Fire Prevention in the Operating Room" is an available, helpful tool.

A "fire map" can be used as an orientation tool—the new employee identifies the location of the extinguishers, exits, pull alarms, evacuation devices, and fire doors and places them on a map. This is also a very effective method of educating new staff in fire safety geography.

CONDUCTING FIRE DRILLS

Evidence supports simulation training for increased retention of information and performance response afterward. A fire drill should occur annually, followed by a debriefing. Drills for evacuating the OR in the event of a major fire and surgical team drills are an important component of patient safety and should include as many staff as possible from every department that works in the perioperative environment. Everyone who works in the environment needs to be included. Evacuation routes should be posted in every operating room and every patient area and checked annually for accuracy.

Meeting fire safety training requirements in an effective, realistic, and capable manner is difficult because of the many demands on the OR staff. However, having a preplanned method of fighting a surgical fire so that every team member knows what to do is critically important. Simulation should include the inevitable problems that arise during emergencies, such as exits that are blocked, equipment that is not working, rooms that are crowded with people and equipment, and surgical tables that are difficult to move. Simulation and training should include the following:

- Understanding the fire alarm and communication systems
- Knowing the location and proper use of firefighting tools; medical gas valves; heating, ventilation, and air-conditioning controls; and electrical supply switches
- Recognizing the chain of command and one's responsibilities within the chain
- Keeping minor fires from getting out of control
- Managing fires that do get out of control
- Knowing the location of portable oxygen tanks and ventilation equipment in order to safely evacuate patients if necessary

All fires start small. Surgical teams should be trained in and practice drills for quickly stopping small fires that involve drapes, gauze, ointments, and liquids. But fires move quickly, and slow reactions or confusion can allow a small fire to become a large, more dangerous one. Large fires require special drills devoted to developing the team effort needed to deal with sizable volumes of flame and smoke and with burning drapes and plastic in the small space of an OR (ECRI, 1992).

Fire extinguishers are critical to managing fires, and staff should be trained in their proper use.

Drills should identify the location of medical gas, ventilation, and electrical systems and controls and when, where, and how to shut off these systems. The fire-containment design and construction of most hospitals helps to ensure that the staff has enough time to evacuate other patients and staff. The use of the hospital's alarm system and system for contacting the local fire department should also be defined. After a drill, debriefing staff to review errors made in the drills is vital.

The team's actions influence the fire triangle; therefore it is wise to identify a physician champion and a facilitator because the multidisciplinary perioperative team members should participate in the development of the facilities policy and practice guidelines. Identify the individual who will order and who uses the gas shut-off valves for the department or the individual OR. Although evacuation is horizontal, every staff member should know where the patient should be transported to, or identify the location of the evacuation map in their immediate work environment. Developing or reviewing policy or practice guidelines following a drill may be beneficial because the multidisciplinary team members will realize the need for collaboration to develop solutions for potential problems related to surgical fire prevention.

FIRE EXTINGUISHERS

Fire extinguishers are classified according to National Fire Protection Association standards as Class A (for wood, paper, cloth, and most plastics), Class B (for flammable liquids or grease), or Class C (for energized electrical equipment).

Types of Fire Extinguishers

The various types of fire extinguishers available to fight each class of fire are described in the following paragraphs. Knowing where these extinguishers are located, how these devices work, and when to use them minimizes the disaster of an OR or surgical patient fire.

Carbon Dioxide

A 5-lb CO_2 fire extinguisher is the best choice for putting out fires typically encountered in ORs, where the patient is the primary concern. Despite their Class BC rating, CO_2 extinguishers can be used to extinguish small masses of cloth, plastic, or paper (Class A) involved in patient fires, and any flammable liquid (Class B) or electrically energized (Class C) fires that could occur in the OR. Equally important, these extinguishers do not leave residue and will not harm the patient, staff, or equipment. A 5-lb capacity CO_2 extinguisher weighs approximately 7 to 9 kg (15 to 20 lb), fits in a space approximately 23 × 23 × 36 cm (9 × 9 × 14 inches), and is easily handled by most people. For easy access the extinguisher should be mounted inside the OR near the entrance (Rothrock, 2007).

Dry Powder

It is important to understand that Class ABC-rated fire extinguishers are not appropriate for use in the OR. These models disperse a cloud of fine, dry powder (usually ammonium phosphate) that extinguishes the fire. This cloud contaminates all surfaces in the OR, including the patient and any surgical wounds. In addition, the powder is a respiratory irritant, which could affect the staff's ability to aid the patient, is hard to remove from wounds, and requires that all contaminated equipment be thoroughly cleaned. Although dry powder extinguishers should be available in the OR suite (outside individual ORs), they should be used in the OR only as a last resort (ECRI, 1992).

Halon

Halon extinguishers consist of hydrogenated halocarbons and are preferred for laser-unit fires. They were of environmental concern at one time, but an environmentally friendly halon fire extinguisher that does not negatively affect the ozone layer is now available. These units have a unique fire extinguishing action (disrupting the flaming process) and a low weight, making them easy to use (Ball, 2004).

Water

Pressurized-water (PW) fire extinguishers are available, but they are heavy and chiefly effective against Class A fires. A PW extinguisher is more difficult to use than a halon or CO_2 device. To extinguish burning water-repellent drapes with a PW fire extinguisher, users must place a finger partially over the end of the nozzle to produce a fine spray. Water in a stream or tossed from a pan can fan the flames and increase a drape fire. Water from corridor-located fire hoses typically spray 50 gallons of water a minute and can be effective as a last resort when immediate rescue or evacuation is needed.

Water as a fire-extinguishing agent can be used on a wide range of fires; however, a fire involving energized electrical equipment, although rare in the OR, should be extinguished not with water, but with an extinguisher rated for Class C fires (ECRI, 1992).

Proper Use of Fire Extinguishers

Local fire department staff or an institution's facility services staff may provide the OR staff with hands-on practice in extinguishing real fires using the equipment available in the OR. A return demonstration helps build the familiarity and confidence needed to use these devices in a frightening and hectic situation. Fire extinguishers should be small enough to be easily carried and handled by the most likely users, and they should be located in plain view in positions of easy access—near escape routes but away from fire-hazardous areas. Most fire extinguishers are operated according to the following procedure, whose steps are abbreviated by the acronym PASS:

Pull the activation pin.
Aim the nozzle at the base of the fire.
Squeeze the handle to release the extinguishing agent.
Sweep the stream over the base of the fire.

ECRI INSTITUTE RECOMMENDATIONS

Perioperative staff should be familiar with the following ECRI Institute (2006) recommendations:

Staff should question the need for 100% oxygen for open delivery during facial surgery and, as a general policy, use air or fraction of inspired oxygen at less than 30% for open delivery (consistent with patient needs).

Do not drape the patient until all flammable preparations have fully dried.

During oropharyngeal surgery, soak gauze or sponges used with uncuffed tracheal tubes to minimize leakage of oxygen into the oropharynx and keep them wet; moisten sponges, gauze, and pledgets (and their strings) so that they will resist igniting.

When performing electrosurgery, electrocautery, or laser surgery, place electrosurgical electrodes in a holster or other location off the patient when not in active use.

Place lasers in standby mode when not in active use.

In addition, the ECRI Institute recommends that staff participate in special drills and training in the use of firefighting equipment; the proper methods for rescue and escape; the identification and location of medical gas, ventilation, and electrical systems and controls and when, where, and how to shut off these systems; and the hospital's alarm system and the system for contacting the local fire department.

THE JOINT COMMISSION RECOMMENDATIONS

The Joint Commission (2003) recommends that health care organizations help prevent surgical fires by doing the following:

Informing staff members, including surgeons and anesthesiologists, about the importance of controlling heat sources by following laser and ESU safety practices

Managing fuels by allowing sufficient time for patient preparation

Establishing guidelines for minimizing oxygen concentration under the drapes

Developing, implementing, and testing procedures to ensure appropriate response by all members of the surgical team to fires in the OR

Raising awareness and ultimately preventing the occurrence of fires in the future by reporting any instances of surgical fires; reports can be made to The Joint Commission, the ECRI Institute, the FDA, and state agencies, among other organizations

REPORTING SURGICAL FIRES—THE LEGAL REQUIREMENTS

Many states and some professional organizations have regulations or standards requiring hospitals to report fires to their local fire department. From a risk management point of view, the safest course is to notify the fire department and keep records of any fire that occurs in the workplace. Clinical department heads should notify the safety officer, the hospital risk manager, and the hospital administrator in the event of a fire.

In addition, the event should be analyzed to determine whether it must be reported to the FDA under the Safe Medical Devices Act. For example, in the case of a laser-related injury to a patient, a report would be required, and the issue should be discussed with the hospital's risk manager. Many facilities bring in external experts (e.g., the ECRI Institute or Russell Phillips & Associates) to help with the systematic review. The risk manager will have current information about who needs to be or who should be notified in case of a surgical fire. In the report and event analysis, the incident should be broken down to its basic causes so that the entire health care organization can learn from the experience. This transparency is critical to the promotion of patient safety.

CONCLUSION

Surgical, perioperative, and interventional procedures, no matter where they are performed, are never a no-risk situation; the potential for a fire should always be recognized. Freestanding ambulatory surgery centers, endoscopy centers, imaging centers, and physician's offices have gaps in emergency services and response teams. It is essential that all areas have well-understood plans, intense staff orientation, and ongoing annual education to safely protect patients from the risk of surgical fires.

REFERENCES

Association of periOperative Registered Nurses: *Fire safety tool kit: be prepared to prevent and respond*, DVD, Denver, 2006, The Association.

Association of periOperative Registered Nurses: Guidance statement: fire prevention in the operating room. In Association of periOperative Registered Nurses: *Standards and recommended practices*, Denver, 2008, The Association.

Ball KA: Laser biophysics, systems and safety. In Lasers: the perioperative challenge, ed 3, St. Louis, 2004, Mosby.

ECRI Institute: The patient is on fire! A surgical fires primer—medical safety devices report, *Guidance* 21(1):19–34, 1992.

ECRI: A clinician's guide to surgical fires: how they occur, how to prevent them, how to put them out [guidance article], *Health Devices* 32(1):5–24, 2003.

ECRI: Surgical fire safety [guidance article], *Health Devices* 35(2):43–67, 2006.

ECRI: *Part Sherlock Holmes. Part fire fighter. Part Houdini* https://www.ecri.org/40years/Pages/Mark_Bruley_Interview.aspx Accessed June 22, 2009.

Henderson Y: *The hazard of explosion of anesthetics*, *JAMA* 94:1491–1498, 1930.

Mathias J: Scoring fire risk for surgical patient, *OR Manager* 22(1):19–20, 2006.

OR surgical fire training: how to prevent and respond to surgical fires, DVD, Marblehead, Mass, 2005, HCPro.

Rothrock J: *Alexander's care of the patient in surgery*, ed 13, St. Louis, 2007, Mosby.

The Joint Commission: Preventing surgical fires, *Sentinel Event Alert*, issue 29, June 24, 2003. available at http://www.jointcommission.org/SentinelEvents/SentinelEventAlert/sea_29.htm. Accessed June 22, 2009.

Turner K: Fires and explosions, *ASA Newsl* 64(9):2000.

William HB: The explosion hazard in anesthesia, *JAMA* 94:918–920, 1930.

Woodbridge PD: Incidence of anesthetic explosions, *JAMA* 113:2308–2310, 1939.

BLOODLESS SURGERY AND PATIENT SAFETY ISSUES

Jarrell Fox • Sandy L. Brown, RN • Rebecca Vigil, RN

"Bloodless" surgery? "NO BLOOD!" These requests most certainly have an impact on patient safety and quality of care in the surgical setting. Have you wondered why there is increasing international interest in nonblood medical and surgical management of patients? The answer may be surprising. Can those in the health care profession safely and compassionately accommodate patient requests to avoid blood transfusion?

The perception within the medical community is that when patients refuse blood, those patients actually are refusing reasonable medical care. This leaves patients and the medical personnel feeling frustrated. The medical professionals (physicians and nurses) believe they are facing an unnecessary barrier to traditional medical care, whereas patients feel frustrated at a perceived indifference to their personal beliefs (Remmers and Speer, 2006).

Patients who desire nonblood medical care are not limited to those who have a religious objection to its use. The principal reasons include a deeply held religious belief, personal concerns about the perceived risks involved, an increased awareness of available alternative strategies, and inadequate availability of safe blood products.

Blood products, as therapeutic agents, have been used routinely for decades but lack clinical trials and regulatory review by the U.S. Food and Drug Administration (FDA) required for other products used in medicine (Committee on Government Reform and Oversight, 1996). Blood is classified as a specialized form of connective tissue. Therefore a blood transfusion should be viewed as an organ transplant because it is living tissue. Medical professionals often view and prescribe it, however, more like a pharmaceutical agent. The most common published risk from blood transfusion is blood delivery error, which supports the notion that blood is handled as a pharmaceutical agent.

Over the past few decades the risk for associated complications with blood transfusion has raised safety concerns in the public, medical, and regulatory arenas. At the same time, data from clinical trials and medical practice have been collected looking at the outcomes of patients who refused blood versus those who received blood transfusion. This has brought to light positive outcomes achieved by using alternative modalities in the perioperative setting to reduce or avoid blood transfusions. These results include improved patient outcomes (Day, 2008; Nowak, 2008), shorter lengths of hospitalization (Vamvakas and Carven, 1998), reduced infection rates (Hill et al, 2003; Blachman, 2005), and significant cost savings (Shander et al, 2007).

These data also reveal a variance in transfusion practice between individual physicians and hospitals and demonstrate the need to standardize blood use protocols and procedures. Time and again in research and clinical experience, justification is found for revisiting a professional point of view on the use of blood transfusions.

The American Association of Blood Banks' *Circular of Information for the Use of Human Blood and Blood Components* (2002) states, "red cell–containing components should not be used to treat anemia that can be corrected with specific medications." Dr. Paul Hébert, critical care specialist at Ottawa General Hospital, Canada, agreed, after completing a landmark study on the effectiveness of blood transfusion practices on critically ill patients suffering from anemia. The study compared patients treated with liberal transfusion policies and those treated with more restrictive ones. He summarizes, "We've been transfusing blood for 50 years and no one's ever bothered to find out how much to give. Now we know it's safe to transfuse less" (Farmer and Webb, 2000).

It is increasingly apparent that, at the very least, less-risky options should be considered before resorting to the use of blood, but the question is, are they? Ask, what is the medical facility's standard of care for treating anemia? What is my reaction when I see a patient's laboratory report of a hemoglobin (Hgb) level of 8 or 9 g/dL? How do I react when a patient makes a request for alternatives to a professional recommendation of transfusion? This may require a paradigm shift within a health care institution and among individual health care professionals. Education is a key factor in accomplishing this. The purpose of this chapter is to provide insight into this emerging and fascinating field.

Major medical centers around the world have successfully implemented nonblood strategies and techniques with dramatic and even impressive results. A successful approach incorporates the collective efforts of a multifaceted team, including skilled physicians and surgeons, capable and compassionate nurses, supportive hospital administration, and appropriately equipped medical facilities.

MEDICAL ETHICS

Medical professionals are committed to applying their knowledge, skills, and experience in fighting disease and death. What health care providers believe is in the best interest of patients may not be what patients believe is best. Patients may have more holistic concerns that include their emotional, psychologic, social, spiritual, and physical well-being. Whether or not we agree with patients' decisions to refuse blood, we have the responsibility to support patients in their constitutional right to refuse medical care just as if it were an aspirin or chemotherapy agent that they were refusing (Smith, 1997). According to Appelbaum and Roth (1983), 19% of patients at teaching hospitals refused at least one treatment or procedure, even though 15% of such refusals "were potentially life endangering."

As John Stuart Mill (1952) aptly wrote, "No society in which these liberties are not, on the whole, respected, is free, whatever may be its form of government… Each is the proper guardian of his own health, whether bodily, or mental and spiritual. Mankind are greater gainers by suffering each other to live as seems good to themselves, than by compelling each to live as seems good to the rest."

CASE STUDY

An otherwise healthy 57-year-old woman presents to an emergency department with right-sided abdominal pain and flulike symptoms of 5 days' duration. Diagnostic laboratory results indicate a hemoglobin (Hgb) level of 10.5 g/dL, hematocrit (Hct) of 31%, and mildly elevated white blood cell count. Computed tomography (CT) scan confirms suspected appendicitis. The patient is prepared for emergent appendectomy. The on-call general surgeon, on seeing the patient and learning that she is one of Jehovah's Witnesses, refuses to do the surgery because of her religious objection to the use of blood transfusions. The physician neither contacts another surgeon to transfer patient care nor writes an order for pain medication. The hospital's house supervisor is not able to find an alternate surgeon on staff to accept the case. Their affiliated hospitals are contacted, and their on-call surgeons also decline the case.

Was this case handled ethically? Did the physician have a reasonable concern? Was there a way to accommodate the patient's request without violating the surgeon's personal ethics?

Ultimately the patient was medicated by an anesthesiologist, and a nurse arranged transfer by ambulance to a local facility with a transfusion-free medicine program. This facility's on-call general surgeon consulted with the patient and her family and proceeded to surgery promptly. During the laparoscopic surgery it was discovered that the appendix had ruptured. The patient subsequently recovered from surgery and was discharged on postoperative day 2.

Thankfully, the views of the first surgeon are not shared by all surgeons. When discussing medical care of the Jehovah's Witness patient population, Remmers and Speer (2006) highlighted that surgical and medical procedures once considered too risky for Witness patients "are now performed routinely with few complications." The referenced literature includes reports of successful complex cardiac surgeries and pancreas, liver, and bone marrow transplantation. The authors note that the willingness of physicians to accommodate Witness patients' request for "bloodless medicine" has led to great medical progress in transfusion medicine and blood conservation.

First Do No Harm

It is the goal of ethically responsible health care professionals to help and to heal people, not to inflict harm. Therefore we must always ask ourselves, does the benefit outweigh the risk? Does the informed patient agree?

ASSOCIATED RISKS FROM TRANSFUSION

Rachel Nowak (2008) recently reported in *New Scientist*, "Over the past decade a number of studies have found that, far from saving lives, blood transfusions can actually harm many patients. The problem is not the much-publicized risk for blood-borne infectious agents, such as HIV and hepatitis, but the blood itself." Study after study has shown that transfusions, particularly those containing red blood cells (RBCs), are linked to higher death rates in patients who have had a heart attack, have undergone heart surgery (Murphy et al, 2007), or are in critical care. The exact nature of the link is uncertain, but it seems likely that chemical changes in aging blood, their impact on the immune system, and the blood's ability to deliver oxygen are key factors.

Most experts now agree that the risk posed by the transfused blood itself is far greater than that of a blood-borne infection. "Probably 40 to 60 per cent of blood transfusions are not good for the patients," says Bruce Spiess, a cardiac anesthesiologist at Virginia Commonwealth University in Richmond (Nowak, 2008). "There is virtually no high-quality study in surgery, or intensive or acute care—outside of when you are bleeding to death—that shows that blood transfusion is beneficial, and many that show it is bad for you," says Gavin Murphy, a cardiac surgeon at the Bristol Heart Institute (Nowak, 2008).

Disease Transmission

Although blood transfusion is considered "safer than it has ever been" (Goodnough et al, 2003), making a safer end product has meant increased cost and reduced supply of "acceptable" blood products. These "safer" transfusions still carry an inherent, although minimal, risk for transfusion-transmitted infections and an ever-more-apparent risk for emerging pathogens.

Immunomodulation

Neil Blumberg, MD, an authority on transfusion medicine and hematology, estimated that 10,000 to 50,000 persons in the United States die each year as a result of transfusion-related immunomodulation. Clinical trials consistently demonstrate an association between the number of transfusions and an increased number of nosocomial infections and multiple organ failures (Blumberg, 2004). Although causation has not yet been proved, the evidence to date gives us reason to proceed with caution (Shorr et al, 2005).

Human Error

A greater and less-appreciated risk than acquiring disease is human error, which reportedly occurs in close to 1 in 1000 transfusions. This error can be fatal if it results in the hemolytic reaction associated with ABO incompatibility, which reportedly occurs in 1 in 100,000 transfusions (Fauci et al, 1998).

Limitations of the Screening Tests

Screening is only as reliable as donors are in answering a screening questionnaire honestly. In an effort to make the blood supply safe, nucleic acid testing has helped in reducing the period in which some of the markers for human immunodeficiency virus (HIV)/acquired immunodeficiency syndrome (AIDS) and hepatitis C virus cannot be detected. The risk, however, is not zero. One need only review the FDA blood product recall lists to see that blood donated by high-risk individuals still makes it into the blood supply.

PROFESSIONAL CONSIDERATIONS

Given the ethical considerations and associated risks from transfusion, how can health care professionals safely deliver care to this patient population? For bloodless or transfusion-free care to be accomplished safely and successfully, three phases of patient care must be integrated vigilantly: (1) preoperative evaluation and preparation, (2) intraoperative strategies and techniques, and (3) postoperative monitoring and care.

It has been said that the most important roles of a nurse are to listen carefully and be observant. This could not be truer or more critical than in the perioperative setting. Some things that otherwise might tend to go unnoticed could be indicators that patients are in danger. In each of the three phases, it is imperative to continually assess the patient's condition and alert the team to possibly significant changes. Assessing and managing anemia throughout these phases is discussed, and associated recommendations could be considered in each phase. Relying on nurses' knowledge, experience, and instinct is a vital factor in caring for these patients safely and integral to avoiding unnecessary complications.

PREOPERATIVE CONSIDERATIONS

Medications/Supplements/Herbs

Is a patient on anticoagulants (e.g., warfarin) or antiplatelet drugs (e.g., clopidogrel or ticlopidine)? Many patients often do not mention taking Alka-Seltzer, because they do not realize that it contains aspirin.

Is a patient currently taking any of the following supplements or herbs that may contribute to increased bleeding times: ginkgo biloba (Rosenblatt and Mindel, 1997), garlic, cayenne, ginger, ginseng, and quinine (Cupp et al, 1999)? Table 7-1 lists herbal supplements and their corresponding complications.

Physical and Medical History

A thorough history and physical should be performed well in advance of the surgery. Do patients have any personal or family history of bleeding

TABLE 7-1 How Herbal Supplements Can Interfere With Surgery

Herbal Supplement	Possible Complications
Aloe vera	May cause increased intestinal muscle movement to digest food (peristalsis), may decrease effectiveness of water pills (diuretics) given after surgery
Bromelain	May cause bleeding or interact with antibiotics such as amoxicillin or tetracyclines
Danshen	May cause bleeding
Dong quai	May cause bleeding
Echinacea	May interfere with immune functioning, may alter effectiveness of immunosuppressant drugs given after transplant surgery
Ephedra	May cause abnormal heartbeat, may cause extreme high blood pressure and coma if combined with certain antidepressants and anesthesia
Feverfew	May cause bleeding
Garlic	May cause bleeding, may interfere with normal blood clotting
Ginger	May cause bleeding
Ginkgo	May cause bleeding
Ginseng	May cause bleeding, may cause rapid heartbeat, may cause high blood pressure
Goldenseal	May cause or worsen swelling and high blood pressure
Kava	May enhance sedative effects of anesthesia
Licorice (not including licorice candy)	May increase blood pressure
Omega-3 fatty acids	May cause bleeding if taken in doses greater than 3 grams a day
Senna	May cause electrolyte imbalance
St. John's wort	May increase or decrease the effects of some drugs used during and after surgery
Valerian	May prolong the effects of anesthesia

From *Herbal supplements: how they can interfere with surgery*, available at http://www.mayoclinic.com/health/herbal-suppements/SA00040. Accessed on August 3, 2009.

disorders or risk factors that might increase bleeding tendency? Contraindications to an elective surgery might include acute infection, anemia, or clotting disorders. Just as an elective surgery likely would be cancelled for an acute infectious process, consideration should be given to rescheduling when patients have an uncontrolled clotting disorder or an anemia. Ideally these would be identified and treated well before the day of surgery. Nevertheless, if first noted on the day of surgery, a nurse has a responsibility, as patient advocate, to notify the surgeon or anesthesiologist of the concern and possibly recommend rescheduling. The physician then would weigh the expected blood loss in light of the patient's hematologic status (Hgb, Hct, platelet count, iron studies) and determine the patient's ability to accommodate the blood loss safely. If it is determined that surgery should be postponed, what can be implemented to optimize the patient's condition for a future surgery?

Active Bleeding

If patients have gross active bleeding, surgery may be warranted emergently. If comorbidities exist, however, that cause slow bleeding, for example, peptic ulcer disease, menstruation, or kidney stones, the risks and benefits of performing surgery must be weighed thoughtfully to determine if a case should be postponed until bleeding has stopped or blood counts return to normal.

Observe Patients, Not Only Laboratory Results

Are patients symptomatic (tachycardic, short of breath with exertion, diaphoretic, or lightheaded), possibly indicative of an acute anemia? Are other nonspecific clues to chronic anemia displayed, such as complaints of being tired all the time, complaints of chest pain, increase in falls, poor eating and sleeping, increased irritability or confusion, bleeding gums, and pale or cool skin? One or more of these may indicate anemia and the need for further assessment.

Chronic anemias may be well tolerated by some patients; however, attempts should still be made to optimize a patient's hematologic status in preparation for surgery. At times this may mean not achieving the ideal "normal" values, but maximizing this patient's potential for a safe surgical course. The importance of questioning the accuracy of results when they do not seem to correspond with the patient "picture" is demonstrated in the following case study.

CASE STUDY

A 59-year-old woman presents to an emergency department by ambulance with multiple episodes of hematemesis and complaints of feeling weak and lightheaded. She has no prior history of peptic ulcer disease, no melena, and no heartburn or indigestion; is positive for arthritis; and is currently taking aspirin (650 mg per day) for hip and knee pain. Laboratory results indicate Hgb, 5.4 g/dL, and Hct, 16%, which triggers an emergent call for gastrointestinal (GI) physician consultation. The consultation is completed quickly, and an upper endoscopy is performed in the emergency department. No active bleeding is found.

What is a reasonable course of treatment in this situation? The patient was typed and crossmatched for transfusion, at which time she expressed her request for nonblood medical management. This made the immediate response and follow-up of the on-call GI physician vital to ensure the safest outcome possible for this patient. Would you have done something differently? Likely few of us would have.

In this patient's case, abnormal critical laboratory results were rechecked and showed her actual Hgb and Hct results were 8.9 g/dL and 26%, respectively. She was admitted for observation and, although mildly symptomatic, never felt as though she were in imminent danger. She was alert and oriented, and her vital signs remained within normal limits. The urgent response was appropriate based on the laboratory values. She was subsequently discharged home in stable condition. This case study demonstrates the need to confirm results while acting quickly to appropriately treat a potentially life-threatening condition.

Managing Anemia

Iron deficiency anemia is common, and simply supplementing with iron and dietary changes often corrects the anemia. If expedience is indicated, intravenous (IV) iron has proved effective. In the authors' practice, iron sucrose (Venofer) has been well tolerated by a majority of patients. If oral iron is ordered, patient compliance should be evaluated, because often it is discontinued by patients as a result of GI side effects (nausea or constipation). A newer oral therapy produced by Colorado Biolabs, heme iron polypeptide with or without folic acid (Proferrin and Proferrin Forte), also is being used and has proved advantages over other oral therapies. It is not altered by taking with food (Uzel et al, 1998), has reduced GI side effects comparable to IV iron (Nissenson et al, 2003), and is highly absorbed (Seligman et al, 2000). Only the formula with folic acid (Proferrin Forte) requires a prescription.

In more severe anemias erythropoietin (Epogen or Procrit) or darbepoetin alfa (Aranesp) perhaps is beneficial. They typically are given in conjunction with iron, unless patients have adequate iron stores. Although an initial response to erythropoietin/darbepoetin alfa (EPO) can be seen within a week, it usually takes several weeks to see the full benefit. Elective surgeries should allow the necessary time for adequate response to this treatment as confirmed by laboratory test results. In emergent cases, initiating EPO treatment concurrently with other medical or surgical intervention facilitates maximum patient benefit. Unfortunately, despite its worldwide approval in the surgical setting beginning in 1993, acceptance of EPO therapy as an alternative to blood transfusion has been slow (Goodnough et al, 1997).

Diet

Dietary measures that may be recommended to patients who are anemic to better prepare themselves for surgery may include increased intake of meat protein, almonds, leafy green vegetables, brown rice, peanut butter, beans, and dried fruits. Supplementation with oral iron, vitamin C, folic acid, and vitamin B complex also may improve RBC counts and health.

Thrombocytopenia

Low platelet counts might warrant use of IV immunoglobulin or oprelvekin (Neumega), which can stimulate platelet production, particularly in preparation for a procedure. IV immunoglobulin typically brings platelet counts to a safe level within 1 to 3 days. The effect, however, is temporary and may last only as long as several weeks. It is used to treat idiopathic thrombocytopenic purpura (George et al, 1996), other thrombocytopenic conditions, life-threatening bleeding, and in preparation for surgical procedures.

Oprelvekin is used for the short-term treatment of thrombocytopenia and may take an average of 2 weeks to reach a safe platelet count. Labeled use is prophylaxis for or treatment of severe thrombocytopenia. Its purpose is to reduce the need for platelet transfusions after myelosuppressive chemotherapy in adult patients who have nonmyeloid malignancies and who are at high risk for severe thrombocytopenia. It also is used off label to increase platelet counts preoperatively and in select other medical conditions of severe thrombocytopenia.

MEDICATIONS TO CONTROL BLEEDING

Is it possible to avoid an invasive surgery or continued blood loss with the use of a medication? Coagulation factor VIIa (NovoSeven) currently has indications for treatment in hemophilia, but its off-label use is rapidly growing and is greater than its indicated use in hemophilic patients (De Gasperi, 2006). It has been reported to control bleeding in other situations when conventional treatment has been unsuccessful, such as major trauma (Gowers and Parr, 2005; Chiara et al, 2006), thrombocytopenia (Goodnough, 2004), warfarin overdose (Lin et al, 2003), obstetric bleeding (Heilmann et al, 2006), and intracranial bleeding (Karadimov et al, 2003).

Vitamin K may be another inexpensive and effective treatment in a bleeding situation. A patient's response to treatment is easily tracked to determine efficacy.

When medical management is not an option or is not a sufficient treatment in itself, minimally invasive procedures may allow mitigating blood loss while treating patients.

PREOPERATIVE AUTOLOGOUS BLOOD DONATION—GOOD MEDICINE?

Studies show that preoperative autologous blood donation (PAD) may not prevent patients from receiving an allogeneic blood transfusion. In fact, 50% of patients who donate blood before surgery present with anemia on the day of surgery (Forgie et al, 1998). PAD did not optimize these patients for surgery. When considering risks associated with transfusion, it is important to remember that

PAD is autologous banked blood. This means that, similar to allogeneic blood, it may be subject to clerical errors (Mackey and Lipton, 1995) and does not therefore eliminate the risk for transmission of disease. Being a banked product, it also carries the risk for bacterial contamination and transfusion reactions, such as immunomodulation from leukocyte activation, depletion of nitrous oxide during storage, and changes in the structure of the red cell flexibility, making it incapable of efficiently delivering oxygen to the microcirculation.

INTRAOPERATIVE CONSIDERATIONS

Minimally Invasive Procedures

When complications are not encountered, minimally invasive options yield significantly less blood loss than open surgeries. There always is an associated risk for bleeding that needs to be addressed by converting to an open approach. This may delay treatment of the bleed and in the end cause greater blood loss. Surgeons must take all of these factors and comorbidities into consideration.

Endoscopy

Endoscopy may be used in conjunction with cautery, fibrin sealants, or other therapies to identify and control bleeding. Typically patients recover quickly and are able to return home within a short period of time.

Cell Tagging

Cell tagging is used to locate a source of bleeding, source of infection, or abnormal vascular conditions. Historically surgeons have resorted to exploratory surgery, with its higher risk for bleeding, to identify the problem. This technology can minimize the need for more invasive procedures.

Interventional Radiology/Selective Arterial Embolization

Selective arterial embolization can be used to cut off blood supply to a tumor, organ, aneursm, or uterine fibroid or to quell postpartum hemorrhage (Roman and Rebarber, 2003). The next two case studies present examples of successful use of this procedure.

CASE STUDY

A 76-year-old man arrives at the emergency department by ambulance with acute onset of sharp, constant left flank pain, followed by a bloody bowel movement. Flank pain is increased upon movement and palpation. Patient denies blood in urine or recent trauma. Patient is mildly hypertensive, but otherwise vital signs are within normal limits. Patient does not appear pale, diaphoretic, or disoriented. There is a medical history of atrial fibrillation and recent history of ischemic cerebrovascular accident for which he was prescribed warfarin. International normalized ratio is 5.3, and initial Hgb level is 13.4 g/dL. CT scan shows a left renal cystic mass with hematoma. The patient is found in hemorrhagic shock secondary to intra-abdominal bleeding resulting from overcoagulation and renal mass. The patient is given fluid resuscitation and activated factor VII (to control bleeding) and taken to radiology, where he has successful multiple embolizations of the left renal artery. The patient responds well to treatment and shortly thereafter returns home without further problems to await possible future removal of the embolized kidney.

CASE STUDY

A 55-year-old woman who has known chronic myelomonocytic leukemia presents to the hospital with increasing abdominal distention and shortness of breath. The patient has a history of progressive splenic enlargement, which has gone untreated because none of the physicians in her locality were willing to approach her care with the restriction on the use of blood or blood replacement therapy in her management. Being unaware that there were other options available, she and her family were resigned to a probable adverse outcome. Presenting laboratory results are as follows: white blood cells, 25.8; Hgb, 10.2 g/dL; Hct, 31%; and platelet count, 38,000. CT scan shows massive splenomegaly with areas of possible early infarction of the spleen and increasing abdominal pain consistent with impending splenic rupture. Splenic artery embolization is completed by an interventional radiologist, and 4 days later a nearly 8-lb spleen is removed. After splenectomy, platelet count rises to 40,000 and continues to rise until at discharge on day 14, the patient's platelet count is 189,000 and Hgb and Hct are stable at 6.3 g/dL and 19%, respectively.

Selective arterial embolization has proved to be an underutilized, minimally invasive, effective option for treating many patients safely and avoiding transfusion.

Laparoscopic or Robot-Assisted Laparoscopic Surgery

Blood loss and complications typically are reduced in laparoscopic and robot-assisted laparoscopic surgeries versus open surgical approaches. Risk factors with both include unexpected bleeding and the need for conversion to an open procedure. Robot-assisted procedures, primarily because they use a new technology and a learning curve is involved, also often mean longer anesthesia times. The significant reduction in blood loss associated with robot-assisted laparoscopic radical prostatectomy (RALRP) versus open prostatectomy is well documented (Tewari et al, 2003; Ahlering et al, 2004). This blood loss reduction also was quantified in a study completed by Miller et al (2007) at the University of North Carolina, in which they found that RALRP reduced blood loss on average from 490 mL with open surgical techniques to 232 mL with robotic techniques. In most published series, complication rates range from 8% to 20% versus 4% to 10%, respectively, in radical prostatectomy (Basillotte et al, 2004). Similar results have been seen in cardiothoracic and gynecologic surgeries using laparoscopic and robot-assisted technology. Smaller incisions typically mean reduced recovery time, pain, and trauma (Intuitive Surgical, 2005).

Surgical Techniques

Many of the surgical techniques pioneered in an effort to provide transfusion-free care have now become the standard of care. Surgeons recognize the need for meticulous surgical technique to maintain hemostasis, especially with increasing numbers of patients requesting treatment without the use of blood products. Constant awareness of patients' coagulative state can prevent unnecessary blood loss. Simple measures can be implemented, such as positioning patients in a way that elevates the surgical site to reduce arterial pressure and facilitates venous drainage away from the surgical wound (Schneeberger et al, 1998), applying tourniquets or local vasoconstrictors to the surgical wound, and using topical hemostats. Anesthesia techniques, such as hypotensive anesthesia and maintaining normothermia, also play a vital role.

Surgical Equipment and Procedures

Hemostasis

Blood loss can be reduced by means of everything from older technology, such as electrocautery and argon beam coagulation, to newer technology, such as fibrin sealants and the Aquamantys System (Transcollation technology, Salient Surgical Technologies, Dover, New Hampshire [formerly TissueLink Medical])

Blood Salvage and Autotransfusion

Blood can be salvaged preoperatively in the case of acute normovolemic hemodilution (ANH), intraoperatively with cell salvage, or postoperatively by means of wound drainage, and later reinfused into patients. These methods virtually remove the risk for transmission of foreign pathogens and allow patients to benefit from the oxygen-carrying capacity of their own blood cells.

Perioperative autologous cell salvage, also known as intraoperative autotransfusion, suctions all lost blood possible from the surgical wound and, in the case of moderate to severe blood loss, can separate, wash, and reinfuse the RBCs into patients.

ANH is used in cases with expected high-volume blood loss. Shortly after a patient's arrival to the operating room, several units of blood are diverted from the patient into blood bags, and the volume then is replaced with colloid or crystalloid solution. The diverted blood volume is kept anti-coagulated in the operating room awaiting reinfusion. Volume loss during surgery remains approximately the same but contains fewer RBCs. When bleeding is controlled or at the end of surgery, the blood diverted preoperatively is reinfused. Because this process is completed at the patient's bedside, there is no storage or screening involved, costs are kept to a minimum, and the risk for human error is virtually eliminated, making this an advantageous procedure compared with PAD (Monk et al, 1995). Although the risks for ANH are not quantified, they seem minimal (Shander and Rijhwani, 2004). Given the reported results of clinical trials completed to date, scientists are fairly confident that ANH does not pose a major risk for patients.

Diversion of Blood From the Surgical Site

The heart-lung pump, or extracorporeal circulation, allows surgeons to perform open heart surgeries that otherwise are impossible. Among the risks associated with this procedure are increased bleeding risk, resulting from high-volume anticoagulation and platelet damage, and inflammatory processes. Because of this, there is a new trend among cardiothoracic surgeons toward off-pump or beating-heart coronary artery bypass grafting (CABG). With this procedure, cell damage that inherently occurs with use of the heart-lung pump is avoided, and less anticoagulant is needed, thereby reducing the bleeding risk and need for allogeneic transfusion. Off-pump CABG is not an option in all situations, such as valve replacement. Minimally invasive CABG is another emerging technique that ideally reduces the risk for bleeding, scarring, and infection, but, as with other minimally invasive procedures, benefits must be weighed against risks and in the light of comorbidities.

Modified ultrafiltration (Moskowitz et al, 2006) was introduced in the early 1990s as a technique to hemoconcentrate the residual blood in the extracorporeal circuit along with the patient's existing blood volume following cardiopulmonary bypass. It carried with it inherent risks, including hemodynamic instability, difficulty purging the entire extracorporeal circuit without redilution of the patient volume, and loss of residual blood that is left in the modified ultrafiltration system at its completion. The Hemobag (Global Blood Resources, Somers, Connecticut) is a modification of this system used by a perfusionist to accomplish hemoconcentration without the associated risks.

Many strategies have been discussed that can be used preoperatively and intraoperatively to facilitate a safer surgical experience for patients who refuse blood products. The care of patients, who have returned to the floor after a successful surgery with no more than the expected blood loss, perhaps with drains in place, is discussed. What can nurses look for and implement to support patients through a safe and uneventful recovery period as well?

POSTOPERATIVE CONSIDERATIONS

A key to a safe and successful postoperative experience is monitoring patients and intervening early rather than adopting a wait-and-see attitude when there is some concern. Advocate for patients. Early intervention averts adverse medical events and crisis management. Trust professional instincts. Look at patients; listen to patients; if there is a negative trend in a patient's condition, act rather than wait. Advocating for patients may mean contacting an attending physician or specialist at times other than regular office hours. This may require persistence.

Have there been significant changes in the appearance of a wound, drainage, patient pain level, or vital signs that might indicate a decline in a patient's hematologic condition? Several aspects of caring for transfusion-free patients are discussed.

Wound Assessment

Monitor wound drainage: is it greater than expected for this type of procedure? Is the patient experiencing greater-than-normal swelling or discoloration of the wound site? Is the patient complaining of unmanaged pain? Swelling and pain may indicate internal bleeding. Are the laboratory results trending in a negative direction? Has the surgeon been made aware, and have appropriate orders been received?

Is reinfusion of wound drainage an option for the patient? Depending on a particular hospital's policy, there typically is a 4- to 6-hour window to reinfuse wound drainage that has been collected into a sterile reservoir. Discuss this option with the physician and then with the patient. Some patients requesting nonblood management require that wound drainage devices be set up in a continuous circuit, meaning that the drain was placed and the line from the reservoir back to the patient IV was primed during surgery.

Supportive Measures—Diet and Exercise

Often underestimated is the importance of diet and exercise in healing and anemias. A high-protein diet promotes healing. Nutritional supplements, including vitamins C and B_{12}, folic acid, and iron, are necessary for healthy RBC production. This is especially important in patients who may be anemic. Adequate activity promotes an appropriate bone marrow response to increase RBC production and minimizes the risk for thrombophlebitis.

Phlebotomy

It is not uncommon to see patients return from surgery with laboratory samples ordered to be drawn anywhere from every few hours to once a day thereafter during their hospital stay. Are they truly necessary to provide quality health care to individuals? Or are patients jeopardized by removing vital resources that could be better used in the healing process? Dr. Howard Corwin, a respected leader in bloodless medicine strategies, chief of Critical Care Medicine and medical director of the intensive care setting at Dartmouth-Hitchcock Medical Center, concluded that patients who stay in an intensive care setting for more than a week often require a blood transfusion solely because of the volume of blood removed by phlebotomy (Corwin et al, 1995; Chant et al, 2006). When dealing with a patient population in which blood transfusions are not an option, every drop of blood counts. It is imperative to modify phlebotomy practices. Limiting phlebotomy to necessary tests and using point-of-care devices, short-fill, or pediatric tubes can help to that end.

Vital Signs

Monitor vital signs closely, including oxygenation. Remember that if patients are anemic, even if their oxygen saturation seems adequate per pulse oximetry, they are likely not perfusing tissues adequately and could benefit from oxygen. If patients are not symptomatic (short of breath or lightheaded), this is a modality that often is overlooked.

Address hypertension immediately. It stands to reason that increased pressure causes patients to be more prone to bleeding.

Hydration

Monitor hydration. If patients are dehydrated, Hct, which indicates percentage of RBCs in the circulating volume, may seem adequate when patients actually are anemic. On the other end of the spectrum, patients who are fluid overloaded appear more anemic than they actually are.

Medications

If antiplatelets and anticoagulants are ordered, continue to closely monitor patients for signs of bleeding. Assess for warning signs, such as bleeding gums, IV sites, increased wound bleeding, or blood-tinged urine.

Promptly addressing changes in a patient's condition can facilitate their safe return home. In a bleeding or anemia situation, time is of the essence. Do not hesitate to report concerns to a physician. You just might save a life.

CONCLUSION

An increasing number of patients and medical professionals are expressing an interest in bloodless medicine or blood conservation. Successful implementation of nonblood strategies and techniques has led to dramatic and impressive results. Each year more studies are published that indicate that the treatment methods held as standard for decades, almost religiously, may not be the safest and most appropriate approach in treating patients. The evidence consistently indicates that preventive measures to reduce bleeding and anemias and judicious use of blood products is simply the best medicine. Medical studies confirm that patients who are treated with these methods have fewer infections, shorter hospital stays, and even reduced mortality when compared with patients who receive blood transfusions.

A successful approach incorporates the collective efforts of a multifaceted team. Skilled physicians and surgeons play a key role on the successful team. They take the necessary precautions and time, using procedures, pharmaceuticals, and medical technology to avoid the need for transfusions. Many physician-based organizations have been formed to educate and publish recommendations for improved practice regarding blood use. The Society for the Advancement of Blood Management, Network for Advancement of Transfusion Alternatives, and Association of American Blood Banks are just a few such organizations.

Capable and compassionate nurses provide the best medical care possible within the parameters of patients' expressed and informed wishes. Nurses are the eyes and ears that can identify a trend and activate a prompt response to avert adverse medical outcomes. A supportive hospital administration upholds patient rights and provides appropriately equipped facilities and trained medical professionals as a center of excellence for patient care.

Regardless of the reason why patients choose to decline blood transfusions, safe and effective alternatives are available. The authors believe that transfusion-free medicine and blood conservation are the future of medicine and will continue to prove themselves the gold standard.

REFERENCES

Ahlering TE, et al: Robot assisted versus open prostatectomy: a comparison of one surgeon's outcomes, *Urology* 63:819–822, 2004.

American Association of Blood Banks et al: *Circular of information for the use of human blood and blood components*, Bethesda, Md, 2002, American Association of Blood Banks.

Appelbaum PS, Roth LH: Patients who refuse treatment in medical hospitals, *J Am Med Assoc* 250:1296–1301, 1983.

Basillotte J, et al: Laparoscopic radical prostatectomy: review and assessment of an emerging technique, *Surg Endosc* 18:1694–1711, 2004.

Blachman MA: Transfusion immunomodulation or TRIM: what does it mean clinically? *Hematology* 10(Suppl): 208–214, 2005.

Blumberg N: *Transfusion-alternative strategies*, Brooklyn, 2004, Watchtower Bible and Tract Society of New York, Inc.

Chant C, et al: Anemia, transfusion, and phlebotomy practices in critically ill patients with prolonged ICU length of stay: a cohort study, *Crit Care* 10(5):R140, 2006.

Chiara O, et al: Treatment of critical bleeding in trauma patients, *Minerva Anesthesiol* 72:383–387, 2006.

Committee on Government Reform and Oversight: *Protecting the nation's blood supply from infectious agents: the need for new standards to meet new threats*, Washington, DC, 1996, U.S. Department of Health and Human Services.

Corwin H, et al: RBC transfusion in the ICU is there a reason? *Chest* 108:767–771, 1995.

Cupp MJ: Herbal remedies: adverse effects and drug interactions, *Am Fam Physician* 59:1239–1244, 1999.

Day M: *Two week old blood no good for transfusion*, 2008, available at http://www.newscientist.com/article/dn13501-twoweekold-blood-no-good-for-transfusions.html. Accessed July 12, 2008.

De Gasperi A: Intraoperative use of recombinant activated factor VII (r-FVIIa), *Minerva Anesthesiol* 72:489–494, 2006.

Farmer S, Webb D: *Your body, your choice*, Media Masters, 2000, Singapore.

Fauci A, et al: Transfusion biology and therapy. In *Harrison's principles of internal medicine*, ed 14, New York, 1998, McGraw-Hill.

Forgie M, et al: Preoperative autologous donation decreased allogeneic transfusion but increases exposure to all red cell transfusion: results of a meta analysis, international study of perioperative transfusion (ISPOT) investigators, *Arch Intern Med* 158:610–616, 1998.

George JN, et al: Idiopathic thrombocytopenic purpura: a practice guideline developed by explicit methods for the American Society of Hematology, *Blood* 88(1):3–40, 1996.

Goodnough LT: Experiences with recombinant human factor VIIa in patients with thrombocytopenia, *Semin Hematol* 41(1 Suppl 1):25–29, 2004.

Goodnough LT, et al: Erythropoietin therapy, *N Engl J Med* 336:933–938, 1997.

Goodnough LT, et al: Transfusion medicine: looking towards the future, *Lancet* 361(9352):161–169, 2003.

Gowers CJD, Parr MJA: Recombinant activated factor VIIa use in massive transfusion and coagulopathy unresponsive to conventional therapy, *Anaesth Intensive Care* 33:196–200, 2005.

Heilmann L, et al: Successful treatment of life-threatening bleeding after cesarean section with recombinant activated factor VII, *Clin Appl Thromb Hemost* 12:227–229, 2006.

Hill GE, et al: Allogeneic blood transfusion increases the risk of postoperative bacterial infection: a meta-analysis, *J Trauma* 54:908–914, 2003.

Intuitive Surgical: The da Vinci® Surgical System, 2005, available at http://www.intuitivesurgical.com/corporate/newsroom/mediakit/da_Vinci_System_Backgrounder.doc. Accessed October 16, 2009.

Karadimov D, et al: Use of activated recombinant factor VII (NovoSeven) during neurosurgery, *J Neurosurg Anesthesiol* 15:330–332, 2003.

Lin J, et al: The use of recombinant activated factor VII to reverse warfarin-induced anticoagulation in patients with hemorrhages in the central nervous system: preliminary findings, *J Neurosurg* 98:737–740, 2003.

Mackey J, Lipton KS: *Association Bulletin 95-4: AABB position on testing of autologous units*, Bethesda, Md, 1995, American Association of Blood Banks.

Mill JS: On liberty. In Adler MJ, editor: *Great books of the Western world*, vol 43, Chicago, 1952, Encyclopedia Britannica, Inc.

Miller J, et al: Prospective evaluation of short-term impact and recovery of health related quality of life in men undergoing robotic assisted laparoscopic radical prostatectomy versus open radical prostatectomy, *J Urol* 178(3):854–859, 2007.

Monk TG, et al: Acute normovolemic hemodilution is a cost-effective alternative to preoperative autologous blood donation by patients undergoing radical retropubic prostatectomy, *Transfusion* 35:559–565, 1995.

Moskowitz D, et al: Use of the Hemobag for modified ultrafiltration in a Jehovah's Witness patient undergoing cardiac surgery, *JECT* 38:265–270, 2006.

Murphy G, et al: Increased mortality, postoperative morbidity, and cost after red blood cell transfusion in patients having cardiac surgery, *Circulation* 116:2544, 2007.

Nissenson A, et al: Clinical evaluation of heme iron polypeptide: sustaining a response to rHuEPO in hemodialysis patients, *Am J Kidney Dis* 42(2):325–330, 2003.

Nowak R: Blood transfusions found to harm some patients, *New Sci* 2653:8–9, 2008.

Remmers PA, Speer AJ: Clinical strategies in the medical care of Jehovah's Witnesses, *Am J Med* 119(12):103–108, 2006.

Roman AS, Rebarber A: Seven ways to control post-partum hemorrhage, *Contemp Ob Gyn* 48(3):34–53, 2003.

Rosenblatt M, Mindel J: Spontaneous hyphema associated with ingestion of ginkgo biloba extract, *N Engl J Med* 336:1108, 1997.

Schneeberger AG, et al: Blood loss in total hip arthroplasty: lateral position combined with preservation of the capsule versus supine position combined with capsulectomy, *Arch Orthop Trauma Surg* 117(1–2):47–49, 1998.

Seligman P, et al: Clinical studies of HIP: an oral heme-iron product, *Nutr Res* 20(9):1279–1286, 2000.

Shander A, Rijhwani TS: Acute normovolemic hemo-dilution, *Transfusion* 44(Suppl 12):26S–34S, 2004.

Shander A, et al: Estimating the cost of blood, past, present, and future directions, *Best Pract Res Clin Anaesthesiol* 21(2): 271–289, 2007.

Shorr A, et al: Transfusion practice and blood stream infections in critically ill patients, *Chest* 127:1722–1728, 2005.

Smith ML: Ethical perspectives on Jehovah's Witnesses' refusal of blood, *Cleve Clin J Med* 64(9):475–481, 1997.

Tewari A, et al: A prospective comparison of radical retropubic and robot-assisted prostatectomy: experience in one institution, *BJU Int* 92:205–210, 2003.

Uzel C, et al: Absorption of heme iron, *Semin Hematol* 35:27–34, 1998.

Vamvakas EC, Carven JH: Allogeneic blood transfusion, hospital charges, and length of hospitalization: a study of 487 consecutive patients undergoing colorectal cancer resection, *Arch Pathol Lab Med* 122:145–151, 1998.

PERIOPERATIVE PATIENT SAFETY AND PROCEDURAL SEDATION

Jan Odom-Forren, PhD, MS, RN, CPAN, FAAN

The concept of patient safety was brought to the forefront in 1999 when the Institute of Medicine published *To Err Is Human: Building a Safer Health System* (Kohn et al, 2000). The authors of the report focused on the impact of medical or health care errors occurring in patients and delineated patient safety as a priority for the health care community The report pointed out that error was the property of a system of care as opposed to individual health care providers and that those systems should provide well-designed processes of care that result in prevention, recognition, and early recovery from errors to ensure that patients remain safe and unharmed (Donaldson, 2008).

The use of sedation administered by nonanesthesia providers for procedures has increased exponentially over the past decade. The term *procedural sedation* is used interchangeably with *moderate sedation. Procedural sedation* is a term that is considered by many to be a more comprehensive description of the actual techniques applied. Procedural sedation "refers to the techniques of managing a patient's pain and anxiety to facilitate appropriate medical care in a safe, effective, and humane fashion" (Brown, 2005). Procedural/moderate sedation is performed in the perioperative environment and in other nonsurgical environments such as the endoscopy suite, the cardiac catheterization laboratory, the radiology department, the labor and delivery suite, physician offices, emergency departments, and dental offices. This use of procedural or nurse-monitored sedation has partially been driven by economic factors, because some insurance companies are unwilling to pay anesthesia providers for monitored anesthesia care during many routine procedures, and by the need to move patients quickly through the procedural area—a more difficult process when scheduling anesthesia (Meltzer, 2003).

The safety of the patient is the primary concern for perioperative registered nurses (RNs) involved in administering sedation or monitoring the patient who has received procedural/moderate sedation (Odom-Forren, 2005). Procedural/moderate sedation is safe, but has potential adverse reactions such as hypoxemia, apnea, hypotension, airway obstruction, and cardiopulmonary arrest (Gross et al, 2002; Vargo, 2007). As a member of the Dartmouth Summit stated, "the side effects of the procedure can traumatize you; the side effects of the sedation can kill you" (Blike and Cravero, 2000). However, the RN alone cannot guarantee the safety of the patient. Patient safety is the responsibility of every person on the perioperative team and relies on an effective sedation delivery system to keep the patient from harm.

SEDATION ISSUES RELATING TO PATIENT SAFETY

Sedation on a Continuum

Sedation falls on a continuum from minimal sedation to deep sedation. Typically, nurse-monitored sedation falls under the definition of moderate sedation. Minimal sedation is used to decrease anxiety but should not affect the patient's respiratory or cardiovascular functions; however, the patient is under the influence of the medication administered and should be treated as such. The patient receiving moderate sedation should be able to maintain respirations without significant cardiovascular changes. With this type of sedation the patient is able to respond to verbal or mild tactile stimulation. The risk for complications increases as the patient moves on the continuum from minimal to moderate sedation. The patient who is receiving moderate sedation has the potential to move into deep sedation and thus become at higher risk for complications. A patient receiving deep sedation should be able to respond to repeated or painful stimulation. The patient receiving deep sedation also is at an increased risk for respiratory compromise, although cardiovascular status is usually preserved. If the patient receiving sedation at any time becomes unresponsive, that patient is receiving general anesthesia with risk for respiratory compromise, cardiac compromise, or both (Blike and Cravero, 2000; Gross et al, 2002; The Joint Commission, 2008). The further the patient moves on the continuum, the greater the risk for the patient (Table 8-1).

The RN monitoring a patient during procedural sedation must be able to rescue a patient who inadvertently moves from one level of sedation to the next level of sedation. Therefore the RN monitoring the patient who is receiving moderate sedation should be prepared to rescue the patient who moves into deep sedation, and the nurse monitoring the patient during deep sedation must be prepared to rescue a patient who has respiratory or cardiovascular compromise and who has moved on the continuum into general anesthesia.

Adverse Reactions

Respiratory depression is the most common adverse reaction to procedural sedation. One panel discussing the risks of sedation noted that sedation complications are related to underuse, overuse, or misuse. Underuse complications cause patients to suffer unnecessary pain and stress, whereas overuse complications can result in respiratory depression or apnea. Misuse complications involve errors in drug administration (e.g., administering sufentanil instead of the ordered medication fentanyl) (Blike and Cravero, 2000).

Cote et al (2000) studied adverse sedation events in pediatric patients. In this critical incident analysis, there were 60 events that resulted in death or permanent central nervous system injury. Respiratory depression was the first event in 80% of the patients. Poor outcome was associated with inadequate resuscitation, inadequate monitoring, inadequate initial evaluation, and inadequate recovery phase.

In a report of adverse events during pediatric sedation and anesthesia outside the operating room, 26 institutions submitted data on 30,037 patients for a period of 17 months. Serious adverse events were rare, with no deaths and cardiopulmonary resuscitation being required only once. Less serious events occurred, such as oxygen desaturation below 90% for more than 30 seconds (157 times per 10,000 sedations), unexpected apnea (24 times per 10,000 sedations), and vomiting (47.2 per 10,000 sedations). Even with a low incidence of serious adverse reactions to pediatric sedation, the number of events that had potential to harm was significant, occurring once in every 89 sedations (Cravero et al, 2006). Because events with the potential to compromise patient safety are so common, it is imperative that personnel

TABLE 8-1 Levels of Sedation

	LEVEL OF SEDATION			
Function	**Minimal**	**Moderate**	**Deep**	**General Anesthesia**
Responsiveness	Normal response to verbal stimulation	Purposeful response to light stimulation	Purposeful response to pain stimulation	Unarousable, even to painful stimulation
Airway	Unaffected	No intervention	Possible intervention	Probable intervention
Ventilation	Unaffected	Adequate	May be inadequate	Often inadequate
Cardiovascular	Unaffected	Usually maintained	Usually maintained	May be impaired

Data from Blike GT, Cravero JP: *Pride, prejudice, and pediatric sedation: a multispecialty evaluation of the state of the art: report from a Dartmouth summit on pediatric sedation*, 2000, available at http://www.npsf.org. Accessed June, 2008; Gross JB et al: American Society of Anesthesiologists Task Force on Sedation and Analgesia by Non-anesthesiologists: ASA practice guidelines for sedation and analgesia by non-anesthesiologists, *Anesthesiology* 96:1004–1017, 2002; Vargo JJ: Minimizing complications: sedation and monitoring, *Gastrointest Endosc Clin N Am* 17:11–28, 2007.

involved in sedation be competent to manage an airway obstruction, emesis, hypoventilation, and apnea (Hertzog and Havidich, 2007).

Adverse reactions to sedation are an international problem. From a questionnaire sent to nonanesthesia providers to assess sedation practices in Ireland, Fanning (2008) found that 22% of respondents reported events including respiratory depression, hypoxia, loss of consciousness, prolonged sedation, and nausea and vomiting. Two events required the presence of an anesthesia provider (Fanning, 2008). Sedation was the cause of most complications that occurred in a study conducted in Germany to determine complications in outpatient gastrointestinal endoscopy patients (Sieg et al, 2001).

In 121 monitored anesthesia care cases pulled from the American Society of Anesthesiologists (ASA) Closed Claims database (1990–2002), the severity of complications was similar to that found with general anesthesia (Bhananker et al, 2006). Twenty-one percent of the claims were caused by respiratory depression secondary to the sedative medications. These events were associated with older age (70 years or older), ASA physical status III and IV, and obesity. Propofol or benzodiazepines used alone were associated with oversedation in 9% of the patients. Propofol with the use of another medication was responsible for 50% of the patients diagnosed with oversedation (Bhananker et al, 2006). This information about patients receiving monitored anesthesia care can be assumed to also apply to patients receiving sedation and analgesia from nonanesthesia providers such as the perioperative RN.

The low percentages of serious complications such as aspiration or hypoxia with resulting neurologic impairment or death require that larger studies be undertaken than have been conducted to date. Surrogate markers are typically used in studies to determine the potential for serious adverse reactions. A surrogate marker commonly used in sedation studies is respiratory depression, with an operational definition for the study such as apnea longer than 30 seconds or oxygen saturation falling below 90%. The occurrence of cardiopulmonary complications is used as a surrogate marker of the risk for occurrence of a significant adverse event (Vargo, 2007). Studies conducted with surrogate markers are able to use lower numbers of patients but have unclear clinical significance (Miner and Krauss, 2007; Vargo, 2007). In summary, although the severe complication rates are low for procedural sedation, failure to recognize or immediately treat these patients can lead to morbidity or even death. Of great importance are patient risk assessment and rescue capabilities (Cravero et al, 2006).

Patient Risk Factors

Preprocedure assessment and identification of high-risk patients is the key to the prevention or successful management of sedation-related events (Hooper, 2005b). Patients at high risk for complications should be evaluated during the preprocedure assessment for appropriateness of nurse-monitored sedation (Table 8-2). Patients at risk for a difficult airway are important to identify because respiratory complications are commonly associated with sedation. Risk factors associated with a difficult airway include a history of problems with anesthesia or sedation, advanced rheumatoid arthritis, chromosomal abnormalities (e.g., trisomy 21), and stridor, snoring, or sleep apnea (Gross et al, 2002; ASA, 2008).

SEDATION PRACTICE ISSUES

It is accepted practice for the competent and educated RN to administer the medication and monitor patients who are undergoing a procedure that requires moderate sedation. For any state Board of Nursing (BON) or governing body that has specifically addressed the issue of moderate sedation, all have agreed that the practice is within the scope of practice for a competent and educated RN. Those BONs or governing bodies that have addressed the issue typically have a position statement, declaratory ruling, advisory opinion, and/or policy statement. Some BONs or governing bodies do not specifically address the issue, but respond with a decision tree or other procedure to address practice questions.

The role of the RN administering deep sedation is more controversial. Currently no consensus exists among state Boards of Nursing or governing bodies regarding the role of the RN administering deep sedation. Many times when asked to provide deep sedation, the RN is required to administer a drug labeled as an anesthetic agent (e.g., propofol). (See section later in chapter on propofol administration.) In other

TABLE 8-2 Patients at High Risk for Sedation-Related Complications

Risk Factor	Intervention
Presence of airway abnormalities	Evaluate airway before sedation. Evaluate for presence of sleep apnea.
ASA classification status of III or greater	Evaluate a class III patient on an individual basis. Consult with anesthesia provider for classes IV or V.
Chronic obstructive pulmonary disease	Administer bronchodilators before procedure. Titrate sedatives in small increments.
Obesity	Pretreat with oral H_2 antagonist. Titrate sedatives in small increments.
Coronary artery disease	Prevent oversedation or undersedation. Allow routine cardiac medications to be taken on day of procedure. Administer supplemental oxygen.
Chronic renal failure	Avoid long-acting opioids. Administer small incremental doses of sedatives.
Drug addiction	Use short-acting sedatives with incremental dosing. Avoid use of reversal agents.
Extremes of age (pediatric and older adult patients)	Administer individual and incremental dosing.

ASA, American Society of Anesthesiologists.

Data from American Society of Anesthesiologists: *Practice guidelines for management of the difficult airway,* available at http://www.asahq.org/publicationsAndServices/Difficult%20Airway.pdf. Accessed August 13, 2008; Gross JB et al: American Society of Anesthesiologists Task Force on Sedation and Analgesia by Non-anesthesiologists: ASA practice guidelines for sedation and analgesia by non-anesthesiologists, *Anesthesiology* 96:1004–1017, 2002; Hooper VD: Management of complications. In Odom-Forren J, Watson D, editors: *Practical guide to moderate sedation/analgesia,* ed 2, St. Louis, 2005, Mosby; Martin ML, Lennox PH: Sedation and analgesia in the interventional radiology department, *J Vasc Interv Radiol* 14:1119–1128, 2003.

cases, deep sedation requires a higher dosage of a typical sedative than the dosage required for moderate sedation. In both cases, the safety of the patient should be the first and most important concern. It is prudent for the RN who is requested to administer deep sedation to know the position of the specific state BON or governing body in the specific state where the practice will occur. If deep sedation is considered to be an acceptable practice in the state, then the individual health care facility should have an educational process in place with a method for determining competency of the RN that is required to care for the patient receiving sedation (Odom-Forren, 2005; Odom-Forren and Watson, 2005). Guidelines are available that differentiate care for the patient undergoing moderate sedation from the one undergoing deep sedation. Any policy outlined by a health care facility for deep sedation should include parameters set by the state BON or governing body and available guidelines, such as those published by the American Society of Anesthesiologists (Gross et al, 2002). It is significant to note that the Association of periOperative Registered Nurses (AORN) (2009) offers "Recommended Practices for Managing the Patient Receiving Moderate Sedation/Analgesia," which is an excellent resource for the perioperative RN. The AORN recommended practices state that certain patients are not appropriate candidates for monitoring by the perioperative nurse, and in those situations it is more appropriate to have the monitored anesthesia care provided by an anesthesia provider (AORN, 2009).

Use of Propofol for Sedation

The use of propofol by nonanesthesia providers in sedation and analgesia has been fraught with controversy (Odom-Forren, 2005; Odom-Forren and Watson, 2005). The advantages of propofol (over benzodiazepines) include less nausea, more-rapid onset, and shorter duration of action, facilitating faster recovery and discharge (Patterson, 2004;

Kremer, 2005; Odom-Forren, 2005; Institute for Safe Medication Practices, 2008). Zed et al (2007) evaluated the efficacy, safety, and patient satisfaction with the use of propofol for procedural sedation for 113 patients in the emergency department. One patient experienced vomiting, 0 experienced apnea, 9 experienced hypotension, and 7 felt pain on injection. All patients and most physicians were satisfied with the use of propofol. The investigators concluded that as part of a standardized protocol, propofol appears to be safe and effective, with high patient and physician satisfaction (Zed et al, 2007). In three other studies that were conducted using nurse-administered propofol sedation (NAPS) with a total of 11,000 patients undergoing gastrointestinal procedures, the investigators found no major complications (Rex et al, 2002; Heuss et al, 2003; Walker et al, 2003). In an article from a university setting where NAPS is used on a regular basis, Overly and Rex (2004) discussed the use of NAPS as cost-effective and satisfying for physicians and nurses. In one study of 33,743 endoscopic procedures using NAPS (Rex et al, 2005), no cases of endotracheal intubation, death, neurologic sequelae, or other permanent injury occurred. Temporary bag-mask ventilation was required by 49 patients. The three centers with a training program conducted by anesthesiologists had a center-specific rate of complications from 9 per 10,000 to 19 per 10,000 (Rex et al, 2005).

Opponents of the use of NAPS point out that the good outcomes of these studies conceal the risks with the use of propofol. Those risks include the tendency to attain deep sedation or even general anesthesia on the sedation continuum, with the resulting problems of airway obstruction and apnea. No reversal agent for propofol is available when these events occur (Gross et al, 2002). Anesthesia providers are quick to note that the absence of morbidity or mortality in a smaller sample of patients should be moderated by the fact that morbidity and mortality for healthy patients undergoing anesthesia is only 1 in 300,000 (Philip, 2008). Vargo (2007), who believes that the safety and efficacy of propofol for use in sedation has been established, goes on to state that the current data in randomized controlled trials do not sufficiently answer the question of its safety compared with standard sedation and analgesia.

The jury is out on the widespread use of propofol for sedation until regulatory agencies, third-party payers, and professional societies come to the same conclusion about propofol's safety. One concern related to nurse-monitored sedation includes propofol's strict product labeling as an anesthetic agent to be used by persons trained in the administration of general anesthesia (Meltzer, 2003). State Boards of Nursing have varying positions regarding the use of propofol administered by nurses, with some boards (e.g., Indiana) stating that it is within the scope of nursing practice for a competent and educated nurse to administer propofol for sedation, and others (e.g., Florida) stating that is not within the scope of practice for a registered nurse to administer propofol (Odom-Forren and Watson, 2005). In 2005 the AORN board of directors endorsed the American Association of Nurse Anesthetists (AANA) and ASA joint statement indicating that only health care professionals trained in general anesthesia should administer propofol (AORN, 2009; ASA, 2009).

If a perioperative nurse is asked to administer propofol for sedation, the nurse needs to ensure that the state Board of Nursing or governing body in that particular state does not have a position statement denoting that propofol is not within the scope of practice for a registered nurse. The health care facility should also have a strict education program that not only determines cognitive knowledge but also uses mentoring to determine competence.

In December 2008 a new drug, fospropofol sodium, was approved for monitored anesthesia care sedation. Fospropofol is a water-soluble prodrug of propofol and is used by determining a weight-based bolus (Vargo, 2007). While undergoing studies, it was unknown whether the increased plasma half-life would mean prolonged recovery, but it was hoped that the drug would be able to maintain a patient at the level of moderate sedation. For short-duration procedures, it is possible that patients may require only a single dose (American Society for Gastrointestinal Endoscopy, 2008). However, the U.S. Food and Drug Administration (FDA) used the same wording with fospropofol as with propofol, requiring use only by persons trained in the administration of general anesthesia, and further states that all patients should be continuously monitored by persons not involved in the conduct of the procedure (FDA, 2009).

Guidelines for the ASA and the American Society for Gastrointestinal Endoscopy (ASGE) have specific criteria for monitoring patients who are under deep sedation, including a committed, qualified practitioner administering the sedation and the evaluation of ventilatory function with consideration of capnography (Gross et al, 2002; ASGE, 2008). The ASA and the ASGE have determined components of a training program for any health care facility that uses NAPS with resultant deep sedation. The ASGE includes an initial phase of training, including didactic material that discusses the sedative agents to be used, contraindications for specific agents, and certification in advanced cardiac life support or the equivalent. Other components of the ASGE program include a written test on didactic material, airway assessment, observation, and administration under supervision (Rex, 2006). Contraindications to propofol administration by nonanesthesia providers at Indiana University, where NAPS is widespread, include increased aspiration risk (e.g., acute upper gastrointestinal bleeding, achalasia, delayed gastric emptying, bowel obstruction); difficult airways (e.g., sleep apnea requiring continuous positive airway pressure, marked obesity, abnormal airway assessment); extreme comorbidities; and allergy to propofol (or to eggs or soybeans) (Rex, 2006). Although the ASA is opposed to NAPS, the ASA has developed criteria that address the safe use of propofol when used by nonanesthesiologists (Box 8-1).

BOX 8-1 Safe Use of Propofol

RESPONSIBLE PHYSICIAN

Must have education and training to manage complications
Must be proficient in airway management
Must have advanced cardiac life support training
Must understand pharmacology of drugs

PRACTITIONER ADMINISTERING PROPOFOL

Must have education and training to identify and manage airway and cardiovascular changes of patient who enters state of general anesthesia
Must have ability to assist in management of complications
Must be present throughout procedure, with no other responsibilities other than monitoring patient
Must monitor patient, assessing level of consciousness, ventilation, oxygen saturation, heart rate, and blood pressure, with monitoring of exhaled carbon dioxide when possible
Must identify early signs of hypotension, bradycardia, apnea, airway obstruction, oxygen desaturation
Must have age-appropriate equipment immediately available
Must not be involved in conduct of surgical/diagnostic procedure

From Odom-Forren J: The evolution of nurse monitored sedation, *J Perianesth Nurs* 20:385–398, 2005 with permission.

VanNatta and Rex (2006) conducted a randomized clinical trial to compare recovery time and patient satisfaction with propofol administered alone titrated to deep sedation versus propofol plus fentanyl, propofol plus midazolam, or propofol plus a combination of midazolam and fentanyl titrated to moderate sedation in 200 outpatients undergoing colonoscopy. Patients who received a combination regimen were discharged more quickly. There were no significant differences in pain or satisfaction among the groups. This randomized controlled trial was the first to titrate propofol to moderate sedation in a combination therapy. The investigators stated that recognition among anesthesia providers of propofol as an agent that can be used for moderate sedation would be helpful in gaining acceptance of use by nonanesthesia personnel. The investigators also noted the importance of a defined training protocol, even when propofol is used for moderate sedation.

Mandel et al (2008) conducted a randomized controlled trial that compared two groups of patients using midazolam plus fentanyl or propofol plus remifentanil delivered by way of patient-controlled sedation (PCS). The patients who received propofol plus remifentanil recovered significantly faster than the group who received midazolam plus fentanyl. In the group administered propofol plus remifentanil, however, two patients required intervention by an anesthesiologist because of the safety end point that was designed for the study of arterial desaturation below 85% for 60 seconds. The investigators stated that those who use this form of sedation must be prepared to administer resuscitative efforts immediately.

Computer-assisted personalized sedation (CAPS) is a method whereby continuous physiologic monitoring is combined with delivery of propofol sedation with the assistance of a computer interface and software. Twenty-four subjects were included in the stage I trial to assess the safeguard software. One subject experienced oxygen saturation below 90%, and seven subjects experienced apnea longer than 30 seconds. All eight responded to automated device actions without intervention by an anesthesiologist. This initial study of an investigational device showed the viability of this technology to deliver propofol sedation to patients in the endoscopy suite (Pambianco et al, 2006).

The importance of propofol and its relation to patient safety for the perioperative patient is its ability to move the patient quickly to deep sedation, with the resulting risk for respiratory compromise. To decrease those risks, studies have been conducted to assess for dosages of propofol that can be titrated to moderate sedation, new drugs are under development, and other methods of delivery systems (e.g., PCS and CAPS) are in process to determine whether those methods would be safer for the patient.

SAFE SEDATION PRACTICE

In discussing vital issues that would decrease the harm associated with pediatric sedation, an expert panel identified the following priorities: the characterization of existing sedation care strategies across specialties, with data collected from multiple institutions; the proactive identification of hazards and vulnerabilities; improved sedation provider and team training with core competencies; systems research; and a patient-centered focus (Blike and Cravero, 2000). Performing safe and effective sedation involves several aspects of sedation, including (1) the persons administering the sedation, (2) the educational processes involved, (3) the environment in which the sedation is conducted, (4) patient-specific information processes, and (5) guidelines and protocols of the institution.

Qualified Individuals

The Joint Commission (TJC) (2008) requires that the "qualified individual" who administers sedation must possess education, training, and experience in evaluating patients before moderate or deep sedation, in rescuing patients who slip into a deeper level of sedation, and in managing a compromised airway or cardiovascular system during a procedure. It is essential that those involved in procedural sedation have compiled in advance and practiced plans for respiratory events (Blike and Cravero, 2000). Examples of responses prepared in advance are basic life support and advanced cardiac life support. Panel members during one summit stated, "any failure to rescue is a marker for a flawed sedation care system that has not trained providers adequately" (Blike and Cravero, 2000). One possible solution for hands-on rescue management is the use of human simulators. Simulators can re-create thousands of common or unusual events that clinicians learn to manage. Shavit et al (2007) conducted a prospective, observational study in two university teaching hospitals in Israel to evaluate the impact of simulation-based education on patient safety during procedural sedation. Nonanesthesiologists who had training in simulation-based education were compared with those who did not receive the simulator-based education. A nine-criteria Sedation Safety Tool was used for evaluation. Significant differences in performance related to patient safety were found between the two groups of nonanesthesiologists. The researchers believed that the patient safety training was the reason for the superior performance of the physicians who had received the training and recommend simulation-based training in sedation safety for all nonanesthesiologists who practice pediatric procedural sedation. Knowing that death and failure to rescue have been determined to be more frequent when care was not delivered by an anesthesia provider is impetus to determine the education necessary to provide safety for patients undergoing nurse-monitored procedural sedation (Silber et al, 2000).

Education and Competence

Competence involves skill, knowledge, action, and critical thinking. Individualized competency-based practice in the sedation environment develops as a result of education, professional literature, and practice (Hooper, 2005a). Competencies of all sedation providers should include knowledge of medication administration and interaction, skill in airway management, and competence in dysrhythmia recognition and management (Box 8-2). All health care providers who perform or monitor the patient undergoing procedural sedation should complete an educational program that includes competencies. Nonanesthesiologist physician providers should also provide evidence of

BOX 8-2 Recommended Airway Management Competencies

BASIC AIRWAY ASSESSMENT

Oral cavity inspection
Mallampati classification
Presence of a patent airway
Monitoring of the rate, depth, and general quality of respiratory effort

PULSE OXIMETRY

Basic use and monitoring
Troubleshooting

BASIC AIRWAY MANAGEMENT

Airway maneuvers
Lateral head lift
Chin lift/support
Jaw thrust
Airway adjuncts
Nasal airway insertion
Oral airway insertion
Endotracheal tube insertion
Oxygen delivery devices

ADVANCED AIRWAY MANAGEMENT

Use of a positive pressure ventilation device
Establishment of an airway by way of intubation

From Hooper V: Competence in patient management. In Odom-Forren J, Watson D: *Practical guide to moderate sedation/analgesia,* ed 2, St. Louis, 2005, Mosby.

competency. It is unfortunate that credentialing does not always relate to competency and is based on a professional title instead of demonstrated competency in skills needed (Blike and Cravero, 2000). Patient safety requires that the nurse providing the sedation recognize any problem, identify the cause, and take immediate and appropriate action to resuscitate the patient and rescue the patient from harm (Blike and Cravero, 2000).

Sedation Environment

The Joint Commission requires that health care facilities address the appropriate equipment for care, resuscitation, and monitoring of vital signs (TJC, 2008). It is fortunate that serious adverse reactions do not occur on a routine basis. Therefore current recommendations for monitoring the patient during sedation are based on surrogate markers (softer outcomes) such as transient hypoxemia or on expert opinion (Vargo, 2007). Pulse oximetry and capnography are objective physiologic measures. The relationship of these monitors to clinical interventions needs to be determined in relationship to interventions and the effect of the intervention (Miner and Krauss, 2007).

Pulse oximetry, used to assess oxygenation, is an adjunct to clinical assessment for detecting hypoxemia. Pulse oximetry provides a noninvasive measure of the arterial hemoglobin oxygen saturation. Oxygen saturation occurs in direct proportion to the partial pressure of oxygen and provides an early indication of emergent hypoxemia (Odom-Forren and Watson, 2005).

The use of pulse oximetry during sedation procedures has not been linked to a reduction in risk for cardiopulmonary complications (Vargo, 2007). Despite the lack of data linking pulse oximetry to fewer complications, however, guidelines of nursing and physician organizations (e.g., ASA, ASGE, AORN, American Society of PeriAnesthesia Nurses [ASPEN], Society of Gastroenterology Nurses and Associates [SGNA]) require the use of pulse oximetry for all cases and suggest availability of supplemental oxygen (Blike and Cravero, 2000; Vargo, 2007; ASGE, 2008; ASPAN, 2008; SGNA, 2008; AORN, 2009). The use of pulse oximetry is required by these guidelines based on studies that have identified respiratory depression with resulting hypoxemia as the precipitating factor in adverse events for adult and pediatric patients (Vargo, 2007). Monitoring oxygenation by use of a pulse oximeter is not a replacement for monitoring ventilatory function (Gross et al, 2002; Odom-Forren and Watson, 2005).

Ventilatory function should be assessed apart from the use of pulse oximetry. Ventilatory function can be assessed by observing depth and rate of respirations or more accurately by auscultation of breath sounds (Odom-Forren and Watson, 2005). Capnography measures ventilation (end-tidal carbon dioxide [CO_2]) by determining the amount of CO_2 in every breath and provides a graphic representation of exhaled CO_2 levels with a tracing called a capnogram (Odom-Forren and Watson, 2005). The advantage of capnography is that it is a real-time display of the patient's ventilatory status and reflects apnea immediately. In one study of 80 patients undergoing colonoscopy procedures, researchers randomized patients into two groups: one group received supplemental oxygen, and the other did not receive supplemental oxygen. Respiratory activity was monitored with a pretracheal stethoscope and capnography, and the staff was blinded to end-tidal CO_2 data. The investigators not only discovered that supplemental oxygen did not prevent apnea but also found that more patients who had apnea in the supplemental oxygen group went undetected by caregivers and received sedation following an apneic episode (Zuccaro et al, 2000). Vargo et al (2002) found that capnography was an excellent indicator of respiratory rate compared with auscultation. Of 54 episodes of apnea or disordered respiration occurring in 28 patients, only 50% of the episodes were detected by pulse oximetry. More important, no episode was detected by visual assessment.

Soto et al (2004) studied the use of capnography to determine whether it accurately detected apnea during monitored anesthesia care. In the study 26% of 39 patients developed apnea of at least 20 seconds. These episodes were undetected by the anesthesia provider but were reliably detected by capnography and respiratory plethysmography, with no difference in detection rates between the two methods. Lightdale et al (2006) published the first randomized controlled trial of capnography in pediatric patients undergoing endoscopy procedures during moderate sedation. The researchers sought to discover whether intervention based on capnographic evidence of alveolar hypoventilation would reduce the incidence of hypoxemia in these patients. Hypoventilation was defined as a pulse oximetry value of less than 95% for more than 5 seconds. In the control group, the sedation team was notified when alveolar hypoventilation lasted longer than 60 seconds. In the intervention group, the sedation team was notified when hypoventilation lasted longer than 15 seconds. When notified, the team would stimulate the patient by repositioning the patient's head and encouraging deep breaths. Patients in the intervention group were significantly less likely to experience hypoxemia compared with the control group. The researchers concluded that the use of capnography during moderate sedation decreased the incidence of arterial desaturation (Lightdale et al, 2006).

Evidence that capnography is of assistance in the prevention of hypoventilation with a resulting decrease in hypoxemia is accumulating. At the present time, guidelines advocate the use of capnography any time a patient undergoes deep sedation (Gross et al, 2002, ASGE, 2008). It remains to be seen whether guidelines in the future will require monitoring of end-tidal CO_2 during moderate sedation. More research is needed to determine the clinical relevance and relationship to clinical interventions (Miner and Krauss, 2007).

Even with insufficient evidence to link hemodynamic monitoring to lack of complications, hemodynamic assessment is required because early detection of hemodynamic changes can result in early intervention, thus preventing a significant adverse event (Vargo, 2007). It is of interest that some organizational guidelines require the use of electrocardiogram (ECG) monitoring on all patients receiving sedation (ASPAN, 2008; AORN, 2009), whereas other organizations require the use of ECG monitoring on those who are receiving deep sedation or who have significant cardiopulmonary disease (Gross et al, 2002; ASGE, 2008; SGNA, 2008). At a minimum, ECG monitoring should be considered when deep sedation is anticipated and in patients who have significant cardiac or pulmonary disease (Gross et al, 2002; ASGE, 2008; SGNA, 2008).

The nurse involved in moderate sedation should have immediate access to suction equipment; supplemental oxygen; airway equipment, including oral and nasal airways and a bag-valve mask device; reversal agents to counteract the effects of the benzodiazepines or opioids; and an emergency cart with a defibrillator. Alarms need to be set on monitors, and all equipment needs to be in working order.

Patient-Specific Information

The patient should receive a procedure-specific history and physical examination. The primary purpose of a preprocedure nursing assessment is to gain baseline health information and to determine whether the patient has any illnesses or conditions that might preclude nurse-monitored sedation (Odom-Forren and Watson, 2005). The history should include the medical diagnoses, any past experiences with sedation or anesthesia, current medications and herbals taken by the patient, and allergies (including medication and latex).

The physical evaluation by the monitoring registered nurse includes an assessment of the heart and lungs and an evaluation of the airway. Physical assessment includes baseline vital signs, height, weight, age, and oxygen saturation. The airway may be assessed using the Mallampati technique, which can be used to determine possible intubation difficulty (Mallampati et al, 1985). The patient should be in a sitting position and directed to open the mouth as wide as possible. When the tongue is protruded, the faucial pillars and uvula should be visible (Figure 8-1). When the faucial pillars, soft palate, and uvula are not visible, the physician should be notified to determine the appropriate plan of action. Some facilities use a simple technique of observing for craniofacial abnormalities—asking the patient to stick out the tongue, open the mouth, and flex the neck to determine the potential for a difficult airway (Box 8-3). An appropriate preprocedure assessment can decrease the risk of adverse

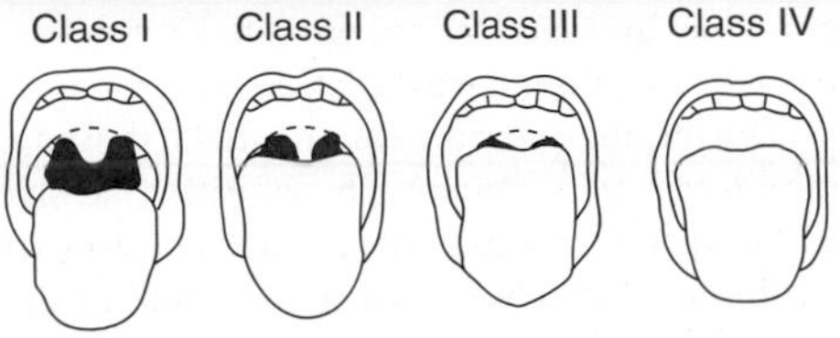

Class I Class II Class III Class IV

FIGURE 8-1 Modified Mallampati classification of pharyngeal structures. *Class I*, Soft palate, tonsillar fauces, tonsillar pillars, and uvula visualized. *Class II*, Soft palate, tonsillar fauces, and uvula visualized. *Class III*, Soft palate and base of uvula visualized. *Class IV*, Soft palate not visualized.
(From Samsoon GL, Young JR: Difficult tracheal intubation: a retrospective study, *Anaesthesia* 42:487–490, 1987.)

BOX 8-3 Presedation History and Physical Evaluation by a Registered Nurse

GENERAL HEALTH
Height and weight
Obesity or recent weight loss
Current infection
Current medications (prescription or over-the-counter)
Current herbal use
Last food intake (fasting history)
Physical handicaps and level of mobility
Baseline vital signs and temperature
History of tobacco or alcohol use
Pain assessment (chronic or acute)

CARDIOVASCULAR
History of cardiovascular disease
Recent cardiac surgery or myocardial infarction
Angina, aortic stenosis, congestive heart failure
Presence of a pacemaker or implantable cardioverter defibrillator

RESPIRATORY
Smoking history
Chronic cough
History of lung surgery or emphysema
Shortness of breath
History of tuberculosis, pneumonia, asthma, or bronchitis
Baseline oximetry reading
Airway assessment
Mallampati assessment or other, such as having patient open mouth, stick out tongue, and flex neck
Craniofacial abnormalities
History of sleep apnea

NEUROLOGIC
General affect, including behavior, speech patterns, gait
Level of consciousness and orientation
History of seizures, headaches
Motor abilities
Preexisiting neurologic deficit

MUSCULOSKELETAL
Muscle strength, mobility, range of motion
Use of orthopedic devices or prostheses
History of arthritis, scoliosis, fractures

INTEGUMENTARY
Color (cyanosis or jaundice)
Temperature and texture
Skin turgor
Integrity of skin
Piercings

GASTROINTESTINAL
Chronic diarrhea or constipation
Predisposition to nausea and vomiting
Time of last oral intake
Previous surgery or procedures

RENAL/HEPATIC
Kidney function (e.g., end-stage renal disease for revision of arteriovenous fistula)
Liver disease, including cirrhosis, hepatitis, anemia

ENDOCRINE
Diabetes (most common abnormality)

From Odom-Forren J, Watson D: *Practical guide to moderate sedation/analgesia*, ed 2, St. Louis, 2005, Mosby.

outcomes and increase patient safety for patients receiving sedation (Gross et al, 2002).

During the procedure, the patient should be monitored on an ongoing basis, with vital signs and oxygen saturation documented at least every 5 minutes. Any adverse reactions should be documented, and the nurse monitoring the patient should be alert to any changes in the patient's condition and immediately communicate that information to the provider. The level of consciousness should be assessed and the medication titrated in increments until the desired level is achieved (TJC, 2008). Back-up personnel who are experts in airway management should be available in the event of a crisis. This availability is typically not as much of a problem in the perioperative area of the hospital as it is in non–operating room environments. When sedation is administered at night or during a weekend, however, help should be as easy to obtain as during busy times of the week.

The same monitoring parameters used during the procedure are used for postprocedure monitoring, with documentation at least every 15 minutes. Immediately after the procedure, the patient is at risk for respiratory depression because noxious stimuli have been removed, and the patient is allowed to rest without interference. The patient who received moderate sedation should be discharged using objective discharge criteria. An important aspect of discharge to keep the patient safe is to ensure that a responsible adult escort is present to assist the patient home and care for the patient after discharge. Even patients who have received minimal sedation with the use of oral sedative agents should have a confirmed escort and the patient advised not to drive, make important decisions, or consume alcohol for at least 24 hours after the procedure (Donaldson et al, 2007). Chung and Assmann (2008) conducted a case review of litigations after ambulatory surgery that spanned a 10-year period. There were three malpractice cases of car accidents identified in patients who did not have an escort. In one case, the patient who was scheduled for a dilation and curettage under local anesthesia received lorazepam (1 mg orally) for antianxiety. The patient refused an offer for a ride home by a friend who worked in the postanesthesia care unit and drove herself home. On the drive home she had a car accident, incurring serious injury, and sued the gynecologist and preoperative nurse who gave her the medication. The gynecologist and preoperative nurse were found negligent for allowing the patient to drive herself home. The injured parties in the second car also sued and were compensated. The investigators go on to state, "patients require escorts to go home regardless of the type of anesthesia" (Chung and Assmann, 2008). Safe patient care requires that the caregiver cancel the case, admit the patient, or arrange a ride home for the patient.

Guidelines and Recommended Practices

Guidelines are "systematically developed recommendations that assist the practitioner and patient in making decisions about health care" (Gross et al, 2002). Recommended practices represent the association's official position on technical and professional practice. Guidelines and recommended practices are advisory and intended to guide practice while allowing for deviation when necessary (Odom-Forren and Watson, 2005). During legal proceedings, however, guidelines, position statements, recommended practices from national organizations, and recommendations from pharmaceutical companies can be presented as expected and acceptable standard of care.

Guidelines can decrease the number of adverse events. Variation in sedation practices prompted The Joint Commission to expand its sedation standards in 2001. These standards were updated in conjunction with the ASA and reflect the ASA's guideline for management of sedation by nonanesthesiologists (Gross et al, 2002). Pitetti et al (2006) examined the efforts of one institution to implement The Joint Commission's guidelines and how the guidelines affected adverse events during sedation. Procedural sedation was then monitored over a 3-year period with 14,386 cases. Adverse events occurred in 7.6% of patients. The most common adverse event was hypoxemia, defined as an oxygen saturation level of 90% or lower for more than 1 minute. The incidence of adverse events decreased significantly over time during the study. Further research is needed to evaluate whether a standardized approach to sedation will reliably decrease adverse events (Pitetti et al, 2006).

CONCLUSION

Serious adverse events with permanent sequelae or death are rare during nurse-monitored sedation; however, to reduce the risk for sedation-related complications that lead to adverse events, practitioners should follow the guidelines in Box 8-4.

BOX 8-4 Steps to Reduce the Risk of Serious Complications

1. Perform and document a thorough presedation evaluation, including a history and physical examination.
2. Use appropriate patient selection by assigning an ASA score to determine those who need further workup.
3. Obtain training in basic and advanced cardiac life support.
4. Follow organizational guidelines, policies, and protocols.
5. Know the pharmacology of the sedative and reversal agents.
6. Titrate sedative dosing in each patient to the desired effect.
7. Obtain and maintain continuous intravenous access, which is an emergency lifeline.
8. Assess the level of sedation, vital signs, and oxygen saturation periodically, and document every 5 minutes during the procedure.
9. Use oxygen supplementation on all patients, or consider its use with moderate sedation and require its use with deep sedation effect.
10. Use ECG monitoring in all patients or, at a minimum, in all patients who have known cardiovascular disease.
11. Consider capnography for patients who are undergoing deep sedation or prolonged procedures.
12. Turn on alarms, and keep them on.
13. Use standardized discharge criteria to determine readiness for discharge.
14. Follow guidelines to enhance patient safety effect.
15. Explore learning opportunities to maintain competencies and keep patients safe.

ASA, American Society of Anesthesiologists; *ECG*, electrocardiogram.

Data from American Society for Gastrointestinal Endoscopy: Sedation and anesthesia in GI endoscopy, *Gastrointest Endosc* 68:205–216, 2008; American Society of PeriAnesthesia Nurses: *2008–2010 Standards of perianesthesia nursing practice*, Cherry Hill, NJ, 2008, The Society; Association of periOperative Registered Nurses: *Perioperative standards and recommended practices*, Denver, 2009, The Association, available at http://72.3.142.35/dxreader/jsp/StartReading.jsp?filenumber=1249877361325588&url=http://72.3.142.35/dxreader/jsp/BookLoader.jsp. Accessed August 13, 2009; Gross JB et al: American Society of Anesthesiologists Task Force on Sedation and Analgesia by Non-anesthesiologists: ASA practice guidelines for sedation and analgesia by non-anesthesiologists, *Anesthesiology* 96:1004-1017, 2002; Odom-Forren J, Watson D: *Practical guide to moderate sedation/analgesia*, ed 2, St. Louis, 2005, Mosby; Shepard S, Lofsky AS: Patient safety tips: conscious sedation (moderate sedation) in the office, *The Doctor's Company*, 2009, available at http://www.thedoctors.com/ecm/groups/public/@tdc/documents/web_content/con_id_002761.pdf. Accessed August 8, 2009; Society of Gastroenterology Nurses and Associates: *Statement on the use of sedation and analgesia in the gastrointestinal endoscopy setting*, available at http://www.sgna.org/resources/Sedation-pos.html, accessed May 2008; Vargo JJ: Minimizing complications: sedation and monitoring, *Gastrointest Endosc Clin N Am* 17:11–28, 2007.

Future areas of research in clinical studies include safety and efficacy studies (e.g., new agents, postdischarge adverse events, and definition of successful sedation); applications of new technology; and procedural sedation and analgesia adjuncts (Miner and Krauss, 2007). Research efforts must continue to determine the diagnosis of scenarios that can lead to adverse events (Soto et al, 2004). No consensus exists on optimal dosing strategies, target depth of sedation, or definition of complications (Miner and Krauss, 2007). Large multicenter trials are needed that have standardized sedation protocols, standardized adverse event reporting, and standardized outcome measures. These trials have the potential to establish the true complication rate for each sedation level, drug, and procedure to determine the best way to manage the patient and provide optimal patient safety (Miner and Krauss, 2007). In the meantime, perioperative nurses would do well to follow multidisciplinary guidelines that are available and to ensure proper education and competency to respond quickly to adverse events. The facility should support a sedation system that has prewritten scenarios of response with practiced personnel.

REFERENCES

American Society of Anesthesiologists: *Practice guidelines for management of the difficult airway*, available at http://www.asahq.org/publicationsAndServices/Difficult%20Airway.pdf. Accessed August 13, 2008.

American Society of Anesthesiologists: *AANA-ASA joint statement regarding propofol administration*, available at http://www.asahq.org/news/asaaanajointstmnt.htm.Accessed August 8, 2009.

American Society for Gastrointestinal Endoscopy: Sedation and anesthesia in GI endoscopy, *Gastrointest Endosc* 68: 205–216, 2008.

American Society of PeriAnesthesia Nurses: *2008–2010 Standards of perianesthesia nursing practice*, Cherry Hill, NJ, 2008, The Society.

Association of periOperative Registered Nurses: *Perioperative standards and recommended practices*, Denver, 2009, The Association, available at http://72.3.142.35/dxreader/jsp/StartReading.jsp?filenumber=1249877736132558&url=http://72.3.142.35/dxreader/jsp/BookLoader.jsp. Accessed August 13, 2009.

Bhananker SM, et al: Injury and liability associated with monitored anesthesia care: a closed claims analysis, *Anesthesiology* 104:228–234, 2006.

Blike GT, Cravero JP: *Pride, prejudice, and pediatric sedation: a multispecialty evaluation of the state of the art—report from a Dartmouth summit on pediatric sedation*, available at http://www.npsf.org2000. Accessed June, 2008.

Brown T, et al: Procedural sedation in the acute care setting, *Am Fam Physician* 71(1):85–90, 2005.

Chung F, Assmann N: Car accidents after ambulatory surgery in patients without an escort, *Anesth Analg* 106:817–820, 2008.

Cote CJ, et al: Adverse events and risk factors in pediatrics: a critical incident analysis of contributing factors, *Pediatrics* 105:805–814, 2000.

Cravero JP, et al: Incidence and nature of adverse events during pediatric sedation/anesthesia for procedures outside the operating room: report from the pediatric sedation research consortium, *Pediatrics* 118:1087–1096, 2006.

Donaldson M, et al: Oral sedation: a primer on anxiolysis for the adult patient, *Anesth Prog* 54:118–129, 2007.

Donaldson MS: An overview of *To Err Is Human*: reemphasizing the message of patient safety. In Hughes RG, editor: *Patient safety and quality: an evidence-based handbook for nurses*, vol 1, Rockville, Md, 2008, U.S. Department of Health and Human Services AHRQ Publication No. 08-0043, Agency for Healthcare Research and Quality.

Fanning RM: Monitoring during sedation given by nonanaesthetic doctors, *Anaesthesia* 63:370–374, 2008.

Gross JB, et al: ASA practice guidelines for sedation and analgesia by non-anesthesiologists, *Anesthesiology* 96:1004–1017, 2002.

Hertzog JH, Havidich JE: Non-anesthesiologist provided pediatric procedural sedation: an update, *Curr Opin Anaesthesiol* 20:365–372, 2007.

Heuss LT, et al: Risk stratification and safe administration of propofol by registered nurses supervised by the gastroenterologist: a prospective observational study of more than 2000 cases, *Gastrointest Endosc* 57:664–671, 2003.

Hooper V: Competence in patient management. In Odom-Forren J, Watson D, editors: *Practical guide to moderate sedation/analgesia*, ed 2 , St. Louis, 2005a, Mosby.

Hooper V: Management of complications. In Odom-Forren J, Watson D, editors: *Practical guide to moderate sedation/analgesia*, ed 2 , St. Louis, 2005b, Mosby.

Institute for Safe Medication Practices: *Propofol sedation: who should administer?* available at http://www.ismp.org/Newsletters/acutecare/articles/20051103.asp?ptr=y. Accessed August 13, 2008.

Kremer MJ: Pharmacology. In Odom-Forren J, Watson D, editors: *Practical guide to moderate sedation/analgesia*, ed 2, St. Louis, 2005, Mosby.

Kohn LT, et al: *To err is human: building a safer health system*, Washington, DC, 2000, National Academy Press.

Lightdale JR, et al: Microstream capnography improves patient monitoring during moderate sedation: a randomized, controlled trial, *Pediatrics* 117:1170–1178, 2006.

Mallampati SR, et al: A clinical sign to predict difficult tracheal intubation: a prospective study, *Can Anaesth Soc J* 32: 429–434, 1985.

Mandel JE, et al: A randomized, controlled, double-blind trial of patient-controlled sedation with propofol/remifentanil versus midazolam/fentanyl for colonoscopy, *Anesth Analg* 106:434–439, 2008.

Meltzer B: RNs pushing propofol, *Outpatient Surg* 4(7): 24–37, 2003.

Miner JR, Krauss B: Procedural sedation and analgesia research: state of the art, *Acad Emerg Med* 14:170–178, 2007.

Odom-Forren J: The evolution of nurse monitored sedation, *J Perianesth Nurs* 20:385–398, 2005.

Odom-Forren J, Watson D: *Practical guide to moderate sedation/analgesia*, ed 2, St. Louis, 2005, Mosby.

Overley CA, Rex DK: A nursing perspective on sedation and nurse-administered propofol for endoscopy, *Gastrointest Endosc Clin N Am* 14:325–333, 2004.

Pambianco DJ, et al: Feasibility assessment of computer assisted personalized sedation: a sedation delivery system to administer propofol for gastrointestinal endoscopy, *Gastrointest Endosc* 63:AB189, 2006.

Patterson P: Should RNs be giving propofol in GI lab? *OR Manager* 20:24–30, 2004.

Philip BK: Sedation with propofol: a new ASA statement, *ASA Newsl* 69(2):2005, available at http://www.asahq.org/Newsletters/2005/02–05/whatsNew02–05.html. Accessed July 2008.

Pitetti R, et al: Effect on hospital-wide sedation practices after implementation of the 2001 JCAHO procedural sedation and analgesia guidelines, *Arch Pediatr Adolesc Med* 160: 211–216, 2006.

Rex DK: Review article: moderate sedation for endoscopy—sedation regimens for non-anaesthesiologists, *Aliment Pharmacol Ther* 24:163–171, 2006.

Rex DK, et al: Safety of propofol administered by registered nurses with gastroenterologist supervision in 2000 endoscopic case, *Am J Gastroenterol* 97:1159–1163, 2002.

Rex DK, et al: Trained registered nurses/endoscopy teams can administer propofol safely for endoscopy, *Gastroenterology* 129:1384–1391, 2005.

Shavit I, et al: Enhancing patient safety during pediatric sedation: the impact of simulation-based training of nonanesthesiolgists, *Arch Pediatr Adolesc Med* 161:740–743, 2007.

Sieg A, et al: Prospective evaluation of complications in outpatient GI endoscopy: a survey among German gastroenterologists, *Gastrointest Endosc* 53:620–627, 2001.

Silber JH, et al: Anesthesiologist direction and patient outcomes, *Anesthesiology* 93:152–163, 2000.

Society of Gastroenterology Nurses and Associates: *Statement on the use of sedation and analgesia in the gastrointestinal endoscopy setting*, available at http://www.sgna.org/resources/Sedation-pos.html. Accessed May 2008.

Soto RG, et al: Capnography accurately detects apnea during monitored anesthesia care, *Anesth Analg* 99: 379–382, 2004.

The Joint Commission: *Hospital accreditation standards*, Oakbrook Terrace, Ill, 2008, The Joint Commission.

U.S. Food and Drug Administration: *FDA approves Lusedra*, available at http://www.drugs.com/newdrugs/fda-approves-lusedra-fospropofol-disodium-monitored-anesthesia-care-mac-sedation-1205.html. Accessed June 27, 2009.

VanNatta ME, Rex DK: Propofol alone titrated to deep sedation versus propofol in combination with opioids and/or benzodiazepines and titrated to moderate sedation for colonoscopy, *Am J Gastroenterol* 101:2209–2217, 2006.

Vargo JJ: Minimizing complications: sedation and monitoring, *Gastrointest Endosc Clin N Am* 17:11–28, 2007.

Vargo JJ, et al: Automated graphic assessment of respiratory activity is superior to pulse oximetry and visual assessment for the detection of early respiratory depression during therapeutic upper endoscopy, *Gastrointest Endosc* 55:826–831, 2002.

Walker JA, et al: Nurse administered propofol sedation without anesthesia specialists in 9152 endoscopic cases in an ambulatory surgery center, *Am J Gastroenterol* 98:1744–1750, 2003.

Zed PJ, et al: Efficacy, safety and patient satisfaction of propofol for procedural sedation and analgesia in the emergency department: a prospective study, *CJEM* 9:421–427, 2007.

Zuccaro G, et al: Routine use of supplemental oxygen prevents recognition of prolonged apnea during endoscopy, *Gastrointest Endosc* 51:AB141, 2000.

INCIDENCE OF DEEP VENOUS THROMBOSIS IN THE SURGICAL PATIENT POPULATION AND PROPHYLACTIC MEASURES TO REDUCE OCCURRENCE

Jennifer S. Barnett, MSN, ARNP, FNP-BC, NP-C • Linda J. DeCarlo, MBA, MSN, RN, RNFA, CNOR, ARNP, FNP-BC

An astounding 200,000 to 600,000 people in the United States develop deep venous thrombosis (DVT) and pulmonary embolism (PE) annually. As many as 60,000 to 200,000 individuals will die of PE, making this more deadly in the United States than motor vehicle accidents, breast cancer, or acquired immunodeficiency syndrome (AIDS). DVT has been called a silent epidemic; about half the time the condition causes no symptoms. All too frequently, people die of PE without ever knowing they had a DVT (American Public Health Association, 2003).

Public awareness of DVT increased in the United States after seeing Vice President Dan Quayle experience a DVT (American Public Health Association, 2003). The death of David Bloom, a 40-year-old NBC news correspondent, who died while covering the war in Iraq, heightened awareness even further. His sudden death after experiencing leg cramps with associated pulmonary embolism increased public awareness of DVT and PE (Nutescu, 2007). Despite this growing awareness, approximately two thirds of Americans know nothing about DVT, and more than half of individuals who are aware of DVT are unaware of risk factors, preexisting conditions, or signs and symptoms of DVT (American Public Health Association, 2003).

More than 23 million surgeries are performed in the United States yearly (Agency for Healthcare Research and Quality, 2009), and every surgical patient is at risk for developing DVT or PE. DVT and PE are jointly referred to as venous thromboembolism (VTE). Although all surgical patients are at risk for VTE, many remain at higher risk because extensive operative procedures are being performed on those with greater medical comorbidities and advancing age (Agnelli, 2004). The type of procedure and patient risk factors determine the potential for postsurgical VTE development (Agency for Healthcare Research and Quality, 2009). As many as one half of DVTs associated with surgery start intraoperatively (Kearon, 2003a). Most hospitalized patients who develop symptomatic VTE are diagnosed after discharge from the hospital. What follows is a costly diagnostic and treatment process with the possibility of readmission. Complications are related to anticoagulation and/or long-term morbidity and may result in death (Geerts et al, 2008). Problems associated with VTE could be avoided by the use of simple, cost-effective measures. Nurses participating in a surgical patient's continuum of care are in a unique position to ensure patient safety by increasing the level of awareness of DVT among patients, physicians, and hospital staff. Aggressively following existing recommendations for VTE prevention can decrease the chance of the deadly complication of pulmonary embolism.

This chapter reviews the background and the incidence of VTE in the surgical patient by surgical specialty, prophylactic measures to reduce occurrence, and nursing implications for practice. Some helpful definitions of common terms can be found in Table 9-1.

PATHOPHYSIOLOGY

In 1856 Rudolph Ludwig Karl Virchow, a German pathologist, identified a triad of factors that lead to intravascular coagulation (Figures 9-1 and 9-2). The factors of stasis, vessel wall injury, and hypercoagulability are as pertinent today as they were 150 years ago when identifying the pathogenesis of DVT formation (Crowther and McCourt, 2004; Kucher and Tapson, 2004; Summerfield, 2006).

DVT occurs when a thrombus consisting of red blood cells, platelets, and leukocytes forms in a large vein. Areas of slow or disturbed blood flow are the most likely location for a thrombus to either partially or completely block circulation.

TABLE 9-1 Helpful Definitions

Term	Definition
Deep venous thrombosis (DVT)	Blood clot in a deep vein
Pulmonary embolism (PE)	Blood clot or fragment of a blood clot breaks loose from the wall of a vein and migrates to the lung, where it blocks a pulmonary artery or one of its branches
Venous thromboembolism (VTE)	The manifestation of a DVT or PE
Thrombus	A stationary blood clot adhered to a vessel wall
Embolus	A thrombus that has separated from a vessel wall and is traveling in the bloodstream to another location

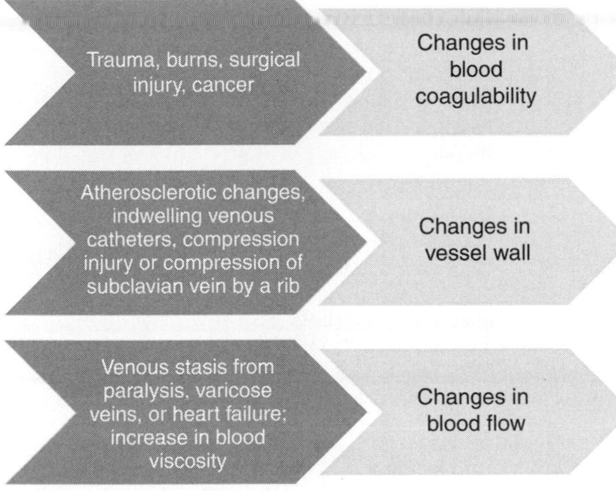

FIGURE 9-1 Virchow's triad: coagulation factors. (From Barnett J, DeCarlo L: Incidence of deep venous thrombosis in the surgical patient population and prophylactic measures to reduce occurrence. *Perioper Nurs Clin* 3(4):367-382, 2008.)

Thrombi can form where a vessel wall injury occurs intraoperatively. Injury can occur from the use of a tourniquet or insertion of an indwelling catheter or during mobilization of vessels to create exposure. Coagulation can be enhanced, or fibrinolysis may be impaired. The result is a hypercoagulable state. Hypercoagulability can be caused by deficiencies in factors that inhibit coagulation (antithrombin III, protein C, protein S) (Woods et al, 2005).

Secondary hypercoagulable states may result from endothelial activation by cytokines, leading to a loss of the normal anticoagulant surface functions of the vessel wall. The vessel wall converts to proinflammatory thrombogenic functions. Vasoconstriction causes venous stasis. The resulting increase in blood viscosity is the precursor to thrombus formation (Woods et al, 2005).

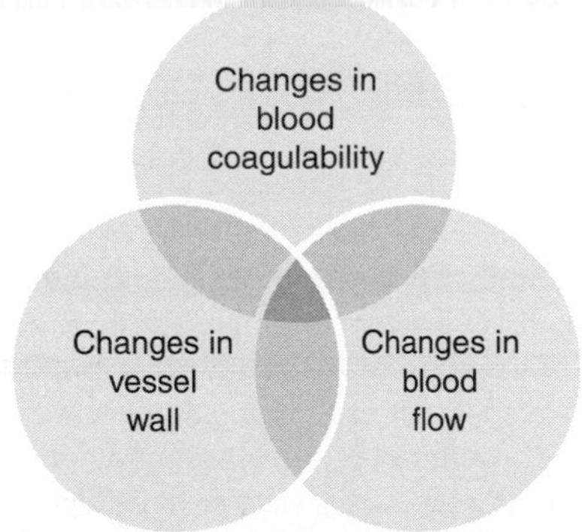

FIGURE 9-2 Virchow's triad: relationship between coagulation factors. (From Barnett J, DeCarlo L: Incidence of deep venous thrombosis in the surgical patient population and prophylactic measures to reduce occurrence. *Perioper Nurs Clin* 3(4):367-382, 2008.)

BOX 9-1 Deep Venous Thrombosis Risk Factors

ACQUIRED RISK FACTORS

Female
Smoking
Age >40 years
Obesity (body mass index >29)
Hypertension
Malignancy/chemotherapy
Prior history of DVT
Prior major surgical procedure (within 3 months)
Trauma (especially pelvis, hip, or leg fracture)
Respiratory failure
General versus neuraxial anesthesia
Anesthesia >3½ hours
ASA classification status >III
Indwelling venous catheters/CVP/arterial line
Surgery
Tourniquet >50 min
Total hip/knee replacement
Planned postoperative admission to ICU
Immobilization (within 30 days)
Acute infection (urinary, respiratory)
Paralysis/paraplegia
Venous stasis/varicose veins
Congestive heart failure
Myocardial infarction
Atrial fibrillation
Diabetes mellitus
Inflammatory bowel disease
Pregnancy (especially third trimester)
Postpartum
Oral contraceptives
Hormone replacement therapy (highest risk during first year of treatment, 45 to 64 years old)
Long plane trips (>5000 km) and automobile trips
Intravenous drug abuse
Nephrotic syndrome
Thrombocytopenia
Antiphospholipid antibody syndrome (lupus)
Polycythemia

INHERITED RISK FACTORS

Ethnicity (white, African American)
Sickle cell trait
Factor V Leiden
Protein C deficiency
Protein S deficiency
Prothrombin gene defect
Dysfibrinogenemia
Plasminogen disorders
Hyperhomocysteinemia
Elevated factor VIII
Elevated factor XI
Thrombophilia

ASA, American Society of Anesthesiologists; *CVP,* central venous pressure; *DVT,* deep venous thrombosis; *ICU,* intensive care unit.

Data from American Public Health Association: *Deep vein thrombosis: advancing awareness to protect patient lives,* white paper, Public Health Leadership Conference on Deep-Vein Thrombosis, 2003:1–12; Chapman MW et al: *Chapman's orthopaedic surgery,* ed 3, Philadelphia, 2000, Lippincott Williams & Wilkins; Ginzberg E et al: Thromboprophylaxis in medical and surgical patients undergoing physical medicine and rehabilitation, *Am J Phys Med Rehabil* 85(2):159–166, 2006; Kearon C: Duration of venous thromboembolism prophylaxis after surgery, *Chest* 124:386S-392S, 2003; Kucher N, Tapson VF: Pulmonary embolism. In Fuster V et al, editors: *Hurst's the heart,* ed 11, New York, 2004, McGraw-Hill; Race TK, Collier PE: The hidden risks of deep vein thrombosis—the need for risk factor assessment, *Crit Care Nurs Q* 30(3):245–254, 2007; Summerfield D: Decreasing the incidence of deep vein thrombosis through the use of prophylaxis, *AORN J* 84(4):642–645, 2006.

Thrombi may form at any point along the vein wall, but most originate in valve pockets. A thrombus may extend retrograde, further proximally, or expand to completely fill the vessel. Thrombosis is often asymptomatic and resolves spontaneously via the fibrinolytic system through the mechanisms of recanalization, organization, and lysis. Resolution of the thrombosis can be partial or complete (Kucher and Tapson, 2004).

Fifty percent of DVTs start intraoperatively with approximately 50% of these resolving spontaneously within 72 hours. The risk for symptomatic VTE is highest 2 weeks after surgery and remains elevated for 2 to 3 months (Kearon, 2003a). When the condition persists, it can develop into a DVT and lead to a life-threatening PE.

Risk factors for developing a DVT can be divided into two categories: acquired and inherited (Box 9-1). The combination of patient risk factors plus the type of surgery determines risk for developing a DVT. The American College of Chest Physicians (ACCP) has compiled data from prospectively validated evidence-based research studies to define risk groups of low, moderate, high, and highest to recommend prophylaxis either by category of risk or by surgical specialty (Nutescu, 2007).

Cancer increases the risk for DVT. Intrinsically tumor production can affect coagulation parameters. Extrinsic factors that contribute to the pathogenesis of thromboembolism are indwelling access catheters used for chemotherapeutic agents, the chemotherapeutic agents, and venous stasis occurring because of weakness and decreased ambulation. Pancreatic, lung, gastrointestinal tract, and breast cancers are associated with a higher risk for DVT (Kucher and Tapson, 2004). The Eighth ACCP Conference on Antithrombotic and Thrombolytic Therapy guidelines have been used by The Joint Commission to create performance standards for VTE risk assessment and prophylaxis (Summerfield, 2006; Race and Collier, 2007).

Nutescu (2007) describes a study using a computer-based VTE screening tool for patients on admission to the hospital. An electronic alert is sent to the patient's physician notifying him or her of the patient's risk for VTE. The ideal system would go one step further. It not only would identify a patient's risk for VTE, but would also specify the AACP recommended prophylaxis based on risk factors and type of surgery scheduled. To be successful, a VTE risk assessment tool must be easy to understand and implement. A combination risk assessment tool and prophylaxis order sheet in the patient's medical record could be completed collaboratively by the nursing staff and the medical staff.

SIGNS AND SYMPTOMS OF DVT AND PE

The clinical manifestations of DVT vary based on the size of the thrombus, the affected vein, and the adequacy of collateral circulation (Woods et al, 2005). The classic symptoms of DVT include swelling, pain, and discoloration of the affected extremity (Ramzi and Leeper, 2004). Calf tenderness, low-grade fever, fatigue, tachycardia, and diaphoresis are also symptoms of DVT (Brunicardi et al, 2004). Physical examination may reveal a palpable cord of thrombosed vein, unilateral edema, warmth, or superficial venous dilation (Ramzi and Leeper, 2004). Because the clinical manifestations of DVT are so variable, objective testing and a thorough history and physical examination should be obtained (Woods et al, 2005). The cardinal signs and symptoms of PE are shortness of breath, pleuritic chest pain, and mental status changes (Brunicardi et al, 2004).

METHODS OF PROPHYLAXIS

Despite risk factors being identified, VTE prophylaxis is underused because of a lack of awareness of DVT risk, variation in the perception of risk factors, and concerns about the risk for bleeding with prophylaxis (American Public Health Association, 2003; Broughton et al, 2007). The most recent recommendations from the American College of Chest Physicians for antithrombotic and thrombolytic therapy were published in 2008 from the eighth ACCP conference (Geerts et al, 2008). The ACCP recommendations for VTE prophylaxis are developed using comprehensive literature searches of evidence-based research. Prevention of VTE falls into two categories: mechanical and pharmacologic prophylaxis.

Mechanical Prophylaxis

Mechanical measures are simple to implement and do not increase the risk for bleeding. People who are low-risk for developing VTE or have contraindications for the use of pharmacologic measures are good candidates for mechanical prophylactic measures, including early ambulation, foot and ankle exercises, passive range of motion, graduated compression stockings (GCS), and intermittent pneumatic compression (IPC) devices (Kehl-Pruett, 2006). All of these measures improve venous return and reduce venous stasis in leg veins during the immediate postoperative period when patients have decreased mobility because of pain (Pearse et al, 2007). Refer to Figure 9-3 for examples of intermittent pneumatic compression devices.

The advantages of using GCS, IPC, and foot pumps are that they carry no risk for bleeding or drug interactions. The disadvantages are that they require virtually constant use and that compliance is difficult to assess. The evidence of efficacy is limited because of variations in equipment design, and they are often used in combination

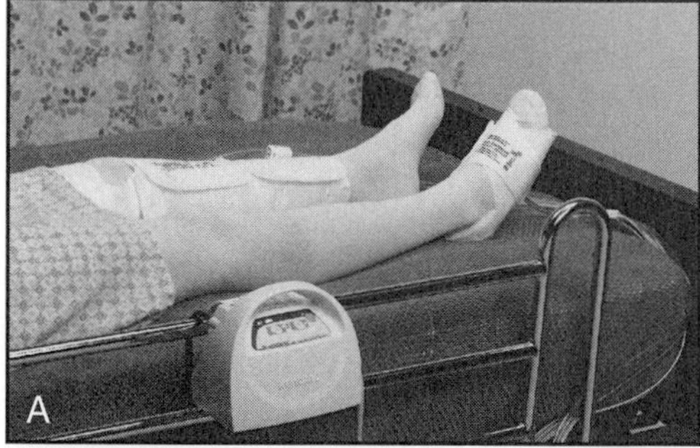

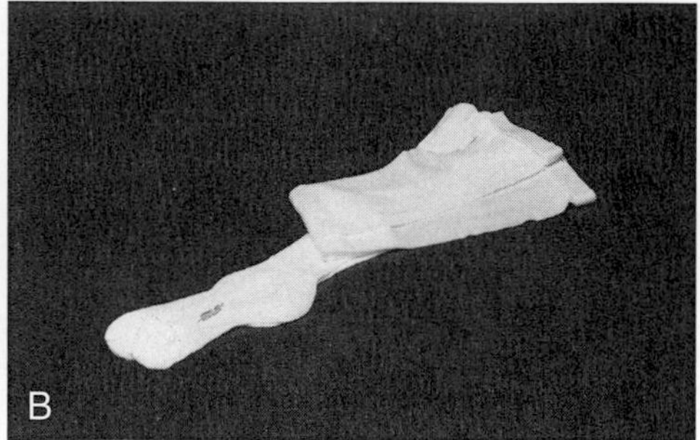

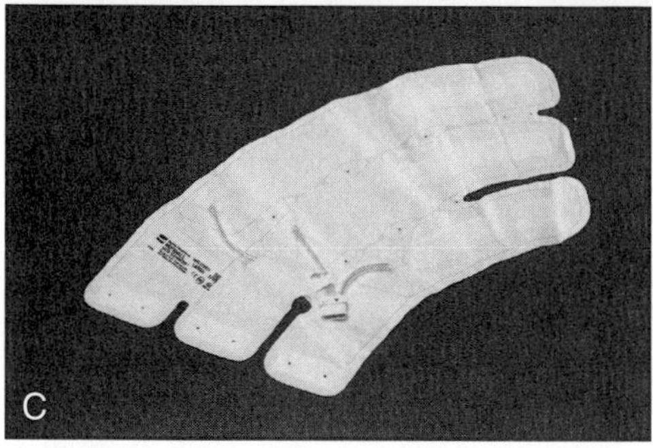

FIGURE 9-3 Examples of external pneumatic compression devices used to promote venous return and prevent deep venous thrombosis (DVT). **A,** SCD machine, sleeves, and TED stockings (courtesy of Covidien, Cincinnati, Ohio); **B,** Kendall TED antiembolism stocking (courtesy of Covidien, Cincinnati, Ohio); **C,** Kendall SCD Express knee sleeve (courtesy of Covidien, Cincinnati, Ohio).

with pharmacologic treatment. Nevertheless, mechanical methods of thromboprophylaxis are safe and useful adjuncts to pharmacologic approaches (Ginzberg et al, 2006).

Graduated Compression Stockings

Graduated compression stockings may reduce the risk for DVT by multiple mechanisms. Compressing the leg reduces the size of the veins, resulting in increased blood velocity, thereby reducing stasis. Reducing the size of the veins also improves the function of the venous valves and decreases pooling. GCS provide greater compression at the ankle and augment the effect of the calf muscle pump. All of these mechanisms cause a reduction of venous pooling, which can result in an alteration in the levels of clotting factors that may lead to thrombus formation (Mazzone et al, 2008). The use of GCS enhances the protective effect of low-dose unfractionated heparin (LDUH) against DVT by an additional 75% compared with LDUH alone (Geerts et al, 2008).

Proper fit is necessary to prevent a tourniquet effect from GCS that are too tight. They should be removed once a shift for 30 minutes to assess underlying skin (Kehl-Pruett, 2006). Contraindications for using GCS are certain dermatologic diseases, peripheral arterial disease, and diabetic neuropathy. Compression stockings have the potential to cause ischemic necrosis of the legs in patients with peripheral arterial disease (Mazzone et al, 2004).

Intermittent Pneumatic Compression

Intermittent pneumatic compression simulates the effects of walking and weight bearing. Several studies have shown that mechanical devices (continuous passive movement and IPC devices) increase the velocity of blood flow, reduce venous stasis, and reduce the incidence of DVT (Pearse et al, 2007). In addition to the mechanical process of increasing blood flow through the femoral veins, IPC has an antithrombotic effect on the components in the coagulation cascade (Eisle et al, 2007).

Devices vary by site of application, rate of inflation/deflation, pressure amplitude, and chamber inflation sequence (Eisle et al, 2007). Successful use depends on proper sizing and application of the sleeve containing the air chambers. Calf devices inflate and deflate to mimic the calf muscle pump (Crowther and McCourt, 2004). The effect is simulation of the calf muscle stretching rather than simulating muscle contraction. Elongation of the muscles in dorsiflexion of the foot increases the flow of blood in the superficial femoral vein fourfold (Eisle et al, 2007).

Early calf IPC devices used low pressure and slow inflation of a single air bladder. More recent devices have multiple air chambers that produce graduated, sequential, and rapid inflation. The newer technology has been shown to improve hemodynamic response compared with the slower, low-pressure inflation of previous devices (Eisle et al, 2007).

Venous plexus foot pumps mimic the action of walking. The devices intermittently compress and relax the sole of the foot, causing muscle contraction and improving venous blood flow (Crowther and McCourt, 2004). Calf IPC has been proved to be superior to IPC of the foot (Eisle et al, 2007). Calf IPC or venous plexus foot pumps should not be used on patients with acute DVT; peripheral vascular ischemia; large, open wounds; skin grafts; or cancer of the extremity. If compression devices are not applied at the onset of bed rest or in surgery, an ultrasound examination should be performed to rule out DVT before initiating compression therapy (Day, 2003).

Intermittent compression devices are the safest and least invasive intervention used to decrease the incidence of DVT; however, the effectiveness is limited by poor compliance rates. To be effective, they must be used for the duration of bed rest—not just a few hours a day. The factors negatively affecting compliance include the following: doctors, nurses, and patients not understanding the importance of IPC; no formal documentation system for the use of IPC devices; and nurses not noticing if an IPC device is ordered or if it is in good working condition (Kehl-Pruett, 2006; Stewart et al, 2006).

Common patient complaints about IPC include a feeling of warmth or having difficulty sleeping with the continuous inflation and deflation (Kehl-Pruett, 2006). Patients most likely to fail IPC prophylaxis include those with cancer or a past history of DVT and those who are older than 60 years old. This higher-risk group should be considered for more intensive prophylaxis (Clarke-Pearson et al, 2003).

Inferior Vena Cava Filters

The most invasive mechanical prophylactic measure to prevent VTE is the placement of an inferior vena cava (IVC) filter. There are multiple indications for placement of an IVC filter. For example, patients who are not good candidates for chemical anticoagulation but need PE prevention may be considered for IVC placement. Preoperative placement of an IVC filter may be appropriate in patients with a history of DVT or PE who are about to undergo a lengthy neurosurgical procedure and have a risk for postoperative bleeding (Agnelli, 2004; Epstein, 2005). Patients with a prior history of DVT who are undergoing a Roux-en-Y gastric bypass procedure for weight loss are also considered candidates for an IVC filter (Prystowsky et al, 2005).

Pharmacologic Prophylaxis

The clinical importance of administering anticoagulant therapy is to decrease the risk for long-term symptomatic VTE and prevent postthrombotic syndrome (Kearon, 2003b). Anticoagulation therapy includes low-dose unfractionated heparin (LDUH), low-molecular-weight heparin (LMWH), synthetic pentasaccharides, warfarin, vitamin K antagonists, and aspirin.

Bleeding is the greatest concern when choosing anticoagulant therapy as a prophylactic measure to prevent VTE. However, multiple studies have shown no increase in major bleeding with LDUH or LMWH. There is a slightly higher risk for minor bleeding with LDUH compared with LMWH (Broughton et al, 2007).

Heparin

Heparin works as a catalyst, activating and binding to antithrombin III, an endogenous antagonist against several coagulation factors. The main effect of LDUH on the coagulation cascade is blocking thrombin and fibrin formation (Woods et al, 2005; Ginzberg et al, 2006). Dosing is based on weight and requires monitoring of partial thromboplastin time (PTT). Dose adjustments are made based on laboratory results. Low-dose unfractionated heparin can be administered intravenously or subcutaneously depending on whether effects are needed immediately or within approximately 1 hour (Woods et al, 2005; Kehl-Pruett, 2006).

Low-molecular-weight heparin activity is more focused than LDUH. The main effect of LMWH is inhibition of factor Xa, thus interfering with the coagulation cascade one step earlier than the action of LDUH (Ginzberg et al, 2006). The advantage of LMWH is it does not bind to plasma proteins. The result is a more predictable anticoagulant dose (Woods et al, 2005). Low-molecular-weight products are eliminated through the kidneys. Therefore patients who have renal impairment, are obese, or are older adults should be considered at high risk for complication with the use of LMWH (Nutescu, 2007). Patients with a higher risk for bleeding should be started on LMWH rather than LDUH (Kehl-Pruett, 2006). Compared with LDUH, LMWH offers comparable or superior efficacy and a similar or lower risk for bleeding (Ginzberg et al, 2006). Low-molecular-weight heparin (enoxaparin, dalteparin, tinzaparin, reviparin, and nadroparin) can be administered once or twice daily on an inpatient or outpatient basis without coagulation monitoring (Kehl-Pruett, 2006). Low-molecular-weight heparin has a higher acquisition cost but is more cost-effective because it does not require PTT testing (Chapman et al 2000; Ginzberg et al, 2006).

There should be special consideration of patients receiving neuraxial anesthesia (epidural and spinal anesthesia) with the use of LMWH or other heparinoids. These patients have risk for the development of epidural or spinal hematoma, which can lead to paralysis (Morrison, 2006). Although the risk for serious complications is low (Rowlings and Hanson, 2005), the risk is increased when the patient has an indwelling epidural catheter or is receiving concomitant nonsteroidal anti-inflammatory drugs, platelet inhibitors, or other forms of anticoagulation (Morrison, 2006). The risk for hematoma versus the benefit of regional anesthesia must be taken into account when considering appropriate patient care (Rowlings and Hanson, 2005). However, the 2003 Consensus Conference of the American Society of Regional Anesthesia (Rowlings and Hanson, 2005) clearly indicates that regional anesthesia can be safely used with LMWH prophylaxis with careful attention to calibration of total daily dose and timing of the initiation and continuance of LMWH in relation to neuraxial anesthesia.

Fondaparinux

Fondaparinux is a synthetic pentasaccharide that binds to antithrombin III. It accelerates the action of antithrombin III to inhibit factor Xa (Ginzberg et al, 2006; Nutescu, 2007). As with LMWH, there is no need to monitor PTT. Fondaparinux should not be used in patients with renal impairment, and with fondaparinux there is a risk for hematoma with spinal anesthesia (Ginzberg et al, 2006; Kehl-Pruett, 2006). There is a concern that, unlike heparin, it cannot be reversed with protamine sulfate.

Fondaparinux has been shown to be more effective than LMWH for the first 7 to 10 days after joint replacement surgery. However, it is associated with an additional risk for bleeding if administered less than 6 hours postoperatively. If anticoagulant therapy is stopped after 7 to 10 days, an additional month of aspirin prophylaxis should be considered in high-risk patients. The effectiveness of fondaparinux is similar to warfarin, whereas aspirin is less effective (Kearon, 2003b).

Warfarin

Warfarin is an oral anticoagulant that has a different mechanism of action than LDUH, LMWH, or fondaparinux. Whereas heparin products block activated coagulation factors, warfarin alters hepatic synthesis of vitamin K–dependent coagulation factor precursors, making them resist activation (Ginzberg et al, 2006). The result is depletion of clotting factors II, VII, IX, and X. Dicumarol, another oral anticoagulant, is used less frequently because of erratic absorption and gastrointestinal side effects. Dosage regulation of warfarin and dicumarol is based on laboratory monitoring of prothrombin time (PT) and international normalized ratio (INR) (Woods et al, 2005).

Warfarin has the convenience of oral administration for both inpatient and outpatient use. It also has a low acquisition cost. However, the narrow therapeutic range requires frequent monitoring. In addition, its effectiveness is affected by a large number of foods, antibiotics, and disease processes (Kehl-Pruett, 2006). There is also a long list of serious interactions with other drugs (Ginzberg et al, 2006). These influences make it difficult to regulate (Kehl-Pruett, 2006). The slow onset of action and widely variable responses are disadvantages. It can take greater than 3 days for the INR results to reach the recommended range of 2.0 to 3.0 (Ginzberg et al, 2006).

There are no controlled studies evaluating the effectiveness of warfarin as VTE prophylaxis. In literature there is discussion of warfarin being associated with less bleeding, yet there is also information published stating that warfarin may cause more bleeding than LMWH during extended prophylaxis. Evidence suggests that warfarin and LMWH have similar efficacy in preventing symptomatic VTE within 3 months of hip and knee replacement (Kearon, 2003b).

Aspirin

Aspirin decreases platelet aggregation and is effective in prophylactic treatment of arterial thrombi. Venous thrombi are composed of fibrin and red blood cells. This is why aspirin is not considered an effective method of preventing VTE. The Eighth ACCP Conference on Antithrombotic and Thrombolytic Therapy advises that aspirin alone is not recommended as prophylaxis in any surgical patient (Kehl-Pruett, 2006). More specifically, aspirin is not recommended for prevention of VTE after orthopedic surgery. It is less effective than LMWH or warfarin. Despite its ineffectiveness in preventing VTE, it is simple to administer, inexpensive, and safe. However, there is a risk for gastrointestinal bleeding (Kearon, 2003b).

The decision about the best prophylactic therapy for a patient should be based on efficacy, safety, and cost (Nutescu, 2007). The efficacy of treatment with GCS, IPC, LDUH, LMWH, warfarin, and aspirin vary significantly by patient populations. The value of reviewing the data from different trials is to provide insight into the overall problem of VTE and the importance of thromboprophylaxis in high-risk situations (Ginzberg et al, 2006).

ECONOMIC IMPLICATIONS

The price of VTE prevention includes the cost of mechanical devices, pharmacologic therapy, and diagnostic procedures. Although prevention may seem costly, it is much more cost-effective than delayed discharge or readmission due to VTE. It is impossible to quantify all of the economic issues involved, especially the cost of loss of life as a result of PE. The impact on a family cannot be assigned a dollar figure (Chapman et al, 2000).

A dollar figure can be assigned to the debilitating effects of venous postthrombotic syndrome. The quality of a patient's life can be affected by chronic leg swelling, pain, leg ulcers, or amputation. The medical resources consumed as a result of these complications in addition to the ongoing costs to the patient in the form of lost income are limitless (Chapman et al, 2000).

INCIDENCE AND PROPHYLAXIS OF VTE IN SURGERY

Two approaches to VTE prophylaxis are an individual patient risk-assessment model versus a model based on surgical specialties. The risk-assessment model ascribes prophylaxis by considering patient-specific risk factors and then providing recommendations based upon risk-factor stratification. The most important drawback to the risk-assessment approach is that this model has not been adequately validated. In addition, it is difficult to determine exactly where an individual patient lies within the continuum of thromboembolic risk factors in order to assign effective prophylactic care. As a result, this method becomes logistically complex and may lead to substandard treatment (Geerts et al, 2008). Prophylaxis based upon a risk-assessment model is seen in Table 9-2.

The second method used to implement VTE prophylaxis categorizes patients based on the surgical specialty providing care for the patient's primary disorder; the American College of Chest Physicians supports this model. Assigning patients to appropriate surgical groups is straightforward, and interventions are recommended using evidence-based guidelines (Geerts et al, 2008). Throughout the remainder of this section, please refer to Table 9-3 for a synopsis of guidelines according to surgical specialty. A majority of the guidelines were obtained from recommendations from the Eighth ACCP Conference on Antithrombotic and Thrombolytic Therapy.

Orthopedic Surgery

It is well documented that patients undergoing orthopedic surgeries are at particularly high risk for developing DVT and PE (Agnelli, 2004;

TABLE 9-2 Surgical Patient Risk Assessment Model for VTE Prophylaxis*

Risk Category	Risk Factors	DVT Incidence Without Prophylaxis (%)	Prevention Strategies
Low risk	Minor surgery in mobile patient	<10	No specific prophylaxis other than early ambulation
Moderate risk	• Majority of general, open gyn, or urologic surgery patients • High bleeding risk	10–40	LMWH given at recommended doses, LDUH every 12 or every 8 hrs, fondaparinux Mechanical thromboprophylaxis
High risk	• Hip or knee arthroplasty, hip fracture surgery • High bleeding risk	40–80	LMWH at recommended doses, fondaparinux, VKAs keeping INR 2–3 Mechanical thromboprophylaxis

DVT, Deep venous thrombosis; *INR,* international normalized ratio; *LDUH,* low-dose unfractionated heparin; *LMWH,* low-molecular-weight heparin; *VKA,* vitamin K antagonist; *VTE,* venous thromboembolism.

From Geerts WH et al: Prevention of venous thromboembolism: antithrombotic and thrombolytic therapy 8th edition: ACCP guidelines, *Chest* 133:381S–453S, 2008.

TABLE 9-3 Surgical Specialty Model VTE Prophylaxis*

Surgical Interventions	Recommended Prophylaxis	Prophylaxis Duration
ORTHOPEDIC		
Total hip replacement (THR)	Usual high-risk dose LMWH 12 hours before surgery or 12-24 hours after surgery, or one-half the usual high-risk dose 4-6 hours after surgery then increase to usual high-risk dose on POD 1 or Fondaparinux 2.5 mg started 6-8 hours after surgery or Dose-adjusted warfarin started preoperatively on the eve of the day of surgery (INR target 2.5, range 2.0-3.0)	At least 10 days with a recommendation to extend up to 35 days
High risk for bleeding	Mechanical thromboprophylaxis. Start on pharmacologic treatment once bleeding risk has decreased	
Total knee replacement	Same as for THR Appropriate IPC use is a beneficial alternative to anticoagulation prophylaxis	At least 10 days and up to 35 days postoperatively
Hip fracture repair	Fondaparinux, LMWH, dose-adjusted warfarin or LDUH	At least 10 days with a recommendation to extend up to 35 days
Contraindication secondary to high risk for bleeding	Appropriate mechanical thromboprophylaxis use is a beneficial alternative to anticoagulation prophylaxis	
Delayed surgery	Initiate LMWH or LDUH between admission and surgery	

TABLE 9-3 Surgical Specialty Model VTE Prophylaxis—cont'd

Surgical Interventions	Recommended Prophylaxis	Prophylaxis Duration
Isolated lower extremity fracture repair (distal to knee)	No routine use of thromboprophylaxis	N/A
ELECTIVE SPINE SURGERY		
No additional risk factors	Early, persistent mobilization	†
Patients with known malignancy, advanced age, neurologic deficit, previous VTE, or anterior approach	Postoperative LDUH, LMWH, or perioperative IPC; alternative consideration for GCS	
Patients with multiple risk factors	LDUH or LMWH with GCS and/or IPC	
KNEE ARTHROSCOPY		
No additional risk factors	No routine use of thromboprophylaxis other than early ambulation	†
For those at higher-than-usual risk for VTE following a prolonged or complex procedure	LMWH is recommended	
GENERAL SURGERY		
Low-risk, minor surgery with no additional risk factors	Early, aggressive mobilization	Those undergoing major surgery should have treatment continue until discharge form hospital
Moderate-risk undergoing major surgery for benign disease	LMWH, LDUH, or fondaparinux	Selected high-risk general surgery patients, including those who undergo major cancer surgery or have a history of VTE, continue prophylaxis with LMWH following hospital discharge for up to 28 days
Higher-risk undergoing major surgery for cancer	LMWH or LDUH every 8 hr or fondaparinux	
Multiple risk factors	LMWH or LDUH every 8 hr or fondaparinux combined with mechanical methods	
High risk for bleeding	Mechanical methods until risk decreases, then substitute or add pharmacologic methods	
Laparoscopic surgery No additional risk factors	Aggressive, early ambulation. (patients with additional risk factors may consider LMWH, LDUH, IPC, or GCS)	†
Inpatient bariatric surgery	Routine LMWH, LDUH every 8 hr, fondaparinux or combine one of these with IPC Higher doses of LMWH or LDUH than usual for nonobese patients	†

Continued

TABLE 9-3 Surgical Specialty Model VTE Prophylaxis—cont'd

Surgical Interventions	Recommended Prophylaxis	Prophylaxis Duration
CARDIOTHORACIC SURGERY		
Major thoracic surgery	Routine use of LMWH, LDUH, or fondaparinux	†
Coronary artery bypass surgery	LMWH, LDUH, GCS, or IPC (LMWH is preferred over LDUH)	
Major cardiothoracic surgery with high risk for bleeding	GCS and/or IPC	
VASCULAR SURGERY		
Patients with no additional risk factors	No routine thromboprophylaxis	†
Major vascular surgery with additional risk factors	LMWH or LDUH or fondaparinux	
Cancer surgery patients	As per specific surgery recommendation	Continue up to 4 weeks after discharge (Institute for Clinical Systems Improvement, 2008)
NEUROSURGERY		
Major neurosurgery	IPC Acceptable alternative is postoperative LMWH or LDUH	
High-risk patients	Combination mechanical and LMWH or LDUH	
GYNECOLOGIC SURGERY		
Surgery ≤ 30 min, benign disease, no additional risk factors; laparoscopic procedures with no additional risk factors	Early, persistent mobilization	Patients undergoing major procedures should continue prophylaxis until discharge
Laparoscopy with additional VTE risk factors	LDUH, LMWH, IPC, or GCS	
Major surgery, benign disease, no additional risk factors	LMWH, LDUH, or IPC started just before surgery continued until patient is ambulatory	Particularly high-risk patients (major cancer surgery or previous VTE) continue prophylaxis up to 28 days after discharge with LMWH
Extensive surgery for malignancy, and for those with additional VTE risk factors	LMWH or LDUH three times daily Alternative is IPC alone until ambulatory or combo of LMWH or LDUH plus GCS, IPC, or fondaparinux	
TRAUMA		
No major contraindication	Start all trauma patients with LMWH as soon as safely possible Acceptable alternative is combination of LMWH and mechanical thromboprophylaxis	Continue until discharge

TABLE 9-3 Surgical Specialty Model VTF Prophylaxis cont'd

Surgical Interventions	Recommended Prophylaxis	Prophylaxis Duration
If LMWH is contraindicated due to active or high risk for bleeding	IPC or GCS alone; start pharmacologic means when bleeding risk has decreased	
High risk for VTE (spinal cord injury, lower extremity or pelvic fracture, major head injury) who has not had optimal prophylaxis	Doppler ultrasound screening Recommend against the use of IVC filters as primary prophylaxis	Patients with major impaired mobility or who undergo inpatient rehabilitation, continue with LMWH or warfarin
UROLOGY		
Transurethral or other low-risk procedures	Persistent, early ambulation	Continuation of treatment has not been evaluated in these patients
Major, open procedures	LDUH 2 times per day to 3 times per day; GCS and/or IPC started just before surgery until patient is ambulatory; fondaparinux; or combination of pharmacologic method with mechanical method	
At very high risk for or actively bleeding	GCS and or IPC until bleeding risk decreases	
Plastic surgery	Intervention based upon individual patient risk factors	†

GCS, graduated compression stockings; *INR*, international normalized ratio; *IPC*, intermittent pneumatic compression; *LDUH*, low-dose unfractionated heparin; *LMWH*, low-molecular-weight heparin; *POD*, postoperative day; *THR*, total hip replacement; *VTE*, venous thromboembolism.

* Guidelines serve as a reference point and are intended to be applied with clinical judgment by the prescribing provider. Individual patient circumstances should be taken into consideration when prescribing.

† No specific guidelines regarding duration of therapy were provided in this surgical specialty by Eighth ACCP Conference on Antithrombotic and Thrombolytic Therapy.

All recommendations are taken from Geerts WH et al: Prevention of venous thromboembolism: antithrombotic and thrombolytic therapy, 8th edition: ACCP guidelines, *Chest* 133:381S–453S, 2008, except where noted.

Bjornara et al, 2006; Summerfield, 2006; Agency for Healthcare Research and Quality, 2009). The Agency for Healthcare Research and Quality (2009) affirms that when prophylaxis is not used, over 50% of patients undergoing major orthopedic surgeries will experience DVT and up to 30% will develop PE postoperatively. Even when appropriate preventive treatment is initiated, VTE is still clinically evident in almost 3% of orthopedic surgery patients. Hospital readmission after hip replacement is most frequently caused by VTE (Agnelli, 2004). A significant factor associated with the high incidence of VTE in orthopedic surgery is that the nature of the surgery often renders the orthopedic surgical patient immobile (Summerfield, 2006). Another concern is the evidence that the use of tourniquets for more than 50 minutes leads to a greater incidence of DVT (Chapman et al, 2000).

Total Hip Replacement

Approximately 1 in 1000 people undergo elective total hip replacement (THR) yearly. Of THR patients who do not receive DVT prophylaxis, 42% to 57% develop DVT detectable by venography, and 0.9% to 28% develop PE. Fatal PE develops in 0.1% to 2.0% of patients who do not receive DVT prophylaxis (Geerts et al, 2008).

Mechanical methods of VTE prevention used in patients undergoing THR, such as GCS and IPC, do reduce DVT, but are not as effective as anticoagulant-based regimens. There is strong evidence against the use of aspirin, dextran, LDUH, GCS, IPC, or venous foot pump as the sole method of VTE prophylaxis in hip-replacement patients. Low-molecular-weight-heparin, fondaparinux, and warfarin have been found to be effective pharmacologic prophylaxis options (Geerts et al, 2008).

Total Knee Replacement

There is a higher overall risk for DVT with total knee replacement (TKR) compared with THR. Literature suggests that between 41% and 85% of TKR patients without prophylaxis develop postoperative DVT (Agnelli, 2004; Summerfield, 2006; Broughton et al, 2007; Geerts et al, 2008; Agency for Healthcare Research and Quality, 2009). Fatal PE occurs in 0.1% to 1.7% of TKR patients (Geerts et al, 2008). Recommendations for prophylactic treatment for TKR are similar to those for THR. Low-molecular-weight heparin is favored over warfarin, but, again, there may be an increased incidence of postoperative bleeding with LMWH, particularly if started early in the postoperative period (Agnelli, 2004; Geerts et al, 2008). When IPC devices are used reliably, they are a beneficial alternative to anticoagulants when anticoagulation therapy is contraindicated (Geerts et al, 2008).

Hip Fracture Repair

Advanced age and delayed surgery are two factors that place individuals undergoing hip fracture repair at particular risk for VTE (Geerts et al, 2008). Rates of DVT after hip fracture without prophylaxis are approximately 50%. Fatal PE occurring 3 months after hip fracture repair is between 0.4% and 7.5% (Geerts et al, 2008). Patients should receive DVT prophylaxis with LMWH or LDUH during the preoperative period if surgery is going to be delayed (Geerts et al, 2008). The appropriate use of VTE prophylaxis appears to reduce the overall risk for DVT by about 60% (Agnelli, 2004).

Lower-Extremity Fracture Repair

Information is scarce regarding the incidence and prevention of VTE after lower-extremity fracture repair. However, several studies have documented an incidence of DVT at 4% and 17% in patients who did not receive prophylaxis. The closer the fracture is to the knee, the higher the risk for DVT. Uncertainty exists regarding the efficacy and cost-effectiveness of VTE prophylaxis in cases of isolated fracture repair regarding clinically significant VTE. Therefore, until further information is available, it is recommended that clinicians decide on a case-by-case basis regarding treatment. It is reasonable in cases of isolated lower-extremity fracture that thromboprophylaxis not be used routinely (Geerts et al, 2008).

Elective Spine Surgery

The limited data available regarding incidence of VTE in patients undergoing elective spine surgery indicate rates of 3.7% for overt DVT and 2.2% for PE. The following are risk factors for these patients: surgery on the cervical spine versus the lumbar spine, advanced age, anterior or combined anterior/posterior approach, malignancy, prolonged surgery, neurologic deficit, and reduced preoperative and postoperative mobility. Elective spinal surgery patients without additional risk factors need no other preventive care other than early, persistent mobilization. The 2008 ACCP recommendations for patients with multiple risk factors include LDUH or LMWH combined with GCS and/or IPC (Geerts et al, 2008).

Joint Arthroscopy

Knee arthroscopy is a very common orthopedic procedure performed in the United States, and over 3 million are performed each year globally (Hoppener, 2006). Without prophylaxis, studies support that asymptomatic DVT occurs in approximately 9% of knee arthroscopy patients (Geerts et al, 2008). Compared with major orthopedic surgery, the risk is relatively low. A paucity of evidence regarding the usefulness of thromboprophylaxis in this population makes it necessary for treatment to be decided individually. Early ambulation, when suitable, should be encouraged with LMWH used for patients with higher-than-usual risk (Geerts et al, 2008).

General Surgery

Studies that estimate incidence of VTE in general surgery patients without the use of thromboprophylaxis are no longer performed. Therefore there is no current research that provides accurate estimates of incidence in this patient group. Screening studies performed in the 1970s and 1980s reported an incidence of DVT and fatal PE ranging from 15% to 30% and 0.2% to 0.9%, respectively. It is possible that rapid postoperative mobilization, extensive use of thromboprophylaxis, and advanced perioperative care has reduced current incidence. On the other hand, the incidence could be higher than previously reported because surgical patients are older, often have multiple comorbidities, and undergo more extensive procedures. In addition, the trend toward shorter hospital stays results in insufficient length of time for recommended VTE prophylaxis. Low-dose-unfractionated heparin and LMWH have been found to reduce the incidence of VTE by at least 60% in general surgical patients and are recommended as routine thromboprophylaxis. Patients undergoing major general surgery should receive routine thromboprophylaxis with the use of LDUH or LMWH according to manufacturers' recommendations. Patients at high risk for bleeding should use mechanical prophylactic measures (Geerts et al, 2008).

Laparoscopic surgical interventions have become used more widely over the past several decades. Uncertainty exists in relation to the use of DVT prophylaxis with laparoscopic surgery. Laparoscopic procedures usually entail fewer traumas and have similar to slightly less activation of the coagulation system compared with open procedures. However, incidence of DVT after laparoscopy is generally small at 1.2%. The Eighth ACCP Conference on Antithrombotic and Thrombolytic Therapy (Geerts et al, 2008) claims that there is not enough evidence to recommend the routine use of thromboprophylaxis in laparoscopic patients. If a particular patient is deemed at high risk, a brief prophylaxis with a current prophylactic routine could be considered (Geerts et al, 2008).

Bariatric surgery has become popular over the past 15 years. Over 100,000 weight-loss surgeries are performed yearly in the United States. The National Bariatric Surgery Registry reports a 0.2% incidence of PE and 0.1% incidence of DVT among 14,641 registered patients undergoing bariatric surgery between 1986 and 1996. The use of LMWH or LDUH three times daily, fondaparinux, or a combination of one pharmacologic method with IPC is recommended. A higher-than-usual dose of LMWH or LDUH is recommended for obese patients (Geerts et al, 2008).

Cardiothoracic Surgery

Few studies are available that deal with VTE in patients who undergo cardiothoracic surgery. The majority of patients undergoing cardiothoracic surgery are in the high-risk category. Patients who undergo thoracic surgery are at similar risk for VTE as those who undergo major general surgery. These patients should be given thromboprophylaxis as recommended for general surgery patients (Geerts et al, 2008).

The overall risk for clinically important VTE for patients undergoing coronary artery bypass graft (CABG) is low. Coronary artery bypass graft surgery is typically performed with the administration of heparin intraoperatively. In addition, CABG patients routinely take aspirin, clopidogrel, or oral anticoagulation after surgery, and early ambulation is a standard of care. Therefore VTE after cardiac surgery is not considered a significant medical dilemma. A lack of empirical data produces an uncertainty regarding the administration of routine thromboprophylaxis to all CABG patients. These patients have multiple risk factors and often have prolonged hospital stays with limited mobility. Therefore it is reasonable to treat CABG patients postoperatively with LMWH, LDUH, IPC, or GCS (Geerts et al, 2008).

Vascular Surgery

The occurrence of VTE in the vascular surgical patient is difficult to assess. This is because during vascular surgery patients routinely receive perioperative antithrombotic agents such as aspirin or clopidogrel as well as heparin or dextran intraoperatively. However, vascular surgery patients remain at high risk for VTE because of advanced age, limb ischemia, extended surgical time, and possible venous trauma. In addition, it is felt that atherosclerosis may be considered an independent risk factor for VTE. One study reported a 1.7% to 2.8% incidence of clinically significant VTE within 3 months of vascular surgery. Open resection of an abdominal aortic aneurysm or aortofemoral bypass seems to have a higher incidence of DVT than leg bypass surgery (Geerts et al, 2008).

A study performed by vanRij et al in 2004 showed that patients undergoing varicose vein surgery had a DVT incidence of 5% despite the use of thromboprophylaxis. Surgical management in this study included general anesthesia for saphenofemoral junction flush ligation, long saphenous vein stripping, and phlebectomies. There is a higher risk for DVT when patients undergo bilateral versus unilateral varicose vein surgery. Extended prophylaxis is recommended for varicose vein surgery patients who have multiple risk factors (vanRij et al, 2004).

The consensus is (Geerts et al, 2008) that patients without additional thromboembolic risk factors who undergo vascular surgery do not need routine prophylaxis. Patients should be encouraged to ambulate early and frequently. However, those undergoing major vascular surgery with additional risk factors should begin prophylaxis with LMWH, LDUH, or fondaparinux after surgery (Geerts et al, 2008).

Neurologic Surgery

Neurosurgical patients have an approximately 22% risk for developing DVT (Agnelli, 2004; Agency for Healthcare Research and Quality, 2009). Intracranial surgery carries a higher risk than spinal surgery. Length of surgery, surgery for malignancy, lower limb paralysis, and advanced age also increase the risk for VTE perioperatively and up to 15 months after surgery (Geerts et al 2008; Agency for Healthcare Research and Quality, 2009). Therefore it is necessary for this patient group to receive some form of VTE prophylaxis. Mechanical prophylaxis is commonly used in neurosurgical patients because of the concern for intracrancial or spinal hemorrhage. Craniotomy patients do have a reduction in DVT by 82% when given LDUH. However, pharmacologic prophylaxis should be used with caution in these patients. Studies show that postoperative intracranial hemorrhage is 2.1% in patients receiving postoperative LMWH, compared with 1.1% in those with mechanical or no prophylaxis. Current recommended treatment options include optimal use of IPC intraoperatively and LDUH or LMWH postoperatively. High-risk neurosurgery patients should have a combination of mechanical (GCS and/or IPC) and LDUH or LMWH (Geerts et al, 2008).

Gynecologic Surgery

Rates for VTE are similar for patients undergoing major gynecologic surgery and those undergoing general surgical procedures. Advanced age, malignancy, previous VTE, prior pelvic radiation, and an abdominal approach are risk factors for gynecologic surgery patients. Early and persistent ambulation is recommended for those undergoing brief (less than 30 minutes) procedures and those undergoing laparoscopic gynecologic interventions who have no additional VTE risk. Gynecology patients with additional VTE risk undergoing laparoscopic procedures should be treated with LMWH, LDUH, IPC, or GCS. Venothromboembolism prophylaxis for patients undergoing major gynecologic surgery is patient specific. See Table 9-3 for current recommendations made by the American College of Chest Physicians (Geerts et al, 2008).

Urologic Surgery

Major urologic surgery carries a risk of 1% to 5% for VTE. Fatal PE is the most common cause of postoperative death in these patients, occurring in less than 1 in 500 patients (Agnelli, 2004; Geerts et al, 2008). Multiple risk factors such as advanced age, malignancy, and lithotomy surgical position are factors in the development of VTE in urologic surgery patients. The risk, however, for patients undergoing transurethral prostatectomy appears to be low. Therefore in these patients early ambulation is the only recommendation. Those undergoing more extensive open procedures (radical prostatectomy, cystectomy, and nephrectomy) should have LDUH, LMWH, or fondaparinux plus GCS and/or IPC worn before surgery and after surgery until they are ambulatory. Patients who are actively bleeding or are at very high risk for bleeding should be started on IPC and/or GCS until bleeding risk is diminished; then pharmacologic prophylaxis may be added or substituted (Geerts et al, 2008).

Trauma Surgery

Major trauma patients have the highest risk for developing VTE. DVT risk exceeds 50%, and PE is the third leading cause of death for those who survive past day 1 (Geerts et al, 2008; Agency for Healthcare Research and Quality, 2009). An increased number of injuries correlates with an increased incidence of DVT (Stawicki et al, 2005). Many of these trauma patients require surgical intervention, and therefore appropriate perioperative thromboprophylaxis should be initiated. The absence of major contraindications allows for the initiation of LMWH as soon as is considered safe.

If pharmacologic treatment must be delayed because of active bleeding, IPC with GCS may be used as an alternative. Patients at high risk for VTE who have had a delay in prophylaxis or suboptimal prophylaxis should be screened for DVT by Doppler ultrasonography. Inferior vena cava filters are not recommended as a primary method of prophylaxis. Treatment should be continued at least until discharge or after for those with major immobility issues (Geerts et al, 2008).

Plastic Surgery

Few publications report rates of VTE with plastic surgery (Broughton et al, 2007). The risk for DVT and PE in facelifts has been reported to be around 0.39% and 0.16%, respectively (Davison et al, 2004; Broughton et al, 2007). Abdominoplasty patients appear to run a 1.1% risk for DVT and 0.8% risk for PE (Davison et al, 2004). The Practice Advisory on Liposuction advises that IPC and LMWH be used for "higher-risk" plastic surgery patients (Broughton et al, 2007). Unfortunately, further specific guidelines do not exist for thromboprophylaxis in the plastic surgery patient (Broughton et al, 2007). Until more studies provide evidence-based guidelines, intervention must be considered on a case-by-case basis taking into consideration individual patient risk factors.

NURSING IMPLICATIONS

Regardless of the knowledge of the incidence of VTE and the effectiveness of VTE prophylaxis, appropriate preventive measures are frequently underutilized. A survey of surgeons revealed that up to 14% of patients undergoing general surgery, 12% of patients undergoing hip fracture repair, and 3% to 5% of THR and TKR patients do not receive VTE prophylaxis (Agency for Healthcare Research and Quality, 2009). According to the Association for periOperative Registered Nurses (2009), "The safety of patients undergoing operative or other invasive procedures is a primary responsibility of the perioperative registered nurse". Therefore VTE prophylaxis of the perioperative patient is an area of opportunity for nurses to make a significant impact on patient safety.

Knowledge is the key to identifying patients at risk for VTE. Venous thromboembolism can be prevented by risk stratification, identifying appropriate measures, and knowing when and how to apply the appropriate measures in a timely manner. Risk stratification begins when nurses perform an in-depth history preoperatively and should be ongoing throughout the patient's hospital stay, particularly if conditions change. Once individual patient risk factors and surgical specialty have been identified, the nurse has the responsibility to advocate for appropriate prophylaxis (Chapman et al, 2000).

Nurses have the responsibility to educate patients and family about VTE. Educating patients about why they are at risk and why specific prevention measures are chosen improves compliance and acceptance of treatment (Kehl-Pruett, 2006). Education should start with basic postoperative teaching topics such as the importance of leg exercises, early ambulation postoperatively, maintenance of hydration, and the avoidance of prolonged periods of inactivity and constrictive clothing. In addition, the nurse must emphasize frequent turning, coughing, and deep breathing, along with not raising the knee gatch on the bed to avoid popliteal pressure (Woods et al, 2005). Patients need to be reminded to avoid standing or sitting for extended periods of time and sitting with knees bent or crossed for long periods (Day, 2003). An explanation of how elevating legs when sitting promotes venous return and prevents venous pooling may create a lasting picture in a patient's mind (Woods et al, 2005).

If elastic stockings or intermittent pneumatic compression is ordered, an explanation of how the calf muscle pump works may reinforce the importance of compliance with these measures. Signs posted on the wall at the foot of the bed in patient rooms have been used in an attempt to increase compliance (Stewart et al, 2006). A similar sign could be used for patients with IPC devices. The signs can serve as a reminder to patients, as well as nursing staff (Figure 9-4).

When anticoagulant therapy is prescribed, patients need to understand the importance of postdischarge follow-up. Specifically, arrangements should be made so patients are clear about where and when to go for follow-up once they leave the hospital. It is important to stress the need to continue the medication after discharge, the laboratory monitoring required, and the risk factors for bleeding (Chapman et al, 2000; Day, 2003; Crowther and McCourt, 2004). Patients need to be alert to signs of bleeding and know

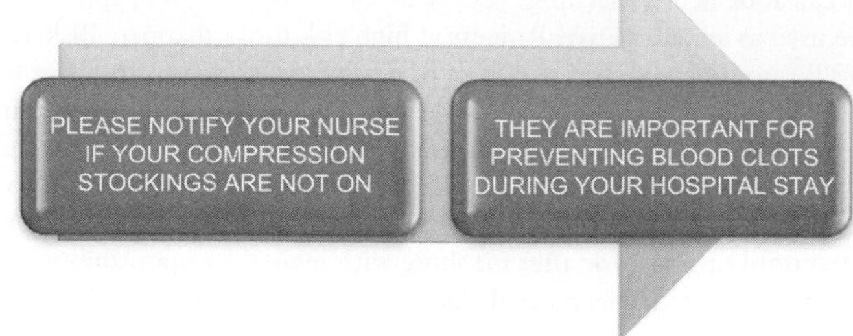

PLEASE NOTIFY YOUR NURSE IF YOUR COMPRESSION STOCKINGS ARE NOT ON
THEY ARE IMPORTANT FOR PREVENTING BLOOD CLOTS DURING YOUR HOSPITAL STAY

FIGURE 9-4 Patient cues for DVT prophylaxis. (From Barnett J, DeCarlo L: Incidence of deep venous thrombosis in the surgical patient population and prophylactic measures to reduce occurrence. *Perioper Nurs Clin* 3(4):367-382, 2008.)

to notify their care provider if they experience unusual bruising, nose or gum bleeding, blood in the urine or stool, vomiting blood, abdominal pain, joint pain or swelling, back pain, headaches, or a change in level of consciousness (Day, 2003; Crowther and McCourt, 2004; Woods et al, 2005; Kaplan, 2007).

Nurses need to discuss prevention of bleeding while on anticoagulant therapy. Patients should be reminded not to use salicylates, ibuprofen, or other over-the-counter products that affect coagulation without consulting their physician. They should use a soft toothbrush and an electric shaver rather than a razor. Contact sports should be avoided, and night-lights should be used to prevent falls. A medical alert bracelet stating the medication being taken should be worn to alert emergency medical personnel. The patient also needs to remind other health care providers that he or she is on anticoagulant therapy (Kaplan, 2007).

Patients taking warfarin should be provided with a list of foods and medications that can alter their INR. They need to know the importance of following up with ordered laboratory tests to prevent excessive bleeding or blood clot formation (Crowther and McCourt, 2004). Patients on warfarin need to know that tissue necrosis can occur from bruising at sites of fatty tissue such as the abdomen, breast, buttocks, and thighs (Day, 2003).

Teaching patients the signs and symptoms of DVT and PE is essential. They need to notify their health care provider immediately if there is redness, swelling, tenderness, pain, discoloration, or asymmetry of their legs or arms. They need to be instructed to call 911 if they experience unexplained shortness of breath, chest pain or palpitations, anxiety or sweating, or coughing up blood.

CONCLUSION

Venous thromboembolism is an important patient safety concern. Nurses are in a key position to raise awareness of VTE prevention in the health care community and implement recommended prophylactic measures. Nurses can ensure that the most up-to-date recommendations are being followed to prevent VTE in surgical patients by being involved in developing VTE prophylaxis guidelines in their facilities. Using the surgical specialty model as the primary method of determining VTE prophylaxis for surgical patients supports the recommendation of the Eighth ACCP Conference on Antithrombotic and Thrombolytic Therapy. The use of appropriate VTE prophylaxis prevents significant mortality, morbidity, and resource expenditures while ensuring patient safety.

ACKNOWLEDGMENTS

The authors would like to acknowledge Joanne E. Peterson, BEd, MAEd in Guidance and Counseling, for her thoughtful critique of the manuscript and Neal Van Der Voorn, MLS, MultiCare Health System Medical Librarian, for his assistance in researching multiple databases to provide an extensive source of references.

REFERENCES

Agency for Healthcare Research and Quality: Prevention of venous thromboembolism, available at http://www.ncbi.nlm.nih.gov/books/bv.fcgi?rid=hstat1.section.61086. Accessed June 5, 2009.

Agnelli G: Prevention of venous thromboemblism in surgical patients, *Circulation* 110(24 Suppl 1):IV4–IV12, 2004.

American Public Health Association: In *Deep vein thrombosis: advancing awareness to protect patient lives*, 2003 White paper, Public Health Leadership Conference on Deep-Vein Thrombosis, 2003:1–12.

Association of periOperative Registered Nurses: AORN position statement: statement on patient safety, available at http://www.aorn.org/PracticeResources/AORNPositionStatements/Position_PatientSafety/ Accessed on June 1, 2009.

Bjornara BT, et al: Frequency and timing of clinical venous thromboemolism after major joint surgery, *J Bone Joint Surg Am* 88:386–391, 2006.

Broughton G, et al: Deep vein thrombosis prophylaxis practice and treatment strategies among plastic surgeons: survey results, *Plast Reconstr Surg* 119(1):157–174, 2007.

Brunicardi FC, et al: *Schwartz's principles of surgery*, ed 8, New York, 2004, McGraw-Hill.

Chapman MW, et al: *Chapman's orthopaedic surgery*, ed 3, Philadelphia, 2000, Lippincott Williams & Wilkins.

Clarke-Pearson DL, et al: Thromboembolism prophylaxis: patients at high risk to fail intermittent pneumatic compression, *Obstet Gynecol* 101(1):157–163, 2003.

Crowther M, McCourt K: Get the edge on deep vein thrombosis, *Nurs Manag* 35(1):21–30, 2004.

Davison SP, et al: Prevention of venous thromboembolism in the plastic surgery patient, *Plast Reconstr Surg* 114: 43e–51e, 2004.

Day MW: Recognizing and managing DVT, *Nursing* 33(5): 37–41, 2003.

Eisle R, et al: Rapid inflation intermittent pneumatic compression for prevention of deep vein thrombosis, *J Bone Joint Surg Am* 89(5):1050–1056, 2007.

Epstein N: Intermittent pneumatic stocking prophylaxis against deep vein thrombosis in anterior cervical spine surgery, *Spine* 30(22):2538–2543, 2005.

Geerts WH, et al: Prevention of venous thromboembolism: antithrombotic and thrombolytic therapy 8th edition: ACCP guidelines, *Chest* 133:381S–453S, 2008.

Ginzberg E, et al: Thromboprophylaxis in medical and surgical patients undergoing physical medicine and rehabilitation, *Am J Phys Med Rehabil* 85(2):159–166, 2006.

Hoppener MR: Low incidence of deep vein thrombosis after knee arthorscopy without thromboprophylaxis: a prospective cohort study of 335 patients, *Acta Orthop* 77(5):767–771, 2006.

Institute for Clinical Systems Improvement: *Health care guideline: venous thromboembolism prophylaxis*, ed 5, 2008. available at http://www.icsi.org/venous_thromboembolism_prophylaxis/venous_thromboembolism_prophylaxis_4.html. Accessed June 5, 2009.

Kaplan R: Deep vein thrombosis: prevention—an overview, Cinahl Nursing Guide, Glendale, Calif, October 12, 2007, Cinahl Information Systems, available at http://search.ebscohost.com/login.aspx?direct=true&db=nrc&AN=5000003405&site=nrc-live. Accessed February 26, 2008.

Kearon C: Duration of venous thromboembolism prophylaxis after surgery, *Chest* 124:386S–392S, 2003a.

Kearon C: Natural history of venous thromboembolism, *Circulation* 107(23 Suppl 1):I22–I30, 2003b.

Kehl-Pruett W: Deep vein thrombosis in hospital patients, *Dimens Crit Care Nurs* 25(2):53–59, 2006.

Kucher N, Tapson VF: Pulmonary embolism. In Fuster V et al: editers: *Hurst's the heart*, ed 11 New York, 2004, McGraw-Hill.

Mazzone C, et al: Physical methods for preventing deep vein thrombosis in stroke. *Cochrane Database of Systematic Reviews*, 2004, Issue 4, Art. No.: CD001922. DOI: 10.1002/14651858.CD001922.pub2.

Morrison R: Venous thromboembolism: scope of the problem and the nurse's role in risk assessment and prevention, *J Vasc Nurs* 24(3):82–90, 2006.

Nutescu EA: Assessing, preventing, and treating venous thrombo-embolism: evidence-based approaches, *Am J Health Syst Pharm* 64(Suppl 7):S5–S13, 2007.

Pearse EO, et al: Early mobilization after conventional knee replacement may reduce the risk of postoperative venous thromboembolism, *J Bone Joint Surg Br* 89(3):316–322, 2007.

Prystowsky JB, et al: Prospective analysis of the incidence of deep vein thrombosis in bariatric surgery patients, *Surgery* 138(4):759–765, 2005.

Race TK, Collier PE: The hidden risks of deep vein thrombosis—the need for risk factor assessment, *Crit Care Nurs Q* 30(3):245–254, 2007.

Ramzi DW, Leeper KV: DVT and pulmonary embolism. I. Diagnosis, *Am Fam Physician* 69(12):2829–2836, 2004.

Rowlings JC, Hanson PB: Neuraxial anesthesia and low-molecular-weight heparin prophylaxis in major orthopedic surgery in the wake of latest American Society of Regional Anesthesia guidelines, *Anesth Analg* 100:1482–1488, 2005.

Stawicki SP, et al: Deep vein thrombosis and pulmonary embolism in trauma patients: an overstatement of the problem? *Am Surg* 71(5):387–391, 2005.

Stewart D, et al: A prospective study of nurse and patient education on compliance with sequential compression devices, *Am Surg* 72(10):921–923, 2006.

Summerfield D: Decreasing the incidence of deep vein thrombosis through the use of prophylaxis, *AORN J* 84(4):642–645, 2006.

vanRij AM, et al: Incidence of deep vein thrombosis after varicose vein surgery, *Br J Surg* 91:1582–1585, 2004.

Woods SL, et al, editors: *Cardiac nursing*, ed 5, Philadelphia, 2005, Lippincott Williams & Wilkins.

PREVENTIVE MEASURES FOR WRONG-SITE, WRONG-PERSON, AND WRONG-PROCEDURE ERROR IN THE PERIOPERATIVE SETTING

Sharon A. McNamara, MS, RN, CNOR

Newspaper headlines inform the public about the wrong leg amputated on a Florida man, a child who has burr holes on the wrong side, and an adult with a subdural hematoma who has a craniotomy performed on the wrong side. These are some of the high-profile cases that have the public questioning the safety of hospitals and that have generated a flurry of activity in the U.S. health care system to put preventive measures into place to maintain quality, safe patient care. Certainly none of the professional practitioners participating in the procedures on these patients willfully performed these wrong-site/side surgeries. However, in our current health care system, which is currently under development for a radical culture change, one of those practitioners could be blamed. The evolution in process is a change in philosophy of not pointing to the people, but taking a broader view to look at the processes or systems in place to support those practitioners in doing the right thing every time. There have been recommendations and campaigns by professional associations on techniques to prevent wrong-site surgeries, but it was not until the Institute of Medicine brought medical errors to the forefront that we came to a more serious consideration of how to prevent wrong-side/site/person/procedure errors. This chapter will review wrong-site surgery prevention in the past, the scope of the problem, risk factors, prevention strategies, and performance measurement. Safe perioperative processes, culture change, and involving the patient are important aspects that will be examined.

HISTORICAL REVIEW OF PATIENT SAFETY AND WRONG-SITE SURGERY PREVENTION

In 1994 the Canadian Orthopaedic Association implemented "Operate Through Your Site." This was an educational program for their surgeons targeted at reducing wrong-site procedures (WSPs) (Canadian Orthopaedic Association Committee on Practice and Economics, 1994). Leading the way in the United States, the Council on Education of the American Academy of Orthopaedic Surgeons (AAOS) organized a task force in 1997 to research data on wrong-site surgery. The task force's charge was to determine the prevalence of wrong-site surgery and to develop recommendations for preventing it. Data from the report demonstrated that from 1985 to 1995, 225 orthopaedic wrong-site surgeries and 106 other surgical specialty insurance claims were filed. These wrong-site surgeries averaged payouts of $48,087 to orthopaedic patients and $76,167 to patients in other specialties (Canale, 2005). Outcomes from this initiative resulted in the *Advisory Statement on Wrong-Site Surgery,* which stated, "The American Academy of Orthopaedic Surgeons (AAOS) believes that a unified effort among surgeons, hospitals and other health care providers to initiate preoperative and other institutional regulations can effectively eliminate wrong-site surgery in the United States" (AAOS, 2008).

The advisory statement spelled out effective methods for eliminating wrong-site surgery (AAOS, 2008):

> *Wrong-site surgery is preventable by having the surgeon, in consultation with the patient when possible; place his or her initials on the operative site using a permanent marking pen and then operating through or adjacent to his or her initials. Spinal surgery done on the wrong level can be prevented with an intraoperative X-ray that marks the exact vertebral level (site) of surgery. Similarly, institutional protocols should include these recommendations and involve operating room nurses and technicians, hospital room committees, anesthesiologists, residents and other preoperative allied health personnel.*

This advocates strongly for having the patient involved, marking of the surgical site, involvement of the surgical team, and specific organizational policies to mandate the preventive measures. The AAOS did not stop there; they also advised that the surgical team should take a time-out and confirm the patient's identity, correct procedure and site, equipment, implants and devices, and an additional check of the patient's medical record and radiologic studies plus addressing discrepancies before starting the procedure. This pause must include all members of the surgical team and leave time to ask questions if necessary. In 1998 the AAOS established the "Sign Your Site" campaign, which issued the advisory statement and created a logo, audiovisual programs, exhibits, and a mail campaign that delivered 20,000 informational flyers to orthopaedic surgeons and operating room committees. The concepts for correct-site surgery were also incorporated into the academy's surgical skills courses, instructional courses, and their specialty day meetings.

In 1998 The Joint Commission International Center for Patient Safety published *Sentinel Event Alert,* issue 6—Lessons Learned: Wrong Site Surgery. This publication identified factors that may contribute to increased risk for wrong-site surgery, and it highlighted communication issues as the leading root cause. Three strategies for reducing the risk of wrong-site surgery were suggested (The Joint Commission International Center for Patient Safety, 2008): (1) marking of the operative site, (2) oral verification of the site by the surgical team, and (3) use of a safety checklist to include all aspects of verification.

The 1999 Institute of Medicine (IOM) report *To Err Is Human: Building a Safer Health System* dealt a serious blow to the U.S. health care system. The purpose of the report was to promote safer processes in our health care systems and to bring out into the open those serious concerns often hidden or discussed behind the closed doors of operating rooms and interventional units. This landmark publication, through its staggering numbers of reported patient deaths from preventable medical errors, heightened the awareness of patient safety issues for health care providers, patients, legislators, regulatory agencies, and the media. Media coverage quickly spread the word that the IOM report suggested that between 44,000 and 98,000 patients die in the United States every year as a result of medical errors. This exceeds the deaths attributable to motor vehicle accidents, breast cancer, and acquired immunodeficiency syndrome (AIDS). The report also put a dollar value on the errors, stating that the national cost was estimated at $37.6 billion to $50 billion for adverse events and that between $17 billion and $29 billion was for preventable adverse events (Kohn et al, 2000). One of the issues stated in the report is the lack of standardized nomenclature. The study used a definition for error from Gaba et al (1994): "An error is defined as a failure of a planned action to be completed as intended (i.e., error of execution) or the use of a wrong plan to achieve an aim (i.e., error of planning)." An adverse event is defined as an injury caused by medical management rather than the underlying condition of the patient. An adverse event attributable to error is a "preventable adverse event" (Brennan et al, 1991). The report is built around a four-tiered approach with recommendations to create health care environments that advocate for the following (Kohn et al, 2000):

> *Establishing a national focus to create leadership, research, tools and protocols to enhance the knowledge base about safety; identifying and learning from errors through immediate and strong mandatory reporting efforts, as well as the encouragement of voluntary efforts, both with the aim of making sure the system continues to be made safe for patients; raising standards and expectations for improvements in safety through the actions of oversight organizations, group purchasers, and professional groups; and creating safety systems inside health care organizations through the implementation of safe practices at the delivery level. This level is the ultimate target of all recommendations.*

The North American Spine Society (NASS) entered the safety campaign in 2001 through design of their SMaX Campaign, which encouraged surgeons to ***S***ign, ***M***ark ***a***nd ***X***-ray surgical sites (Wong et al, 2001). The x-ray step related to an additional safety check of a radiograph of the spinal level for site verification before beginning procedures on the vertebrae.

In 2001 a second report from the IOM's Committee on the Quality of Health Care in America was published. *Crossing the Quality Chasm: A New Health System for the 21st Century* focused on a call to action to redesign the health care delivery system. The movement is directed toward an efficient, cost-effective, quality, and patient-centered system in which the patient is actively involved—a system that promotes an environment that supports patient and professional safety. The report advocated new skills and new approaches with integration of information technology and alignment of payment policies that included addressing quality improvement and outcomes. Six aims for improvement will drive the needed changes in key dimensions of the current health system. These aims establish that health care should have the following characteristics (Committee on Quality of Health Care in America, Institute of Medicine, 2001):

- Safe—avoiding injuries to patients from the care that is intended to help them
- Effective—providing services, preferences, needs, and values based on scientific knowledge to all who could benefit and refraining from providing services to those not likely to benefit (avoiding underuse and overuse, respectively)
- Patient-centered—providing care that is respectful of and responsive to the individual patient and ensuring that patient values guide all clinical decisions
- Timely—reducing waits and sometimes harmful delays for both those who receive and give care
- Efficient—avoiding waste, including waste of equipment, supplies, ideas, and energy
- Equitable—providing care that does not vary in quality because of personal characteristics such as gender, ethnicity, geographic location, and socioeconomic status

In 2002 the National Quality Forum (NQF) published *Serious Reportable Events in Healthcare.* This report identified 27 never events—events that were considered preventable and should never happen. Surgery performed on the wrong body part was on the list. Surgery on the wrong patient and the wrong procedure were listed with additional specifications and implementation guidance for each.

In 2003 The Joint Commission held a Wrong Site Surgery Summit. The Joint Commission collaborated with numerous professional associations: the American Hospital Association, the American College of Surgeons, the American Academy of Orthopaedic Surgeons, the Association of periOperative Registered Nurses, the American Medical Association plus more than 20 other organizations. The goal of the summit was to achieve consensus on the adoption of a standard protocol for preventing wrong-site, wrong-procedure, and wrong-person surgery. The result of input, specific recommendations, and consensus on the principles for prevention was the Universal Protocol for preventing wrong-site surgery.

In October 2003 AAOS produced the "Sign-Your-Site: A Checklist for Safety" tool (Canale, 2005). On June 20, 2004, the Patient Safety First Campaign of the Association of peri-Operative Registered Nurses (AORN) spearheaded its inaugural National "Time Out" Day. The observance was endorsed by the American College of Surgeons, the American Society of Anesthesiologists, the American Society for Healthcare Risk Management, and the American Hospital Association. The purpose of the day was to increase awareness of The Joint Commission's *Universal Protocol for Preventing Wrong Site, Wrong Procedure, Wrong Person Surgery.* Concurrently the AORN's *Correct Site Surgery Tool Kit* was rolled out to 40,000 members. In addition, 50,000 copies of the tool kit were sent to chief executive officers and risk managers across the United States to emphasize the importance of standardizing the implementation of the Universal Protocol. The kit contained tools to assist with implementation: an educational CD-ROM, free independent study activity, copy of the Universal Protocol and the Frequently Asked Questions, a plasticized pocket reference guide for implementing The Joint Commission Universal Protocol, and The Joint Commission *Speak Up* safety initiative patient safety brochure. AORN (2008) continues to hold National Time Out day every year and to provide free resources to reinforce the necessity to implement and monitor the Universal Protocol for prevention of wrong-site procedures and improved care for our patients.

In 2006 The Joint Commission International Center for Patient Safety developed the International Patient Safety Goals. Six goals were created, of which the fourth goal is eliminate wrong-site, wrong-patient, wrong-procedure surgery. The goal includes the criteria to mark the site, conduct a time-out, and use checklists. These requirements are mirrored in the Universal Protocol's best practices (The Joint Commission International Center for Patient Safety, 2008). In July 2007 the Council on Surgical and Perioperative Safety (CSPS) (2008), a coalition of seven U.S. national organizations that represents the perioperative care team, endorsed as one of its core principles "that all measures will be used to ensure correct patient, correct site, correct procedure surgery, including implementation of the Universal Protocol of The Joint Commission is recommended and support of the Time-Out prior to surgery or initiation of an invasive procedure." The coalition consists of the following member organizations: the Association of periOperative Registered Nurses, the American College of Surgeons, the American Society of Anesthesiologists, the American Association of Nurse Anesthetists, the Society of PeriAnesthesia Nurses, the Association of Surgical Technologists, and the American Association of Surgical Physician Assistants. Convening this group of practitioners for the select goal of safety in the surgical and interventional areas is groundbreaking, and it is anticipated that the collaborative work will support consensus among the practitioners in our health care system to create, maintain, and monitor processes to prevent WSPs.

In June 2008 the World Health Organization (WHO) held the Second Global Patient Safety Challenge, Safe Surgery Saves Lives. The WHO Surgical Safety Checklist was launched, which will provide to surgical teams across the globe an international tool "to ensure that patients undergo the right operation at the correct body site, with safe anesthesia, established infection prevention measures and effective teamwork for safer care" (WHO, 2008).

STATEMENT OF THE PROBLEM AND IMPACT

The importance of a concerted effort to examine wrong-site procedures and the effects is substantiated by the fact that these are considered preventable adverse events. The NQF includes wrong-site surgery events on its list of serious reportable events, frequently referred to as never events. WSPs include wrong person, wrong side or site, wrong spinal level, wrong organ, wrong implant, wrong nerve block. These WSPs can occur in any area of the hospital or ambulatory setting; they are not limited to the surgical areas. The risks are also present in the procedural areas such as the cardiac catheterization laboratory or interventional radiology, procedures performed on patient units, in ambulatory care facilities, or in the physician's office, where more complex procedures are being performed routinely. Despite the ambitious efforts of many professional organizations, agencies, individual facilities, and practitioners to eliminate WSPs, the numbers have not declined. For example, The Joint Commission database recorded 88 wrong-site surgeries in 2005, compared with 116 in 2008 (TJC, 2009). WSP is the most frequently reported category of sentinel events, and communication is the number one area of risk (TJC, 2008).

In Pennsylvania all hospitals and ambulatory surgical centers are mandated to report wrong-site surgeries and near misses. From June 2004 through December 2006 there were 427 reports filed—253 near misses and 174 surgical interventions started on the wrong patient, procedure, side, or part. Eighty-three patients' incorrect procedures were carried out to completion (Clarke et al, 2007). This leaves the following questions: (1) Is reporting improving because secure, anonymous, and mandatory sites to facilitate reporting are provided and the punitive culture is changing, or is the number of cases actually increasing? (2) Are these incidents still being underreported? As we move forward toward a culture of safety in which we examine processes instead of punishing individuals, we have the potential for continued improvement in practice and reporting. However, it is obvious we have not eliminated WSPs.

RISK FACTORS FOR WRONG-SITE SURGERY

Inability to understand the full scope of the problem is not reason for inaction because many of these sentinel events are preventable. In addition, these occurrences are detrimental to the patient, the practitioner, and the organization. The patient initially appears to be the only victim with the possibility of emotional and/or a permanent physical injury or death. However, the practitioners take an oath to do no harm—there is an altruistic facet to their choice of profession, and causing harm to a patient can be devastating to the individual when the error is actually related to process or culture, thus creating another victim. The organization risks loss of trust not only from the patient, his or her family, and the community, but also from the practitioners depending on the culture in which the evaluation of the incident is completed. There are many who fall victim in potentially preventable adverse events.

Identification of risk factors for individual procedures can assist in development of preventive methods and herald particular circumstances or events that increase the potential for a WSP. The Joint Commission (2008) has identified multiple factors in its reviews of WSPs, including multiple surgeons involved in the procedure, multiple procedures being performed, time pressures, unusual patient characteristics, failure to involve the patient in identification of the correct site, poor communication among the perioperative team caring for the patient, and reliance solely on the surgeon for determining the correct site. Other contributing factors that could lead to a WSP include two patients with the same name, emergency procedures, morbid obesity, and unusual patient anatomy.

The American College of Surgeons targeted key high-risk processes from actual root cause analyses that related to WSP. Communication breakdown among team members and with the patient and family ranked highest. Cultural factors such as hierarchy and intimidation were included. The patient preparation process demonstrated issues with incomplete patient assessments, including not checking the medical record, x-ray films, and other reports. The procedure for preparation of the operating room illuminated numerous issues such as unavailable patient information, staffing levels and competency, resident supervision, lack of safety policies and protocols, and distractions, which included the various individuals' emotional and physical status and environmental influences. The surgical scheduling process was also mentioned (Manuel and Nora, 2004). When considering an electronic medical record system, the scheduler and the practitioners must be alert to inadequacies of the system that could support choosing the wrong patient or the wrong visit and thus transferring the current information to the wrong patient's chart. Also, all information coming from an outside source in any form needs to have the patient and information validated.

In their research of the literature and numerous databases to investigate prevalence of WSP, Seiden and Barach (2006) discovered many of the previous findings. The categories they chose to use were human factors such as personnel changes, workload, environment, and lack of accountability; patient factors involving sedation, confusion of the patient about his or her procedure; and procedural aspects related to room change for the patient before surgery, patient position changes, wrong site being prepped or draped, and lack of cross-checks. Incorrect specimen labeling has resulted in a procedure on a wrong patient. Removal from the room of patient stickers for labeling specimens must be completed at procedure end to ensure that the next patient's specimen is not labeled with the previous patient's information. If the pathology results require additional surgery, the wrong patient may fall victim to a WSP.

A discussion on potential barriers to implementation of the Universal Protocol is important because these barriers increase the possibility of risk. The author and other perioperative directors have seen negative first reactions by staff and surgeons concerning the possibility of increasing the workload and decreasing efficiency, which caused a lack of support. Surgeons were hesitant to move toward a standardized approach and "cookie-cutter" medicine; adaptation to the change in culture was slow. Some staff performed the time-out robotically, and the team performed under an assumption of safety. We also discussed diverse staff competency ranging from novice to expert nurses. This variance in competency and experience could create staff hesitancy to challenge the surgeons to do a time-out or question a possible error. These types of behavior are found throughout the literature, along with organizations that appear to put the cost or return-on-investment benefit before the quality and safety benefits. Each of these carries a level of risk for enabling processes, or lack of, that leave room for error.

Two other important considerations for risk in performance of WSP are (1) the pressure to produce and (2) environmental noise and distractions. The constant pressure for efficiency and decreased turnaround time may influence practitioners to take dangerous shortcuts that increase the potential for error. Just the hectic pace at the start of a procedure can have part of the team moving forward without the proper safety checks, such as the surgeon starting the incision before the time-out. Current operating room and interventional suites are frequently outfitted with music systems intended to provide a tranquil atmosphere, but, depending on the surgeon's choice of music and the favored genre of the other professionals, this could be a major aggravation or distraction. In addition to the music there are various alarms that cannot be silenced, numerous pagers and telephones that may need answering, suction, and smoke evacuators, all demanding the attention of the circulating nurse and accosting the ears and senses of the team. All of this takes attention away from the patient and the procedure at hand and leaves room for error.

Certain specialties are rising to the top of the risk list in the literature. Orthopaedic surgery appears to have a higher risk of WSP. As stated earlier, the AAOS has a long history of advocating prevention of WSP, which may affect increased reporting. Opportunities for lateralization errors and the higher volume of cases in orthopaedics may relate to the increased risk and percentage of WSP in orthopaedics (Cowell, 1998). An AAOS task force in their review of claims from 22 insurers found orthopaedic procedures accounted for 68% of WSP (Michaels et al, 2007). The Joint Commission (2008) reported 41% of wrong-site surgeries for orthopaedics in 2001. A survey of 1050 hand surgeons resulted in information that 21% admitted to one wrong-site surgery and that an additional 16% reported near misses. Most frequent locations were hand, wrist, and fingers (Meinberg and Stern, 2003).

The number and variety of possible areas of risk demonstrate that potentially every patient may be exposed to a WSP. Would this information not validate for every practitioner the need for preventive measures in every surgical and interventional arena?

STRATEGIES TO PREVENT WRONG-SITE PROCEDURES

Communication has been identified by The Joint Commission as the number one reason for medical errors. It would then seem fitting that many of the strategies that will be discussed revolve around some form of communication. Transitions or handoffs of the patient's care are areas of high risk for communication breakdowns. Improving teamwork and continuity of care in relation to these transitions, whether from nurse to nurse, physician to nurse, or patient to doctor, as examples, is addressed in Chapter 1 relative to patient safety.

Current tools and strategies being implemented across the world demonstrate increasing awareness of the issue of WSP and the need to come out of the climate of secrecy into a culture of acknowledgment of the error, learning from the investigation, developing creative methods for prevention, and sharing those so that no other patient has to suffer the same devastating events. Movement toward this culture change is not always fluid. Leadership is of extreme importance in creating and maintaining the metamorphosis in culture to eradicate preventable wrong-site procedures. It is obvious from the historical review that many key professional associations have stepped forward to lead the charge. Coming to consensus on criteria for the Universal Protocol was monumental. Administrative support from the individual health care institutions in the policy setting, education, marketing, roll out, and measurement of the quality improvement efforts to prevent WSP is imperative to success. This includes the medical, surgical, interventional, nursing, and allied staffs that are enlightened and can act as peer examples to lead the move to a culture of safety.

Communication Among Physicians

Robert Wachter, MD, speaks to the fact that providing data is useful, but telling error or near-miss stories is key to motivating practitioners to do things differently (Understanding patient safety, 2008). Using analogies from other industries such as the Aviation Safety Reporting System, National Aeronautics and Space Administration, Federal Aviation Administration, or Toyota's Six Sigma is not often convincing to physicians because they see health care as far more complex than flying an airplane or making an automobile. The system/process aspects of these high-reliability organizations may provide valuable insight into systems thinking, but selling them as the main campaign is difficult for physicians. Many physicians have never had a WSP or near miss and find it incomprehensible that this would happen to them. Encouraging well-respected clinicians to share their stories is compelling in creating understanding that a WSP can happen to even the most detailed physician.

Universal Protocol

It appears that the Universal Protocol made mandatory by The Joint Commission in 2004 is becoming the gold standard for processes to prevent WSP. The Universal Protocol, as discussed earlier, grew out of a summit of medical and surgical professional organizations representing a large portion of the practitioners and organizations that may be affected by and have the ability to prevent a WSP. Consensus was reached by this group on the creation of the Universal Protocol, which would facilitate a specific standardized approach to preventing WSP. The protocol contained many of the requirements found in the AAOS and NASS initiatives, but with further emphasis on verification processes, marking the site, and taking a time-out or final verification immediately before starting the procedure (TJC, 2007). Kwan et al (2006) analyzed data compiled from a large malpractice insurer between 1985 and 2004. More than 3 million surgical procedures were evaluated for wrong-site surgeries. Twenty-five wrong-site surgeries were found, not inclusive of spine surgeries. Ten of 13 charts reviewed demonstrated minor injury to the patient, 2 procedures resulted in temporary major injuries, and 1 patient was left with permanent injury. An interesting conclusion by the authors was that The Joint Commission's Universal Protocol might have prevented 8 of these wrong-site surgeries. The numbers in this example also demonstrate the difficulty in establishing rates for WSP.

Currently The Joint Commission, The Joint Commission International, and the World Health Organization (2007) are collaborating on the performance of correct procedure at correct body site issue. There is agreement that an organizational policy describing a standardized approach that correct procedures are consistently performed on correct patients needs be in place in the organization. An informed consent process is in place that advises the patient regarding all aspects of his or her care, including the proposed procedure, alternatives, risks, and benefits in language the patient can understand. Three other areas of agreement that are needed are a preprocedure verification, marking of the procedure site, and conducting a time-out, all aspects of the Universal Protocol.

Verification of Patient Information

As noted in the risks section, the process for preventing WSP should begin with the surgical scheduling of the patient's procedure. Important aspects to be considered for preciseness are the correct name of the patient; correct procedure with correct spelling; and, if laterality is involved, the side is spelled out as left or right, no abbreviations. With the new electronic medical record systems, ensuring that this is the correct person and the correct visit is very important. Other important information at this time would be any special considerations for this unique patient, such as latex allergy, morbid obesity, or special implants that would need to be ordered. This verification process of the correct person, procedure, and site should be a repetitive process, with the patient involved if possible, that follows the patient through the entire continuum of care—when admitted to the facility, before the patient leaves the preoperative area to go to the procedure or operating room, and as care is transferred between caregivers. Once the patient is in the surgical or procedure room, before beginning the procedure, relevant documentation is reviewed, and it is verified that images are labeled and on the viewer correctly or pulled up accurately electronically and that special equipment and implants are immediately available.

Marking the Operative Site

The second requirement of the protocol mandates marking the operative site. The unambiguous, indelible mark is to be placed at or near the incision site so it will be visible after preparation and draping. The intent is to have the person performing the procedure mark the site with the patient participating, awake and aware, if possible. The nonoperative site should not be marked, and the method of marking should be consistent across the enterprise. Single-organ cases do not require marking, but all cases involving laterality or multiple structures such as fingers, toes, lesions, or multiple levels of the spine should be marked. It is expected that in addition to the external spine level mark there should be special intraoperative radiographic techniques used to mark the exact vertebral level. Concern regarding sterility of the mark has been proved unfounded (Cronen et al, 2005).

Time-Out

The third requirement states that a time-out will be conducted immediately before starting the procedure. The time-out takes place in the location where the procedure will be completed, immediately before starting the procedure, and with the entire operative team actively involved. During this time-out the following are agreed on: correct patient, side, site, and procedure; patient position; and that the proper implants and equipment are available. If there is any discrepancy in the processes, there must be a policy and system to reconcile the differences (The Joint Commission, 2007).

Checklists

The process needs to be documented, and checklists are one of the strategies recommended to confirm that a comprehensive, consistent, effective preoperative verification process has been completed. Checklists also act as a good trigger for the practitioner to be sure that all criteria are completed and negating the need to depend on memory systems that can fail. An example is WakeMed Health and Hospitals' enterprise-wide checklist, which meets the 2009 Joint Commission Universal Protocol (Box 10-1). The checklist is used as a visual cue in every operating room and procedure area throughout the facility. This standardization of process reduces the risk for error and ensures standardization of the time-out process in all surgical and procedural areas, including the patient care units and clinics.

Examples of checklists are available in the literature and are frequently accompanied by discussions of implementation in addition to policies and other resources. An excellent article with numerous resources outlining implementation at the Children's Hospital in Boston could assist in development of policies, an education program, documentation suggestions, marketing, and measurement methods. This article has examples of both the preoperative assessment and the time-out checklist criteria (Norton, 2007). At the University of California, San Francisco Medical Center, Charlene Bennett, RN, MS, challenged her staff to come up with an acronym so the staff could remember the elements of the time-out. The staff came up with a creative, catchy acronym, APPLE PIE: ***A***ntibiotics, ***P***atient's name, ***P***rocedure, ***L***aterality, ***E***quipment, ***P***osition, ***I***mplants, ***E***veryone participates. The slogan "The Items for a Time-Out Are as Easy as Apple Pie" made remembering the elements easy and patient safety fun and was more likely to energize compliance (Bennett, 2007).

BOX 10-1 Universal Protocol Patient Safety Checklist

VERBAL VERIFICATION OF EACH SAFETY CHECK MANDATED BY EACH TEAM MEMBER

- Correct patient using two identifiers
- Correct procedure according to consent/medical record
- Correct physician(s) according to consent/medical record
- Correct side and site(s) are properly marked
- Correct patient position verified
- Relevant images and results are properly labeled and appropriately displayed
- Correct special equipment/supplies or implants are available
- Correct antibiotic or fluids for irrigation purposes
- Safety precautions based on patient history or medication use are verified
- Correct information documented on perioperative or procedural/medical record

OPERATIVE AREAS

- Correct medications within sterile field are labeled with name and dosage
- Correct preoperative antibiotics have been administered

Reprinted with permission from WakeMed Health & Hospitals, Raleigh, NC.

University of Massachusetts Memorial Medical Center in Worcester, Massachusetts, uses an electronic record that can create its own challenges for documenting the elements of a time-out verification. Their process involved using laminated cue cards to communicate the new process before implementing the one-page checklist that is completed by the circulating registered nurse. The electronic record contains all the elements, leaving no staff questions about what needs to be agreed on and documented as part of the permanent patient record (Hylka, 2006). The AORN tool kit, which can be accessed and downloaded at http://www.aorn.org, is another example of a checklist that includes sections for preoperative verification, marking the site, and time-out criteria. Posting checklists in the procedure room to act as a memory jogger relieves reliance on memory systems that often fail in the organized chaos of the operating/procedure rooms.

Preliminary findings from the Pennsylvania Patient Safety Reporting System demonstrated that in 16 in-depth queries about near-miss events and 6 wrong-site surgeries, all of the near-miss events used a checklist for documentation of the verification process, but only 4 of the 6 wrong-site events used a checklist. This is statistically significant per chi-square test and suggests that checklists have value in identifying risks in documentation variances that may lead to WSP (Pennsylvania Patient Safety Reporting System [PA PSRS], 2007).

An area that is problematic in complying with the Universal Protocol is procedures completed on the patient units. Lankenau Hospital in Pennsylvania developed a system in which the time-out checklist is attached to the specific instrument trays that would be used in procedures on the patient units. The Central Sterile Processing Department collaborated by placing the checklists and putting a bright green sticker with "time-out" on the cart where the trays are stored. These cues serve to identify the tray for a procedure needing a time-out, and the document becomes the written verification of the process. Lankenau has seen a decrease in bedside events related to WSP (Landmesser, 2007).

The WHO Surgical Safety Checklist (First Edition) and Implementation Guide can be accessed online. The WHO checklist combines some of the human factors of the brief and debrief through the sign in and sign out, team training with inclusion of introductions of all the participants, and assigned roles during the time-out. Surgical site infection considerations such as antibiotic prophylaxis and sterility indicator checks are also included. This checklist varies from the Universal Protocol checklist in that it is not as rigid and structured. In fact, it is intended that individual facilities or organizations will add or modify it to fit their practice. BryanLGH Medical Center has revised the WHO Surgical Safety Checklist to meet its needs and incorporated a section to assess the risk of fire into the time-out portion. Figure 10-1 shows the form; the back has lined space for the debriefing notes. The form is not part of the patient's chart, but is used as a quality improvement tool.

Several mechanisms are being used to reinforce the implementation of a time-out. The Methodist Hospital in Houston developed a bright-colored reprocessable tent with "time-out" printed boldly on it. This device is placed over the first instrument to be used in the procedure to stimulate team participation in and compliance with the Universal Protocol time-out. The hospital has achieved a 95% compliance rate (Charlton, 2004). A number of surgical supply companies have produced disposable scalpels with a cover that slides over the blade and handle with the words "time-out." Removing the sleeve is meant to trigger the verification pause. Some operating room staff keep the scalpel on the back table out of the reach of the surgeon until the time-out is completed.

The staff at Glenbrook Hospital in Illinois has found that scripting gives nurses who are not assertive communicators a tool they can rely on for consistency. They have developed a generic script that lays out the dialogue to verify the six elements of the Universal Protocol. This script has decreased the inconsistencies in the communication process and reduced the risk of errors in surgery (Bloomfield, 2006).

Another strategy is collaboration among hospitals in a geographic region to establish processes to meet the Universal Protocols elements as a community team. At three operative/invasive sites for WakeMed Health and Hospitals in Raleigh, North Carolina, the surgeons also practiced at two other regional competitor hospitals, REX and Duke Raleigh. The surgeons would frequently say that they did not have to do these processes at the other hospitals. This led the directors of surgical services at the five hospitals to come together and standardize the policies, procedures, and roll-out dates for the various stages of the Universal Protocol. It was very effective, and everyone continues to work closely to standardize as many practices as possible to facilitate safer, quality care to the community.

Technology as a Strategy

Technology has not taken a backseat to creating innovative methods to prevent WSP. Richard A. Chole, MD, believed a fail-safe marking system was needed. His invention involves a special wristband, marking pen, and CheckSite alarms. Once the site is marked, the special label on the pen is peeled off and placed on the wrist band. This label in place will block a signal emitted by a chip in the wristband, which is potentially activated as the patient proceeds into the operating room through the threshold fitted with the alarms.

If there is no label, the alarm sounds—it can be set for a gentle sound or a visual clue alerting the staff to the risk (Page, 2006). Another invention similar to the CheckSite system is a radio frequency identification (RFID) technology that encodes patient information on a SurgiChip, which can be electronically read by a handheld reader, thus verifying the correct information before the surgery commences (Tablac, 2007). No matter what process is put into place, the importance of having all practitioners (the surgical team) actively involved and centered on the individual patient and his or her needs to ensure a correct procedure cannot be overemphasized.

BryanLGH Medical Center
SURGICAL SAFETY CHECKLIST

Sign-In: Prior to induction of anesthesia

□ Site Marked □ Not applicable
□ Confirmed patient identity, site, and procedure
□ Anesthesia safety check completed
□ Does patient have:
□Yes □No Known pertinent allergies
□Yes □No Difficult airway
□Yes □No Risk of >500cc blood loss (7ml/kg in children)
□ Essential imaging displayed, implants, equipment □ Not applicable

Time Out: Prior to skin incision

□ Surgeon, nurse, anesthesia, surgical tech stop all activity and verbally confirm patient, site, procedure, position
□ Antibiotic prophylaxis given in last 60 minutes □Yes □No □ Not ordered □ Redosed
□ Essential imaging displayed, implants, equipment □ Not applicable
- Surgeon reviews: What are the critical or unexpected steps, operative duration, anticipated blood loss?
- Anesthesia team reviews: What are critical resuscitation plans, patient-specific concerns, if any?
- Nursing team reviews: What are the equipment issues, other patient concerns?

Alcohol-based prep solution had sufficient time to dry and for fumes to dissipate **Yes___ NA___**	YES	NO
Surgical site or incision less than or equal to 12 inches from oxygen		
Open oxygen source (patient receiving supplemental oxygen via any variety of face mask or nasal cannulas) (head and neck procedures)		
Available ignition source (e.g., electrosurgery unit, laser, fiber optic light source)		
Score: 3 = High risk; 2 = Low risk with potential to convert to high risk; 1 = Low risk; 0 = No risk/action required **Total Fire Risk Score**		

Fire Risk Score 1 to 2: Precautions implemented (mark all that apply)	**Fire Risk Score 3: Precautions implemented** (mark all that apply)
Fire Risk Score equal to 2, low risk with potential to convert to a level 3 risk (e.g., ET tube puncture, surgical intervention in thoracic cavity). Convert to high-risk precautions.	□Titrate deliverable oxygen to 30% or below □Observe prep drying times (minimum of 3 minutes) □Follow appropriate draping protocol (i.e., incise drape) □Use wet sponges □Have basin of sterile saline or water available for suppression purposes only □Greater than 50 ml saline available in bulb syringe/asepto on head and neck procedures □Protect heat sources (cautery pencil holster for electrosurgery, utilize standby mode or turn off heat source with fiber optic light source when not in use) □Minimize electrosurgery settings

FIGURE 10-1 BryanLGH Medical Center in Lincoln, Nebraska, version of the WHO Surgical Safety Checklist. (Reprinted with permission from BryanLGH Medical Center, Lincoln, Neb.)

Continued

Sign-Out: Prior to removal of surgical drape

Surgeon reviews with entire team:
- What procedure was done
- Important intraoperative events

Anesthesia professional reviews with entire team:
- Important intraoperative events
- Recovery plan

Nurse reviews with entire team:
- Instrument and sponge counts
- Specimen labeling (including patient name, copy of pathology report to ____________)
- Important intraoperative events/recovery plan

SIS# ____________ Signature/Date ____________

Record Confidential - The content of this document is related to improving patient care.

Non-EMR
Form 1087d (Rev.10/08)

Patient Sticker:

Debriefing:

____

FIGURE 10-1—cont'd

PERFORMANCE MEASUREMENT

As we move forward toward a culture of safety, there surfaces an increasing awareness of the need for proactive approaches to identifying potential risks, putting preventive measures into place, and evaluating the progress. How do we measure our goal of creating safe systems inside health care organizations and, even more specifically, creating safe practices at the clinical interface to prevent WSP?

Root Cause Analysis

One method of evaluating WSP is to learn from the error and prevent future risk. This can be done by investigating the root cause or the basic reason for the failure of the process through a root cause analysis (RCA). Dattilo and Constantino (2006) define the RCA as "the process of learning from consequences wherein health care providers take a step back and gain knowledge from near-misses, adverse events, or sentinel events in the operating room and all areas of healthcare" and a sentinel event as an "unexpected incident related to a system or process deficiency which leads to death or major enduring loss of function." These authors describe surgical events that become sentinel events including surgery on the wrong body part, surgery performed on the wrong patient, wrong procedure done on the wrong patient, and a surgical procedure performed at the correct operative site but at the wrong level such as in spine surgery.

A WSP RCA should include all participants directly or indirectly involved in the procedure, including surgeon, nurses, surgical technologists, anesthesia providers, managers, directors, vice presidents, the risk manager, and the safety officer. Even the patient and family perspective can reveal contributing factors. Administrators' participation is very important because these leaders have the authority to change systems and the environment to support the necessary improvements in the action plan. The perspective and perceptions of all players illuminate multiple processes and factors that affect disruption of the patient care process, which can potentially result in a WSP. Results of the RCA often do not find just one reason or breakdown that caused the WSP. The process involves using fishbone diagrams to map out the causes and effects related to the WSP. The Joint Commission (2005) has developed a root cause analysis matrix that maps out areas of inquiry for specific sentinel events. The following processes are not all-inclusive but are aspects to be considered in an RCA of a wrong-site procedure:

- Review of information received from the physician's office regarding the patient and procedure
- Consideration of patient identification and the process at every patient handoff
- Assessment of the patient in the preoperative area, including history and physical reassessment, review of the consent for surgery, and marking of the surgical site if applicable
- Intraoperative emphasis on preanesthesia and preincision time-out process
- Intraoperative briefing and debriefing processes if it is policy
- Review of availability of images displayed properly, implants, required equipment and instrumentation in proper functioning order
- Visibility of site marking after draping
- Count procedure and use of safe zone
- Staffing levels, orientation and training of staff, competency assessment/credentialing
- Communication with patient/family, communication among staff members
- Availability of information, and conditions of the physical environment
- Identification of any distraction, such as music, behavior, inappropriate traffic or interruptions

For each area of discovery an action plan is developed, responsible party identified, and implementation time frames set. It is important to allow each of the participants to describe his or her perceptions of the event because each viewpoint may bring different insights into the process failures. The outcome must be to reduce or eliminate the risk to patients in the future, and the mode of measuring this is elimination of WSP.

Universal reporting of medical errors and near misses is another suggested method of measuring improvement in WSP. It is expected that the system meet three basic principles: (1) it is anonymous, (2) it is not discoverable, and (3) it is not punitive. There are numerous reporting systems implemented throughout private and public establishments across the United States with the purpose of monitoring and evaluating the quality of health care. Andrus et al (2003) discuss many of the barriers to implementing such a program. "Error-reporter buy in" heads their list because they believe that "the completeness of any error-reporting process is directly proportional to all the critical elements of anonymity, nondiscoverability, a nonpunitive process and an individual's personal risk." Eliminating the risk is accomplished through a fourth principle of immunity for the committer and reporter of the errors. This principled process would also negate the ability of the patient's right to take legal action, a definite barrier. The authors see this as a practical solution to eliminate all disincentives to report, and they remind us that "error reporting should not be our goal, but only a means of learning from our shortcomings to help improve the future care of our patients."

Enterprise-Wide Policy or Procedure

There is a need for an enterprise-wide policy or procedure with the explicitly defined processes to meet the criteria in the Universal Protocol. Three things can be measured in relation to policy or procedure: (1) whether one exists, (2) staff's knowledge of the policy or procedure, and (3) whether it is being followed accordingly. Existence of the policy should be easy to evaluate, but one may want to examine the content to be sure it includes all aspects of the Universal Protocol criteria to prevent WSP and to determine if it is being used. When assessing use of the policy, direct observation ensures validity and measures both the use and practitioner knowledge. Medical record review can be done, but that is retrospective and only substantiates documentation, not necessarily practitioner knowledge, communication methods, or performance of the policy content. Direct observation provides the opportunity to identify risks introduced by the policy and to revise the policy based on provider feedback. The measurement tool should evaluate practitioner behaviors and knowledge and provide feedback (Michaels et al, 2007).

The Pennsylvania Patient Safety Reporting System (PA-PSRS) has demonstrated decreased frequency of wrong-site surgeries. This is a mandatory reporting structure for all hospitals in Pennsylvania to report wrong-site surgeries and near misses. In 2007 the PA-PSRS conducted an observation of site verification processes at six Pennsylvania facilities. The goal was to understand the variations in interpretation and implementation of the Universal Protocol and how they might relate to WSP. One or more steps were observed for 48 procedures. Significant variation in implementation of the Universal Protocol, as well as verification of information, site marking, and time-out procedures were noted. Noteworthy variations existed in all areas of the operative patient's journey. Both in these observations and in a previous retrospective analysis (Clarke et al, 2007) the wrong-site errors related to misinformation, which usually occurred preoperatively, or misperception, which occurred most frequently intraoperatively. In the retrospective study, incorrect information in preoperative documentation for surgery, schedule, consent, history, and physical resulted in 25 wrong-site procedures out of 155 reviewed, whereas misperception, right/left confusion, resulted in 45 wrong-site procedures. The observation study allowed for real-time information gathering. Breakdowns were noted with incorrect consents when secondhand information was used and when verification of the patient's information was completed with passive acknowledgments. Errors were noted when marking the site did not involve the patient or the mark was not consistent with all documents. Other issues developed when the patient was turned to position, resulting in left/right confusion, and with regional blocks when performed before a time-out was done. There was a correlation found between attention to checking inconsistencies in documents and finding wrong-site errors before the start of the procedure. The more frequently that independent checks were performed, the less opportunity for misinformation to reach the operating room and potentially harm the patient (PA PSRS, 2007).

Pronovost et al (2006a) focus on the fact that health care lacks a structured approach to evaluation of the progress being made in reducing the risk of events that cannot be measured in rates. WSP is one of these risk events. Measurement is an absolute necessity if we are to evaluate improvement. It remains one of the challenges in addressing the problem of WSPs because practitioners and organizations may conduct an internal in-depth evaluation and root cause analysis of the never event, but the results frequently remain private for fear of liability or media attention (Pronovost et al, 2006b). Without a reliable national database, understanding the scope of the problem of WSP is impossible. Without the following, we will not eliminate WSPs: (1) a culture of safety in which practitioners are provided a trusting environment with supportive processes for provision of patient care, (2) the confidence in the team that anyone can stop the process if there is a question of safety, and (3) a "just" response to error.

CONCLUSION

Wrong site, wrong patient, and wrong surgery are preventable events that continue to occur. Historical dealings with these mistakes frequently meant a search for the person to blame and shame. Current methodology demonstrates that often a break in the process or system has caused the error—not the people involved. This chapter examined the initiatives that professional associations and regulatory, private, and public institutions are putting into place to prevent events that should never happen to patients, practitioners, or facilities.

REFERENCES

American Academy of Orthopaedic Surgeons: *Advisory statement on wrong-site surgery*, available at http://www.aaos.org Accessed April 27, 2008.

Andrus CH, et al: "To err is human": uniformly reporting medical errors and near misses, a naive, costly, and misdirected goal, *J Am Coll Surg* 196(6):914, 2003.

Association of Registered periOperative Nurses: *Correct site surgery tool kit: building a safer tomorrow*, 2004. available at http://www.aorn.org Accessed April 25, 2008.

Bennett C: Timeout: it's easy as apple pie!, *OR Manager* 23(7):14, 2007.

Bloomfield C: Scripting for success, *AORN J* 83(5):1127–1128, 2006.

Brennan TA, et al: Incidence of adverse events and negligence in hospitalized patients: results of the Harvard Medical Practice Study I, *N Engl J Med* 324:370–376, 1991.

Canadian Orthopaedic Association Committee on Practice and Economics: *Position paper on wrong-sided surgery in orthopaedics*, Winnipeg, Manitoba, Canada, 1994, Canadian Orthopaedic Association.

Canale TS: Wrong site surgery: a preventable complication, *Clin Orthop Relat Res* 433:26, 2005.

Charlton N: Time out—the surgical pause that counts, *AORN J* 80(6):1121–1122, 2004.

Clarke JR, et al: Getting surgery right, *Ann Surg* 246(3):397, 2007.

Committee on Quality of Health Care in America: *Institute of Medicine: Crossing the quality chasm: a new health system for the 21st century*, Washington, DC, 2001, National Academy Press.

Council on Surgical and Perioperative Safety: Council on Surgical & Perioperative Safety core principles, available at http://www.cspsteam,org/education2.html Accessed May 14, 2008.

Cowell HR: Wrong-site surgery, *J Bone Joint Surg Am* 80:463, 1998.

Cronen G, et al: Sterility of surgical site marking, *J Bone Joint Surg Am* 87(10):2193–2195, 2005.

Dattilo E, Constantino RE: Root cause analysis and nursing management responsibilities in wrong-site surgery, *Dimens Crit Care Nurs* 25(5):221–225, 2006.

Gaba D, et al: *Crisis management in anesthesiology*, New York, 1994, Churchill-Livingston.

Hylka SC: Ensuring consistent time-out in a system, *OR Manager* 22(7):10, 2006.

Insights into preventing wrong-site surgery: PA-PSRS patient safety advisory: available at http://www.psa.state.pa.us Accessed May 14, 2008.

Kohn LT, et al: *To err is human: building a safer health system*, Washington, DC, 2000, National Academy Press.

Kwan MR, et al: Incidence, patterns, and prevention of wrong-site surgery, *Arch Surg* 141:353–358, 2006.

Landmesser S: A time-out tool helps improve compliance at the patient's bedside, *OR Manager* 23(12):15, 2007.

Manuel BM, Nora PF: *Surgical patient safety essential is information for surgeons in today's environment*, Chicago, 2004, American College of Surgeons.

Meinberg RG, Stern PJ: Incidence of wrong-site surgery among hand surgeons, *J Bone Joint Surgery Am* 85:193–197, 2003.

Michaels RK, et al: Achieving the national quality forum's "never events": prevention of wrong site, wrong procedure, and wrong patient operations, *Ann Surg* 245:527, 2007.

Norton E: Implementing the universal protocol hospital-wide, *AORN J* 85(6):1187–1197, 2007.

Page L: System marks new methods of preventing wrong-site surgery, *Mater Manag Health Care* 15(2):55–56, 2006.

Pennsylvania Patient Safety Reporting System (PA PSRS): Insight into preventing wrong site surgery, *Patient Saf Advis* 4(4):109, 112–123, 2007.

Pronovost PJ, et al: Tracking progress in patient safety: an elusive target, *JAMA* 296(6):696–699, 2006a.

Pronovost PJ, et al: A practical tool to learn from defects in patient care, *Jt Comm J Qual Saf* 32(2):102–108, 2006b.

Seiden SC, Barach P: Wrong-side/wrong-procedure, and wrong-patient adverse events: are they preventable?, *Arch Surg* 141:931–939, 2006.

Tablac A: *Doctor's invention aims to prevent surgical mishaps*, available at http://www.stltoday.com. Accessed November 5, 2007.

The Joint Commission: A follow-up review of wrong site surgery, *Sentinel Event Alert*, issue 24, 2001, available at http://www.thejoint commission.org. Accessed May 17, 2008.

The Joint Commission: *Root cause analysis matrix: minimum scope of root cause analysis for specific types of sentinel events*, October 2005, available at http://www.joint commission.org. Accessed June1, 2008.

The Joint Commission: Performance of correct procedure at correct body site, *Patient Safety Solutions* 1(4):2007, available at http://www.thejointcommission.org. Accessed May 12, 2008.

The Joint Commission: *Sentinel event statistics as of June 30, 2009*. June 30, 2009, available at http://www.jointcommission.org/NR/rdonlyres/241CD6F3-6EF0-4E9C-90AD-7FEAE5EDCEA5/0/SE_Stats_6_09.pdf. Accessed September 13, 2009.

The Joint Commission International Center for Patient Safety: Lessons learned: wrong site surgery, *Sentinel Event Alert* issue 6, 1998, available at http://www.jcipatientsafety.org/14791/. Accessed May 8, 2008.

The Joint Commission International Center for Patient Safety: *International patient safety goals created*, 2006, available at http://www.jcipatientsafety.org/show.asp?durki=11753. Accessed April 8, 2008.

Understanding patient safety: a Q&A with Robert Wachter, MD *Infection Control Today*, March 1, 2008. available at http://www.infectioncontroltoday.com/articles/understanding-patient-safety.html. Accessed September 14, 2009.

Wong D, et al: *Prevention of wrong site surgery: sign, mark and x-ray (SMaX)*, LaGrange, Ill, 2001, North American Spine Society. available at http://www.spine.org/smax.cfm Accessed April 27, 2000.

World Health Organization: *Safe surgery saves lives initiative*, June 25, 2008. available at http://www.who.int/patientsafety/challenge/safe.surgery/en/index.html Accessed May 7, 2008.

TO COUNT OR NOT TO COUNT

A Surgical Misadventure

Cecil A. King, MS, RN, CNOR, APRN

On August 1, 2007, in the Inpatient Prospective Payment System Fiscal Year 2008 Final Rule, the Centers for Medicare and Medicaid Services (2008) identified eight hospital-acquired conditions that are (1) high cost or high volume or both, (2) result in the assignment of a case to a diagnosis-related group that has a higher payment when present as a secondary diagnosis, and (3) could reasonably have been prevented through the application of evidence-based guidelines. The first item on that list is a foreign object retained after surgery. For discharges occurring on or after October 1, 2008, hospitals will not receive additional payment for cases in which one of the selected conditions was not present on admission. That is, the case will be paid as though the secondary diagnosis were not present. An unintended retained foreign body (RFB) has become one of the never events in an age in which both quality and efficiency are paramount and becoming more and more linked to pay for performance (Thomas and Caldis, 2007). This then begs the question as to whether or not the Association of periOperative Registered Nurses' (AORN's) "Recommended Practices for Sponge, Sharps, and Instrument Counts" can be considered an evidence-based guideline. Would the routine counting of surgical instruments have prevented leaving behind a 2- by 13-inch malleable retractor? How does one explain that error to the patient, the family, and the public when something this large and obvious is left behind (Figure 11-1)?

NORMALIZATION OF DEVIANCE

What happened in this case that predisposed it to an RFB? Two major patient safety issues became apparent during an internal claims closed-case review. One was the normalization of deviance, whereby there was a drift from the norm to the point that the deviance became the norm (Groom, 2006; Marx, 2008). People cut corners and drifted from the norm (e.g., counting of instruments) because until then nothing bad had happened. It was not the policy, nor was there a procedure in place at this facility for the counting of instruments (Thomas and Caldis, 2007). There was a generalized perception that instruments had never been left in patients at this facility; therefore the counting of instruments was not necessary. James Reason writes, that "All errors involve some kind of deviation. In cases of slips, lapses, and fumbles, actions deviate from the current intention" (Reason, 2005).

RISK FACTORS

There is a growing body of evidence demonstrating risk factors related to RFBs. Gawande et al (2003a), in an analysis of errors reported by surgeons at three teaching hospitals, found that one half to three quarters of adverse events are attributable to surgery and that more than 50% are preventable. The incidence of RFBs has been reported to be somewhere between 1 in 9000 and 1 in 19,000 surgical cases (i.e., 0.0001 to 0.00005), which may be translated to 1 or more a year within a large medical facility (Gawande et al, 2003b). Greenberg (2007) reported that a discrepancy may occur in about 1 out of 8 general surgery cases, with these discrepancies increasing the risk for an RFB. Given the risk and consequences related to RFBs and the fact that AORN's "Recommended Practices" (2008) represent "... what is believed to be an optimal level of practice (i.e., care)," the perioperative nurse has a professional duty and an inherent ethical and legal obligation to prevent harm such as an RFB.

LEGAL STANDARD OF CARE

The law requires only that unintentional foreign bodies not be negligently left in patients.

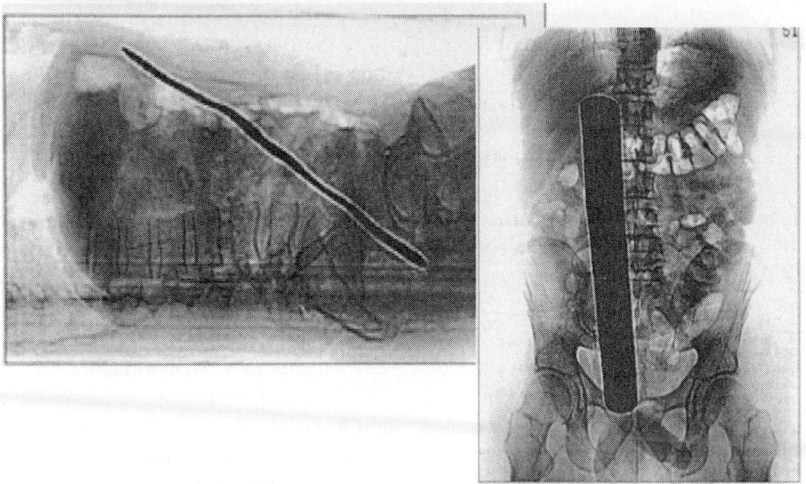

Figure 11-1 Retained malleable rectractor, 2001. (From King CA: To count or not to count: a surgical misadventure. *Perioperative Nurs Clin* 3(4):395–400, 2008.)

"The law does not prescribe how counts should be performed, who should perform them, or even that that they need to be performed" (AORN, 2008). It is the individual perioperative nurse's professional responsibility to act as a prudent nurse would under the same or similar circumstances. It would behoove the prudent perioperative nurse to seek direction from AORN's "Recommended Practices" (2008), which recommends that sponges, needles, instruments, and other items "… be counted on all procedures in which the possibility exists that [an item] could be retained." The employer is responsible for the employee's actions that are taken within the scope of his or her employment. Upon accepting employment, there is an implied agreement between the perioperative nurse and the employer that he or she will perform within the standard of care (i.e., standards of practice). The legal standard of care refers to what any prudent nurse with similar training, experience, or education would do in the same or similar situation. Failure to demonstrate this standard of care is considered negligence. The doctrine of res ipsa loquitur (the thing speaks for itself) applies to RFBs, rendering this sort of litigation almost indefensible (Aiken, 1998). In cases involving an RFB, the retained object presents as prima facie evidence of negligence. Before 1977 the surgeon may have been held ultimately responsible for an RFB under the captain-of-the-ship doctrine. However, in 1977 the Texas Supreme Court ruled in favor of the surgeon, *Sparger v Worley Hospital, Inc.*, 547 SW2d 582 (Tex 1977), refusing to apply the captain-of-the-ship doctrine by finding that the incorrect sponge count was the responsibility of the nursing staff and therefore the hospital (Iyer, 2001). Such a breach in one's duty to deliver the standard of care or the failure to act as a reasonable person would act in a similar situation falls into the category of an unintentional tort or negligence (Aiken, 1998). Although AORN is not a regulatory body and therefore AORN's "Recommended Practices" are not enforceable under the law, an individual's behavior is held up to that of the "Recommended Practices" because they are often cited as what a prudent nurse would do in the same or similar situation. Schroeter (2004) describes the perioperative nurse's ethical obligation as it relates to practice standards by stating, "Nurses must be able to act to ensure that safe, competent, legal, and ethical care is provided to all patients."

REVIEW OF THE LITERATURE

Kaiser et al (1997) studied the frequency of occurrence of retained surgical sponges by examining RFB insurance claims over a 7-year period. Forty-eight percent (n = 40) of this sample involved retained surgical sponges. A falsely correct sponge count was documented in 76% of the abdominal cases in this study. In 1996 the costs were reported at $2,072,319 in total indemnity payments and $572,079 in defense costs. In 3 of the 40 cases the surgeon was found guilty of negligence by the court despite the nursing staffs' admitted liability. In a retrospective study of 24 patients presenting with an RFB after abdominal surgery, Gonzalez-Ojeda et al (1999) reported that RFBs may occur at a rate of 1 in 1000 to 1500 open-abdominal procedures.

Risk Factors

Although there are upwards of 1300 published papers found when using the search term "retained foreign body, surgery" at the PubMed Web site, the first comprehensive study to identify risk factors for RFBs was undertaken between 1985 and 2001. It used a retrospective case-control methodology of reviewing the medical records associated with claims and incidence reports of RFBs. Gawande et al (2003b) concluded that the risk for an RFB significantly increases during emergency procedures, when there are unplanned changes in the procedure, and in patients with a significantly higher body mass index. In patients presenting with an RFB, it was less likely that a surgical count had been performed. Gawande et al recommended that using a counting process similar to AORN's "Recommended Practices," monitoring personnel's compliance with the process, and using radiologic screening of patients at high risk for RFBs are measures that may be implemented to prevent an RFB. Based upon projections of Gawande et al, the ratio of the number of radiographs it would take to detect an RFB is about 300:1 and very dependent on the quality of the film and expertise of the person reading the film. Yet the cost-benefit ratio is about $50,000 paid out in claims versus about $100 for the cost to obtain a plain radiograph to detect an RFB. Given the risk-benefit ratio to the patient, performing a plain radiograph to detect or rule out an RFB would seem a far more prudent practice than to do nothing at all.

SENTINEL EVENT

What happened in the case depicted in Figure 11-1 that contributed to leaving behind a malleable retractor? The superseding causal effect was the normalization of deviance, a cultural-sociologic phenomenon whereby individuals or teams repeatedly accept lower standards of performance until the lower standard becomes the norm. There was a prevailing attitude of complacency about counting instruments because "nothing has happened so far." We see this often in health care. Eventually the attitude that nothing has happened "yet" becomes the norm, and therein lies the danger (Groom, 2006). The facility in which this event occurred did not routinely count surgical instruments because "nothing has happened" and because the prevailing belief was that there were no data supporting the manual counting of instruments as a reliable method of prevention. "This again appears to substantiate the danger of not knowing what one does not know" (Rhodes, 2003). What was lacking was transparency and two-way communication between the risk management and claims departments and the management of the operating room (OR). What would become evident upon closer examination was that there was indeed a problem; the incidence of RFBs averaged about 1.8 per year at this facility.

Community Standard

A benchmark survey of the area hospitals and members of the University Hospital Consortium (UHC) was conducted to assess the community standard related to the counting of surgical instruments. This e-mailed survey has no scientific rigor, reliability, or validity and therefore should not be considered as evidence-based data. UHC was chosen as the comparative national benchmark because the event occurred at a major academic medical center and the investigator had access to the UHC perioperative staff e-mail directory. Of the 13 hospitals contacted within the urban area in which the incident occurred, 62% (8/13) counted instruments in cases as recommended by AORN. A much higher percentage, 95% (20/21) of academic medical centers responding to the survey reported counting instruments as outlined in AORN's "Recommended Practices." The largest response, 34, came from surveying AORN Member-Talk, an electronic interactive bulletin board. This indicated that of the 34 members responding, 82% (28/34) reported counting instruments according to AORN's "Recommended Practices." It was apparent that the community standard at both the local and national levels was to count instruments as outlined in the AORN's "Recommended Practices."

Institutional Incidence of RFB

The case referenced earlier (see Figure 11-1) received local and national media attention. The story, which focused on medical errors, and the patient's radiographs were published in the *New York Times*, and the patient appeared on the television program *Good Morning America.* It was discovered that over the course of 5 years the facility had experienced 9 RFBs, at a rate of 1.8 per year. A comprehensive evaluation of these cases was undertaken. Box 11-1 lists the commonalities identified in a closed-claims review of these cases.

ROOT CAUSE ANALYSIS

The myth that "nothing had happened yet" was dispelled, and work turned to focusing on eliminating barriers to performing instrument counts. The findings of the case-by-case analysis of the closed-claims cases was presented to a multidisciplinary quality improvement team, which performed a root cause analysis (RCA) of the case. The RCA identified the following factors as contributing to the RFB:

- Inappropriate procedure (i.e., not counting instruments on open-cavity procedures)
- Potential for interruptions and distractions
- Sets were too large, with 250 or more instruments

BOX 11-1 Commonalities of RFBs in Nine Cases Over 5 Years

SURGICAL SERVICES
4 Cardiothoracic
3 Gynecologic
2 General Surgery

CAVITY OF INVOLVEMENT
Thoracic or abdominal

OTHER FACTORS
6/9 Involved a retained instrument
5/9 Incision was after 13:00
6/9 Cased finished after 15:00
7/9 Occurred on a Thursday or Friday
3 (on average) changes in nursing personnel between counts
n = 9 (1996–2001)
Incidence rate: 1.8/year

- Lack of experience or competence
- Time of day
- Variations in instrument tray setups
- Variations in the process of counting
- Transcription errors: circulator forgot to document items added or removed from the field
- Lack of cooperation in the count process by the surgeons
- Lack of consistency in assigning staff breaks and handoffs when going on break

Performance Improvement Activities

Two immediate performance improvement (PI) activities were put into place. The first was to work toward standardization and streamlining of instrument sets to facilitate the counting process. The second was to conduct a direct observation of the more common procedures to identify those instruments that were used consistently and those that were rarely used. This provided the team leaders with important data as they met with their respective surgeons and team members in working to reduce the number of instruments in any given set. The departmental patient safety initiative was that no patient was to leave the hospital with a retrained surgical instrument, sponge, or needle. Therefore routine plain radiographs were obtained on all intracavity procedures while the instrument count process and education were being implemented. The following PI activities were put in place:

- Identify procedures requiring instrument counts
- Identify those sets needing reconfiguration
- Reconfigure and reduce the number of instruments per set
- Count instruments on all open-cavity procedures (e.g., chest, abdomen, pelvis)
- Revise surgical count procedure to reflect AORN's "Recommended Practices" (see Appendix A)
- Conduct demonstration and return-demonstration training and competency validation of counting process
- Limit phone calls into the room
- As they are scrubbed, surgeons (e.g., residents) hand off pagers to covering colleagues
- Implement one purposeful PI–risk management communication process
- Develop an interdisciplinary PI process
- Conduct a Failure Mode and Effects Analysis of the count process

In spite of the data supporting the need to implement the manual counting of instruments, it was met with resistance by some of the nursing staff and surgeons who felt it would impede the flow of the case and jeopardize patient safety. Two very important lessons were learned. The first was the impact of normalization of deviance on patient safety. The second was that, without transparency and open communication between the leadership in the OR and risk management (e.g., claims), there are missed opportunities for improvement because every miscount should be viewed as an opportunity for improvement. The danger lies in not knowing what you do not know.

ADJUNCT COUNTING TECHNOLOGY

Over the past 5 years, technologic advances such as bar coding, electronic article surveillance, and radiofrequency identification (RFID) have been applied to the problem of retained sponges. It is worth reiterating that most of these devices have focused on the detection of surgical sponges. Marcario et al (2006) reported 100% accuracy in the detection of tagged sponges using an RFID wand. These findings should be considered with caution given the small sample size (n = 8) and given the limitation associated with the RFID wand. This clinical trial raised important user issues, not unlike the traditional manual counting method: there is always the chance for operator error, and the user must know how to use the device correctly. For the scan to be done correctly it has to be performed farther than a few inches away from the skin, or the device will not read the entire area of the surgical site, and a retained sponge may be missed. Retained sponges could also be missed if the scan is performed too early (e.g., if additional sponges were placed in the wound during closure). An economic analysis of such a device is warranted to justify the additional cost of the device and tagged sponges. The average price for an RFID device is about $144 per case, in addition to the added labor cost and time.

Greenberg et al (2008) conducted a randomized controlled clinical trial to evaluate a computer-assisted method of counting bar-coded sponges. The bar-code method significantly increased the detection of misplaced and miscounted sponges. However, it is important to evaluate the effects of adjunct counting technology on workflow and personnel performance. Greenberg et al reported that the introduction of the bar-coding technology decreased perceived team performance and increased the time dedicated to the sponge count by about 3 minutes. However, by the end of the study, the majority of participants found the system easy to use, were confident in the system's ability to detect sponges, and reported an improvement in patient safety.

The emerging technologic surgical count devices should be developed and investigated in such a manner as to evaluate both their statistical and clinical significance in light of their clinical practicality. Cost should be included in these evaluations and compared with the cost of a count discrepancy as reported by Egorova et al (2008).

EVIDENCE-BASED PRACTICE

In January 2008 two important studies were published in the *Annuals of Surgery* (Egorova et al, 2008; Ponrartana et al, 2008) that finally provided satisfactory evidence suggesting which approaches were more efficacious in the prevention of RFBs. These studies recommended both policy changes and further research as follows:

The current manual counting process as outlined by AORN (2008) in the "Recommended Practices for Sponge, Sharps, and Instrument Counts" plays an important role in the detection of RFBs and should be used consistently. Egorova et al are the first to publish the efficacy of manual counting and reported a sensitivity of 77% and a specificity of 99%. Only 1.6% of the discrepant counts were actually associated with RFBs.

The potential for an RFB is increased 100-fold in the event of a discrepancy (Egorova et al, 2008).

Any time there is a discrepancy in the manual count, a radiograph should be obtained unless the needle is less than 10 mm in size (i.e., a suture of about 5–0 to 6–0) (Ponrartana, 2008).

The manual counting process can be detrimental in some circumstances (Dierks et al, 2005). Each facility should consider when it is in the best interest of the patient to abort the count (e.g., life-threatening emergencies), and a radiograph should be performed routinely before the patient leaves the OR (Egorova et al, 2008).

The routine use of a radiograph before the patient leaves the OR should be considered as an adjunct for all high-risk patients or during high-risk situations (e.g., unplanned change in the procedure, emergency, bariatric patients) (Gawande et al, 2003b; Gibbs et al, 2007).

Further studies to look at the counting process to determine the rate at which discrepancies occur are warranted. Although the projected incidence rates are low, they should be considered within the context that, for the most part, this information is obtained by voluntary reporting and there is a high probability that the incidence of RFBs is highly underestimated. The findings of Egorova et al (2008) suggest the incidence of RFBs is higher than previously thought.

CONCLUSION

An instrument or other surgical item left in the patient is a rare and yet devastating and preventable complication of surgery. Despite the increasing body of knowledge over the past decade, it has been difficult to quantify the frequency of this event and to validate that the manual counting process is an effective preventive method. The manual counting process has been shown to be labor intensive and to negatively affect the progress of the surgical procedure (Christian et al, 2006). Until now there have been no data supporting the accuracy and reliability of manual counting. With the publication of the work of Egorova et al (2008) and Ponrartana et al (2008) in the January 2008 issue of the *Annuals of Surgery*, we are able to better understand the utility of our current approach in the prevention of RFBs. As stated by Gibbs et al (2007), what is needed to further advance any patient safety effort

> *... is a committed management team, inclusive of the chief executive officer and the board of directors, and a dedication to supervision, an educational program within which roles, responsibilities, and expectations are reinforced with all staff, including physicians. A thorough prevention, detection, and correction process must be aimed at eliminating risk but focused enough to detect and then communicate throughout the organization any correction interventions to ensure prevention of a future event.*

REFERENCES

Aiken TD: Standards of care in legal nurse consulting: principles and practice. In Bogart JB, editor: *Legal nurse consulting: principles and practice*, Boca Raton, Fla, 1998, CRC Press.

Association of periOperative Registered Nurses: AORN recommended practices for sponge, sharps, and instrument counts. In Association of periOperative Registered Nurses: *Perioperative standards and recommended practices*, Denver, 2008, The Association.

Centers for Medicare & Medicaid Services: *Hospital-acquired conditions*, available at http://www.cms.hhs. gov/HospitalAcqCond/06_Hospital-Acquired%20 Conditions.asp#TopOfPage. Accessed June 29, 2008.

Christian CK, et al: A prospective study of patient safety in the operating room, *Surgery* 139:159–173, 2006.

Dierks MM, et al: Healthcare safety: the impact of disabling "safety" protocols, *IEEE SMC Trans A: Syst Hum* 34:693–698, 2005.

Egorova NN, et al: Managing the prevention of retained surgical instruments. What is the value of counting? *Ann Surg* 247(1):13–18, 2008.

Gawande AA, et al: Analysis of errors reported by surgeons at three teaching hospitals, *Surgery* 133(6):614–621, 2003a.

Gawande AA, et al: Risk factors for retained instruments and sponges after surgery, *N Engl J Med* 348(3):229–235, 2003b.

Gibbs VC, et al: Preventable errors in the operating room: retained foreign bodies after surgery—part I, *Curr Probl Surg* 44(5):325–329, 2007.

Gonzalez-Ojeda A, et al: Retained foreign bodies following intra-abdominal surgery, *Hepatogastroenterology* 46(26):808–812, 1999.

Greenberg CC: A prospective study of OR counting protocol, *J Am Coll Surg* 205(3S):S73, 2007 (abstract).

Greenberg CC, et al: Bar-coding surgical sponges to improve safety: a randomized controlled trial, *Ann Surg* 247(4):612–616, 2008.

Groom R: Normalization of deviance: rocket science 101, *J Extra Corpor Technol* 38(3):201–202, 2006.

Iyer PW: *Nursing malpractice*, ed 2, Tucson, Az, 2001, Lawyers and Judges Publishing.

Kaiser CW, et al: The retained surgical sponge, *Ann Surg* 224(1):79–84, 1997.

Marcario MD, et al: Initial clinical evaluation of a handheld device for detecting retained surgical gauze sponges using radiofrequency identification technology, *Arch Surg* 141:659–662, 2006.

Marx D: *Patient safety and the "Just Culture": a primer for health care executives*, April 17 2001. available at http://www.mers-tm.net/support/Marx_Primer.pdf. Accessed June 29, 2008.

Ponrartana S, et al: Accuracy of plain abdominal radiographs in the detection of retained surgical needles in the peritoneal cavity, *Ann Surg* 247(1):8–12, 2008.

Reason J: Safety in the operating theatre—part II, *Qual Safe Health Care* 14:57, 2005.

Rhodes RS: Invited commentary: analyzing adverse medical events—it's the system, *Surgery* 133(6):625, 2003.

Schroeter K: Unit 3: patient advocacy. In *Ethics in perioperative nursing practice*, Denver, 2004, Association of periOperative Registered Nurses.

Thomas FG, Caldis T : Emerging issues of pay-for-performance in health care, *Health Care Financ Rev* 29(1):1–4, 2007.

ANESTHESIA AND PERIOPERATIVE SAFETY

Deborah Dlugose, RN, CCRN, CRNA

Safety is the most important consideration in anesthesia care. The risk for death associated with anesthesia care has diminished greatly during the past 50 years. In *To Err Is Human*, the landmark publication that ignited the twenty-first century health care safety revolution, the authors specifically recognize the pioneering role of anesthesiology in advancing patient safety by a dedicated and consistent professional action program (Kohn et al, 2000).

Although each team member in perioperative care has specific profession-related goals, everyone is also invested in the anesthesia provider's patient commitments: maintenance of airway, breathing, circulation, and other physiologic parameters; provision of analgesia, sleep, and amnesia; and optimizing anatomic and physiologic conditions for the surgeon's work. Safety issues become more complicated by factors such as individual patient variability, complex medical and surgical conditions, defined institutional processes, and anesthesia-unique complications. Orkin and Longnecker (2008) relate about 75% of risk to patient-specific characteristics, including age, gender, and comorbidities; surgical issues account for 20% of risk; and 5% of risk is assigned directly to anesthesia-related factors.

With shared commitment to safety, everyone in the operating room (OR) is a member of the anesthesia care team. Complete safe care of the surgical patient cannot be separated from the anesthesia care. Anesthesia providers rely on other team members to help prevent certain complications and to assist with treatment of others. Knowledge about selected anesthesia complications and ongoing communication with anesthesia providers are essential components of perioperative safety. The different vantage point of perioperative nurses in the surgical environment, as well as sharply honed nursing skills and professional intuition (Benner and Tanner, 1987; Rovithis and Parissopoulos, 2005), also link them to the anesthesia team as communicators, patient advocates, resource providers, and hands-on colleagues.

Anesthesia providers, perioperative nurses, surgeons, and other team members share responsibility for many safety protocols and issues. Some of these include positioning, infection control, fire safety, latex allergy, electrosurgery safety, thermal support, and the Universal Protocol/Time Out for Patient Safety. These topics are addressed in other chapters of this book; their importance binds everyone together on the perioperative continuum.

Anesthesia care always has potential for disaster. Anesthesia providers deliver potent medications, interfere with breathing, alter physiology, and perform invasive procedures, often on patients with serious underlying medical and surgical problems, using sophisticated equipment and supplies. There is little or no margin of error. Quick intervention may be necessary, sometimes to the point of full resuscitative efforts. Vital sign changes, airway problems, major bleeding, or other serious intraoperative events sometimes require skilled assistance from other perioperative team members. Although the most serious anesthesia complications are very rare, it is important for the entire team to be prepared for them, just as airline, submarine, and space crews prepare for disasters. The goal of anesthesia care must be to ensure that no patient is harmed (Cooper and Longnecker, 2008). We must constantly remind ourselves that as anesthesia safety has improved during past decades, complacency and overconfidence are frequently our companions. Consider the analogy of Captain "Sully" Sullenberger's safe landing of a large airliner on the Hudson River on January 16, 2009, with no loss of life to 155 passengers, after a bird strike caused complete engine failure (McFadden,

2009). Only a truly well-prepared team with disaster training and a strong leader could manage such a dramatic event. Like Captain Sullenberger and his crew, the perioperative team must be fully prepared for disasters we hope not to experience.

This chapter provides an overview of anesthesia care with an emphasis on selected complications and safety issues that may require perioperative team action. This knowledge will increase the ability of perioperative nurses to assist in minimizing anesthesia-related complications and to maximize team action when unforeseen complications occur. All team members may be required to participate when anesthesia providers must handle complications with rapid assessment, quick prioritization, and immediate intervention. This teamwork challenge may be magnified by the multiple responsibilities carried by perioperative nurses.

The foundation for anesthesia patient safety begins with preanesthetic assessment and planning for each patient, with anesthetic strategy tailored to individual patient needs as well as surgeons' and institutional requirements. That discussion is beyond the scope of this chapter, yet it lies behind every patient's safe care: anticipation of potential problems, planning how to avoid them, and intervening appropriately if problems arise despite best efforts. Some of this preplanning must be closely coordinated between anesthesia providers and perioperative nurses (e.g., latex allergy, unusual blood type). Ideally, potential anesthesia issues should be shared at the time-out before the procedure's beginning; unfortunately, some anesthesia complications arise in an unforeseen manner after procedures are underway.

TYPES OF ANESTHESIA

Although general anesthesia comes first to mind, anesthesia providers deliver a wide spectrum of other techniques, ranging from local anesthesia (with or without sedation and analgesia) to peripheral nerve blocks to central neural blocks (spinal or epidural). Combination techniques may be used for some procedures. Perioperative nurses and team members may assist with any of these techniques at selected points. Significant complications may arise with any anesthetic technique.

General Anesthesia

General anesthesia uses a variety of techniques in which unconsciousness is induced to provide hypnosis (sleep), amnesia (memory loss), and immobility. General anesthesia agents also have significant side effects (and potential complications) on all major body systems. Thus anesthesia providers delicately balance beneficial dosages against side effects and complications, in the dynamic scenario of surgical actions and physiologic responses.

Most commonly, general anesthesia is delivered by an inhalational agent such as desflurane, sevoflurane, or isoflurane, which are liquid agents vaporized in the anesthesia machine. The vaporized agent molecules are delivered to the patient's lungs on carrier gases (oxygen, nitrous oxide, medical air, or some combination) via face mask, endotracheal tube, or laryngeal mask airway (LMA). Although various inhalational agents have been used for about 160 years, the exact mechanism by which they cause general anesthesia when they reach the brain is unknown.

Intravenous narcotics, neuromuscular blocker drugs, and other adjuncts such as antiemetics, antibiotics, and steroids may also be provided. General anesthesia may also be delivered completely as total intravenous anesthesia (TIVA) in selected situations, such as known or suspected malignant hyperthermia, when inhalational agents must be avoided.

Anesthesia providers carefully titrate all medications and agents throughout the anesthetic course, based on information from the patient's vital sign monitors and the surgical field, as well as knowledge of physiology and pharmacology. The anesthesia provider is the most important monitor; all of the machines are simply extensions of the individual's ability to gather information about the patient's physiologic status. As technology has advanced, sophisticated monitoring devices have increased our assessment ability. However, safe anesthesia care requires vigilant prepared human providers with engaged brains. In the event of serious complications or crises, support from other anesthesia providers and perioperative team members is necessary.

Induction and Emergence

Induction of anesthesia may be one of the most taxing times for anesthesia providers, with multiple crisis opportunities in this brief period, much like the takeoff of an airliner. Although this challenging period coincides with the perioperative nurse's own demanding responsibilities at the beginning of the case, true commitment to patient safety requires that anesthesia providers have hands-on colleagues available to assist in case of difficulty. If another anesthesia provider is available, the perioperative nurse should still maintain vigilance on the induction situation, in case even more help is needed.

As surgery starts, the anesthesia provider's goal is to match the anesthetic level to the surgical situation, delivering appropriate amounts of medications as surgical stimuli wax and wane, as well as handling physiologic reactions that may result from underlying disease or from drug interactions. All doses are titrated exactly to the individual patient and the surgical moment; there are no standard "cookbook" anesthesia recipes. Although it may appear that identical anesthetic courses are delivered to various patients, decisions are actually matched to individuals and circumstances. Although perioperative team members may assume that "nothing is happening" during a quiet anesthesia period as uncomplicated surgery progresses, the anesthesia provider is gently adjusting medications, fluids, and techniques for smooth maintenance as well as a timely emergence at the end of surgery. Although smooth anesthesia maintenance (like a smooth airline flight) is everyone's goal, development of any of the complications reviewed in this chapter (and others) will rapidly shift the anesthesia provider into a high-activity mode. The whole team may be called into assistance, including surgeons, perioperative nurses, and ancillary personnel.

As surgery draws to an end, the anesthesia provider starts the process of emergence, much as an airline captain starts final descent. The anesthesia provider takes multiple steps that aim to awaken the patient very shortly after the dressing is placed, in stable condition, ready for transport to the postanesthesia care unit (PACU). Reduction of percentage of inhalational agent, reversal of neuromuscular blockade, and return to 100% oxygen (with agent finally turned off) bring the patient back to consciousness, with strong spontaneous breathing, strong protective airway reflexes (cough, gag, swallow), excellent muscle strength (indicated both by peripheral nerve stimulator and motor activity), as well as the ability to follow commands, which confirms return of higher brain function. At this point the trachea may be extubated or the LMA removed after oropharyngeal suction, with face mask oxygen immediately applied. Every step in this process has profound safety implications because significant crises can easily arise during emergence, just as problems may arise during airline landings. Some of these potential crises will be discussed later.

In this emergence period, perioperative nurses are also taxed with end-of-case responsibilities, yet first allegiance to patient safety requires presence and engagement during the emergence process. Besides increasing safety, participation with anesthesia providers during the most critical parts of anesthesia care increases the ability of perioperative nurses to provide meaningful reports to the next registered nurse (RN) in the PACU or the intensive care unit. A structured communication tool such as the SBAR (***s***ituation, ***b***ackground, ***a***ssessment, ***r***ecommendation) report developed by the Institute for Healthcare Improvement (2009) and adapted by others allows coherent organization of the information to be transmitted. Although anesthesia providers deliver the full anesthesia care report, the perioperative nurse's responsibility for the whole patient should include a brief description of the anesthetic course, especially if there were untoward events or crises. Reports that focus only on surgical drains, dressings, and names of procedures diminish the role of the perioperative nurse as a professional participant in whole-patient care. Communication and interaction among the anesthesia provider, surgeon, and perioperative nurse during events of the procedure are then summarized at the end-of-procedure sign-out, as recommended by safety groups such as the World Health Organization (2008).

Transport from OR to the next unit requires supplemental oxygen and—for some patients—hemodynamic monitoring. Whether or not perioperative nurses accompany patients to the next unit, nursing care should be finalized with brief, clear communication and documentation of the anesthetic course, surgical procedure, and nursing-related concerns.

Safety and General Anesthesia

Safety issues for general anesthesia may be related to anesthesia techniques, patient variability, underlying medical conditions, and surgical situations. This section will review some of the most common acute perioperative safety concerns.

Airway Problems

Airway maintenance is paramount. Many airway issues are only mildly complicated. Anesthesia providers may cope with patient anatomy that creates difficult mask ventilation or difficult intubation, but both may be achieved without danger, often with the help of other team members and airway adjuncts, such as oral airways, nasal airways, LMAs, various laryngoscopes, and videolaryngoscopes.

However, despite best efforts, complete inability to oxygenate and ventilate a patient by any means may occur, creating a "lost airway." This critical airway situation requires the full attention of everyone in the operating room because nothing else matters if the airway is lost. Failure to deliver oxygen and remove carbon dioxide from organs and tissues will quickly result in serious injury to tissues and organs, followed by death (Hagberg et al, 2005). As technology, training, and crisis anticipation have improved during recent decades, deaths associated with airway problems at induction have decreased. However, difficult airway problems during maintenance, emergence, and recovery have not decreased. (Peterson et al, 2005).

The American Society of Anesthesiologists (ASA) has developed *Practice Guidelines for Management of the Difficult Airway* (Figure 12-1). As part of the ASA Difficult Airway Algorithm, anesthesia providers aim to avoid problems with careful preanesthetic assessment to allow safe planning for potentially difficult airways identified in advance (ASA, 2003).

The Mallampati classification of oral opening (Mallampati, 1983) has become well established as one of the simplest elements of airway evaluation, although it is not a stand-alone assessment. Perioperative nurses should be familiar with the Mallampati classification for their own planning at the beginning of a case when word arrives of a patient with a class III or class IV airway, or if they participate in preoperative evaluations themselves (Figure 12-2). Preliminary airway evaluation has moved into the realm of nursing practice (Odom-Forren and Watson, 2005).

Some other conditions that may be associated with difficult intubation and airway management include obesity; obstructive sleep apnea (OSA); inadequate neck extension related to arthritis, ankylosing spondylitis, or fusion; tumors; epiglottitis; neck abscesses; postoperative hematomas; airway trauma; and foreign body. The classic difficult airway, often associated with obesity and obstructive sleep apnea, includes a short thick neck, large tongue, and generous submandibular tissue, which reflects redundant tissue in the oropharyngeal and laryngeal areas. Prominent upper incisors ("buck teeth") and receding mandible also make laryngoscopy difficult. Men with full beards may be difficult for mask ventilation, although not necessarily for intubation, unless it is discovered that the beard was grown to disguise an anomaly such as an extremely receding mandible.

The results of preanesthetic airway evaluation are not completely reliable. Occasionally an airway that has been deemed easy by examination parameters results in unanticipated difficulty; conversely, a planned difficult airway may turn out to be surprisingly easy to manage. However, most anesthesia providers experience that classic predictors of difficult airway management are usually true, and conservative action is the standard of care. Knowledge of a difficult airway allows planning for safe management to secure the airway, often with techniques such as awake, sedated fiberoptic-assisted intubation after topical local anesthetic (LA) has been applied to the mucosa of the airway to reduce gag and cough reflexes. Recent introduction of videolaryngoscopes to clinical practice has improved ability to visualize airway structures in many patients whose intubation pathways in the past may have included fiberoptic-assisted technique. However, the videolaryngoscope is only a major step forward in safety, not a guarantee for every patient airway.

Unanticipated difficult airway management may arise from several situations, such as difficult tracheal intubation despite preoperative evaluation deemed adequate; oversedation during a planned "awake" intubation; unrecognized esophageal intubation; airway obstruction by laryngospasm or edema; postoperative bleeding in neck surgery; tumor; vomitus or foreign body; or failure to establish a surgical airway quickly when conventional airway maneuvers fail. It is important to note that patients with OSA have a high incidence of difficult intubation and that patients with difficult intubations have a high incidence of sleep apnea (F. Chung et al, 2008). OSA patients require extra care and planning both for airway management and for their increased postoperative risk for easy oversedation with analgesics (ASA, 2006b). Many cases have been reported of postoperative hypoventilation

1. Assess the likelihood and clinical impact of basic management problems:
   A. Difficult ventilation
   B. Difficult intubation
   C. Difficulty with patient cooperation or consent
   D. Difficult tracheostomy

2. Actively pursue opportunities to deliver supplemental oxygen throughout the process of difficult airway management

3. Consider the relative merits and feasibility of basic management choices:

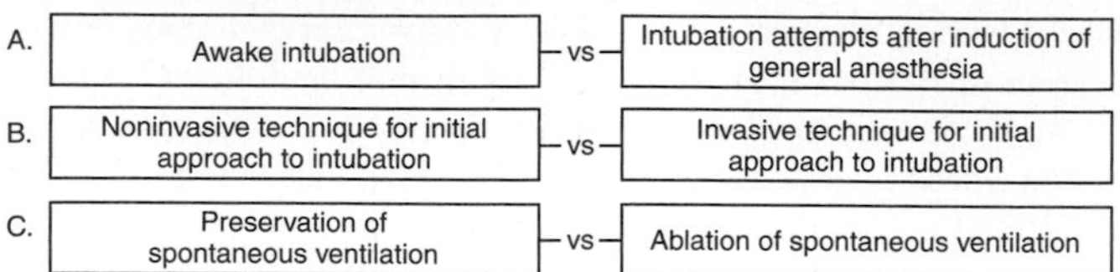

4. Develop primary and alternative stategies:

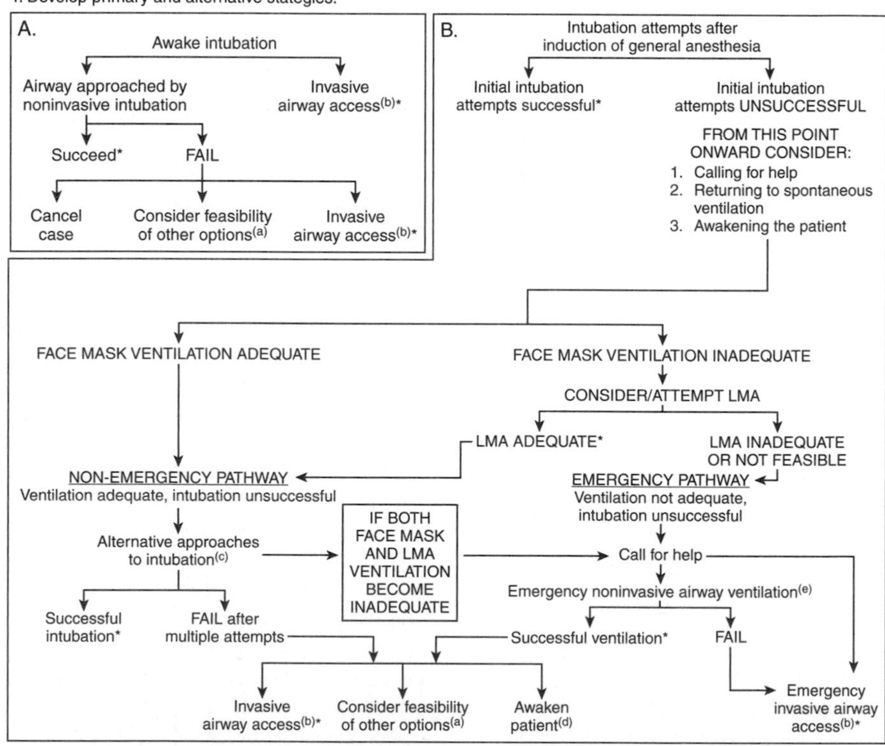

*Confirm ventilation, tracheal intubation, or LMA placement with exhaled CO_2

a. Other options include (but are not limited to) surgery utilizing face mask or LMA anesthesia, local anesthesia infiltration, or regional nerve blockade. Pursuit of these options usually implies that mask ventilation will not be problematic. Therefore, these options may be of limited value if this step in the algorithm has been reached via the Emergency Pathway.
b. Invasive airway access includes surgical or percutaneous tracheostomy or cricothyrotomy.
c. Alternative noninvasive approaches to difficult intubation include (but are not limited to) use of different laryngoscope blades, LMA as an intubation conduit (with or without fiberoptic guidance), fiberoptic intubation, intubating stylet or tube changer, light wand, retrograde intubation, and blind oral or nasal intubation.
d. Consider re-preparation of the patient for awake intubation or canceling surgery.
e. Options for emergency noninvasive airway ventilation include (but are not limited to) rigid bronchoscope, esophageal-tracheal Combitube ventilation, or transtracheal jet ventilation.

FIGURE 12-1 The American Society of Anesthesiologists (ASA) Difficult Airway Algorithm. (From ASA Task Force on Management of the Difficult Airway: Practice guidelines for management of the difficult airway: an updated report, *Anesthesiology* 98:1269–1277, 2003.)

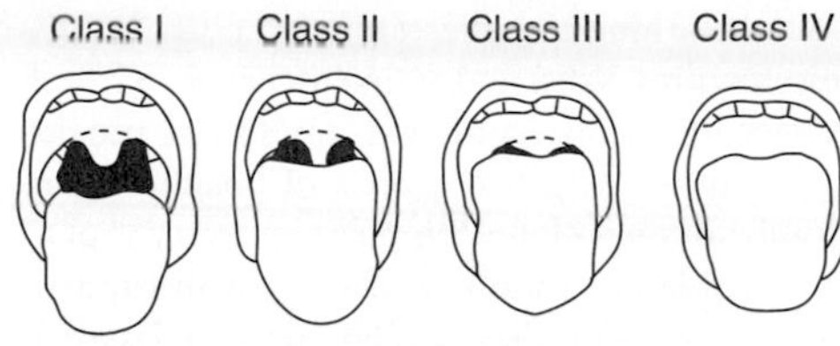

FIGURE 12-2 Modified Mallampati classification of pharyngeal structures. *Class I,* Soft palate, tonsillar fauces, tonsillar pillars, and uvula visualized. *Class II,* Soft palate, tonsillar fauces, and uvula visualized. *Class III,* Soft palate and base of uvula visualized. *Class IV,* Soft palate not visualized. (From Samsoon GL, Young JR: Difficult tracheal intubation: a retrospective study, *Anaesthesia* 42:487–490, 1987.)

or respiratory arrest in OSA patients with emergency treatment ending up with a difficult-to-impossible airway by providers unfamiliar with appropriate airway rescue techniques. Although the serious nature of obstructive sleep apnea is recognized by anesthesia providers (S.A. Chung et al, 2008), it is important for all team members to understand its acute and chronic implications.

Any difficult airway situation quickly requires help from other team members. Everyone in the operating suite should know the exact location of the difficult airway cart, what to unplug to transport it to the bedside, and what its various components include. Perioperative nurses provide valuable leadership in this process as well as hands-on skill for assistance with mask-ventilation, airway suction, cricoid pressure, opening and testing of airway devices, and documentation of events, medications, vital signs, and times during an airway crisis.

Familiarity with airway techniques such as LMA, intubating laryngeal mask airway (ILMA) (Liu et al, 2008), lightwands (Massó et al, 2006), and videolaryngoscopes allow perioperative nurses to assist anesthesia providers with airway rescue attempts and to document these techniques appropriately. Although such documentation may not be part of formal perioperative nursing notes, they may be considered analogous to Code Blue records; even informal notes and times can be helpful to the anesthesia provider who must later create a detailed report of the crisis.

Difficult Airway Classification. If intubation cannot be achieved, but oxygenation and ventilation can be maintained by face mask or LMA, the airway is classified as difficult. However, if the situation deteriorates to the situation of "cannot ventilate (by mask/LMA) and cannot intubate," the airway is declared lost. The clock is ticking as oxygenation falls, CO_2 rises, and tissue and organ damage become imminent.

The steps for handling such a crisis are outlined in the ASA Difficult Airway Algorithm (ASA, 2003). Although perioperative nurses do not perform airway rescue, they must be familiar with basic knowledge of the algorithm's steps. With the possibility that movement through the algorithm's steps may fail to secure the airway by various endotracheal intubation techniques, perioperative nurses must anticipate and prepare for a rapid surgical airway.

The decision for an immediate surgical airway (cricothyroidotomy or tracheostomy) cannot be delayed; worsening hypoxemia and hypercarbia that occur with a lost airway may lead to cardiopulmonary arrest. Full advanced life support should be anticipated before it is needed. Concurrent airway rescue and advanced cardiac life support may be required.

Any airway difficulty at the beginning of a procedure sets the stage for extra caution at the end of the procedure, when extubation is considered (and may possibly be delayed for safety reasons). Premature extubation in a difficult airway patient may result in a repeat difficult airway situation, with chance of rescue reduced the second time around, because of airway edema, trauma related to prior attempts, or intrinsic pathologic conditions such as obstructive sleep apnea (Isono, 2009). The airway danger during this period cannot be minimized. Fully awake extubation in the sitting position is mandatory; some suggest extubating over an airway exchange catheter, which is left in the trachea as a conduit to allow rapid blind reintubation if deterioration occurs (Mort, 2007). Transfer planning, documentation, and nursing report must emphasize the critical airway status, which may overshadow an uncomplicated surgical course.

Patients who have had a difficult airway experience should be notified in writing, including a description of what technique finally worked to secure the airway. There is also a Medic-Alert Registry for Difficult Airway.

Dental Injury

Dental injury is one of the most common anesthesia complications (Hagberg et al, 2005).

All patients should be advised of this risk before anesthesia care, personalized to their own dental status (Anderson and Abbey, 2008). Perioperative nurses should be aware of dental status, as well as dental prostheses. However, every anesthesia provider has anecdotes about dental prostheses discovered after induction of general anesthesia, related to patient's denial of appliances, staff overlook of prostheses, or some combination of circumstances.

Teeth are easily damaged during airway manipulation and laryngoscopy, particularly when loose or in poor condition as a result of periodontal disease or caries. Although most patients with poor dentition seem to show minimal concern with tooth loss during airway manipulation, a dislodged tooth that tumbles into the airway creates danger by airway obstruction. To prevent this problem, the anesthesia provider may deliberately remove a very loose tooth just before laryngoscopy; it must be properly labeled in a specimen cup for the patient. A tooth that is unintentionally loosened and falls down the airway must be retrieved by bronchoscopy or esophagoscopy. Young children with loose teeth should have any removed teeth saved both to protect their airways and to provide to parents or guardian.

Even smooth endotracheal intubation technique may elicit physiologic complications related to patient comorbidities. Hypertension, dysrhythmias, or myocardial ischemia may be provoked by the sympathetic stimulation of laryngoscopy and intubation. Patients with poor respiratory status may develop hypoxemia and/or hypercarbia, as well as laryngospasm and bronchospasm. Increased intracranial pressure and increased intraocular pressure from the stimulus of laryngoscopy are serious concerns for neurosurgical and ophthalmology patients. Tissue damage to lips, tongue, uvula, vocal cords, esophagus, or other laryngeal structures is always possible. Cervical spine or temporomandibular joint injuries may also occur during airway manipulation. Some of these complications may be readily evident and serious enough to cause cancellation of surgery (e.g., myocardial ischemia); some may be noted later with minor effect (e.g., postintubation sore throat); and some may be noted later with potentially critical results (e.g., esophageal tear).

Breathing Problems

The patient with a clear and patent airway (natural, endotracheal tube, or tracheostomy) may risk other breathing complications. Successful breathing requires satisfactory maintenance of both oxygenation and ventilation. Anesthesia providers monitor these two aspects of breathing very closely: oxygenation with pulse oximetry (SpO_2) and ventilation (removal of CO_2) with capnography. Every anesthesia technique has risks that could interfere with oxygenation, ventilation, or both (Morgan et al, 2006).

In some situations, difficulties with falling oxygenation may be temporarily overridden by increasing oxygen flow to the patient while ascertaining the problem's source. Although every operating room denizen is familiar with loss of pulse-oximetry signal with certain artifacts (such as cautery), a true decrease in the SpO_2 is a critical event. If oxygenation falls to the point where cells cannot maintain oxygen-based aerobic metabolism, cellular switch to anaerobic metabolism will create lactic acid byproducts. This increased acid environment and falling pH disrupts cellular and organ function, creating a critical downward physiologic spiral that must be reversed before death ensues.

If the breathing problem includes difficulty in removing CO_2 (hypoventilation), the increased CO_2 adds to the bloodstream's acidity with potential for further cellular insult. In addition, rising CO_2 contributes to decreasing level of consciousness ("CO_2 narcosis"). An understanding of arterial blood gases in respiratory crisis helps perioperative nurses predict future steps likely to be requested by anesthesia providers, as well as the likelihood that a breathing problem could turn into a full arrest scenario. Anesthesia providers aim to prevent breathing issues, but accept that early recognition and treatment are essential when respiratory problems arise.

Laryngospasm. The classic description of laryngospasm as vocal cords snapping shut in spasm if the patient's larynx becomes irritated in the light stages of anesthesia has been shown to also include other laryngeal structures (such as arytenoids and aryepiglottic folds) infolding upon themselves with the epiglottis covering these structures. An occluded airway results.

Laryngospasm can be provoked by secretions, sudden stimulation, pain, and airway manipulation. In patients who are most at risk for laryngospasm, such as children with airway surgery, many airway providers try to avoid the problem by extubating the child in a deeper plane of anesthesia, after return of spontaneous ventilation; they support the airway by face mask with 100% oxygen until the child awakens (Morgan, 2006).

First treatment for laryngospasm is a firm jaw thrust, which elevates the hyoid bone at the top of the trachea, unfolding the epiglottis and aryepiglottic folds; 100% oxygen is also delivered through a tightly fitting face mask with positive pressure. If the spasm does not break, a small dose of a short-acting neuromuscular blocker (succinylcholine) may be given, with ventilation assisted appropriately. Gentle suction of the oropharynx should ensure that no blood, secretions, or gastric contents are present to reirritate the larynx.

Perioperative nurses who are present during laryngospasm should be prepared to help with mask seal, as well as to communicate vital signs from the monitor (likely to be behind the anesthesia provider, who is concentrating on maintaining the airway).

A sputtering cough and gasp indicates the breaking of the spasm. However, the patient requires mask oxygenation and close monitoring until full return to consciousness. In an infant or child, a cry or yell for "Mommy" indicates both air movement and return to a higher level of consciousness. Laryngospasm may also occur in adults, although it is less common. After laryngospasm, patients must be monitored for development of negative-pressure pulmonary edema, as discussed later (Mirshab, 2002).

Stridor. Postintubation stridor (commonly called croup in children) is caused by edema of vocal cords or trachea. It is most common in children ages 1 to 4 years, appearing within 3 hours of extubation. The work of breathing is greatly increased by even a few millimeters of edema in a toddler's airway, which mandates immediate treatment with nebulized racemic epinephrine. Intravenous dexamethasone may be given for prevention (Morgan et al, 2006). The condition is occasionally seen in adults and treated with the same regimen.

Bronchospasm. Bronchospasm can occur just from the insult of placing an endotracheal tube into the trachea of a susceptible patient. Wheezing is the sound of air moving through narrowed airways, much like a whistle. Although wheezing is considered the classic sign of bronchospasm, the most dangerous presentation is a "silent spasm" in which the spasm is so intense that no air can be moved. This intense bronchospasm is most likely to occur with an asthmatic patient during intubation under general anesthesia, when a combination of factors related to disease, medications, and mechanical insult (laryngoscopy and intubation) combine to result in bronchospasm. Severe bronchospasm may result in reduced ability to oxygenate or ventilate the patient. The anesthesia provider will treat the bronchospasm with 100% oxygen and aerosol or metered-dose beta-adrenergic agents into the breathing circuit. The inhalational anesthetic agents are also bronchodilators. Steroid-dependent asthmatics may also receive a dose of intravenous hydrocortisone (Morgan et al, 2006). The severity of the episode and its response to treatment will be evaluated by the anesthesia provider and the surgeon before proceeding with surgery or for postoperative care planning. New postoperative arrangements for an intensive care bed may be required.

Aspiration of Gastric Contents. Many patients believe that nothing by mouth (NPO) status is imposed to prevent the inconvenience and discomfort of postoperative nausea and vomiting. They have not been educated about the serious morbidity and mortality that can follow aspiration of gastric contents; the low acidic pH of gastric acid may create a chemical pneumonitis that can be widely spread through the lungs if the aspirated volume is greater than 0.4 mL/kg and the pH is less than 2.5 (Morgan et al, 2006). If food particles, blood, small objects, or teeth are aspirated, severe hypoxemia can follow because of airway obstruction, development of atelectasis, and pneumonitis. In the most-dreaded scenario, the pathologic response accelerates into full-blown respiratory distress syndrome, which may culminate in death.

Patients who have received induction doses of sedative or anesthetic medication no longer have airway reflexes (cough, gag, swallow) to protect their airways. Others are at risk for aspiration because of emergency surgery shortly after eating or drinking or because of blood in the upper gastrointestinal (GI) tract or GI obstruction. Some patients are identified preoperatively to be at extra risk for aspiration of gastric contents. These include patients with reduced airway reflexes (drug or alcohol intoxication, central nervous system diseases, neuromuscular diseases, pregnancy, uncontrolled gastroesophageal reflux, or large hiatal hernia). These patients are often treated with medications to increase gastric emptying (e.g., metoclopramide), to reduce gastric acid (e.g., an H_2 blocker such as ranitidine or famotidine), or to raise gastric pH (a clear antacid such as Bicitra). These medications reduce the chance for passive regurgitation of gastric contents into the larynx during induction of general anesthesia, before the airway is secured with a cuffed endotracheal tube.

In addition to the aforementioned medications to reduce risk, anesthesia providers will choose a technique to secure the airway in a manner that minimizes risk, if general anesthesia is required. If the patient's airway has been assessed as potentially difficult to manage, the anesthesia provider may opt for awake intubation. This process includes topical LA to the airway by nebulizer, spray, or gargle, with the patient sitting upright. Small amounts of sedation may be given, but patient cooperation must be maintained as the fiberoptic bronchoscope is used to secure the airway with a cuffed endotracheal tube before induction of general anesthesia and placing into supine position for surgery. Perioperative nurses' understanding of the anesthesia plan will include recognition of the twofold safety goal of difficult airway management and prevention of aspiration of gastric contents.

If the patient's airway has been deemed non-difficult ahead of time, the anesthesia provider is likely to choose a rapid-sequence induction with the Sellick maneuver (i.e., cricoid pressure). Perioperative nurses are frequently called upon to provide cricoid pressure without recognizing that this simple act may have critical implications for patient safety.

It is essential to know how to identify the cricoid ring (which is the only tracheal ring that is a full circle; all the others are C-shaped, with the open section toward the spine). The large shield-shaped thyroid cartilage ("Adam's apple") is the most prominent landmark of the upper trachea with its bottom midmargin at the top of a small, soft elliptical space (Figure 12-3). This indentation is the cricothyroid space (where emergency cricothyroidotomy is done). The strip of cartilage just below the cricothyroid space is the cricoid ring. In a supine unconscious patient, firm pressure on this circular cricoid cartilage will occlude the esophagus and prevent regurgitation of gastric contents into larynx and lungs.

The person applying cricoid pressure to reduce chance of aspiration must know to hold the pressure until the laryngoscopist announces that it is time to let go. This announcement will be delivered only when there is confirmation that the tube

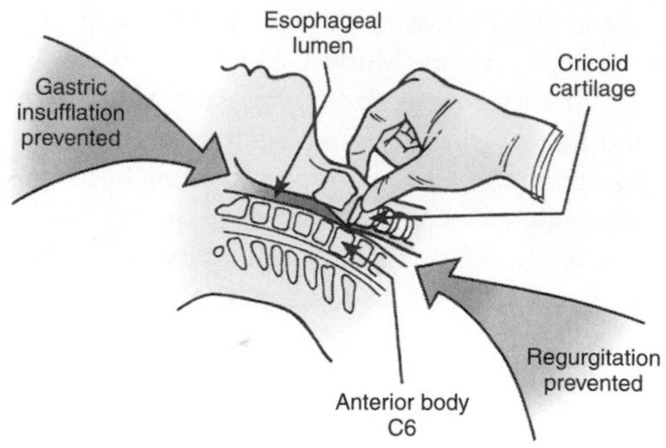

FIGURE 12-3 Applying cricoid pressure. (From Grande CM: *Textbook of trauma anesthesia and critical care,* St. Louis, 1993, Mosby.)

has been placed into the trachea and the cuff has been inflated appropriately. There must be bilateral chest rise and fall, bilateral breath sounds, and an appropriate and sustained end-tidal CO_2 waveform must also be clearly witnessed before cricoid pressure can be safely released. If there is any doubt, the anesthesia provider may complete further assessments, such as gastric auscultation or a second laryngoscopy to re-view the tube's presence between the cords, while the assistant continues to hold cricoid pressure. Premature release of cricoid pressure could result in a pool of gastric contents roiling up into the trachea if the endotracheal tube had been an unrecognized esophageal intubation, with potentially disastrous results.

Negative Pressure Pulmonary Edema. The term *pulmonary edema* brings to mind an image of fluid overload or poor heart function. However, the perioperative airway situation occasionally gives rise to negative-pressure pulmonary edema (NPPE). It is sometimes called postobstructive pulmonary edema (POPE). This noncardiogenic pulmonary edema occurs after upper airway obstruction while a patient is still generating intrathoracic pressure trying to take a breath (Lowery and Myers, 2008). This reversed pressure gradient causes fluid to be pulled from capillaries into the alveoli, resulting in an overflow of secretions, which can be dramatic enough to cause severe hypoxemia (Davidson et al, 2004). NPPE is more likely to happen in adults with obstructive sleep apnea, patients with airway lesions, and patients for any nasal, oral, or pharyngeal procedure. Pediatric patients have extremely compliant chest walls that can generate large amounts of negative pressure if they are trying to breathe against any obstruction, such as laryngospasm, or if they are biting their endotracheal tubes. Strong young males who awaken with immense strength and empty the anesthesia breathing bag to a flat position also create an airway obstruction against which negative pressure is being generated.

The onset of NPPE is usually sudden as copious frothy pink secretions appear and oxygen saturation falls. However, onset may also be delayed for up to several hours. Rales and wheezes, tachycardia, hypertension, and diaphoresis indicate sympathetic stress (Kesimci et al, 2007).

Reversing hypoxemia and reducing the fluid in the lungs to increase oxygen transport are top priorities. For many patients, close monitoring while maintaining a clear airway, in a sitting position, with 100% oxygen is adequate. If the patient is still intubated, positive end-expiratory pressure (PEEP) may be added to improve alveolar reexpansion. If the patient has already been extubated, failure to improve will require reintubation and positive-pressure ventilation with PEEP. Care must be taken to ensure that the patient cannot bite the endotracheal tube to create more obstruction and worsen the situation. Use of a diuretic such as furosemide is controversial, particularly if there is any possibility that the patient is already hypovolemic.

Weakness After Neuromuscular Blockade. The goal of every anesthesia provider is prompt emergence and extubation, but there are times when the patient's breathing does not meet extubation criteria; sometimes this is related to incomplete reversal of neuromuscular blockade. Anesthesia providers use a peripheral nerve stimulator (PNS) to show return of function after reversal of neuromuscular blockade, but most commonly used PNS devices are qualitative, with some potential for error (Donati and Bevan, 2009). More accurate PNS measurement is coming into clinical practice that allows actual measurement of the return of neuromuscular function (Rizzi, 2004; Murphy et al, 2008). However, no matter which device is used, patients must meet clinical criteria to prove sustained return of full muscle strength.

Even with the full dose of anticholinesterase reversal medication (along with its protective anticholinergic), some patients remain weak and unable to maintain adequate respiratory volumes, despite being awake and responsive. They may have shown positive results on the PNS, indicating full reversal by that criterion. Yet they exhibit uncoordinated jerky movements, which are classically referred to as "floppy fish motions," reflecting inadequate muscle strength for spontaneous ventilation. These patients are not ready for extubation, for reasons related to individual variability, drug interactions, underlying disease, or other factors that may not be discernible. Although this situation may be regarded by some as a complication, slow return from anesthetic medications usually reflects the continuum of patient variability and sensitivity. However, when patients are extubated prematurely while weak and unable to maintain adequate ventilation, complications will definitely occur, as the consequences of hypoxia and hypercarbia ensue. These awake patients are also burdened with anxiety associated with being too weak to breathe effectively. Therefore anesthesia providers are bound to the rule of safe practice, which requires that no extubation occurs until patients have proved the ability to maintain strong spontaneous ventilation, with excellent strength, strong airway reflexes, and return of consciousness.

In another neuromuscular blockade problem, patients intubated with succinylcholine at the beginning of the case experience unexpected prolonged paralysis from the drug. Rather than the 3- to 5-minute expected drug duration, the paralysis lasts for 3 to 5 hours, because of a rare genetic condition (atypical pseudocholinesterase) in which limited amount of the enzyme is available to break down the succinylcholine and allow return of muscle function. There is no reversal for this situation. These patients must receive mechanical ventilation until muscle function returns to allow adequate respiratory function and safe extubation (Rosenberg et al, 2009). For short surgeries such patients must be transferred still intubated to the PACU for mechanical ventilation (along with sedation for amnesia to minimize memory of the postoperative paralysis). This is a noncrisis event that is usually recognized before the end of surgery; the anesthesia provider and perioperative nurse have time to communicate effectively, with postoperative plans for ventilation. Because atypical pseudocholinesterase is a genetic trait, the patient and family members should be notified about it in writing to notify future anesthesia providers about the event. An "allergy" or adverse drug warning for succinylcholine should be placed on the chart.

Circulation Problems

Anesthesia providers must focus on control of the circulatory system. However, patient variability, comorbidities, medications, anesthesia techniques, and surgical scenarios bring circulation challenges that range from minor to massive. Intraoperative hypotension, hypertension, heart rate changes, and dysrhythmias are common events, which may be short-lived and easily treated. They may be related to a patient's underlying disease, surgical problems, anesthesia issues, or some combination. Most circulation changes are mild, and their appearance requires timely but gentle treatment. However, any circulation change may become critical, leading to potential damage to heart, brain, and other vital organs. Maintaining adequate perfusion is an essential part of anesthesia care. Standard monitoring of circulation by noninvasive devices (blood pressure, electrocardiogram [ECG], pulse oximeter wave) is supplemented by invasive monitoring (arterial line, central venous pressure line, urinary output, pulmonary artery catheter) in situations where circulation extremes are expected or develop.

Anesthesia providers manipulate circulatory physiology with medications and fluids, including blood products and artificial fluid expanders. When massive bleeding occurs, the challenge to maintain perfusion becomes acute, as profound hypotension and loss of circulatory volume insults cellular metabolism, resulting in development of metabolic acidosis. This acidosis further degrades cellular and organ function, resulting in a downward physiologic spiral that must be reversed with resuscitation before cardiac arrest occurs. Massive transfusion requires great teamwork, with careful attention to identification and verification of blood product units.

When vital signs become unstable, anesthesia providers immediately begin treatment while seeking possible underlying causes. Many emergency situations may be avoided by early identification and treatment. Vigilant providers may detect early clues of complications such as hidden bleeding, slow-onset pneumothorax, gradual development of pulmonary edema, or insidious onset of malignant hyperthermia. Early detection and immediate treatment may be lifesaving. On the other hand, some events may present without warning as full cardiac arrest or fulminant crisis.

Pneumothorax. Air or gas in the pleural space during anesthesia or surgery may create a critical cardiorespiratory situation. It may be difficult to diagnose (Gaba et al, 1994) because early symptoms are nonspecific, unless there is an indicator for suspicion. Hypotension and tachycardia, hypoxemia and hypercarbia, increased peak inspiratory pressure and decreased lung compliance are early signs. More specific signs include asymmetric breath sounds, tracheal deviation from midline, and distended neck veins.

These developing signs and symptoms may follow such procedures as placement of a central line, regional nerve block, or surgery near the pleural cavity. Pneumothorax may also occur during laparoscopy due to CO_2 insufflation or during oral and dental procedures when high-speed drills are used. Bilateral tension pneumothoraces may present suddenly as an unexpected cardiac arrest, requiring immediate surgical and nursing teamwork for resuscitation.

Treatment may include simple aspiration technique for uncomplicated pneumothorax; however, a large pneumothorax or one that is complicated by hemothorax, empyema, or persistent air leaks will require tube thoracostomy with drainage to a water-seal suction pleural drainage device (Naik, 2008).

Pulmonary Embolism. Pulmonary embolism results when any foreign material enters the venous system. This includes blood clots from the legs and pelvic areas, fat, air, and amniotic fluid. When the foreign material reaches the lung circulation, it increases dead space and pulmonary vascular resistance. The result is hypoxemia along with hypotension, decreased end-tidal CO_2, and ECG changes of right heart strain, ST-T wave changes, or bradycardia. Diagnosis of venous embolism may be difficult because these changes are nonspecific. However, a massive pulmonary embolus may present as a sudden cardiac arrest with pulseless electrical activity or asystole. Prevention of clot-related pulmonary emboli with low-molecular-weight heparin and prophylactic use of sequential compression devices has now become routine nursing care for surgical patients.

Other embolic substances must always be kept in mind according to the type of surgery. In major orthopedic procedures, the possibility of fat emboli should be considered if the patient becomes unstable, because marrow fat or other debris may move into the venous circulation through bony medullary veins. A recent theory suggests that symptoms of fat emboli are an inflammatory response rather than mechanical obstruction of pulmonary circulation (Gutsche, 2008). Fat emboli are usually accompanied by widespread petechiae. Clotting abnormalities, dyspnea, and confusion are also present. These symptoms usually occur within 72 hours after long bone fractures. Reports with more advanced technology have been able to identify perioperative fat microemboli that travel to the brain; this phenomenon may explain rare cases of prolonged coma (Byrick et al, 2001) and fatal cerebral embolization (Weiss et al, 1996) after major orthopedic procedures.

Air Embolus. Vascular air embolism is the entrainment of air or exogenously delivered gas into the bloodstream. Although an air embolus has potential to be fatal, the main factors that create morbidity and mortality are the volume of air entrained and the rate of accumulation. It is believed that 200 to 300 mL is the adult lethal volume (Mirski et al, 2007). Any surgical procedure in which the wound is higher than the heart or where there are large, venous channels on the field carries risk for air embolism. Historically the sitting craniotomy has always been considered the classic case for this risk; however, other positions where the wound is above the heart should also be considered (such as lateral thoracotomy, urology cases in Trendelenburg position). There is also significant risk for air embolism with laparoscopic insufflation of gas under pressure, exteriorization of the uterus at cesarean section, and insertion and removal of central venous lines (Mirski et al, 2007). Sudden decrease in end-tidal CO_2 and the appearance of nitrogen in end-tidal gases serve as first alerts to the anesthesia provider that air embolus may be occurring (Morgan et al, 2006). The use of a precordial Doppler ultrasound is the most sensitive noninvasive monitor to discern an air embolus, capable of noting 0.25 mL of air with sound change to "mill-wheel murmur."

Rapid teamwork from everyone is essential if an air embolus is identified during surgery. It is likely that diagnosis will not be made until a substantial amount of air has been entrained (Morgan et al, 2006). The first action is to stop entrainment of air or gas by flooding the field with saline-soaked sponges. One hundred percent oxygen should be delivered. Placing the patient into the partial left lateral decubitus position may help to relieve the "air-lock" created by the embolus bubble on the right side of the heart. Closed-chest compressions may also help to move smaller air bubbles forward through the lungs to reduce embolic obstruction. Success rates with aspirating air from the right atrium have not been high (Mirski et al, 2007). Hemodynamic support will be provided with dobutamine, norepinephrine, or ephedrine. The diagnosis is particularly serious if the patient is in the 10% to 25% of people with who have a probe-patent foramen ovale, which can facilitate bubble passage into arterial circulation, resulting in stroke or coronary vessel occlusion.

Amniotic Fluid Embolus. According to Leighton (2009), amniotic fluid embolism is the second leading direct cause of maternal death in the United States, although it is still rare. Its cause is unknown, although newer evidence suggests its nature may be more anaphylactoid than embolic (Moore, 2008a). Eighty percent of mothers with this condition die. Symptoms include acute hypoxia, dyspnea, acute hypotension or cardiac arrest, and coagulopathy or severe hemorrhage without other explanations. Fetal bradycardia ensues; after delivery, uterine atony results in excessive bleeding. Seizures and altered mental status may occur. Perioperative nurses participating in obstetric surgeries must always be ready to join the anesthesia provider and surgeon during resuscitation during this catastrophe, which may include rapid surgical delivery of the infant to facilitate maternal intensive care. Extreme teamwork for both mother and infant is required in this situation.

Malignant Hyperthermia. Malignant hyperthermia (MH) is actually a syndrome of uncontrolled skeletal muscle metabolism with potentially fatal outcome. Its onset may be muted or delayed after exposure to triggering agents (Gronert et al, 2005). Elevated temperature is a late finding (Opton, 2008). Genetically susceptible individuals who receive inhalational agents or succinylcholine may have MH triggered at any time during anesthesia or in the postanesthesia period. A specific ryanodine receptor gene mutation has now been identified with malignant hyperthermia (Anderson et al, 2008; Kaufmann, 2008). Because of genetic transmission, it is essential to query every patient about bloodline relatives who may have experienced MH. Progress in understanding and treating this disease is essential as anesthesia providers and teams are also expected to recognize and treat MH, even though it is a rare disease.

Genetically susceptible individuals have abnormal function of the ryanodine receptor in skeletal muscle; triggering agents cause uncontrolled calcium release and muscle metabolism. The first sign is increased end-tidal CO_2, which may be substantial, often accompanied by tachycardia. Masseter spasm at the time of intubation may also signal MH. Other symptoms that develop from the effects of uncontrolled muscle metabolism include hypertension or unstable blood pressure (BP), dysrhythmias, cyanosis or mottling, whole-body rigidity, myoglobinuria, rhabdomyolysis, and disseminated intravascular coagulation. When diagnostic suspicion for MH arises, arterial blood gases are drawn; results that show both respiratory and metabolic acidosis indicate fulminant MH. By this point, temperature rises, even above 43° C. Profound acidosis and/or hyperkalemia from muscle metabolism may trigger cardiac arrest and death, unless rapid and coordinated treatment ensues.

At this point in perioperative safety history, every team member should be familiar with the MH syndrome and its teamwork, although many professionals may never see a case in their careers. Although MH was formally identified only in 1960 (Denborough and Lovell, 1960; Denborough, 2008), availability of a swine model that also experienced MH allowed relatively rapid development of dantrolene, which was brought to clinical use in 1979. Dantrolene and well-planned treatment algorithms have reduced the mortality rate for MH from 80% to less than 10% (Baker et al, 2007).

Although MH often presents in the pediatric population, it can occur in any age group. Some musculoskeletal conditions may have an increased association with MH, including Duchenne muscular dystrophy, central core disease, and osteogenesis imperfecta.

Ongoing challenges with MH include identification of susceptible individuals by history, with blood testing for the abnormal ryanodine receptor (RYR1) now available when indicated (Malignant Hyperthermia Association of the United States [MHAUS], undated). This testing is used for selected individuals with high suspicion for the genetic abnormality rather than serving as a widely available screening tool (MHAUS, 2009).

Every surgery suite should have the MH treatment algorithm prominently posted, along with the hotline telephone number to reach a consultant at the Malignant Hyperthermia Association of the United States (MHAUS). The team approach to MH safety should include mock drills, checklists, and worksheets with specific task assignments for team members. MHAUS provides resources such as slide shows to ensure that guidelines and algorithms are in place. True case histories are available to enrich educational planning for everyone in perioperative, surgical, and anesthesia services (Rosenberg and Rothstein, 2006).

All of the medications and treatment supplies must be organized in a central location for easy access. A stock of 36 vials of dantrolene is recommended, available within 5 minutes, for initial stabilization. With adult doses starting at 2.5 mg/kg, up to 10 mg/kg and sometimes higher, arrangements for additional supply must also be in place.

Perioperative nurses who have never participated in an MH event may not be aware that dantrolene powder is difficult to reconstitute. Each vial contains only 20 mg of the drug, requiring 60 mL of preservative-free sterile water, with the particulate somewhat resistant to dissolving. Baker et al (2007) created a warming system to facilitate more rapid dissolution of dantrolene in sterile water. Planning for MH treatment includes the labor-intensive work of preparing the dantrolene, which requires its own team who know how to reconstitute this unique medication. An essential safety consideration is the large amount of sterile water for injection that is needed for reconstitution; 1-L bags of sterile water for injection may be designated for this use, but they must be clearly flagged in some manner to ensure that they are used only as diluents, lest a bag of water be attached erroneously to a patient's intravenous line. Sterile water given intravenously can cause fatal hemolysis (Pennsylvania Patient Safety Authority, 2008).

Delayed Emergence

Delayed emergence from general anesthesia may be a safety concern, or it may reflect individual patient variability, depending on the length of the delay and results of differential diagnosis. Residual drug effect is the most common cause of delayed emergence. Anesthetics, sedatives, and analgesics may individually or in combination result in slow awakening in certain patients. If the delay raises excessive concern, gentle titration of flumazenil and/or naloxone reverses effects of benzodiazepine and narcotics. Hypothermia may also delay emergence, because low core temperatures potentiate central nervous system depressants (Morgan et al, 2006).

Hypoxemia and hypercarbia may be readily excluded with blood-gas analysis; hypoglycemia is also easily measured at the bedside and treated. Other metabolic possibilities must be sought, including electrolyte imbalances such as hypernatremia and hyponatremia. Because medication error must always be considered, the case's syringes and vials should be reviewed. New safety recommendations encourage saving all vials and syringes until safe case completion (Eichorn, 2009).

Perioperative stroke is extremely rare, except after neurosurgery, cardiac procedures, and cerebrovascular procedures. Radiologic imaging and neurology consultation may be required.

The possibility of secret ingestion of herbals or other depressants before surgery must always be considered.

Emergence Delirium

Agitated emergence requires careful consideration after the patient's physical safety is ensured, along with that of the care team, who may be at risk for injury. Although patients may awaken enough to meet extubation criteria, they may not be clear enough to express pain lucidly.

A trial of analgesia may be helpful, as long as it is ensured that restlessness is not a sign of hypoxemia (easily proved by pulse oximetry). However, other physiologic events such as bladder distention or intra-abdominal bleeding may be the cause of agitation beyond "normal" incisional discomfort. Delirium risk is higher in older adult patients; approximately 10% may experience it. Risk is also higher for patients who have baseline low cognitive function, dementia, depression, and general debility (Rooke, 2009).

An essential team consideration in providing a smooth emergence is reducing noise in the room when patients are being awakened, to minimize the amount of unfamiliar stimuli bombarding them. Only one person should be speaking to the patient (usually the anesthesia provider), and no one should shout at the patient unless he or she is known to be deaf. Even patients awakening smoothly often admit that they are somewhat disoriented; therefore reduction of agitation also includes an obligation to maintain professional decorum and quiet. Efforts to reduce instrument noise, overhead announcements and other disconcerting stimuli should be considered.

Safety considerations become even more urgent when the patient moves beyond agitated to delirious, which can occur as a side effect of medications such as atropine or scopolamine, which may cause central anticholinergic syndrome. This syndrome shows physical anticholinergic signs ("Mad as a hatter; blind as a bat [pupils dilated]; red as a beet; dry as a bone"). Treatment with physostigmine will usually reverse delirium and symptoms. Delirium after ketamine is also possible. Although most patients who receive ketamine receive midazolam concurrently to minimize disruptive dreams or hallucinations, further doses of midazolam may be required. Patients with serious psychiatric illness such as posttraumatic stress disorder or panic attacks may also require postemergence sedation. Finally, the possibility of undivulged substance abuse (alcohol, street drugs) must also be considered if agitation becomes extreme. In all agitated patients the priority of safety for patient and staff must be maintained.

Eye Injury and Blindness

Reports of perianesthesia eye problems range from corneal abrasions to blindness. Care must be shown for the anesthetized patient's eyes, because of reduced tear production and inability to blink. Even momentary loss of vigilance by team members could contribute to a corneal abrasion. However, the ASA Closed Claims Project review of eye injury was rarely able to identify a specific cause for corneal injuries (Morgan et al, 2006). Corneal abrasions or other injury may occur from the face mask or other manipulations during airway management. A perioperative nurse assisting at induction stands in a position to identify any unintentional ocular encroachment as the anesthesia provider manipulates the airway. On awakening, the patient's tendency to reach for his or her face may contribute to eye injury, especially when wearing a pulse oximeter and dragging intravenous lines. It is possible that postoperative complaints of corneal abrasion may even occur in the recovery period.

Recent closed-claim studies have identified postoperative vision loss (POVL) as a devastating ocular complication. Vision loss may range from partial field deficit to complete blindness, presenting immediately after surgery or up to several days later. POVL has been categorized into two subgroups: central retinal artery occlusion (CRAO) and ischemic optic neuropathy (ION). CRAO is probably embolic and is mostly likely to happen after cardiopulmonary bypass. However, it may also occur after prolonged spine surgery with the headrest producing direct pressure on the orbits. CRAO is usually unilateral. Prognosis for return of vision after CRAO is poor. Ischemic optic neuropathy is more common than CRAO after complex spine surgery. Although the mechanism of ION is poorly understood, patient risk factors have been identified, including diabetes, atherosclerosis, anemia, intraoperative hypotension, and long surgery with large blood loss. ION is more likely to be bilateral than CRAO, and it has a better prognosis for return of some vision (Moore, 2008b).

The American Society of Anesthesiologists (2006a) has published a practice advisory about POVL in spine patients. Recommendations include close arterial BP monitoring, maintenance of euvolemia, maintenance of an adequate hemoglobin level, and avoidance of pressure on the orbits. If POVL is suspected, ophthalmologic consultation should be requested immediately. All of these recommendations require team participation, particularly safe positioning for prolonged procedures. Anesthesia providers will check and document facial pressure points frequently during the procedure. Surgeons may consider staged procedures for patients who are at high risk for POVL (Moore, 2008b). The ASA is following this issue closely with an ongoing case report registry for POVL (Lee et al, 2006).

Thermal Safety

Although patients describe the discomfort of being cold during surgery, it is well known that perioperative hypothermia is physiologically unsafe (Sessler, 2008). Chapter 15 discusses details of this issue. Anesthesia contributes significantly to heat loss with vasodilation that occurs with inhalation agents or regional anesthesia, as well as other perioperative factors, such as cool room, exposed skin, evaporating preparation agents, and open wounds. As discussed in Chapter 15, perioperative nurses' collaboration with anesthesia providers in thermal support adds to patient safety.

Regional Anesthesia

Regional anesthesia uses LA medications to block conduction of nerve (pain) signals to the brain. Because both motor and sensory functions are reduced or eliminated for the duration of the block, the patient is unable to move areas affected by the anesthetized nerves. This blockade can provide ideal surgical circumstances. However, motor and sensory blockade of the nerves are accompanied by blockade of the sympathetic nerves that maintain blood pressure and heart rate, as well as the nerves that transmit deep touch and pressure. This sympathetic blockade may have great safety implications for vital signs.

Subarachnoid block (spinal anesthesia) and epidural anesthesia are the two forms of neuraxial blockade used for major regional anesthesia. Safety issues can arise with neuraxial block during the perioperative period. Strictest attention to aseptic technique is essential during neuraxial block to minimize the chance of central nervous system infection. Neuraxial block is contraindicated in infection at the injection site, coagulopathy, severe hypovolemia, increased intracranial pressure, and severe cardiac valvular diseases. Other relative contraindications are also considered by anesthesia providers, including patient refusal (Morgan et al, 2006).

Spinal Anesthesia

Spinal anesthesia involves injection of a very small dose (usually 2 mL or less) of a local anesthetic into the cerebrospinal fluid (CSF) of the subarachnoid space, with a small-bore needle (22 to 27 gauge) placed into the patient's lumbar area. The needle is directed under aseptic conditions between lumbar vertebrae until clear free-flowing CSF is returned from the hub of the needle, confirming placement of the needle tip into the subarachnoid space. The level of anesthesia usually depends on dose and baricity of medication injected (Bernards, 2009). Dosage of local anesthetic is selected considering multiple patient factors, aiming for the ideal level of several dermatomes above the surgical site. After injection, the effect of hyperbaric spinal anesthesia is noted first at feet and legs, with the effect moving up the torso as the local anesthetic mixes into CSF and blocks transmission by the spinal nerves.

Anesthesia providers carefully monitor the level of spinal anesthesia because of the risk of the anesthetic level rising too high. The level of anesthesia is estimated by checking response to sharp, cold, or touch stimuli. These dermatome measurements, vital-sign monitoring, and maintenance of verbal contact allow anesthesia providers to anticipate dangerously high levels of anesthesia and be prepared for rescue treatment. An anesthetic level that rises to high thoracic levels weakens respiratory muscles and may impair breathing; if the level creeps to the cervical area, loss of protective airway reflexes and respiratory function may occur. Bradycardia and profound hypotension will also be noted. Cardiorespiratory arrest will occur if the level of anesthesia rises to the brain's CSF to block the cardiorespiratory center of the brainstem. This scenario requires full resuscitative support until the blockade resolves. With appropriate support, the patient should suffer no complications (Bernards, 2009).

The most common complication of spinal anesthesia is hypotension caused by vasodilation and/or bradycardia that occur because sympathetic nerves are blocked along with pain-transmission nerves (Warren and Liu, 2008). Hypotension may be more dramatic in higher-level blockade because a wider area of sympathetic blockade ensues. Closed-claims studies have uncovered cases of sudden bradycardia or asystole during spinal anesthesia that are not related to oversedation or respiratory insufficiency with high block. In the initial landmark study 14 such patients had difficult resuscitations, ending either in death or survival with neurologic damage. Increased vagal tone in patients with low baseline heart rates may be a contributing factor. Successful rescue depends on quick recognition of the deteriorating situation, prompt treatment of the bradycardia, rapid delivery of fluids, and head-down positioning to enhance venous return (Brull and Greengrass, 2008).

Epidural Anesthesia

Epidural anesthesia involves needle placement of local anesthetic into the epidural space to block nerve impulses to the brain. The epidural space is a potential space that lies just outside the subarachnoid space; it is identified by a "loss of resistance" technique with an air-filled glass syringe (Warren and Liu, 2008). Depending on dose and concentration of local anesthetic, an epidural block may be analgesic, as used for labor and delivery or for postoperative pain management, or it may be fully anesthetic for abdominal procedures such as cesarean section. Although epidural block is most commonly placed at the lumbar area, thoracic-level blockade is sometimes used to provide analgesia for upper abdominal or thoracic pain relief.

Epidural injection uses a large-gauge needle (usually 17 to 18 gauge) whose inner diameter allows a catheter to be threaded through for repeat doses of the local anesthetic. Doses of epidural medication are usually larger than those for subarachnoid block, starting at 3 to 5 mL and titrating up to a total dose of 12 to 24 mL (Morgan et al, 2006). Occasionally a single-shot epidural block is provided, usually for pain diagnosis or relief. Epidural anesthesia takes effect like a widening belt, extending both caudally and cranially from the injection level (Bernards, 2009). Its onset is slower than spinal anesthesia because it diffuses more slowly through the epidural spaces and the fibrous and fat coverings of the epidural nerves to exert nerve block action.

The level of epidural block depends on multiple patient and technical factors that are considered by anesthesia providers. However, two serious complications can occur if the epidural needle tip or catheter moves into either the subarachnoid space or into an epidural vein. The perioperative nurse must anticipate either serious complication when epidural anesthesia is being placed because rapid teamwork is required for rescue. Unintentional injection of the larger-dose local anesthetic intended for the epidural space into the subarachnoid fluid quickly creates a "high spinal" with cardiorespiratory arrest very likely. Injection of the larger-dose local anesthetic into an epidural vein can cause seizures and cardiorespiratory collapse by the mechanism of local anesthetic toxicity. Local anesthetic toxicity is discussed later in this chapter.

To minimize risk for these crises, a test dose is given before the larger dose of local anesthetic. The test dose is a small amount of local anesthetic with a small amount of epinephrine, typically 3 mL of 1.5% lidocaine with epinephrine 1:200,000 (Morgan et al, 2006). When the test dose is injected, the patient is closely monitored for the onset of unintended spinal block (legs suddenly numb) or evidence of unintended intravenous injection of the medication (rapid heart rate caused by absorption of the epinephrine, indicating venous dose absorption). Perioperative nurses who assist anesthesia providers with epidural placement must be aware of both elements of the test dose and must be vigilant for the onset of dangerous symptoms that indicate that the epidural needle or catheter is misplaced. Misplacement of the needle is common because of patients' anatomic variations; the critical aspect of safe care is quick recognition of symptoms of subarachnoid or intravenous injection, which allows rapid rescue and avoidance of serious complications.

Onset of epidural anesthesia is slower and less dense than spinal blockade (Morgan et al, 2006). Incremental dosing through the catheter allows titration of anesthesia to the desired level. As with subarachnoid block, hypotension and bradycardia may occur because sympathetic nerves are blocked along with sensory and motor nerves. These symptoms are promptly treated by anesthesia providers with pressors, vagolytics, and fluids.

Peripheral Nerve Blocks

Most peripheral nerve blocks provide longer, more localized analgesia than neuraxial blocks. Patient satisfaction is usually high with localized pain relief that maintains functional capacity of the rest of the body. Peripheral blocks may also be acceptable for some anticoagulated patients for whom neuraxial blockade risks central nervous system hematoma.

Recent addition of continuous catheter techniques to extend duration of peripheral blocks makes them even more attractive after procedures such as major joint replacement (Mulroy, 2006).

Finally, development of ultrasound guidance devices increases accurate delivery of LA and block success rate (Gray, 2006). However, even with the advances in technology, the provider must have considerable training and knowledge in many of these techniques (Tsui and Rosenquist, 2009).

Safe placement of peripheral nerve blocks requires skilled assistance with technique and patient monitoring. The provider must ensure that nerves are not pierced and damaged and that LA is not injected into vessels to cause systemic toxicity. Thus careful monitoring is essential. At the least, after baseline vital signs are obtained, a pulse oximeter is placed to allow instantaneous recognition of heart rate elevation, which may signal intravascular injection when epinephrine is being used. Ongoing BP measurements should be available. All precautions for rapid treatment of LA toxicity should also be available.

Although preparation of equipment and supplies is important, the most important monitor during placement of a nerve block is maintenance of verbal contact with the patient. Although this role may be filled by an anesthesia department member, the perioperative nurse should also be familiar with the rationale for monitoring verbal contact as well as vital signs and providing momentary assistance needed for block insertion. Although very light sedation and analgesia may be given, verbal monitoring must be able to allow two important notifications: nerve trespass and evidence of intravascular injection or systemic absorption of LA. If the needle touches a nerve, the patient will experience a paresthesia; it is important to observe stoic patients to query them if they grimace and to identify if any pain is like an electric shock or "hitting your funny bone," the well-known paresthesia of daily life. If LA is placed into a vessel, the presence of epinephrine will cause a transient rapid rise in heart rate of about 20 beats per minute. If there is no epinephrine in the LA, careful attention must be paid to the development of early toxicity warning signs, such as numbness at lips, ringing in ears, or feeling dizzy. Although the provider makes injections incrementally with aspiration between each injection, there is always the possibility that the needle tip could unintentionally pierce a vessel or nerve. Ongoing monitoring after injection of the full dose of LA is necessary for the possibility of rapid systemic absorption causing toxicity. The potential for block placement to progress to medical emergency if LA toxicity occurs must also be kept in mind.

Arm Blocks

Brachial Plexus Blocks. The entire arm can be anesthetized by injection of local anesthetic into the nerve sheath of the brachial plexus, which provides both motor and sensory function to the arm. Needle placement for this block varies by provider preference; approach may be at axillary, infraclavicular, supraclavicular, or interscalene points. Needle location may be confirmed with a peripheral nerve stimulator or with an ultrasound-guidance device. The trend toward ultrasound guidance is believed to improve accuracy for block placement to reduce the number of failed blocks, as well as the number of unintentional intravenous injections of local anesthetics, which cause serious toxicity (Aziz and Horn, 2008). However, like most technologic advances, it has no guarantee attached (Hadzic et al, 2008). Individual nerve blocks of the arm or hand may also be placed for primary anesthesia or to supplement axillary blocks.

Intravenous Regional Anesthesia. Injection of local anesthesia into a small dorsal hand vein of an exsanguinated arm with a double tourniquet creates anesthesia of the arm for 45 to 60 minutes (Morgan et al, 2006). This Bier block (named after its developing physician, a pioneer in local anesthesia) is ideal for short hand and wrist procedures. The block is time limited, related to uptake and metabolism of the local anesthetic as well as tourniquet discomfort. The tourniquet is shared for retention of anesthetic drug in the arm as well as exsanguination of the surgical field. The double tourniquet allows switching position of the pressure site if the patient's arm becomes uncomfortable. A minimum tourniquet time of at least 20 minutes is recommended, even if the surgery is shorter. Seizures have been reported after premature release of all the LA medication into systemic circulation (Sen and Barts, 2008).

Lower Extremity Blocks. Blockade of the leg can be approached with a variety of techniques with blockades of sciatic, femoral, obturator, and popliteal fossa. Combination techniques may be done. Nerve stimulators or ultrasound-guidance devices may be used to locate the desired nerves.

Other Nerve Blocks

Individual nerve blocks may also be placed to anesthetize specific body areas, such as digits, eyes, or selected areas of skin surface. The foot can be fully anesthetized with a five-injection technique at the ankle level, which blocks all the foot nerves.

Local Anesthetic Toxicity

Local anesthetics are often considered benign medications, yet there are circumstances in which these medications can produce serious morbidity and death. A thorough understanding of local anesthetic toxicity is an essential part of perioperative medication safety.

Anesthesia providers must also know every medication the patient receives at any time. When local anesthetics are injected by the surgeon, the anesthesia provider must know details of time and dose as injection occurs (not an end-of-case total). Full name and dose of the drug and any additive must be announced ("1% lidocaine with epinephrine 1 to 200:000" rather than "lido with epi"). The usual labeling and verification processes for medication safety on the field must be followed. If epinephrine is being added to medications on the field, the potential for calculation errors cannot be overemphasized, caused by the traditional archaic mixture nomenclature for this drug.

As regional anesthesia and nerve blocks become increasingly popular, chances for local anesthetic toxicity increase, either by unintentional intravascular injection or by systemic overdose as a result of gradual absorption of large amounts of infiltrated LA. Anesthesia providers make every effort to prevent local anesthetic toxicity with aspiration, test dosing, and incremental dosing, yet toxicity still occurs in perhaps 20 of every 10,000 blocks (Fallin and Burns, 2008).

Local anesthetic toxicity may start with benign symptoms such as numbness around lips or ringing in ears and then progress to visual disturbances, muscular twitching, seizures, coma, cardiorespiratory arrest and possibly death (Heavner, 2008). Bupivacaine is known to be particularly cardiotoxic (Fallin and Burns, 2008) with low resuscitation success in this situation. The toxicity of bupivacaine is magnified by pregnancy, hypoxemia, and respiratory acidosis (Morgan et al, 2006). Until recently, standard advanced cardiovascular life support (ACLS) resuscitation (support of airway, breathing, and circulation) was the only treatment, often proving inadequate, even with prolonged efforts. Arrhythmias, myocardial depression, severe hypotension, and electromechanical dissociation may be expected (Tasch and Butterwork, 2008).

Lipid Rescue for Local Anesthetic Toxicity. A new rescue technique for systemic injection, overdose, or toxic absorption is the infusion of 20% lipid emulsion (Weinberg, 2006), the same mixture used traditionally as a base for total parenteral nutrition. Every site that uses local anesthetics should include a 500-mL bag of 20% lipid infusion on the block cart or emergency cart.

All other resuscitation is continued while the lipid is infused with an intravenous loading dose of 1.5 mL/kg, followed by infusion of 0.25 to 0.5 mL/kg/min until cardiac symptoms resolve (Fallin and Burns, 2008; Weinberg, 2009). A growing body of evidence supports this practice (Rowlingson, 2008).

Local Anesthesia and Methemoglobinemia. Dramatic oxygen desaturation after administration of topical benzocaine may occur because of the development of methemoglobinemia. In the perioperative setting this event may happen after airway topicalization for awake intubation or endoscopy for GI procedures. Cyanosis is evident, and oxygen saturation does not improve with administration of 100% oxygen because the abnormal methemoglobin gains precedence over oxygen-carrying hemoglobin. The patient may become restless or agitated related to hypoxemia, even though breathing 100% oxygen. An arterial blood gas sample must be drawn to be sent for co-oximetry (Matthew et al, 2008) which will define presence of excessive methemoglobin (greater than 30%, compared with normal 0.5% to 3%). Blood is usually noted to be chocolate brown, indicating presence of methemoglobin.

High levels of methemoglobinemia are treated with intravenous methylene blue 1 mg/kg over 5 minutes, repeated in 1 hour if necessary. Methemoglobinemia may be congenital, with patients presenting with a family history and their own history of cyanosis. Plans must be made for this genetic issue. Other patients may develop methemoglobinemia after administration of topical local anesthetics such as benzocaine, especially if large doses were given. Some institutions have discontinued benzocaine to prevent this problem (Institute for Safe Medical Practices, 2009). However, substitution of topical lidocaine spray in overgenerous doses may create a different form of local anesthetic toxicity.

MONITORED ANESTHESIA CARE (SEDATION AND ANALGESIA)

Anesthesia providers often deliver sedation and analgesia to patients receiving local anesthesia from surgeons in a technique named monitored anesthesia care (MAC). The term MAC arose from a billing classification and does not reflect the careful titration of sedation and analgesia that ensures maintenance of airway, breathing, circulation, and comfort while providing the surgeon with an adequate surgical field. Sedation practice by anesthesia providers lies further along the same continuum as procedural or "moderate" sedation delivered by registered nurses; although anesthesia providers are professionally trained and legally entitled to deliver deeper sedation than RNs, all of the same principles of safe care apply. Studies of sedation care have shown that severe injuries or death can occur during MAC (Harris and Sebel, 2008).

Depth of sedation and analgesia may vary, depending on the patient's physical status and other factors; a critically ill patient may receive only oxygen and monitoring, lest sedative drugs cause unstable vital signs to deteriorate further. On the other hand, a young healthy patient with a clear airway may receive oxygen and deep sedation/analgesia, remaining completely stable.

However, the anesthesia provider is prepared to intervene with all MAC patients if vital signs become unstable or other events occur, such as unexpected regurgitation and aspiration of gastric contents, allergic reaction, or ECG changes indicating cardiac ischemia. Standards of care for any other anesthetic must be followed in MAC cases, which cannot be considered lesser cases (Kirby and Lobato, 2008). In fact, it is often more difficult to deliver a smooth sedation than a general anesthetic. It may be more challenging to maintain the patient's level of consciousness appropriately drowsy while preserving a clear airway and maintaining stable vital signs than to deliver a full general anesthetic in which the patient's physiology is taken over and controlled.

Problems with oxygenation or ventilation are the most common MAC crises. With today's growing population of patients with undiagnosed obstructive sleep apnea, the potential for more crises during MAC is predictable. Patient safety may be reduced by erroneous perception of MAC cases as totally benign events. Closed-claim studies have shown that MAC cases have claim rates for death similar to those for general anesthesia, with claims for brain injury higher for MAC than for general or regional anesthesia (Kirby and Lobato, 2008). Because many MAC patients are older adults with complicated medical histories, every team member must remain vigilant during sedation cases to identify potential developing problems or to serve as an emergency anesthesia team member.

OTHER CAUSES OF ANESTHESIA-RELATED CRISES

Because anesthesia care has become statistically safe, perioperative team members may become lulled into complacency. In addition to the critical topics discussed in this chapter, other crises may suddenly arise to demand immediate rescue by a prepared team. These include events such as anaphylactic reaction, unexpected malfunction of a permanent pacemaker, and vasovagal reactions. Even in the ophthalmology suite, often considered the least likely location for crisis, cardiac arrest may be induced by the oculocardiac reflex or by misplacement of local anesthetic during retrobulbar block (RBB); LA that moves into the subarachnoid space from an intended RBB creates "total spinal anesthesia," which requires full ACLS support until the block wears away (Robicsek et al, 2008).

Crisis Management

This chapter has reviewed selected anesthesia issues. The huge number of combinations of patients, circumstances, techniques, and other individual factors creates an infinite number of potential crises that may arise. However, the basic principles of patient safety and crisis management must remain in action at all times, with critically thinking participants adapting to the moment. Gaba et al (1994) introduced principles of anesthesia crisis resource management, adapted from the aviation model, that are simple and applicable. First on the list is calling for help early and quickly when unusual circumstances arise. Specific team roles should be quickly identified, including the role of event manager. Strong, clear communication is essential; in the potential chaos of a crisis, noise must be kept to a minimum, and all directions must be loud and unambiguous. Follow-through of orders should also be announced and documented by an assigned scribe. Situational awareness must be maintained without fixations on single ideas, lest details become overwhelming and the big picture is lost. Periodic training and practice in crisis events is valuable, particularly because of the rarity of the most serious events. The growing use of simulation promises new opportunities for these types of activities.

CONCLUSION

Keeping our patients safe under anesthesia care is a difficult task. During the past decade anesthesia leaders have been working toward a high reliability organization (HRO) model as a guide to increase patient safety. Among the features of HROs (such as naval aviation, nuclear power, and off-shore oil platforms) is that safety takes top priority over all other concerns, including production pressure (Cooper and Longnecker, 2008). The full analogy of HROs applied to the perioperative environment is still incomplete. Yet, development of a culture of safety, with mindfulness, vigilance, coherent systems, well-planned teamwork, and control for human factors is well underway. Anesthesia providers and perioperative nurses are playing a large role in this movement as part of their commitment to individual patients and health care as a whole.

DEDICATION

This chapter is dedicated to the dozens of perioperative nurses who have shared my 30-year effort to provide our patients with the safest, most comfortable and comforting anesthesia and nursing care possible. Thanks for being on my team. You know who you are.

REFERENCES

American Society of Anesthesiologists: Practice guidelines for management of the difficult airway: an updated report by the American Society of Anesthesiologists Task Force on Management of the Difficult Airway, *Anesthesiology* 98:1269–1277, 2003.

American Society of Anesthesiologists: Practice advisory for perioperative visual loss associated with spine surgery: a report by the American Society of Anesthesiologists Task Force on Perioperative Blindness, *Anesthesiology* 104:1319–1328, 2006a.

American Society of Anesthesiologists: Practice guidelines for the perioperative management of patients with obstructive sleep apnea: a report by the American Society of Anesthesiologists Task Force on Perioperative Management of Patients With Obstructive Sleep Apnea, *Anesthesiology* 104:1081–1093, 2006b.

Anderson AA, et al: Identification and biochemical characterization of a novel ryanodine receptor gene mutation associated with malignant hyperthermia, *Anesthesiology* 108:208–215, 2008.

Anderson DW, Abbey KW: Handle dental injuries as you handle teeth, with care. In Marcucci C, et al: *Avoiding common anesthesia errors*, Philadelphia, 2008, Wolters Kluwer Lippincott Williams & Wilkins.

Aziz M, Horn JL: Incorporate ultrasound guidance for peripheral nerve blockade into your practice. In Marcucci C, et al: *Avoiding common anesthesia errors*, Philadelphia, 2008, Wolters Kluwer Lippincott Williams & Wilkins.

Baker KR, et al: The Icarus effect: the influence of diluents warming on dantrolene sodium mixing time, *AANA J* 75:101–106, 2007.

Benner P, Tanner C: How expert nurses use intuition, *AJN* 87:22–31, 1987.

Bernards CM: Epidural and spinal anesthesia. In Barash PG, et al, editors: *Clinical Anesthesia*, ed 6, Philadelphia, 2009, Wolters Kluwer Lippincott Williams & Wilkins.

Brull SJ, Greengrass RA: Neuraxial anesthesia. In Lobato EB, et al, editors: *Complications in anesthesiology*, Philadelphia, 2008, Wolters Kluwer Lippincott Williams & Wilkins.

Byrick RJ, et al: Prolonged coma after unreamed, locked nailing of femoral shaft fracture, *Anesthesiology* 94:163–165, 2001.

Chung F, et al: Patients with difficult intubation may need referral to sleep clinics, *Anesth Analg* 107:915–920, 2008.

Chung SA, et al: A systematic review of obstructive sleep apnea and its implications for anesthesiologists, *Anesth Analg* 107:1543–1563, 2008.

Cooper JB, Longnecker D: Safety and quality: the guiding principles of patient-centered care. In Longnecker DE, et al, editors: *Anesthesiology*, New York, 2008, McGraw Hill Medical.

Davidson S, et al: Diagnosis and treatment of negative pressure pulmonary edema in a pediatric patient: a case report, *AANA J* 72:337–338, 2004.

Denborough M: Malignant hyperthermia, *Anesthesiology* 108:156–157, 2008.

Denborough MA, Lovell RRH: Anesthetic deaths in a family, *Lancet* 276:45–46, 1960.

Donati F, Bevan DR: Neuromuscular blocking agents. In Barash PG, et al, editors: *Clinical anesthesia*, ed 6, Philadelphia, 2009, Wolters Kluwer Lippincott Williams & Wilkins.

Eichorn J: Syringe swaps in OR still harming patients, *Anesthesia Patient Safety Foundation Newsletter* 23:49–76, Winter 2008–2009.

Fallin HA, Burns DA: Consider lipid emulsion for local anesthetic overdose. In Marcucci C, et al, editors: *Avoiding common anesthesia errors*, Philadelphia, 2008, Wolters Kluwer Lippincott Williams & Wilkins.

Gaba DM, et al: *Crisis management in anesthesiology*, Philadelphia, 1994, Churchill-Livingstone.

Gray AT: Ultrasound-guided regional anesthesia: current state of the art, *Anesthesiology* 104:368–373, 2006.

Gronert GA, et al: Malignant hyperthermia. In Miller RD, et al: *Miller's anesthesia*, ed 6, Philadelphia, 2005, Elsevier Churchill Livingstone.

Gutsche JT, Hanson CW III: Pulmonary embolism. In Lobato EB, et al, editors: *Complications in anesthesiology*, Philadelphia, 2008, Wolters Kluwer Lippincott Williams & Wilkins.

Hadzic A, et al: Ultrasound guidance may reduce but not eliminate complications of peripheral nerve blocks, *Anesthesiology* 108:557–558, 2008.

Hagberg C, et al: Complications of managing the airway, *Best Pract Res Clin Anaesthesiol* 19:641–659, 2005.

Harris RS, Sebel PS: Monitored anesthesia care and conscious sedation. In Longnecker DE, et al, editors: *Anesthesiology*, New York, 2008, McGraw Hill Medical.

Heavner JE: Pharmacology of local anesthetics. In Longnecker DE, et al, editors: *Anesthesiology*, New York, 2008, McGraw Hill Medical.

Institute for Healthcare Improvement: *SBAR technique for communication: a situational briefing model*, available at http://www.ihi.org/IHI/Topics/PatientSafety/SafetyGeneral/Tools/SBARTechniqueforCommunicationASituationalBriefingModel.htm. Accessed July 22, 2009.

Institute for Safe Medical Practices: Benzocaine spray and methemoglobinemia, *Nurse Advise-Err* 7:2. Feb 2009, available at http://www.ismp.org. Accessed February 28, 2009.

Isono S: Obstructive sleep apnea of obese adults: pathophysiology and perioperative airway management, *Anesthesiology* 110:908–921, 2009.

Kaufmann A: Novel ryanodine receptor mutation that may cause malignant hyperthermia, *Anesthesiology* 109: 457–464, 2008.

Kesimci E, et al: Management of unpredicted postoperative negative pressure pulmonary edema: a report of two cases, *Internet J Anesthesiol* 12:1, 2007.

Kirby RR, Lobato EB: Monitored anesthesia care. In Lobato EB, et al, editors: *Complications in anesthesiology*, Philadelphia, 2008, Wolters Kluwer Lippincott Williams & Wilkins.

Kohn LT, et al: *To err is human: building a safer health system, Washington*, DC, 2000, National Academy Press.

Lee L, et al: The American Society of Anesthesiologists Postoperative Visual Loss Registry: analysis of 93 spine surgery cases with postoperative visual loss, *Anesthesiology* 105:652–659, 2006.

Leighton BL: Why obstetric anesthesiologists get sued, *Anesthesiology* 110:8–9, 2009.

Liu E, et al: Success of tracheal intubation with intubating laryngeal mask airways: a randomized trial of the LMA Fastrach and LMA CTrach, *Anesthesiology* 108:621–626, 2008.

Lowery JE, Myers LL: Florid negative pressure pulmonary edema, *Internet J Otorhinolaryngol* 7:2, 2008.

Malignant Hyperthermia Association of the United States: *MHAUS guidelines—testing for malignant hyperthermia (MH) susceptibility: how do I counsel my patients?* n.d., available at: http://medical.mhaus.org/PubData/PDFs/dx_testing_options.pdf. Accessed December 10, 2009.

Mallampati SR: Clinical signs to predict difficult tracheal intubation [hypothesis], *Can Anaesth Soc J* 30:316, 1983.

Massó Eva, et al: Lightwand tracheal intubation with and without muscle relaxation, *Anesthesiology* 104:249–254, 2006.

Matthew L, et al: Consider methemoglobinemia after ruling out the common causes for a low pulse oximeter reading. In Marcucci C, et al, editors: *Avoiding common anesthesia errors*, Philadelphia, 2008, Wolters Kluwer Lippincott Williams & Wilkins.

McFadden RD: Pilot is hailed after jetliner's icy plunge, *New York Times* January 16 2009, available at http://www.nytimes.com/2009/01/16/nyregion/16crash.html?_r=1&pagewanted=print. Accessed July 3, 2009.

Mirshab C: A 19-year-old man with postoperative respiratory insufficiency. In Duke J, editor: *Anesthesia Pearls*, Philadelphia, 2002, Elsevier.

Mirski M, et al: Diagnosis and treatment of vascular air embolism, *Anesthesiology* 106:164–177, 2007.

Moore LE: *Amniotic fluid embolism*, 2008a, available at http://emedicine.medscape.com/article/253068-overview updated August 12. Accessed October 16, 2009.

Moore LE: Remember that loss of vision is one of the most feared and devastating complications of spine surgery. In Marcucci C, et al, editors: *Avoiding common anesthesia errors*, Philadelphia, 2008b, Wolters Kluwer Lippincott Williams & Wilkins.

Morgan GE, et al: *Clinical anesthesiology*, ed 4, New York, 2006, Lange Medical Books/McGraw Hill.

Mort TC: Continuous airway access for the difficult extubation: the efficacy of the airway exchange catheter, *Anesth Analg* 105:1357–1362, 2007.

Mulroy MF: Peripheral nerve blockade. In Barash PG, et al, editors: *Clinical Anesthesia*, ed 3, Philadelphia, 2006, Lippincott Williams & Wilkins.

Murphy GS, et al: Intraoperative acceleromyographic monitoring reduces the risk of residual neuromuscular blockade and adverse respiratory events in the postanesthesia care unit, *Anesthesiology* 109:389–398, 2008.

Naik B: Pneumothorax and barotrauma. In Lobato EB, et al, editors: *Complications in anesthesiology*, Philadelphia, 2008, Wolters Kluwer Lippincott Williams & Wilkins.

Odom-Forren J, Watson DS: *Practical guide to moderate sedation/analgesia*, St. Louis, 2005, Elsevier Mosby.

Opton JC: Remember that elevated temperature is a late finding in malignant hyperthermia. In Marcucci C, et al, editors: *Avoiding common anesthesia errors*, Philadelphia, 2008, Wolters Kluwer Lippincott Williams & Wilkins.

Orkin FK, Longnecker DE: Anesthesia risk. In Longnecker DE, et al, editors: *Anesthesiology*, New York, 2008, McGraw Hill Medical.

Pennsylvania Patient Safety Authority: Sterile water should not be given "freely, *Pennsylvania Patient Safety Advisory* 5:53–56, 2008.

Peterson GN, et al: Management of the difficult airway: a closed claims analysis, *Anesthesiology* 103:33–39, 2005.

Rizzi RR: Neuromuscular monitoring advancement, *Anesthesiology* 100:454, 2004.

Robicsek SA, et al: Cardiac arrest. In Lobato EB, et al, editors: *Complications in anesthesiology*, Philadelphia, 2008, Wolters Kluwer Lippincott Williams & Wilkins.

Rooke GA: Anesthesia for the older patient. In Barash PG, et al, editors: *Clinical Anesthesia*, ed 6, Philadelphia, 2009, Wolters Kluwer Lippincott Williams & Wilkins.

Rosenberg H, Rothstein A: Malignant hyperthermia death holds many lessons, *Anesthesia Patient Safety Foundation Newsletter* 21:32–34, 2006.

Rosenberg H, et al: Malignant hyperthermia and other inherited disorders. In Barash PG, et al, editors: *Clinical anesthesia*, ed 6, Philadelphia, 2009, Wolters Kluwer Lippincott Williams & Wilkins.

Rovithis M, Parissopoulos S: Intuition in nursing practice, *ICUS Nurs Web J* 22:1–10, 2005.

Rowlingson JC: Lipid rescue: a step forward in patient safety? Likely so! *Anesth Analg* 106:1333–1336, 2008.

Sen S, Barts M: Do not overlook the "old-fashioned" Bier block, but beware of the speedy surgeon! In Marcucci C, et al, editors: *Avoiding common anesthesia errors*, Philadelphia, 2008, Wolters Kluwer Lippincott Williams & Wilkins.

Sessler DI: Temperature monitoring and perioperative thermoregulation, *Anesthesiology* 109:318–338, 2008.

Tasch MD, Butterwork JF IV: Adverse reactions to local anesthetics. In Lobato EB, et al, editors: *Complications in anesthesiology*, Philadelphia, 2008, Wolters Kluwer Lippincott Williams & Wilkins.

Tsui BCH, Rosenquist RW: Peripheral nerve blockade. In Barash PG, et al, editors: *Clinical anesthesia*, ed 6, Philadelphia, 2009, Wolters Kluwer Lippincott Williams & Wilkins.

Warren DT, Liu SS: Neuraxial anesthesia. In Longnecker DE, et al, editors: *Anesthesiology*, New York, 2008, McGraw Hill Medical.

Weinberg G: Lipid infusion resuscitation for local anesthetic toxicity: proof of clinical efficacy, *Anesthesiology* 105:7–8, 2006.

Weinberg G: *Lipid rescue resuscitation for cardiac toxicity*, available at http://www.lipidrescue.org. Accessed June 10 2009.

Weiss SJ, et al: Fatal paradoxical cerebral embolization during bilateral knee arthroplasty, *Anesthesiology* 84(3): 721–723, 1996.

World Health Organization: *Surgical safety checklist (first edition)*, 2008, available at http://www.who.int/patientsafety/safesurgery/en. Accessed June 15, 2009.

PREVENTING SURGICAL SITE INFECTIONS

Peter B. Graves, BSN, RN, CNOR

Prevention of surgical site infections (SSIs) is a key risk management and quality improvement issue. A surgical site infection is one of the most common hospital-acquired infections (HAIs) and is a significant cause of morbidity and mortality (Centers for Disease Control and Prevention [CDC], 2009b). SSIs have a significant impact on the patient and place an additional cost burden upon individuals, families, payers, and society. In addition to the financial impact, the physical and psychologic impact on the patient cannot be underestimated. The goal for every facility should be a zero surgical site infection rate; unfortunately, to achieve this goal changes in conventional practices must be supported and implemented. Several factors may be tied to contracting an SSI (Box 13-1).

Today's health care environment is quickly evolving with a commitment and clear focus of payer groups, governmental agencies, health care organizations, and other stakeholders to do something about the spiraling cost burden upon society as a result of these infections. Preventing SSIs requires a team commitment and approach that enlists not just the surgical department, but every practitioner, administrator, organization, and recommending body responsible for delivering or affecting patient care. Initiatives focusing upon pay for performance, never events, and cost containment, driven by both the Centers for Medicare & Medicaid Services (CMS) and Congress, are forcing change upon the health care system.

CHALLENGES

Surveillance

Current epidemiology has met a true challenge with early discharge and outpatient surgical procedures. This challenge is in part a result of a shortened duration of postoperative hospitalization, which is now measured in hours or days, not weeks. This complicates the ability to monitor and observe for the development of a surgical infection. In some cases or situations, infections may go virtually untracked. Although the true number of SSIs may never be known, there are many variables to identify and correct to prevent surgical site infections.

Many organizations use a variety of methods (e.g., risk index) to stratify surgical procedures into groups so that data can be effectively reviewed for infection risk based upon similar patient populations. In addition, active surveillance and self-reported surveys are sent to surgical practitioners as an assessment of surgical site infections identified postoperatively. This is one of the common surveillance strategies used. Unfortunately, this method may not always capture every surgical site infection in every situation. It is important to remember that 96% of superficial surgical site infections occur within the first 28 days of surgery (World Health Organization [WHO], 2008b).

An SSI is commonly defined as occurring at the site of surgery. Surveillance of the surgical sites lasts for 30 days if the operation does not include an implantable device (e.g., pacemaker, heart valve, orthopedic implant). If an implant is involved, then tracking takes place for a year and is conducted by both the surgeon and the infection preventionist.

Across the United States, health care organizations use follow-up interviews for their same-day surgery patients. The phone interview may explore postoperative pain issues, surgical site appearance (if visualized), patient teaching, satisfaction with care received, and reminders for follow-up appointments. This call normally takes place within a prescribed time frame after discharge. In many situations, little actionable information can be gathered from this interview with respect to surgical site infections. Postdischarge

BOX 13-1 Patient and Surgical Factors That May Be Tied to Surgical Site Infection

PATIENT CHARACTERISTICS
Age
Nutritional status
Diabetes
Smoking
Obesity
Microbial colonization
Remote infection
Altered immune response
Perioperative length of stay

SURGICAL ELEMENTS
Preoperative skin preparation
Hair removal (shaving)
Surgical hand antisepsis of surgical team members
Environmental controls
Surgical attire and drapes
Instrument sterilization
Length of operation
Surgical technique
Antimicrobial prophylaxis

Modified from World Health Organization: *WHO guidelines for safe surgery (first edition)*, Geneva, Switzerland, 2008b, available at http://www.gawande.com/documents/WHOGuidelinesforSafeSurgery_001.pdf. Accessed August 17, 2009.

surveillance requires a robust effort to track patients and involves the entire surgical team and the organization. To put this in perspective, consider a methicillin-susceptible *Staphylococcus aureus* (MSSA) infection. A common gram-positive opportunistic pathogen responsible for many wound infections, coagulase-positive *S. aureus* commonly has an incubation period of about 5 days before signs and symptoms become evident. This example highlights the difficulty in tracking some, but not all, hospital-acquired infections when the SSI does not manifest itself until after the patient is discharged or telephonic follow-up is conducted.

Prevalence

More than 50 million procedures are performed per year, and the incidence of SSIs has been reported to be about 300,000 per year, which account for approximately 22% of all the health care–acquired infections each year (CDC, 2009b). The majority of the 300,000 SSIs are not life threatening; however, the CDC estimates that SSI results in approximately 8000 deaths annually (CDC, 2009b). When looking at the prevalence of SSIs, about 70% involve the superficial skin, whereas the other 30% are considered more serious. These numbers place a significant burden on society when considering the estimated average cost of an SSI infection is $35,000 per event (Scott, 2009).

SURGICAL SITE INFECTION GUIDELINES

Although every SSI cannot be blamed on the health care system, one of the important tools being used to identify and prevent the causes of these infections is the Surgical Care Improvement Project (SCIP) initiative (MEDQIC, 2007). SCIP is a national quality partnership of organizations focused on improving surgical care by significantly reducing surgical complications. SCIP is a unique partnership that is proving to be a transformational undertaking in health care. The four goals of SCIP in preventing SSIs to reduce the incidence of surgical complications nationally 25% by the year 2010 are as follows:

1. Antimicrobial prophylaxis
   - Given within 1 hour of surgery
   - Prophylactic antibiotic selection
2. Glycemic control in cardiac patients
   - Controlled postoperative serum glucose level
   - Discontinued within 24 hours (48 hours in cardiac patients)
3. Appropriate hair removal
   - Use clippers rather than razors
4. Immediate postoperative normothermia in colorectal patients

Although SCIP is not the only quality partnership under way in perioperative settings, some of these recommendations found in SCIP can be traced back to the "Guideline for Prevention of Surgical Site Infection" (Mangram et al, 1999). The CDC guideline offered 72 recommendations (Mangram et al, 1999). Using an evidence-based rating system, eight of these recommendations were assigned a 1A rating, which designates the highest level of evidence. Many health care organizations often look to the weight of the evidence to help drive implementation and compliance in the clinical setting. However, with the various practice settings in place today (e.g., hospital, surgical center, office based), not all facilities have universally implemented these recommendations. One such example is the slow implementation of the 1A recommendation to use a clipper, not a razor, if hair removal is required (Edminston, 2007).

There are numerous differences between the SCIP and the CDC "Guideline for Prevention of Surgical Site Infection"; one of the most noticeable differences appears in the data collection tools and the definitions. The data collection tools used by SCIP are much larger and more complex, requiring a significant investment in labor. However, the data collected by SCIP is providing greater insight into the world of infections. This is resulting in evidence-based recommendations that are driving the decision-making process and affecting patient outcomes in a significant way.

In addition to SCIP initiatives and the CDC's guidelines to prevent SSIs, numerous other stakeholders are aggressively promoting the prevention of SSIs. One example is the Society for Healthcare Epidemiology of America, which recently published "A Compendium of Strategies to Prevent Healthcare-Associated Infections in Acute Care Hospitals" (Yokoe et al, 2008). The strategies emphasize the importance of surveillance, the need for feedback and education for the entire health care team, attention to practice issues highlighted in other guidelines, and the development of special approaches for facilities to address specific locations or populations (Yokoe et al, 2008).

SURGICAL ENVIRONMENT

Environmental Hygiene

There is increasing pressure upon organizations to maintain and minimize the risk of transmission of transmissible infections within the health care facility. One of the key factors for prevention of infections is a clean environment (Dancer, 2008). Environmental cleaning is both time consuming and a labor-intensive process. Thorough environmental cleaning requires training and monitoring to validate that cleaning is adequate.

It is well acknowledged that implementation of appropriate hand hygiene practices reduces infections. By targeting environmental cleaning efforts within the health care facility on patient and health care touch points (e.g., door handles, surfaces, phones), the environmental cleaning regimen has been easier to maintain than hand hygiene improvements. As a method to stop the spread of multidrug-resistant organisms (MDROs), this strategy could have significant benefits to the surgical environment, as well as the entire health care facility (Dancer, 2008).

The Association of periOperative Registered Nurses (AORN) in the "Recommended Practices for Environmental Cleaning in the Perioperative Setting" clearly describes the methodology and the rigor needed for environmental cleaning in the surgical setting (AORN, 2009a). The unfortunate aspect is that some facilities may fall short in meeting these recommendations as a result of emphasis upon production (e.g., turnover time). When the surgical environment (surfaces, equipment, or supplies) is not thoroughly cleaned, the transfer of pathogenic organisms becomes a possibility. When individuals do not follow the prescribed application time (wet time) of the surface cleanser—failure to use a product per the manufacturer's written instructions—they achieve less than the desired effects and reduce efficacy of the product. Visual inspection of surfaces does little to guarantee an environment free of pathogenic organisms (Dancer, 2008). This can be seen in the reports of infection outbreaks when incomplete or inadequate environmental surface cleaning takes place within facilities, such as reports of methicillin-resistant *S. aureus* (MRSA) or *Clostridium difficile* transmission from improper or inadequate cleaning. This is a crucial aspect of the prevention of infections within the perioperative environment. An example of an SSI outbreak took place at some ambulatory surgery centers (ASCs) and is described in the following (CDC, 2009a):

> *ASCs in the United States have been the fastest growing provider type participating in Medicare, increasing in number by more than 38% between 2002 and 2007. A 2008 hepatitis C outbreak in Nevada was traced to poor infection control practices at various ASCs (potentially affecting more than 50,000 people). Follow-up surveys throughout Nevada found infection control deficiencies at more than 40% of the ASCs.*

HEALTH CARE PROVIDER ISSUES

Hand Hygiene

Much has been written about hand hygiene being the most important action a health care worker can take to prevent the spread of infections. In surgery the term *sterile conscience,* which describes doing the right thing even when no one is watching, is always applied. It is inconceivable to break sterile technique and not do anything to minimize or remedy the break.

Health care organizations are now being required by The Joint Commission to have stricter policies and performance monitoring in place as a way to improve and maintain hand hygiene practices. Clean hands do save lives by breaking the chain of infection. Hand hygiene should involve hand washing with soap (plain or antimicrobial) and water if hands are visibly soiled. If hands are not visibly soiled, the use of an alcoholic agent is preferred (Boyce and Pittet, 2002; WHO, 2008a). In the surgical environment all health care workers should perform a soap-and-water hand wash initially to ensure that hands are physically clean when arriving to work, before and after using the restroom, before meals, and before going home at the end of one's shift. Scrubbed staff should wash their hands with soap (plain or antimicrobial) and water before their first scrub of the day (AORN, 2009b).

Surgical Hand Antisepsis

In 2002 Parienti et al demonstrated that there was no statistical difference in surgical site infections between the use of surgical hand scrubbing (i.e., scrub brush, antiseptic soap, and water) and the use of surgical hand rubbing (i.e., 1-minute timed wash followed by application of an alcoholic agent) (Table 13-1). There was a noticeable lack of compliance with performance in both groups. This study was a randomized equivalency study over a 17-month period evaluating approximately 4400 patients (Parienti et al, 2002). To increase compliance, operating room leadership should consistently monitor, enforce, and reward proper surgical hand antisepsis behaviors through education, observation, and counseling.

AORN's "Recommended Practices for Hand Hygiene in the Perioperative Setting" (2009b), CDC's "Guideline for Hand Hygiene in Health-Care Settings" (2002), and WHO's *Guidelines on Hand Hygiene in Health Care* (2008a) each recommend that practitioners follow the manufacturer's written instructions for product use and use the recommended amount. If practitioners choose to use a product for less than its prescribed time or amount, the desired efficacy may not be realized (Graves and Twomey, 2006). The intent of the surgical scrub or rub is to eliminate transient flora and to reduce colonizing flora to minimize the potential SSI risk to the patient.

Surgical Attire

In 1883 Gustav Neuber encouraged the use of gown and cap, and in 1897 Mirculiz advocated the use of a mask to reduce organisms from the mouth and nose. Dr. William Halsted, credited by many as the father of modern-day surgery, encouraged the use of surgical gloves along with dedicated surgical attire in 1899. Although gloves were initially worn to protect Dr. Halsted's scrub nurse, it soon became apparent that the surgical glove reduced the patient's exposure to a surgeon's flora and the potential for SSIs. Surgical attire has not made a dramatic design change since that time.

The surgical uniform, or "scrubs," is intended to be worn within the semirestricted and restricted areas that are designed to promote hygiene and

TABLE 13-1 Surgical Hand Antisepsis Comparison

Protocol	SSI Rate (95% Confidence Interval)	Performance Compliance (retrospective, P = 0.008)
Surgical hand rub	55/2252 (2.44%)	44%
Surgical hand scrub	53/2135 (2.48%)	28%

From Graves PB, Twomey CT: Surgical hand antisepsis: an evidence based review, *Perioper Nurs Clin* 1(3):235-249, 2006.

cleanliness. Today surgical attire takes on many different looks and styles, but the basic intent remains unchanged—maintaining a professional hygienic appearance to our patients and the public.

Today there are three types of surgical attire: (1) facility-provided surgical attire (hospital owned and laundered, hospital owned and third-party laundered, or leased [fee per use]); (2) home-laundered surgical attire; and (3) single-use disposable surgical attire, which is gaining in popularity and acceptance as a result of improved nonwoven fabrics.

Many health care organizations and recommending bodies (e.g., AORN, Association for the Advancement of Medical Instrumentation [AAMI], Association for Professionals in Infection Control and Epidemiology [APIC]) have taken different positions on how surgical attire should be laundered, worn, and managed within the surgical environment. This inconsistency has created confusion for health care workers and organizations alike. There is an acknowledged lack of well-characterized studies that demonstrate that laundering of worn surgical attire in the home is a safe and effective practice. Rather, there is emerging evidence that home laundering may not render surgical attire as clean as hospital and commercial third-party laundering processes. Guidelines such as the AORN's "Recommended Practices for Surgical Attire" (2009f) do not recommended home laundering of surgical attire.

Whatever process is chosen by the health care organization to clean the surgical uniform, it should be validated by the organization, as in the case of hospital and third-party commercial laundry facilities. Health care organizations should have a process in place to confirm that the surgical uniform is clean and has met the same criteria used by the facility to validate other linen (process validation). Although there has been no study that links surgical scrubs to infections in patients, it has been demonstrated that MDROs can survive on fabrics for an extended period of time (Neely and Maley, 2000).

Surgical scrubs intended to be worn within the restricted areas should not be worn into the area from outside the health care facility. If scrubs are worn outside, they should be classified as street clothes and changed before entering the semirestricted or restricted environment. Only freshly laundered or single-use disposable surgical attire should be worn in the semirestricted or restricted environment of the surgical department.

Personal Protective Equipment

Surgical Caps and Hoods. The Occupational Safety and Health Administration (OSHA) (2009) requires head covering as a part of universal precautions. In addition to OSHA's mandate, AORN recommends covering all hair in an effort to reduce contamination of the surgical field from exposed hair and scalp. There have been reports of SSI outbreaks traced back to the hair and scalp of surgical personnel (Mastro et al, 1990).

Surgical Masks. OSHA requires the wearing of a surgical mask when in the operating room. Use of fluid-repellant surgical masks may also help protect the practitioner from splash of patient fluids.

Surgical Gowns. OSHA (2009) requires the use of surgical gowns to protect the wearer from exposure to blood and other potentially infectious materials. Although the intent of these devices initially was to protect the patient from organisms brought in to the surgical suite by the surgical team, the shift has moved dramatically to protecting the surgical team from patient fluid contamination. AORN's "Recommended Practices for Maintaining a Sterile Field" (2009c) describes in detail steps that the wearer must consider (e.g., wearing gowns in the natural wrist area).

Surgical Gloves. There are a number of identified issues surrounding surgical gloves and SSI. First, it has been well documented in the literature that absorbable dusting USP cornstarch, used as a donning agent in surgical gloves, contributes to the formation of adhesions and granulomas (Giercksky, 1997; Holmdahl and Risberg, 1997; van den Tol et al, 2001). Next, powder may contribute in yet another way to infections. It was demonstrated that powder in a wound actually decreases local resistance to infection. The study documented that resistance to infection by *S. aureus* bacterium was decreased by a factor of 10 when powder was involved (Jaffray and Nade, 1983). This would apply not only to the surgical suite, but to postoperative wound care as well. Powder on a glove, whether it is latex or synthetic, surgical or examination, can contaminate a wound.

AORN (2009e) recommends in the "Recommended Practices for the Prevention of Transmissible Infections in the Perioperative Practice Settings" that "health care practitioners should double glove during invasive procedures." AORN encourages double gloving as a result of the systematic review of the double-gloving data performed by the Cochrane Collaborative. The Cochrane Collaborative further acknowledged that end users who used a colored underglove were able to more quickly identify barrier breeches and thus take appropriate action (Tanner and Parkinson, 2006). Considering the available data on the failure rates of surgical gloves, it is critical to take appropriate measures to protect both the practitioner and the patient as much as possible.

PATIENT ISSUES

Wound Healing

In response to an injury, healing is a complex physiologic cascade, whether the injury is a result of a burn, penetrating object, or surgical knife. In simplistic terms, an injury can lead to a disruption of the microcirculation that results in platelet aggregation occurring at the wound site with a release of chemical attractants and growth factors. Coagulation occurs by occluding vessels with fibrin, thus preventing further bleeding (but it may also result in a widening of the area of impaired circulation). During the inflammatory phase, additional factors are released: fibrin leads growth factor sequences, mast cells release histamine, leukocytes migrate, and macrophages phagocytize bacteria and dead tissue and stimulate angiogenesis. Angiogenesis incorporates the growth and movement of endothelial cells, and the endothelial response is dependent on blood perfusion and arterial partial pressure of oxygen (PaO_2). Fibroblasts migrate into the area in response to the growth factors and other chemical attractants. Once established in a wound, fibroblasts initiate the cascade for collagen development. Wound strength is ultimately dependent on collagen deposition. Therefore the strength of a wound in the healing stages is dependent on oxygenation and perfusion and vulnerable to respiratory and perfusion complications. Epithelial cells move and replicate in response to growth factors and oxygen tension, so healing occurs most rapidly in hydrated well-oxygenated tissues. In the late stages of healing, contraction of the collagen fibers occurs, which shortens scars and shrinks open wounds. Wound healing can be influenced by growth factors and antiinflammatory steroids produced by the body or given to the patient (Hunt and Hopf, 1997).

Any time there is an interruption in skin integrity, the body is very dependent on its ability to clear foreign material and resist infection. The major pathways involved in these two activities in wounds are nonspecific phagocytosis and intracellular killing. For these defense systems to operate, once again, oxygenation, perfusion, and arterial oxygen tension are critical.

Multidrug-Resistant Organisms

MDROs have received widespread attention in the literature for the past several years. In addition, the development of MDRO infections will increase the patient's length of stay and costs and will affect the morbidity and mortality rates. Common organisms that fall into the MDRO category are MRSA, vancomycin-resistant enterococci, and other gram-negative bacilli (*Acinetobacter baumannii*). Each of these MDROs has unique and sometimes shared risk factors. Health care workers should follow organizational and CDC guidelines in the prevention of these infections. One must use personal protective equipment and isolation guidelines to combat the spread of these sometimes fatal organisms. It is recommended to continue the use of isolation precaution(s) in the surgical setting. Consultation with an infection preventionist is warranted.

As a result of the prevalence of MDROs and the CMS pay-for-performance initiatives, many organizations have begun to culture specific patient populations preemptively. The most common method of culturing patients is through nasal, pharyngeal, or perineal culturing. Although culturing of all patients is not recommended by either the Society for Healthcare Epidemiology of America (SHEA) (Yokoe et al, 2008) or APIC (2008), the number of facilities culturing patients is increasing.

Patient Colonization

In very simplistic terms the CDC (2009b) defines colonization to mean that an "organism is present on or in the body, but not causing an illness." In most cases bacteria may live harmlessly on an individual's skin, but it does, however, set the stage for the opportunistic organism to seek out other weaknesses in the host's defenses. Colonization can also be transient or persistent.

S. aureus colonization is all too familiar in every part of the country. To become nasally colonized with *S. aureus*, four conditions must be met as described by Wertheim et al (2005): (1) contact must occur with *S. aureus* and the nose; (2) within the nose, binding of *S. aureus* with receptors must take place; (3) host defenses must be overcome by the invading *S. aureus*; and, finally, (4) *S. aureus* must be able to grow. This is why both hand hygiene and environmental hygiene are important to break the chain of transmission. There have been increasing reports in the literature of SSIs in patients with a history of MRSA nasal colonization.

Body Colonization Location. Any area of the human body can become colonized. Wertheim et al reported that in respect to *S. aureus* carriage, the nose is the most common location. The other areas where *S. aureus* can be found are the hands, perineum, forearms, chest, and pharynx. Bacterial loads, dispersal, and risk of infection are often higher in persistent carriers than in intermittent carriers (Wertheim et al, 2005). In addition, individuals who are both nasal and perineal carriers not only disperse more *S. aureus*, but also have higher bacterial loads (Wertheim et al, 2005). It is well acknowledged that presence of nasal colonization is a risk factor for SSIs. Identification of pathogenic nasal colonization is taking on a more important role in the prevention of surgical site infections with respect to MRSA.

Patient Hygiene

In the "Recommended Practices for Preoperative Patient Skin Antisepsis," AORN (2009d) identified skin cleanliness as the initial step in preparation for surgery. Showering twice, the evening before and the morning of surgery, with a 4% chlorhexidine gluconate soap was identified as the preferred method, when possible, to accomplish general skin cleansing (AORN, 2009d). APIC (2008) also published a guide for the prevention of mediastinitis surgical site infections following cardiac surgery. Preoperative showering twice was recommended—once the night before and once the morning of surgery—to reduce the bacterial microbe levels to as low as possible. According to the APIC guideline, patients should be instructed to use clean, freshly laundered towels to dry with after showering, wear clean nightclothes after showering, and to sleep in clean, freshly laundered bedding. A similar routine should be followed on the morning of surgery—use a clean, freshly laundered towel to dry with, and wear freshly laundered, clean clothes to the facility. By effectively showering before surgery, the skin is rendered clean, a precursor for surgical skin antisepsis. In addition to clean skin, using 4% chlorhexidine gluconate twice before surgery gives the agent an opportunity to bind to the stratum corneum and provide persistence, thus reducing bacterial counts (Boyce and Pittet, 2002). It is also important to instruct (verbally and in writing) the patient to follow the manufacturer's written and labeled instructions to achieve the level of efficacy desired. Many facilities have developed instructional sheets to assist patients in their native language. In addition, some facilities have developed a verification of use (e.g., verbal questions, return with an empty bottle or packets). Although no system is foolproof, involving patients in their care is an important risk-reduction step.

Surgical Skin Antisepsis

It is well acknowledged that the skin cannot be rendered sterile; rather it can be made to be surgically clean. The perioperative nurse should assess for the cleanliness of the patient's skin before preparation. If the skin has not been cleansed before arrival to the surgical department, then general skin cleansing should take place, particularly if an alcoholic skin preparation agent is chosen. Alcoholic skin preparations are not intended to cleanse the skin or remove soils or spores; rather they are designed to be used on physically clean skin. Preparation agents should be chosen for use based not on the ability to stain the skin or define the prepped area; they should be chosen based on their ability to be fast acting and broad spectrum, to demonstrate persistence, and to be minimally affected by organic materials, such as blood or other body fluids. Using AORN's "Recommended Practices for Preoperative Patient Skin Antisepsis" (2009d) practitioners should pay close attention to patient's skin preparation as a key step in the avoidance of potential surgical site infections.

Patient Hand Hygiene

Much has been written about the importance of hand hygiene for health care workers, but a significant and noticeable gap in the literature exists with respect to the importance of patient hand hygiene. It is common sense that patient hand hygiene should be a cornerstone for every health care organization's infection prevention program. Every patient who is capable should perform hand hygiene by first washing with soap (plain or antimicrobial) and water upon entry into the health care facility. This will leave their skin physically clean. Before surgery, offer the patient the ability to wash the hands again or to use an alcohol-based hand sanitizer to degerm their hands; this follows the same guiding principles we use for health care workers. The objective is to maintain hand hygiene with every surgical patient (all patients for that matter). The rationale of this intervention is to minimize the transient and resident organisms on the patient's hand and to reduce the potential for cross contamination and ultimately infections. Patients' hand hygiene should be continuous throughout their stay. Wash with soap (plain or antimicrobial) and water if hands are soiled, or use an alcohol-based hand sanitizer for skin not soiled (Boyce and Pittet, 2002). This is a nursing intervention that does not require a physician's order.

Oxygenation

In a recent meta-analysis of five randomized controlled trials evaluating the use of supplemental oxygen and SSIs, it was reported that supplemental oxygen did have a beneficial effect on the prevention of SSIs (Qadan et al, 2009). The following are the findings of the meta-analysis:

- Most studies have demonstrated a favorable outcome to supplemental hyperoxia.
- No agreed-upon guideline is available for the use of supplemental oxygen to prevent SSIs.
- Oxygen did exert a statistically beneficial effect on SSI prevention and should be recommended for colorectal surgical patients (Qadan et al, 2009).

In addition, it was recommended to maintain normothermia, careful glycemic control, and intravascular volume (Qadan et al, 2009).

It has been theorized that oxidative killing by neutrophils occurs at the wound site, is a primary defense against surgical pathogens, and is directly related to tissue oxygenation (Ratnaraj et al, 2004). Others have reported similar opinions on oxidative killing by neutrophils. Increasing intraoperative tissue oxygen tension markedly reduces the potential risk of such infections (Akca et al, 2002). Although the practice of using supplemental oxygen during surgery and postoperatively remains controversial, it is nonetheless an important area that deserves further study.

Smoking

Patients who present with a history of smoking should be counseled to cease smoking. There is no clear recommendation for the period of time an individual should cease smoking before surgery. It was reported that, among patients who had reconstructive head and neck surgery, patients who stopped smoking more than 3 weeks before surgery had a reduced impaired wound healing (Kuri et al, 2005). Although more research is needed to identify the ideal time for cessation of smoking, it is clear that smoking slows wound healing and increases the potential for infection.

Normothermia

The importance of normothermia on the prevention of SSIs cannot be emphasized enough. The impact of hypothermia on patient outcomes for the surgical patient has been extensively researched. Some studies indicate a statistically significant difference for the development of a SSI between patients with hypothermia and those with normothermia (Kurz, 1996; Flores-Maldonado et al, 2001; Melling et al, 2001) (Table 13-2). Maintaining the patient's core temperature requires a coordinated effort among all the team members. Normothermia should be initiated before surgery and be continuously monitored throughout the patient's care. In the SCIP initiative, maintaining normothermia in colorectal patients is a core measure. Chapter 15 will address issues related to the importance of maintaining normothermia.

Perioperative normothermia has an impact on SSI and length of stay. It has also been acknowledged that hypothermia can trigger thermoregulatory vasoconstriction, which decreases tissue oxygen tension; as a result of vasoconstriction, reduced oxygen in tissue kills neutrophils and decreases wound strength by reducing the deposition of collagen, ultimately impairing immune function (Edminston, 2007). Several factors that can contribute to patient cooling in surgery are listed in Box 13-2.

TABLE 13-2 Normothermia Studies

Study*	Normothermia SSI Rates (%)	Hypothermia SSI Rates (%)
Flores-Maldonado et al	1.9	11.8
Melling et al	5	14
Kurz et al	6	19

SSI, Surgical site infection.

* Flores-Maldonado A et al: Mild perioperative hypothermia and the risk of wound infection, *Arch Med Res* 32(3):227-231, 2001; Kurz A et al: Perioperative normothermia to reduce the incidence of surgical-wound infection and shorten hospitalization, Study of Wound Infection and Temperature Group, *N Engl J Med* 334(19):1209-1215, 1996; Melling AC et al: Effects of preoperative warming on the incidence of wound infection after clean surgery: a randomised controlled trial, *Lancet* 358(9285):876-880, 2001.

BOX 13-2 Conditions That Contribute to Patient Cooling

SLOW METABOLISM

Presurgical fasting
Anesthesia

CONDUCTIVE COOLING

Skin preparation solutions
Cold OR table
Cool IV solution
Cool irrigation

CONVECTION AND EVAPORATIVE COOLING

Thin gowns (lost insulation)
Body surface exposure
Open wounds
Cool OR air temperature

IV, Intravenous; *OR,* operating room.

Antibiotic Usage

One method for preventing SSI that has stood the test of time and is clearly supported by evidence-based studies is the proper timing and dosing of antibiotic before surgery. "Ensuring the appropriate use and timing of preoperative prophylactic antibiotics has been shown to be efficacious and should be the cornerstone of any good SSI prevention program" (Wong, 1999). As part of the SCIP initiative, it is recommended that preoperative prophylactic antibiotics be administered within 60 minutes of the incision, or longer when indicated, and that the selection of the agent be based on efficacy (MEDQIC, 2007). Timing of the dose should ensure that the optimal therapeutic level is achieved in the blood at the time the incision is made, and that therapeutic level should be maintained throughout the operation and until, at most, the first few hours after closure (Mangram et al, 1999).

Even with numerous studies and national initiatives under way, errors in antibiotic prophylaxis do occur. Error rates in the United States vary from 25% to 40% depending on surgical specialty (Edminston, 2007). Research shows that delivering antibiotics to a patient within 1 hour of beginning surgery can dramatically cut SSI rates, yet this practice is far from universal.

Other Risk Factors

Reviewing the abundant recent literature on SSIs, it becomes apparent that the problem is multifactorial, as is the solution. Clear understanding of risk factors allows the practitioner to control for adverse outcomes. The prevalence rates of SSI in patients with remote infections were 2.7 times higher than in patients without remote infection (Mangram et al, 1999). In a 2003 report, surgical wounds that culture positive for MRSA were associated with a twelvefold increase in postoperative mortality within the first 90 days compared with those without SSI (Engemann, 2003). Other risk factors that have been identified in the CDC SSI guidelines and in the SCIP initiatives are the following:

- Glycemic control has received a great deal of scrutiny of its role in SSIs and slowing wound healing.
- A reduction in SSIs in diabetic patients by controlling blood glucose levels to normal levels has been well documented (Lafreniere, 2001).

- "Postoperative hyperglycemia and previously undiagnosed diabetes are associated with development of SSIs among cardiothoracic surgery patients" (Latham et al, 2001).
- "... preoperative, perioperative, and postoperative control of glucose levels in diabetics and preoperative reduction of weight in obese patients may help to reduce SSIs post-CABG [coronary artery bypass graft] surgery" (Latham et al, 2001).

As discussed earlier, tissue perfusion and oxygenation have a direct effect upon surgical site infections. A number of studies have reported obesity as a risk factor for SSI, particularly when body mass index is greater than 30 (Edminston, 2007).

The evidence on malnutrition and SSI is inconclusive. However, studies have shown serum albumin levels, although not a comprehensive measure of nutritional status, are considered predictive of increased risk for postoperative infection (Sessler and Akca, 2002).

CONCLUSION

Although some surgical complications may be unavoidable, surgical care can be improved through better adherence to evidence-based practice recommendations and more attention to designing systems of care with safety measures. A number of recent, successful projects have shown that institutional implementation of evidence-based practices can have a significant impact on surgical infections and complications. All of the twenty-first century advances are being pushed by the desire for improved patient outcomes and by today's health care economics. Do not wait for SSIs to happen; be proactive about prevention to improve our patients' outcomes.

REFERENCES

Akca O, et al: Hypercapnia improves tissue oxygenation, *Anesthesiology* 97(4):801–806, 2002.

Association of periOperative Registered Nurses: Recommended practices for environmental cleaning in the perioperative setting. In Association of periOperative Registered Nurses: *Perioperative standards and recommended practices, 2009 ed*, Denver, 2009a, The Association.

Association of periOperative Registered Nurses: Recommended practices for hand hygiene in the perioperative setting. In Association of periOperative Registered Nurses: *Perioperative standards and recommended practices, 2009 ed*, Denver, 2009b, The Association.

Association of periOperative Registered Nurses: Recommended practices for maintaining a sterile field. In Association of periOperative Registered Nurses: *Perioperative standards and recommended practices, 2009 ed*, Denver, 2009c, The Association.

Association of periOperative Registered Nurses: Recommended practices for preoperative patient skin antisepsis. In Association of periOperative Registered Nurses: *Perioperative standards and recommended practices, 2009 ed*, Denver, 2009d, The Association.

Association of periOperative Registered Nurses: Recommended practices for the prevention of transmissible infections in the perioperative practice settings. In Association of periOperative Registered Nurses: *Perioperative standards and recommended practices, 2009 ed*, Denver, 2009e, The Association.

Association of periOperative Registered Nurses: Recommended practices for surgical attire. In Association of periOperative Registered Nurses: *Perioperative standards and recommended practices, 2009 ed*, Denver, 2009f, The Association.

APIC: *Elimination guide: the guide for the prevention of mediastinitis surgical site skin infections following cardiac surgery*, Washington, DC, 2008, Association for Professionals in Infection Control and Epidemiology, Inc.

Boyce J, Pittet D: Guideline for hand hygiene in health-care settings: recommendations of the Healthcare Infection Control Practices Advisory Committee and the HICPAC/SHEA/APIC/IDSA Hand Hygiene Task Force, Society for Healthcare Epidemiology of America/Association for Professionals in Infection Control/Infectious Diseases Society of America, *MMWR Recomm Rep* 51(RR-16):1–45, 2002.

Centers for Disease Control and Prevention: *Infectious diseases recovery plan*, 2009. May 15, available at http://www.recovery.gov/?q=content/program-plan&program_id=5259. Accessed May 25, 2009a.

Centers for Disease Control and Prevention: *Surgical site infection (SSI)*, 2009. available at http://www.cdc.gov/ncidod/dhqp/FAQ_SSI.html. Accessed June 14, 2009b.

Dancer S: Importance of the environment in methicillin-resistant *Staphylococcus aureus* acquisition: the case for hospital cleaning, *Lancet Infect Dis* 8(2):101–113, 2008.

Edminston CE: Reducing the risk of surgical site infections—improving surgical outcomes. In APIC grand rounds: protecting patients from the risk of surgical site infections (SSI), Dallas, 2007, Association for Professionals in Infection Control and Epidemiology, Inc.

Engemann JJ, et al: Adverse clinical and economic outcomes attributable to methicillin resistance among patients with *Staphylococcus aureus* surgical site infection, *Clin Infect Dis* 36(5):592–598, 2003.

Flores-Maldonado A, et al: Mild perioperative hypothermia and the risk of wound infection, *Arch Med Res* 32(3):227–231, 2001.

Giercksky KE: Misdiagnosis of cancer due to multiple glove powder granulomas, *Eur J Surg Suppl* 579:11–14, 1997.

Graves PB, Twomey CT: Surgical hand antisepsis: an evidence based review, *Perioper Nurs Clin* 1(3):235–249, 2006.

Holmdahl L, Risberg B: Adhesion: prevention and complications in general surgery, *Eur J Surg* 163:169–174, 1997.

Hunt TK, Hopf HW: Wound healing and wound infection: what surgeons and anesthesiologists can do, *Surg Clin North Am* 77(3):587–605, 1997.

Jaffray D, Nade S: Does surgical glove powder decrease the inoculum of bacteria required to produce an abscess? *J R Coll Surg Edinb* 28(4):219–222, 1983.

Kuri M, et al: Determination of the duration of perioperative smoking cessation to improve wound healing after head and neck surgery, *Anesthesiology* 102(5):892–896, 2005.

Kurz A, et al: Perioperative normothermia to reduce the incidence of surgical-wound infection and shorten hospitalization, Study of Wound Infection and Temperature Group, *N Engl J Med* 334(19):1209–1215, 1996.

Lafreniere R, et al: Infection control in the operating room: current practices or sacred cows? *J Am Coll Surg* 193(4): 407–416, 2001.

Latham R, et al: The association of diabetes and glucose control with surgical-site infections among cardiothoracic surgery patients, *Infect Control Hosp Epidemiol* 22(10):607–612, 2001.

Mangram AJ, et al: Guideline for prevention of surgical site infection, 1999, Hospital Infection Control Practices Advisory Committee, *Infect Control Hosp Epidemiol* 20(4):250–278, quiz 279–280, 1999.

Mastro TD, et al: An outbreak of surgical-wound infections due to group A streptococcus carried on the scalp, *N Engl J Med* 323(14):968–972, 1990.

MEDQIC: *Improving surgical care*, 2007. Surgical Care Improvement Project [cited April 25,], available from http://medqic.org/dcs/ContentServer?cid=1136495755695&pagename=Medqic%2FOtherResource%2FOtherResourcesTemplate&c=OtherResource. Accessed October 16, 2007.

Melling AC, et al: Effects of preoperative warming on the incidence of wound infection after clean surgery: a randomised controlled trial, *Lancet* 358(9285):876–880, 2001.

Neely AN, Maley MP: Survival of enterococci and staphylococci on hospital fabrics and plastic, *J Clin Microbiol* 38(2):724–726, 2000.

Occupational Safety and Health Administration: *Bloodborne pathogens*, 2009. section 1910.1030, 1997, available from http://www.osha.gov/pls/oshaweb/owadisp.show_document?p_table=STANDARDS&p_id=10051. Accessed June 14, 2009.

Parienti JJ, et al: Hand-rubbing with an aqueous alcoholic solution vs traditional surgical hand-scrubbing and 30-day surgical site infections, *JAMA* 288(6):722–727, 2002.

Qudan M, et al: Perioperative supplemental oxygen therapy and surgical site infection, *Arch Surg* 144(4):359–366, 2009.

Ratnaraj J, et al: Supplemental oxygen and carbon dioxide each increase subcutaneous and intestinal intramural oxygenation, *Anesth Analg* 99(1):207–211, 2004.

Scott RD: *The direct medical costs of healthcare-associated infections in U.S. hospitals and the benefits of prevention*, March 2009, Division of Healthcare Quality Promotion, National Center for Preparedness, Detection, and Control of Infectious Disease, Coordinating Center for Infectious Diseases, Centers for Disease Control and Prevention.

Sessler D, Akca O: Nonpharmacological prevention of surgical wound infections, *Clin Infect Dis* 35(11):1397–1404, 2002.

Tanner J, Parkinson H: Double gloving to reduce surgical cross-infection, *Cochrane Database Syst Rev* (3):2006 CD003087.

van den Tol MP, et al: Glove powder promotes adhesion formation and facilitates tumour cell adhesion and growth, *Br J Surg* 88:1258–1263, 2001.

Wertheim HF, et al: The role of nasal carriage in *Staphylococcus aureus* infections, *Lancet Infect Dis* 12(5):751–762, 2005.

Wong ES: The price of a surgical-site infection: more than just excess length of stay, *Infect Control Hosp Epidemiol* 20(11):722–724, 1999.

World Health Organization: *WHO guidelines on hand hygiene in health care (advanced draft): a summary*, 2008a. Geneva, Switzerland, available at http://www.ihatoday.org/issues/quality/whohandguide.pdf. Accessed June 14, 2009.

World Health Organization: *WHO guidelines for safe surgery (first edition)*, 2008b. Geneva, Switzerland, available at http://www.gawande.com/documents/WHOGuidelinesforSafeSurgery_001.pdf. Accessed August 17, 2009.

Yokoe DS, et al: A compendium of strategies to prevent healthcare-associated infections in acute care hospitals, *Infect Control Hosp Epidemiol* 29(Suppl 1):S12–S21, 2008.

PREVENTION OF POSITIONING INJURIES

Chapter 14

Debra Fawcett, PhD, RN

Positioning the surgical patient is a vital component of perioperative nursing practice and must be completed with knowledge and forethought. To safely and correctly position the surgical patient, the entire team must have a thorough understanding of the surgical procedure, the position desired, the physiologic effects of the position, time required in the position, and the anatomic boundaries. To prevent positioning injuries, the perioperative nurse must complete a preoperative assessment that includes such factors as the patient's current health status and identification of comorbidities that will influence the course of the surgical procedure. Assessments should also include, but are not limited to, preexisting skin conditions, age, preexisting nerve conditions, nutritional status, physical/mobility issues, and height and weight (Association of periOperative Registered Nurses [AORN], 2009). Other safety factors such as the use of pressure redistributing surfaces and positioning devices must be considered in advance to safely position the surgical patient. Care should always be taken to have an adequate number of persons available to position and transfer the patient. Postoperative skin assessments should be performed as well. Assessments should include skin condition, areas of tenderness, and complaints of pain, numbness, or tingling in peripheral extremities.

The goals of patient positioning are (1) optimal exposure for the surgical team, (2) maintenance of correct body alignment, (3) support of respiratory and cardiovascular function, (4) protection of neuromuscular function, (5) protection of skin integrity, and (6) to allow for anesthesia access (Heizenroth, 2007).

ADVERSE EVENTS

Despite more than three decades of research on iatrogenic events occurring in operating rooms (ORs) across the country, few identifiable or predictable causes of these injuries have been found (Gwande et al, 1999). Because of the lack of identification, there is a paucity of information regarding complications related to surgical positioning (Warner, 2009). Regardless of the cause, adverse events are expensive to the hospital and patient, may cause permanent disability, and are potentially deadly. Patient safety advocates and the public now hold health care providers and health care workers responsible for adverse events occurring in operating rooms across the United States. Nurses are being held accountable not only for nursing practice, but also for the identification of risk factors for adverse injury, preventive measures, and adherence to standards and recommended practices. Standards and recommended practices for positioning of the surgical patient are set forth by the Association of periOperative Registered Nurses (AORN). Positioning of the surgical patient requires several members of the perioperative team (i.e., surgeon, anesthesia provider, perioperative nurse, surgical technologist, and orderly) to participate in positioning the patient and ensuring implementation of appropriate positioning principles. Each member of the perioperative team must be knowledgeable and comply with the accepted AORN standards and recommended practices specific for proper positioning techniques and provide for the safety of the patient.

Pressure-Related Injuries

The most commonly identified injury related to positioning in the operating room is pressure-related injuries. Pressure-related injuries encompass intraoperatively acquired pressure ulcers, nerve injuries, and the development of DVT (deep vein thrombosis). Many factors lead to the occurrence of intraoperative pressure injuries, but the most detrimental factor is that of decreased blood flow to the dermal layer of skin and all the entities encased within the dermal layer. Decreased blood flow to an area of skin may result from long periods of pressure to a specific area of the body, from twisting or compression of nerves and vessels, or shear and negativity. The more intense the pressure and the longer the duration of the pressure, the greater the possibility of decreased blood flow to the tissues and underlying structures. First, a review of basic anatomy of the skin and musculoskeletal system may be necessary.

Anatomy and Physiology of the Skin

The skin is the largest organ of the human body and protects the internal body from injury, temperature changes, and bacterial invasions (Taylor et al, 2008). The skin also reduces water loss and acts as a permeable barrier to the environment (Boyce and Pittet, 2002). Human skin is made up of two layers, the epidermis (the outer layer) and the dermis (the second layer). The epidermis is generally only 0.1 to 1.5 mm thick (Patton and Thibodeau, 2010). It is made of stratified layers of epithelial cells and forms a waterproof top (Taylor et al, 2008). The epithelial layer is constantly shedding and regenerating each day. The five layers of epithelial cells include the basal cell layer, the squamous cell layer, the stratum granulosum, the stratum lucidum, and the stratum corneum. This layer also houses the hair follicles, sebaceous glands, and pilosebaceous glands (Heizenroth, 2007).

The dermis, or the second layer of skin, contains blood vessels, nerves, and lymphatic vessels (Patton and Thibodeau, 2010). It is also composed of three types of fibrous connective tissues: (1) collagen, (2) elastin and reticulin, and (3) a gel-like, ground substance. The dermis contains blood vessels, nerves, and lymphatic vessels (Figure 14-1). The dermis lies directly below the epidermis and is much thicker. Sweat glands and sensory nerve endings are in rich supply in the dermis. Two layers make up the dermis: the capillary layer and the reticular layer. Nerve endings and blood vessels lie within the reticular layer. Pressure within the dermal layer affects the nerve cell receptors, including receptors that sense pain, heat, cold, itch, and pressure. After injury, the dermal layer does not regenerate as the epidermis does; instead it forms granulation tissue.

Musculoskeletal System

The human musculoskeletal system gives our bodies support, allows for movement, and assists in protecting our body from external harm. Strain and pressure on the musculoskeletal system during a surgical procedure can lead to an unexpected injury. During the surgical procedure the patient is often unconscious and unable to inform the team of pain or discomfort related to the surgical position. The patient cannot reposition for comfort or state if an extremity "has gone to sleep." During the process of positioning, the surgical team should maintain as much correct anatomic alignment as possible; avoid twisting or rotation of limbs if possible, and never force a joint beyond its natural capacity. Do not hyperextend a joint, and always pad the joints and pressure points for protection from pressure injuries. Make sure that all extremities are secure and that no undue pressure will occur during the surgical procedure.

Pressure Ulcers

Pressure ulcers are a major health problem affecting approximately 3 million adults (Ayello and Lyder, 2007). According to the Agency for Healthcare Research and Quality (AHRQ) (Russo, 2008) hospitalizations involving patients with pressure ulcers increased by nearly 80% between 1993 and 2006. Pressure ulcers are defined by the National Pressure Ulcer Advisory Panel (Black et al, 2007) as a localized injury to the skin and/or underlying tissue usually over a bony prominence as a result of pressure or pressure in combination with shear and/or friction. They are staged using the system in Box 14-1. The Institute for Healthcare Improvement (IHI) has made the prevention of pressure ulcers 1 of 12 interventions in its 5 Million Lives Campaign (Ayello and Lyder, 2007).

Millions of surgical procedures are performed each year. During the surgical procedure, patients are anesthetized and often put into positions that may cause pressure or compression to the tissue for long periods of time. Being unconscious and immobile, the patient cannot complain of pain or discomfort. Pressure ulcers develop when capillaries supplying the skin and subcutaneous tissues are compressed enough to slow down perfusion, causing aggregation of blood at the site of pressure, thus leading to ischemia to the area under pressure (Ayello and Lyder, 2007).

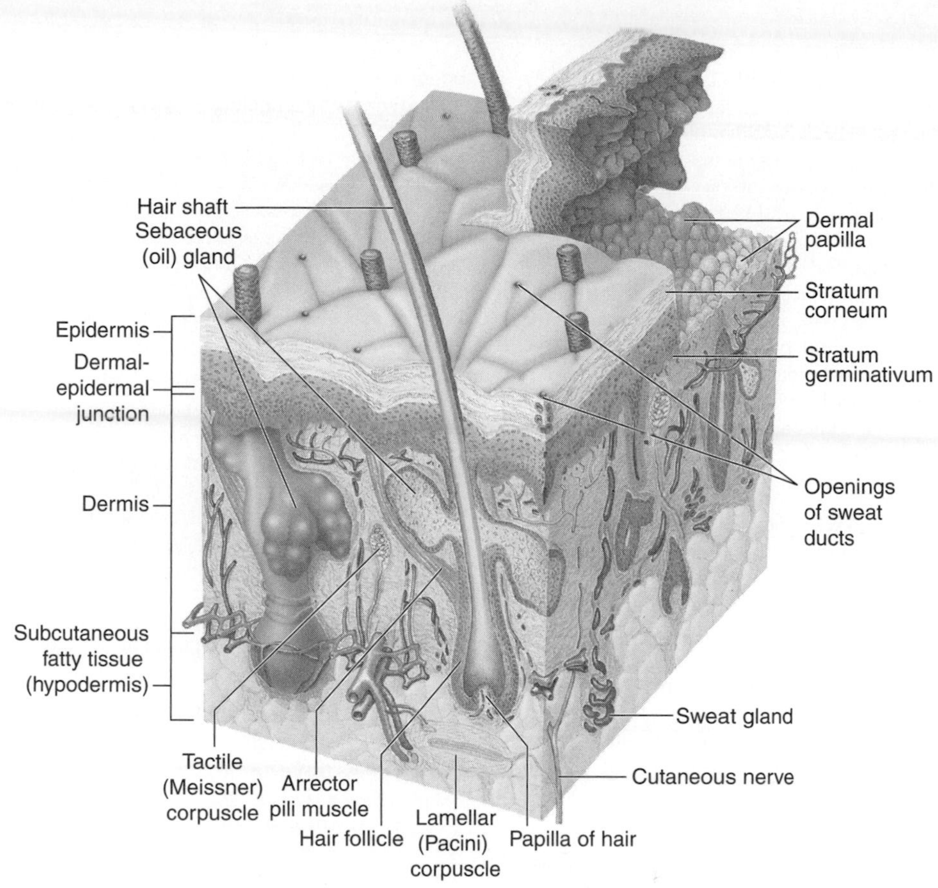

FIGURE 14-1 Microscopic view of the skin. (From Thibodeau GA, Patton KT: *The human body in health and disease*, ed 5, St. Louis, 2010, Mosby.)

Development of pressure ulcers may result in increased patient pain, increased hospital stays, possible disfigurement, and increased cost for the institution. Estimates for treatment of a pressure ulcer can total as much as $100,000 to heal one full-thickness ulcer (Scott-Williams, 2006). Nationally the average cost to treat pressure ulcers is reported to be 2.5 times the cost of preventing them (Ayello and Lyder, 2007). In addition to the cost of treatment, development of a pressure ulcer can leave the institution open to potential litigation. More than 17,000 pressure ulcer–related lawsuits are filed every year, and the settlement involving health care–acquired pressure ulcers is usually about $250,000 (Scott-Williams, 2006).

Pressure ulcers in the OR usually result from improper positioning, inadequate padding and protection, incorrect use of positioning devices, or extended periods of pressure while on the OR bed (Fawcett, 2004). Pressure ulcers acquired in the OR are often mislabeled as burns or as an area of erythema because pressure ulcers acquired in the OR react differently than those acquired in the general hospital or extended care facilities. Operating room–acquired pressure ulcers do not usually present themselves until 3 to 5 days postoperatively and develop from the deep tissue, progressing to the outer surface. Pressure ulcers occurring from the operating room often deteriorate fairly rapidly to a stage III or stage IV (Blackett and Falconio-

BOX 14-1 Pressure Ulcer Definition and Stages

(SUSPECTED) DEEP TISSUE INJURY

Purple or maroon localized area of discolored intact skin or blood-filled blister due to damage of underlying soft tissue from pressure and/or shear. The area may be preceded by tissue that is painful, firm, mushy, boggy, warmer or cooler as compared to adjacent tissue.

Further description

Deep tissue injury may be difficult to detect in individuals with dark skin tones. Evolution may include a blister over a dark wound bed. The wound may further evolve and become covered by a thin eschar. Evolution may be rapid, exposing additional layers of tissue even with optimal treatment.

STAGE I

Intact skin with non-blanchable redness of a localized area usually over a bony prominence. Darkly pigmented skin may not have visible blanching; its color may differ from the surrounding area.

Further description

The area may be painful, firm, soft, warmer or cooler as compared to adjacent tissue. Stage I may be difficult to detect in individuals with dark skin tones. May indicate "at risk" persons (a heralding sign of risk.)

STAGE II

Partial-thickness loss of dermis presenting as a shallow open ulcer with a red pink wound bed, without slough. May also present as an intact or open/ruptured serum-filled blister.

Further description

Presents as a shiny or dry shallow ulcer without slough or bruising. (Bruising indicating suspected deep tissue injury.) This stage should not be used to describe skin tears, tape burns, perineal dermatitis, maceration, or denudement.

STAGE III

Full-thickness tissue loss. Subcutaneous fat may be visible but bone, tendon, or muscle are *not* exposed. Slough may be present but does not obscure the depth of tissue loss. *May* include undermining and tunneling.

Further description

The depth of a Stage III pressure ulcer varies by anatomic location. The bridge of the nose, ear, occiput, and malleolus do not have subcutaneous tissue and Stage III ulcers can be shallow. In contrast, areas of significant adiposity can develop extremely deep Stage III pressure ulcers. Bone/tendon is not visible or directly palpable.

STAGE IV

Full-thickness tissue loss with exposed bone, tendon, or muscle. Slough or eschar may be present on some parts of the wound bed. Often includes undermining and tunneling.

Further description

The depth of a Stage IV pressure ulcer varies by anatomic location. The bridge of the nose, ear, occiput, and malleolus do not have subcutaneous tissue and these ulcers can be shallow. Stage IV ulcers can extend into muscle and/or supporting structures (for example, fascia, tendon, or joint capsule) making osteomyelitis possible. Bone/tendon is visible or directly palpable.

UNSTAGEABLE

Full-thickness tissue loss in which the base of the ulcer is covered by slough (yellow, tan, gray, green, or brown) and/or eschar (tan, brown, or black) in the wound bed.

Further description

Until enough slough and/or eschar is removed to expose the base of the wound, the true depth, and therefore stage, cannot be determined. Stable (dry, adherent, intact with erythema or fluctuance) eschar on the heels serves as "the body's natural (biological) cover" and should not be removed.

This staging system should be used only to describe pressure ulcers. Wounds from other causes, such as arterial, venous, diabetic foot, skin tears, tape burns, perineal dermatitis, maceration, or denudement should not be staged using this system. Other staging systems exist for some of these conditions and should be used instead.

West, 2009). Following the surgical procedure, the perioperative nurse should assess the patient for areas of erythema or blanching on the skin. Particular attention should be paid to the heels, occiput, scapula, and coccyx because these are the most frequent sites for development of pressure ulcers in the OR.

Previous studies have demonstrated that the heels are the most common site for pressure ulcers and that 25% of these start during surgery

BOX 14-2 Common Areas of Pressure

- Heels
- Hips
- Occiput
- Knees
- Shoulders
- Ankles
- Elbows
- Shoulder blades
- Buttocks
- Skin folds
- Sacrum

(Box 14-2) (Huber and Huber, 2009). Furthermore, 83% of these develop during the first 5 days of hospitalization (Bansal et al, 2005; Huber and Huber, 2008). Many pressure ulcers can be prevented with an understanding of the etiology of pressure ulcers and principles of proper positioning, off-loading, and interface pressures. Off-loading is the process of removing or taking off pressure from a pressure point. The surgical team may completely off-load pressure by raising the heel or using heel devices that off-load. Interface pressure is a measurement of the interaction between the surface and the patient. Normal interface pressures are between 25 mm Hg and 32 mm Hg. It must be kept in mind that the interface pressure is a measurement of only one point in time and demonstrates where the pressures are the highest at that time. The incidence of heel pressure ulcers can be reduced or prevented by off-loading the pressure. Care must be taken so that devices used to off-load pressure do not increase the potential for deep vein thrombosis. Maintaining alignment, the correct use of devices, and use of surfaces that redistribute pressure promote patient safety.

Nerve Injury

An iatrogenic nerve injury caused by improper positioning for a surgical procedure, external compression, or twisting is another possible surgical complication (Dillavou et al, 1997). Although the true cause of peripheral nerve injury is unknown, it has been assumed that external pressure/compression against the nerve during the surgical procedure is the primary cause. In 1894 Budinger first recognized that there was a relationship between improper positioning and peripheral nerve injury. Stretching and compression are often identified as the main culprits in position-related nerve injuries (Heizenroth, 2007). Whatever the true cause of these events, it is a reminder to nurses that they must comply with guidelines and standards for safe positioning of the surgical patient.

BOX 14-3 Nerve Injuries

UPPER EXTREMITY NERVE INJURIES

Brachial plexus injuries
Long thoracic nerve dysfunction
Axillary
Radial nerve compression
Median nerve compression
Ulnar neuropathies

LOWER EXTREMITY NERVE INJURIES

Sciatic nerve injury
Obturator nerve
Common peroneal
Femoral nerve

Peripheral nerve injuries that occur during positioning may cause impaired function (Fawcett, 2004; Heizenroth, 2007). Nerve injuries are often broken down into upper extremity nerve injuries and lower extremity nerve injuries (Box 14-3).

MOST COMMON SURGICAL POSITIONS

Supine Position

When positioning the patient in the supine position, the surgical team must provide for protection against pressure injuries. In this position the patient lies on his or her back with a pillow beneath the head (Warner, 2009). The arms may be either at a less than 90-degree angle out to the side or "tucked" in alongside the patient's body. Perfusion to the hands must not be compromised. If the surgical procedure will be long, the team must ensure that the mattress and support devices are designed to redistribute pressure over time. Areas where it is expected that pressure may occur should have additional padding or off-loading when possible.

Upper Extremity Nerve Injury

The occurrence of upper extremity peripheral nerve injury can be reduced by proper use of positioning devices, securing the arms correctly, and appropriate use of padding. In addition, the team must be very careful to not extend the arms more than 90 degrees when on the arm boards. Upper extremity nerve injuries may be caused by the location, improper positioning, or inappropriate use of padding devices and material and may result in untoward patient outcomes (Tables 14-1 to 14-4).

TABLE 14-1 Brachial Plexus Injuries

Causes	Symptoms
Arm abducted more than 90 degrees	Shoulder pain
Arm sags off the bed and externally rotates	Tenderness in supraclavicular area
Head is rotated to opposite side	Numbness or flaccidity
Material used to restrain arms is too tight, causing compression	Motor and/or sensory deficit of arm
Shoulder braces not well padded	Motor and/or sensory deficit of arm and shoulder
Axillary roll improperly placed	Motor and/or sensory deficit of arm and shoulder

TABLE 14-2 Ulnar Nerve Injuries

Causes	Symptoms
Arm extended/ forearm pronated	Weak grip
Arm folded too tightly across chest	Cannot oppose or abduct fifth finger
Inadequate padding of elbows	Impaired adduction
Elbow slipped off the OR bed or arm board	Clawlike hand
Surgical team rests against side of bed and puts pressure on upper extremity	Pain, possible sensory and/or motor deficit
Surgical devices attached to bed rested against the arm	Pain, possible sensory and/or motor deficit
Patient did not fit correctly on the OR bed and arms pressed against metal rail	Pain, possible sensory and/or motor deficit

OR, Operating room.

TABLE 14-3 Radial Nerve Injury

Causes	Symptoms
Table attachment presses against the arm (e.g., metal retractors that may result in pressure)	Numbness or tingling of skin on back of arm, forearm, or hand
Pressure against the proximal forearm during surgery	Wrist drop
In lateral position, the dependent arm may be pushed against position devices, support item	Cannot extend phalangeal joints, weak thumb adduction

TABLE 14-4 Median Nerve Injury

Causes	Symptoms
Arms tucked too tightly	Numbness of palmar surfaces
Surgical team leans on arms	Numbness to thumb and two adjacent fingers
Arms are twisted, causing compression	Motor and/or sensory deficit of hand
Forced elbow extension	Motor and/or sensory deficit of hand

Lower Extremity Nerve Injury

As with the upper extremities, there are positioning risks for the lower extremities in the supine position. It might be assumed that in the supine position there is minimal stress or strain that may result in injury, but that is not the case. The supine position puts undue stress on the vertebral system. Lying on a hard surface for extended periods of time puts pressure on joints and various areas of the body and puts strain on the back. The team must flex the hips about 15 degrees to relieve strain and add to the comfort of the patient postoperatively. Using a bolster under the knees is fine, but the team must make sure that it will not add to the potential for DVTs or add undue pressure to the heels. Bolsters should be made from a soft material, not hard rolled-up bath blankets. Lower extremity nerve injuries may occur because of improper positioning or inappropriate use of padding devices and materials and may result in untoward patient outcomes (Tables 14-5 to 14-7).

TABLE 14-5 Sciatic Nerve Injury

Causes	Symptoms
Inadequately padded OR bed	Paresthesia of muscles below the knee
Lack of support under knees	Numbness lateral half of calf, most of foot
Poor support surface	Foot drop
Thighs and legs externally rotated	Pain radiating down the affected leg

OR, Operating room.

TABLE 14-6 Common Peroneal Nerve Injury

Causes	Symptoms
Thighs externally rotated	Foot drop
Strap across the popliteal space too tight	Decreased loss of dorsal extension
Elastic stocking too tight	Cannot evert the affected foot
Twisting of the knee	No sensation on the dorsum of the foot

Supine Position Overview

Nursing actions and interventions to minimize positioning risk for a patient in the supine position include the following:

- Arms should be supinated (if that is the natural alignment).
- Extend arms *no more* than 90 degrees.
- Avoid using force to restrain arms (firm but not tight).
- Use extra padding at elbows.
- Drawsheet should be at least 2 inches above the elbow and tucked smoothly under the patient.
- Do not lean against the surgical bed.
- Do not use intravenous (IV) bags or rolled towels as axillary rolls if the surgery will be long.
- Check all positioning devices for correct use, proper functioning before use.
- Maintain correct anatomic alignment.
- When using a sled (elbow guard), make sure padding is inside the sled and that padding protects the elbow from pressure on side of bed and that arm cannot get caught between the bed and sled.
- Follow AORN standards for the use of positioning devices and positioning.
- Ensure correct use of all positioning devices according to manufacturer's guidelines and for the distribution of pressure.
- Make sure all positioning devices are in correct working order.
- If the patient is bariatric or large, be sure to place on an OR bed that allows for proper padding and proper restraint of arms as necessary.
- If extra arm boards are being used on the side of the bed, be sure to have adequate padding between the bed and arm, and make sure the arm boards are locked so that the patient's arm cannot drop between the bed and sled or get pinched.
- Elevate patient's hips 15 degrees to relieve back strain.
- Use a soft bolster under the knee.
- Protect the heels.

TABLE 14-7 Femoral Nerve Injury

Causes	Symptoms
Legs stretched in frog-legged position	Difficulty straightening the leg
Pressure directly on the nerve from leaning instruments	Numbness or weakness in the thigh or knee
Pressure directly on the nerve from leaning instruments	Strange sensations on front of thigh or inside calf

Lateral Position

In the lateral position the patient is lying on his or her nonoperative side, surgical side up. The arms are usually extended at a 90-degree angle out in front of the patient. The upper arm may be supported by an elevated arm board, pillows, raised Mayo stand with padding, or special devices for the support of the arm. The patient is held in place with the use of kidney rests, beanbags, rolled towels, pillows, and possibly safety straps. If tape is used to stabilize the patient, make sure it is not causing compression of nerves or vessels and is not adhered to the skin. An axillary roll is placed to protect the brachial plexus region. Do not pull or twist to get the patient's arms in place. A pressure-redistributing mattress should be used.

Pillows or positioning devices should be placed to decrease pressure between patient's knees, and ankles should be protected from undue pressure. Care must be taken to protect the eyes in this position. Use of special headrests is recommended to prevent pressure injuries.

In this position the ulnar nerve, radial nerve, brachial plexus nerve group, and common peroneal nerve are at greatest risks.

Lateral Position Overview

Nursing actions and interventions to minimize positioning risk for a patient in the lateral position include the following:

- Use adequate padding around the elbow; be sure to check both the down arm and the upper arm.
- Check upper arm on support device to make sure there is not pressure around the elbow.
- Stabilize the upper arm in correct anatomic alignment with the elbow free.
- Stabilize the arm under the drapes so that the arm does not slide off the bed.
- Use pressure-reducing OR pads.
- Use correct-size arm boards with pressure-distributing padding. If devices are attached to the bed, make sure the arm does not rest against them.
- Make sure team members do not rest against the arm or arm board.
- Use pressure-distributing axillary rolls.
- Do not use IV bags for positioning.
- Use all assistive devices correctly.
- Use only soft padding between the knees.
- Safety strap must be above the knee away from the lateral head of the fibula.
- Use extra padding at the ankles.
- Head must be maintained in correct alignment, with eyes protected.
- Support wrists as necessary.

Prone Position

In the prone position the patient is lying face down. The arms are either at the side or out on arm boards. Arms on arm boards must have adequate padding around the elbows and be secured so that they will not slip off during the surgical procedure. Remember not to cause peripheral compression with straps and bindings that are too tight. When positioning the prone patient, the nurse must remember that the ulnar nerve arises from the brachial plexus and that pressure, compression, or twisting can result in an injury. The arms should not be forced into position, but allowed to rotate naturally (down and forward) when placed onto the arm board. Pressure in the axillary region, as well as injury at the elbow, can cause ulnar nerve injury.

If the arms are to be at the patient's side, they should be held close to the body and secured with a smooth drawsheet tucked under the patient (Rothrock, 2007). Knees should be well padded, and the toes should be off-loaded to prevent pressure injury. If a safety strap is used, care must be taken to keep pressure from the popliteal space.

Chest rolls should be soft and extend from acromioclavicular joint to the iliac crest. Care should be taken to prevent pressure on breasts and genitals. Potential nerve injuries include ulnar nerve, radial nerve, common peroneal, and brachial plexus (see Tables 14-1 through 14-3 and 14-6).

Prone Position Overview

Nursing actions and interventions to minimize positioning risk for a patient in the prone position include the following:

- Provide adequate padding of elbows.
- Arms should be rotated down and forward to prevent compression or twisting of brachial plexus area.
- Drawsheet should be snug but not tight.
- No one rests on against side of bed or arm.
- Arms are secured onto arm boards and will not fall off during the procedure.
- No attachments rest against the arm.
- Chest rolls are placed so that there is no pressure on the brachial plexus.
- Any positioning device used to position the patient is checked for correct placement *after* the patient is in position.
- After positioning, patient pressure points and placement of all support devices are checked.
- Head is in correct alignment.
- Toes are not resting on bed.
- Safety strap is not in popliteal space.
- Breasts are not crushed.
- Male genitalia are without pressure or compression.
- Eyes and ears are well protected.
- Medial aspect of elbow is well padded.

NOTE: protection of the eyes in this position is very important.

Lithotomy Position

In the standard lithotomy position, the patient is supine with the arms crossed on the trunk or with one or both arms extended (Warner, 2009). Each lower extremity is elevated at the hip and placed into stirrups. The thighs should be flexed to approximately 90 degrees on the trunk. Both extremities are to be lifted simultaneously into the stirrup to prevent injury to the lateral cutaneous nerves and inguinal ligaments (Warner, 2009). When lowering the legs to the supine position, it is imperative that the knees be brought together at the knees and ankles, then lowered to the supine position. This reduces strain on the lower spine (Warner, 2009). It also helps decrease sudden hypotension. There are several variants to standard lithotomy position. Potential nerve injuries in the lithotomy position include obturator (Table 14-8), common peroneal, sciatic, and brachial plexus (with shoulder braces).

Lithotomy Position Overview

Nursing actions and interventions to minimize positioning risk for a patient in the lithotomy position include the following:
- Lift and lower legs simultaneously.
- Keep buttocks even with the end of the bed.
- Check stirrups for stability before use.
- Stirrups are the same height.
- Pressure-relieving surface is used.
- Arms not extended more than 90 degrees.
- Provide padding between stirrups and patient's lower extremities.
- Team does not lean on thighs during procedure.
- Legs are not hyperabducted.
- Patient is secured so as not to slide off.

TABLE 14-8 Obturator Nerve

Causes	Symptoms
Excessive flexion of hip	Weakness or paralysis of thigh
Lifting one leg at a time	Pain on the inner aspect of thigh
Twisting of leg during surgery	Motor and/or sensory deficit of lower extremity
Leaning on the legs during the procedure	Motor and/or sensory deficit of lower extremity

POSITIONING EQUIPMENT AND DEVICES

Every operating room across the country uses positioning devices and surfaces to assist with positioning and prevent injury. The correct use of positioning devices adds to patient safety and can assist in ensuring positive patient outcomes. It is the responsibility of the OR team to purchase devices and surfaces based on evidence about the protection and safety of the patient. For the OR mattresses evidence should demonstrate that the mattress redistributes pressure and continues to redistribute it for extended periods of time through interface pressures, laser Doppler studies, and materials used. It is important to note that interface pressures measure only a moment in time and should not be used as the sole criterion for purchase of surfaces. However, interface pressures can be used as a comparison to identify where pressures are the highest and to identify how well pressure is distributed at that point in time. Evidence of pressure redistribution should be provided for positioning devices as well. It is the responsibility of the OR team to know in advance how the equipment works, make sure it is clean and intact, and know the manufacturer's guidelines for its use.

Devices

In today's health care arena hospitals focus on cost cutting, and one place to cut costs is in the purchase of extra positioning equipment. Items such as axillary rolls are often viewed as unnecessary and an added cost when an IV bag could do just as well and is readily available. Use of IV bags, rolled towels, and sand-filled bags may actually increase the potential for injury and should not be used to position the patient (Scott-Williams, 2006). Use of a device for a purpose other than what it was intended for can leave the OR team open to litigation and the patient open to unexpected injury. All devices should be normothermic (maintain temperature at a normal level for extended periods), flame resistant, lightweight, durable, easily cleaned, nonallergenic, and available in multiple sizes; they should redistribute pressure and meet federal guidelines.

The Big Question: What Do I Use?

Before the team can address this issue it must address the type, number, and general population of the patients. Are they all 2- to 3-hour surgeries, or do you do a lot of short-stay procedures? Do your patients come in with a lot of comorbidities? What is the average weight and size of the patients? Then the team needs to ask, what are our competencies? If the staff does not understand the standards or why a position needs to be done a certain way, then education needs to be a priority. Not understanding the goals of positioning can lead to increased potential for injury to the surgical patient. Make sure the entire team knows the goals of positioning.

Positioning devices come in many shapes and materials with each material component having its positive and negative qualities. The team needs to have a good understanding of the different components of positioning devices as well. The following provides a short synopsis of different materials used. It is important to understand that research has not clearly demonstrated that one is significantly better than another, but has demonstrated that some do *not* have effective pressure-reduction properties over time and that others may increase other potential problems for the surgical patient.

Foam

Of the many types of materials now on the market, perhaps the most common and cost-efficient is foam. Foam support surfaces are made of two types—closed cell foam and open cell foam (Brienza and Geyer, 2005). Foam has what we like to call "memory"—it will return to its nominal shape or thickness. Foam is often used because it is lightweight, readily available, and can shape into many positions. Foam can be very useful in short-term procedures. One drawback of foam is that it tends to "bottom out"—flatten and provide no support after a period of time—and can actually increase the pressure (Goodman, 2003; Brienza and Geyer, 2005; Scott-Williams, 2006). Soft foams are better than the more sturdy foams, but must be much thicker to reduce the potential to "bottom out." Foam also has the ability to raise the patient's temperature after a short period, therefore making them sweat and increasing the potential for maceration and skin breakdown. Foam also holds moisture from body fluids, preparation solutions, irrigation, and other sources. As foam becomes wet, it will also bottom out more quickly.

Viscoelastic foam. Viscoelastic foam is open cell foam that is temperature sensitive (Brienza and Geyer, 2005). As the body warms the surface, the surface becomes more pliable and better able to redistribute pressure. The surface contours itself around the patient because of an elastic response (Brienza and Geyer, 2005). This is called immersion. Viscoelastic foam also has the ability to return to its shape after use. There are some older studies that demonstrate that viscoelastic foam is more effective at pressure redistribution than the traditional foam mattresses used in many ORs.

Gel

Gel is a chemical compound encased in a durable, leak-proof membrane (Goodman, 2003). Most gel products are heavy by nature and have been shown to increase the moisture next to the patient after 1 hour (Goodman, 2003). In addition, many gel products have not proved the ability to provide controlled pressure redistribution over time. When using gel, the team must carefully evaluate for leaks, tears, and cleanliness. More evidence on pressure redistribution using gel is needed.

Air

Air is another mode that is being used with a variety of positioning devices. Air overlays and air-filled devices serve as extra positioning aids. The research is still ambiguous regarding the use of air overlays, but more research is being conducted. There are many different names for support surfaces using air as a distribution process. The surface may be referred to as a static support surface or as a waffle overlay. When considering air, the team must answer the following questions: (1) Will the device support the patient? (2) Will it bottom out? (3) Is it durable? (4) What is the stability of the surface? Products using air must also meet federal regulatory guidelines.

Linens

Everyday items are used to position a patient for a surgical procedure. Pillows, towels, and blankets are folded, molded, taped, and rolled to provide the extra support needed to position the surgical patient. Linens are not designed for positioning the surgical patient and have no inherent pressure redistribution properties. Linens bottom out over time and hold moisture. In addition, linens can become wrinkled and bunched under the patient during the initial positioning process, adding to the potential for pressure injuries. When linen gets wet from irrigation fluids, preparation solution, body fluids and a myriad of other products used during a procedure, it will hold the moisture next to the skin, leading to maceration and skin breakdown. Linen is not normothermic. That is not to say that linen cannot be used for short surgical procedures, but the potential for unwarranted injury must be weighed in advance. For long procedures the team must look for products that redistribute pressure, wick moisture away from the skin, are normothermic in nature, and are designed for the purpose that they will be used for.

Combination of Devices

In practice the OR team will see a combination of many types of materials being used to position the patient. Gel because of its weight may be combined with foam, making it lighter and easier to use. Viscoelastic foam is being used in mattresses and in positioning devices. Some institutions have used fluidized surfaces in an effort to reduce the occurrence of pressure ulcers. Other institutions are using overlays on their current mattress system. Whatever decisions the OR team makes, they should be based on the recommended practices set forth by AORN for the selection of positioning devices in the OR and on the evidence-based practices that are available.

CONCLUSION

Positioning of the surgical patient is a team effort; all must participate. The surgical team must focus on the safety of the patient first and do everything possible to prevent adverse outcomes. The safety of the patient depends on the preparedness of the operating room team. This must include using evidence-based practice and following guidelines in the purchase of surfaces and positioning devices. Assessments both preoperatively and postoperatively must be completed that include skin assessment and awareness of potential nerve injury to the patient. All assessments must be well documented. Special needs of each patient must be identified and complied with, as well as documented. All comorbidities must be documented and attended to. The team members must continually improve their knowledge, skills, and competencies. They must have a through understanding of the anatomy, physiology, and surgical positions. Thorough understanding of the devices used and the manufacturer's guidelines is imperative. Special populations (e.g., bariatric) must be addressed for their specific needs, and equipment must be able to withstand and redistribute the weight. The team must provide a safe and efficient environment for the surgical patient. Documentation must be completed, and policies for proper positioning must be developed and followed.

REFERENCES

Association of periOperative Registered Nurses: *Perioperative standards and recommended practices*, Denver, 2009, The Association.

Ayello E, Lyder C: *Protecting patients from harm: preventing pressure ulcers, Nursing*, 2007, available at http://www.nursing2007.com. Accessed January 2009.

Bansal C, et al: Decubitus ulcers, *Int J Dermatol* 44:805–810, 2005.

Black J, et al: National Pressure Ulcer Advisory Panel's updated pressure ulcer staging system, *Adv Skin Wound Care* 20(5):269–274, 2007.

Blackett A, Falconio-West M: IHI campaign zeros in on pressure ulcers, 2009, Institute for Healthcare Improvement, available at http://www.Fivemillionlives/safety.com. Accessed January 2009.

Boyce J, Pittet D: Guideline for hand hygiene in health-care settings: recommendations of the Healthcare Infection Control Practices Advisory Committee and the HICPAC/SHEA/APIC/IDSA Hand Hygiene Task Force, Society for Healthcare Epidemiology of America/Association for Professionals in Infection Control/Infectious Diseases Society of America, *MMWR Recomm Rep* 51(RR-16):1–45, 2002.

Centers for Disease Control and Prevention: Guideline for hand hygiene in health-care settings: recommendations of the Healthcare Infection Control Practices Advisory Committee and the HICPAC/SHEA/APIC/IDSA Hand Hygiene Task Force, *MMWR*, 2002:51(No. RR-16). See also *Infect Control Hosp Epidemiol* 2002:23[suppl]:S3-S40; *Am J Infect Control* 2002;30(8):1–46.

Brienza D, Geyer M: Using support surfaces to manage tissue integrity, *Adv Skin Wound Care* 18:151–157, 2005.

Budinger K: Ueber lahmunger nach chloroformnarkosen, *Arch Klin Chirc* 47:121–145, 1894.

Dillavou E, et al: Lower extremity iatrogenic nerve injury due to compression during intraabdominal surgery, *Am J Surg* 173:504–508, 1997.

Fawcett D: *A comparison of three pressure reducing surfaces using interface pressures*, unpublished dissertation, 2004.

Goodman T: *Positioning; a patient safety initiative*, Denver, 2003, ConMed.

Gwande A, et al: The incidence and nature of surgical adverse events in Colorado and Utah in 1992, *Surgery* 126(1):66–75, 1999.

Heizenroth P: Positioning the patient for surgery. In Rothrock JC, editor: *Alexander's care of the patient in surgery*, ed 13, St. Louis, 2007, Mosby.

Huber D, Huber J: Popliteal vein compression under general anesthesia, *Eur J Vasc Endovasc Surg* 37(4):464–469, 2009.

Patton KT, Thibodeau GA: *Anatomy and physiology*, ed 7, St. Louis, 2010, Mosby.

Rothrock J: *Alexander's care of the patient in surgery*, ed 13, St. Louis, 2007, Mosby.

Russo CA, et al: *Hospitalizations related to pressure ulcers, 2006,* 2008, available at HCUP Statistical Brief #64. Agency for Healthcare Research and Quality, Rockville, Md, December 2008, http://www.hcup-us.ahrq.gov/reports/statbriefs/sb64.pdf. Accessed October 16, 2009.

Scott-Williams S: Prevent patient positioning problems, *Outpatient Surgery Magazine* 7(12):50–54, 2006.

Taylor C, et al: *Fundamentals of nursing*, Philadelphia, 2008, Lippincott.

Warner M: Patient positioning and related injuries. In Cahalan M, Stock C, eds: *Clinical anesthesia,* ed 6, Philadelphia, 2009, Lippincott.

NORMOTHERMIA MANAGEMENT

Prevention of Harm From Perioperative Hypothermia

V. Doreen Wagner, PhD, RN, CNOR

Perioperative temperature management is an important and proactive patient safety initiative because it may have tremendous impact on surgical patient outcomes, especially in high-risk patients. Over the past few decades, research on temperature homeostasis has illuminated a wide range of adverse pathophysiologic effects of perioperative hypothermia on surgical patients. Hypothermia, defined as a core body temperature below 36.0° C or 96.8° F, is a potentially harmful event that warrants assessment and intervention during each phase of perioperative care (Association of periOperative Registered Nurses [AORN], 2009). Box 15-1 lists the known consequences of hypothermia.

By a combination of behavioral and physiologic responses, the human body normally maintains a steady internal core temperature close to 37° C (98.6° F) despite significant environmental temperature changes. When a patient undergoes general anesthesia for longer than 30 minutes or a major procedure under neuraxial anesthesia (e.g., spinal or epidural anesthesia) for longer than 1 hour, hypothermia is to be expected. All general anesthetics produce a dose-dependent decrease in core temperature because of the disruption of both behavioral and physiologic mechanisms of thermoregulation. Neuraxial anesthesia approaches also impair temperature regulation, although to a lesser degree than does general anesthesia (Sessler, 2008).

Perioperative hypothermia occurs in either a planned or unplanned manner. Therapeutic hypothermia, a planned temperature management event, is used during surgeries that have tissue hypoxia and ischemia risks such as in cardiac surgery, neurosurgery, and organ transplantation; the maintenance of hypothermia lowers basal metabolic rates and oxygen consumption effects. Planned hypothermia is also used to reduce the risk for malignant hyperthermia development in potential surgical candidates. In planned hypothermia the rewarming of the patient is also planned and monitored (Kumar et al, 2005; Sessler, 2008). Conversely, unplanned hypothermia results from anesthesia-induced thermoregulation impairment, heat loss inherent during surgery, and the cold perioperative environment. As the duration of anesthesia time increases, the risk for unplanned hypothermia increases for all patients. These risk factors associated with the development of unplanned perioperative hypothermia are provided in Box 15-2. Unfortunately, unplanned hypothermia remains a patient safety problem because the use of routine prevention measures is not the standard of care for all patients undergoing surgery.

The maintenance of a normal core body temperature, or normothermia, is a persistent challenge for the perioperative team. Research evidence supports that normothermia maintenance is an effective way to avoid and/or treat many of the complications that occur with unplanned perioperative hypothermia (Wagner, 2006; AORN, 2009). This chapter will review both the physiology of temperature regulation and the etiology of unplanned perioperative hypothermia, the relationship between surgical complications and hypothermia, as well as approaches to prevent and treat unplanned hypothermia. Therapeutic hypothermia is briefly discussed to clarify the similarities and differences between the two types of hypothermia.

Awareness of the risks for developing hypothermia is the first step to prevention of harm from the complications that may occur from perioperative hypothermia. Given the availability of temperature monitoring and warming technology, the simplicity of interventions for prevention and treatment of hypothermia, demonstrated cost savings, and the decades' worth of scientific evidence, it would seem that normothermia management would be an easy and proactive approach to

BOX 15-1 Consequences of Hypothermia

- Thermal discomfort from shivering
- Impaired platelet function
- Increased cardiac ischemia
- Altered drug metabolism
- Impaired immune response
- Increased risk for infection
- Delayed recovery from anesthesia

BOX 15-2 Risk Factors Associated With Perioperative Hypothermia

Preoperative/preexisting hypothermia
Preoperative medications (sedatives, anxiolytics)
Duration and type of procedure
- Longer than 30 minutes
- Type of anesthesia
  - General anesthesia
  - Regional anesthesia
- Open cavity surgery

Age of patient
- Neonate or infant
- Geriatric adult

Low body weight
Traumatic injury
Extensive burn injury
Central nervous system dysfunctions
Cardiovascular diseases
Metabolic disorders
- Hypothyroidism
- Hypopituitarism
- Diabetic neuropathies

Chronic antipsychotic or antidepressant use
Use of pneumatic tourniquet
Cold surgical environment
Cool irrigation solutions
Cool infusions of fluids, blood, and blood products

the protection of surgical patients from the harm of complications. The achievement of normothermia throughout the patient's surgical experience is both a worthwhile perioperative goal and a patient safety initiative. An understanding of how the body maintains and manages its temperature is necessary.

PHYSIOLOGY OF TEMPERATURE REGULATION

Human body temperature is a tightly controlled physiologic parameter that is normally controlled within 0.2° C (0.4° F). The normal core temperature ranges from 36° C to 38° C (96.8° F to 100.4° F), with every individual recognized as having a unique baseline core temperature within this range. Values less than 36° C (96.8° F) or greater than 38° C (100.4° F) usually indicate a loss of thermoregulatory control or an extreme thermal environment that overwhelms thermoregulatory defenses (Sessler, 2008). Even small variations in the core body temperature stimulate antagonistic thermoregulatory defenses, because maintenance of normothermia is necessary for life.

Thermoregulatory thresholds and control are similar in men and women, but notably decline in older adults. Thermoregulatory control is intact in slightly premature infants, but is presumed immature in the less-developed infant, such as those weighing less than a kilogram (Mestyan et al, 1964). Thresholds vary daily by 0.5° C to 1° C (0.9° F to 1.8° F) in both sexes because of circadian rhythm and by approximately 0.5° C (0.9° F) with menstrual cycles in women. Infection, thyroid disease, drugs (including sedatives, nicotine, and alcohol), exercise, nutrition, and thermal adaptation will all alter threshold temperatures; however, these alterations are small compared with the profound impairment that general anesthesia creates (Tayefeh et al, 1998; Sessler, 2008).

The major autonomic thermoregulatory mechanisms in humans are vasodilation, vasoconstriction, shivering, and sweating. The hypothalamus, which is the controlling center for the autonomic nervous system, acts as a thermostat to maintain body temperature within the narrow physiologic range of only 0.2° C to 0.4° C (0.4° F to 0.7° F). Vasodilation and sweating are mechanisms of heat dissipation, whereas vasoconstriction and shivering are the main heat-conserving mechanisms. Each of these defenses has a threshold or set point that involves an incremental temperature change due to response as a maximum intensity response. Sweating and vasoconstriction thresholds are separated only by a few tenths of a degree Celsius, whereas the shivering threshold is a full degree Celsius below the vasoconstriction threshold. This interthreshold range defines the normal range of body temperature (Sessler, 2008).

Thermoregulation is the balance between heat loss and heat gain, which determines core temperature of the human body. The thermoregulatory system consists of a sensory component, a control center, and effector mechanisms. The hypothalamus control center maintains normothermia by balancing heat production, heat conservation, and heat loss hormonally. Peripheral thermoreceptors in the skin and central thermoreceptors in the hypothalamus, spinal cord, abdominal organs, and other central locations provide the hypothalamus with regulatory information about skin and core temperatures. If skin and core temperatures are low, the hypothalamus responds by triggering heat-production and heat-conservation mechanisms. Increased heat production is initiated by a series of hormonal mechanisms involving the hypothalamus and its connections with the endocrine system. The heat-producing mechanism begins with a hypothalamic hormone, thyrotropin-stimulating hormone–releasing hormone (TSH-RH). TSH-RH in turn stimulates the anterior pituitary to release thyroid-stimulating hormone, which acts on the thyroid gland, stimulating release of thyroxine, one of the thyroid hormones. Thyroxine then acts on the adrenal medulla, causing the release of epinephrine into the bloodstream. Epinephrine causes vasoconstriction, stimulates glycolysis, and increases metabolic rates, thus increasing heat production (Silva, 2005).

The hypothalamus also triggers heat conservation. The mechanisms of heat conservation involve stimulating the sympathetic nervous system, which is responsible for stimulating the adrenal cortex, increasing skeletal muscle tone, initiating the shivering response, and producing vasoconstriction. The hypothalamus also functions in raising body temperature by relaying information to the cerebral cortex (Silva, 2005). Awareness of cold provokes voluntary responses such as increased body movement. Behavioral responses require a conscious perception of body temperature. Minute changes in skin surface temperature are easily perceived; however, changes in central temperature are poorly sensed by humans. In fact, behavioral thermoregulation is half mediated by skin temperature, whereas the actual mean skin temperature contributes only 10% to 20% to the autonomic control of thermoregulatory defenses (Frank et al, 1999).

The body can also be described as two thermal compartments: a core compartment and a peripheral compartment. The core compartment houses the central nervous system and the organs in the skull, chest, and abdominal cavity. The peripheral compartment surrounds the core and includes the skin, fat, and muscles—tissues in which temperature is nonhomogeneous. A chief characteristic of the peripheral compartment is that heat content and distribution change significantly over time and as a function of environmental exposure. This is in striking contrast to the core compartment, for which temperature is usually precisely regulated. The peripheral compartment temperature ranges from 31° C to 35° C (87.8° F to 95° F), with skin temperature at 28° C to 32° C (82.4° F to 89.6° F). The core compartment is kept constant at about 37° C (98.6° F), irrespective of the environmental temperature. The peripheral compartment functions as a thermal buffer—either absorbing or releasing heat to the environment—protecting the core compartment by maintaining a constant temperature for the vital organs. This peripheral thermal buffer is largely controlled by arteriovenous shunts located in the extremities (Sessler, 2008).

The skin of the upper portion of the chest, as well as the skin on the face, is the most sensitive to temperature. The widespread belief that much of the body heat is lost through the head is untrue (Sessler, 2008). Remember, the head encases the brain and is part of the core compartment.

PERIOPERATIVE HYPOTHERMIA RISK FACTORS

General Anesthesia

General anesthesia obliterates behavioral adaptive responses and impairs vasoconstriction, and direct peripheral vasodilation effects cause the patient's core temperature to drop up to 1.6° C (2.7° F) during the first hour of anesthesia. This drop in core temperature can be explained by redistribution of heat from the body's core to the periphery. Redistribution occurs because anesthetics inhibit thermoregulatory control and disrupt the tonic vasoconstriction that normally maintains a core-to-peripheral temperature gradient. Anesthesia agents decrease vasoconstriction thresholds by 2° C to 4° C (3.6° F to 7.2° F) with the opening of arteriovenous shunts (Matsukawa et al, 1995; Sessler, 2008). Figure 15-1 depicts the decrease in body temperature that occurs when heat is redistributed from the body's core compartment to the peripheral tissues. Not a clear exchange of heat with the environment, this redistribution is a heat flow from the actual core to the periphery, resulting in decreased core temperatures. Anesthetics inhibit thermoregulation in a dose-dependent manner and inhibit vasoconstriction and shivering approximately three times more than they inhibit sweating (Sessler, 2008).

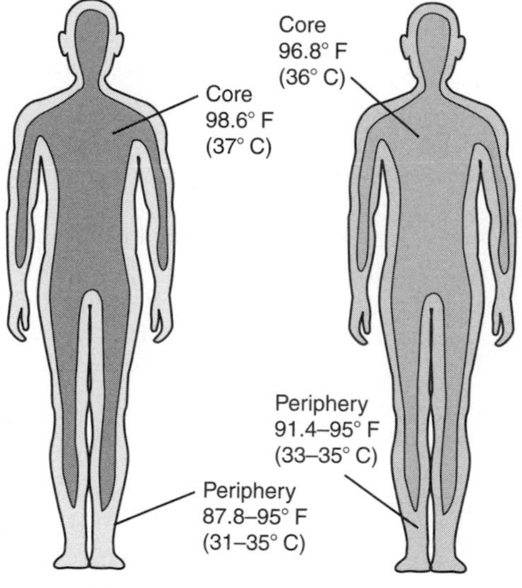

FIGURE 15-1 Core-to-peripheral redistribution of heat after anesthesia administration. (From Sessler DI: Perioperative heat balance, *Anesthesiology* 92:583, 2000.)

The next phase of the hypothermic action is a slower, linear decrease in core temperature with heat loss exceeding heat production. This phase lasts approximately 2 to 3 hours and depends on the difference between loss and metabolic heat production. During this time, core temperature continues to decrease an additional 1.1° C (2° F). Approximately 90% of heat loss is through the skin surface, with convection and radiation usually contributing more to the process than evaporation or conduction. Heat from the patient is transferred to the environment in four ways: radiation, convection, conduction, and evaporation (Figure 15-2) (Kurz et al, 1995). Box 15-3 lists heat loss mechanisms that occur in the perioperative setting. If patients are actively warmed during this phase, the heat loss can be effectively limited.

After 3 to 5 hours of anesthesia, there is a plateau phase that may reflect a steady state of heat loss equaling heat production and is seen in patients who are well insulated. However, if a patient is quite hypothermic, an arrested temperature decline results from activation of thermoregulatory vasoconstriction, which decreases cutaneous heat loss and acts to hold metabolic heat in the body core. Typically this happens when the patient's core temperature is about 34° C (93.2° F) (Sessler, 2008).

Regional Anesthesia

Regional anesthesia decreases the vasoconstriction and shivering to a slighter loss, approximately

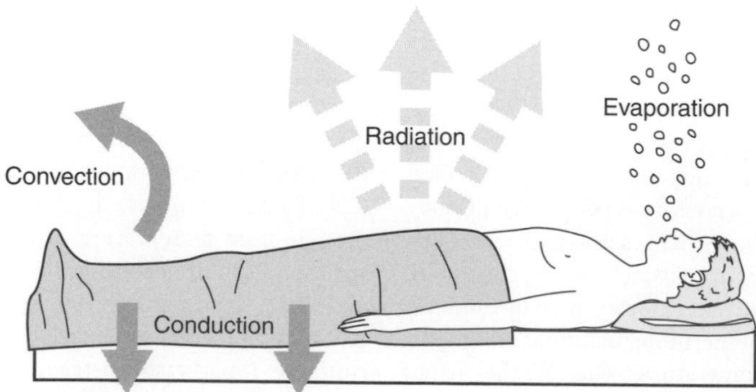

FIGURE 15-2 Mechanisms of heat loss. (From Sessler DI: Perioperative heat balance, *Anesthesiology* 92:583, 2000.)

0.6° C (1° F), and is dependent on the level of the block. Although the magnitude of response is less, the pattern of thermal impairment is similar to that of general anesthetics. This similar pattern of impairment suggests an alteration in central rather than peripheral control of temperature (Heier and Caldwell, 2006; Sessler, 2008). Core hypothermia during regional anesthesia may not be recognized by the patient. The reason is that thermal perception and behavioral regulation are mainly determined by skin rather than core temperatures. During regional anesthesia, skin temperature may increase even when there is core hypothermia present. The patient often has the perception of warmth, but will have autonomic thermoregulatory responses, including shivering (Sessler, 2008).

BOX 15-3 Heat Loss Mechanisms

RADIATION

- Accounts for approximately 40% of heat loss
  - May account for up to 65% of heat loss in cool environments
- Heat loss in the form of infrared heat rays—a type of electromagnetic heat transfer wave

CONVECTION

- Accounts for approximately 32% of heat loss
- Loss to air and water vapor molecules circulating around the body
  - Heat removed from body when air moves across the skin surface
- As ambient temperature rises, the amount of heat dissipated by convection decreases
  - Once air temperature exceeds mean skin temperature, heat is gained by the body

EVAPORATION

- Accounts for approximately 28% of heat loss
- Occurs when wet surfaces (e.g., open abdomen, diaphoretic patient) evaporate into atmosphere and take heat along
  - Conversion of a liquid to gaseous phase

CONDUCTION

- Accounts for a minute amount of heat loss in perioperative arena
- Transfer of heat energy from warmer to cooler objects by direct physical contact

Sedatives and analgesics also impair thermoregulatory control to some degree (Sato et al, 2009). If combined with the impairment of regional anesthesia and other factors, such as a preexisting illness, the thermoregulatory impairment would be severe (Sessler, 2008).

Other Risk Factors

Besides anesthesia agents, there are numerous factors that place surgical patients at a higher risk for the development of unplanned hypothermia during surgery. To see a compilation of the risk factors, see Box 15-2. The ambient temperature of the operating room environment determines the rate at which metabolic heat is lost from the skin through radiation, convection, and evaporation. Skin preparation methods may also contribute to hypothermia through evaporative loss (Sessler et al, 1993). There is a greater risk for hypothermia during procedures in which large body surface areas are left exposed, in situations where the peritoneal cavity is opened, and during longer surgical procedures (Roe, 1971). Infusions of cool fluids, blood, and blood products have been shown to increase risk for hypothermia. A unit of refrigerated blood decreases mean body temperature approximately 0.25° C (0.45° F) in a 70-kg (154-lb) patient (Sessler et al, 1993; Camus et al, 1996; Hasankhani et al, 2007). Use of a pneumatic tourniquet helps prevent hypothermia while inflated; however, when deflated, an abrupt hypothermia occurs. Upon release of the cuff pressure, a redistribution of heat from the core compartment to the peripheral compartment results in a rapid decline in core temperature (Sanders et al, 1996; Akata et al, 1998). The use of cool irrigation solutions into the abdomen, pelvis, or chest cavity enhances heat transfer from the core and decreases body temperature with the increased heat loss (Moore et al, 1997).

Numerous clinical studies have found that hypothermia increases the risk for death in trauma patients. The trauma patient has predisposing factors from injuries and preexisting hypothermia from exposure in the field, blood loss and shock, rapid infusions of cool fluids, removal of clothing, and impaired heat production. Hypothermia depresses ventilatory, renal, and hepatic functions (Moore, 2008). In one large study more than 50% of the trauma patients known to be hypothermic died (Rutherford et al, 1998).

In patients with extensive burns there is a loss of body heat from radiation from the burned tissues and from convection when the tissues are exposed to air currents. Because of the extreme heat loss through the burned tissues, these patients are at high risk for developing perioperative unplanned hypothermia (Corallo et al, 2008; AORN, 2009).

Factors that place patients at an intrinsic risk for developing hypothermia include patient physical status and comorbidities. Endocrine diseases, in particular, cause patients to be more prone to hypothermia (Sessler, 2008). Cardiovascular diseases may cause peripheral vasoconstriction and preemptive hypothermia (Frank, 1995). Thin or small-stature patients with a lack of tissue mass are more likely to become hypothermic. Obese patients generally have low core-to-peripheral temperature gradients and little redistribution hypothermia development. Infants and children cool more quickly because of their high ratio of surface area to weight, which leads to more heat loss through the skin (Kurz et al, 1995). Increased age is considered a predictive risk factor for perioperative unplanned hypothermia. Older adult patients have decreased thermoregulatory efficiency, decreased muscle mass, and changes in vascular tone that inhibit vasoconstriction and decrease heat production (Ayres, 2004).

HYPOTHERMIA AND COMPLICATIONS

Any level of hypothermia can cause serious patient problems. Even mild hypothermia (i.e., temperature less than 36° C [96.8° F]) has been consistently linked with perioperative complications. Randomized clinical trials have found increased adverse events associated with hypothermia ranging from those that affect basic comfort levels to effects on molecular interactions and cellular functions in a number of systems, including the cardiovascular, integumentary, hematologic, immune, renal, hepatic, and neuroendocrine systems (Wagner, 2006; AORN, 2009). Of course, the more at risk the patient and the more significant the level of hypothermia, the greater the chance of adverse outcomes. A discussion of complications from perioperative hypothermia follows.

Thermal Discomfort

Whether negative or positive in nature, memories of thermal comfort after surgery have an impact on overall patient satisfaction with surgical care. Thermal comfort may have more effects on surgical patient outcomes than nurses formally recognize. Even patients with normal core temperatures may experience thermal discomfort because of a low skin temperature that significantly contributes to thermal sensations. The need for thermal comfort is responsible for the initiation of behavioral thermoregulation (Wagner et al, 1996; Sessler, 2008). Thermal comfort measures may be used throughout all phases of perioperative care; however, during both the intraoperative and immediate postoperative phases of care the patient will need more than a thermal comfort intervention. When a patient is unable to relate in a subjective manner while in a surgical environment, thermal comfort measures become thermal protective or prevention measures during the intraoperative and immediate postoperative phase of care. Thermal protection is an appropriate term or concept that reflects the practice of perioperative nurses especially during the intraoperative and postoperative phases of care. Perioperative nurses frequently use preoperative warmth measures both for prevention of hypothermia and to provide comfort.

In a study examining the relative contribution of core and skin temperatures to thermal comfort and autonomic responses in humans, it was noted that thermal comfort was responsible for the initiation of behavioral thermoregulation and that humans are usually able to control both ambient temperature and the level of body-surface insulation. Findings show skin temperature contributed greatly toward subjective thermal comfort, whereas core temperature predominately regulates the autonomic and metabolic responses (Frank et al, 1999).

Of all the complications of hypothermia reported, shivering is the most frequent and probably the most familiar. It is how the body tries to correct hypothermia and usually occurs in the recovery phase following surgery. Even though shivering is the body's attempt to generate heat, it actually produces little heat, especially when a patient has received anesthesia. Shivering is metabolically valuable to the patient in that it increases oxygen requirements with the increased metabolic rate and carbon dioxide (CO_2) production. Shivering can lead to double or triple the oxygen consumption and carbon dioxide production in postanesthesia patients, although the increases are normally much smaller. Increases in metabolic requirements might predispose patients to further complications if limitations with cardiac or respiratory reserves already exist. Shivering also has been found to increase overall myocardial work and decrease arterial oxygen saturation, mixed venous saturation, and glycogen stores. The stress from shivering frequently results in elevated heart rate, labored breathing, and muscle spasms. Severe shivering may also result in tachycardia, hypertension, and myocardial ischemia, which could lead to cardiac arrest (Sessler, 2008). In addition, shivering increases incisional pain and is often remembered by patients as a fearful experience.

Body System Complications

Neuroendocrine System

Therapeutic hypothermia is used as a method of cerebral protection during periods of reduced cerebral blood flow by decreasing the metabolic demands of the brain tissue. However, it can also have unfavorable sequelae on the neurologic system. Cerebral blood flow is very sensitive to changes in temperature, with 1° C (1.8° F) drop in the core temperature resulting in a 6% to 7% drop in cerebral blood flow (Bay et al, 1986; Moore, 2008). Hypothermia can result in slowed mental functioning, delayed emergence from anesthesia, and blunted reflexes. These negative effects can increase the length of postoperative recovery, delay or inhibit assessment of neurologic status of the patient, and, if prolonged hypothermia is allowed, can lead to permanent neurologic deficits (Panagiotis et al, 2005).

Decreased blood flow that occurs during hypothermia may also increase the risk for metabolic acidosis. Epinephrine and norepinephrine levels have also shown increases in hypothermic patients. These increased levels of catecholamines could affect the neuroendocrine responses to surgical stress. Activation of complement and C-reactive proteins are seen in hypothermic events. In one study hypothermic patients had three times the incidence of myocardial ischemia and twelvefold higher incidence of angina postoperatively (Frank et al, 1995; Kumar et al, 2005).

Cardiovascular System

In mild hypothermia, activation of the sympathetic nervous system releases increased catecholamines, which lead to vasoconstriction. Hypothermia-induced vasoconstriction has been shown to reduce leg blood flow, cause venous stasis, and result in greater desaturation of venous blood. There is a potential contribution to increased thrombus formation and serious cardiac output, rate, and rhythm disturbances when hypothermic, which may be manifested as hypertension, bradycardia, or premature ventricular contractions (Scott and Buckland, 2006). Meta-analysis showed that normothermic patients had a 44% lower myocardial infarction (MI) rate. The decreased incidence of MI represents a potential average cost savings of between $68 and $90 per surgical patient. In contrast, the costs of a patient experiencing cardiovascular complications from hypothermia could be quite high, depending on the patient outcome (Mahoney and Odom, 1999). The resulting cardiac morbidity and mortality may seriously impact recovery in these patients when imbalance occurs between myocardial oxygen supply and demand. In fact, the most common cause of postoperative morbidity, hypothermia, has been associated with a greater incidence of cardiac complications, such as unstable angina/ischemia, cardiac arrest, and MI.

Another problem that occurs is coagulopathy, a condition in which the blood does not clot properly. Hypothermia has the effect of prolonging both the prothrombin time and partial thromboplastin times. Hypothermia induces coagulopathy because it reduces platelet function and affects both the intrinsic and extrinsic pathways in the clotting process. The body's normal clotting mechanisms become altered, causing increased bleeding and blood loss. With a 2° C (3.6° F) drop in temperature, blood loss increases by approximately 500 mL (Schmied et al, 1996). Even with less than 1° C (1.8° F) decrease, there is significant increase in blood loss, by approximately 16% (4% to 26%), and increased relative risk for transfusion by approximately 22% (3% to 37%) (Rajagopalan et al, 2008). Normothermic patients require 86% fewer units of red blood cells, 79% fewer units of plasma, and 78% fewer units of platelets than hypothermic patients. Cost savings related to maintaining perioperative normothermia with resulting reduction in the use of blood products are estimated to be $227 to $344 per patient (Mahoney and Odom, 1999).

Respiratory System

Hyperventilation is the initial response to hypothermia, followed by hypoventilation and irregular breathing patterns. Hypothermia causes a shift in the oxygen-hemoglobin dissociation curve that makes the hemoglobin have a greater affinity for oxygen. As a result, inhibition of oxygen release occurs, and oxygen delivery decreases with resulting tissue hypoxia, anaerobic metabolism, and lactic acidosis. Arterial blood gas values typically show hypoxia with respiratory alkalosis. Another problem during hypothermic events is the decreased bronchial arterial blood flow, which further retards oxygen uptake and delivery to the periphery.

Renal and Hepatic Systems

Hypothermia slows metabolic processes with resulting prolonged and altered drug actions. Hypothermia causes decreased renal flow and clearance. The enzymes that moderate organ function, primarily the liver and kidneys, are temperature sensitive and thus susceptible to hypothermia. The resultant decrease in blood flow to the kidneys leads to impaired glomerular filtration, delayed drug metabolism, and accumulation of drug products. There are also increased blood urea nitrogen and creatinine serum levels. In addition, slowed blood flow interferes with hepatic and pancreatic activities, further increasing the risk for drug accumulation. The delay of opiate and sedative clearance can contribute to a delayed emergence from anesthesia. Opiates and anesthetic agents may have prolonged action, which may lead to hypoventilation that can further complicate the patient's recovery. Muscle relaxants can be reactivated during recovery as the patient starts to rewarm and metabolize medications. In addition, the decrease in metabolism as a result of hypothermia significantly prolongs the length of stay in the postanesthesia care unit (PACU) and increases overall patient cost (Leslie and Sessler, 2003; Heier and Caldwell, 2006).

Immune System

Hypothermia is immunosuppressive, as demonstrated by decreased resistance to wound infections in numerous studies. In vitro studies have shown a reduction in phagocytic capacity of neutrophils (Wenisch et al, 1996; Beilin et al, 1998). Surgical incisions expose the patient to exogenous and endogenous pathogens. The patient's susceptibility to surgical site infections (SSIs) is increased by hypothermia because of vasoconstriction, which in turn decreases tissue oxygenation. A good blood supply is essential to bring oxygen, cellular nutrients, and leukocytes to promote wound healing. The primary defense against surgical pathogens is oxidative killing by neutrophils. Hypothermia reduces the production of superoxide radicals and other oxygen intermediates at a given level of tissue oxygenation. In this way hypothermia hampers neutrophil oxidative killing by making less oxygen available to the tissues, and thus neutrophils cannot undergo oxidative burst. Even mild decreases in temperature (1° C [1.8° F]) depress lymphocyte, phagocytic, and cytokine activity and production (Wenisch et al, 1996; MacFie et al, 2005). One study showed that hypothermic patients with core temperatures just 1.5° C to 2.0° C (2.7° F to 3.6° F) below normal—35.5° C to 35.0° C (95.9° F to 95° F)—had three times as many culture-positive surgical wound infections as normothermic patients (Kurz et al, 1996).

Patients with SSIs stay an average of 1 week longer in the hospital compared with those without SSIs. A meta-analysis of the effect of hypothermia on SSI rates revealed that nosocomial wound infections occurred 64% less often in normothermic patients. By maintaining normothermia, it is estimated that up to $1700 per patient could be saved through improved infection rates (Mahoney and Odom, 1999).

Delayed Recovery

Delayed recovery is potentially expensive because the PACU charges are similar to those in intensive care units. As mentioned above, numerous studies have been conducted with results that show hypothermia may delay recovery by enhancing anesthetic potency, delaying drug metabolism, producing hemodynamic instability, or depressing cognitive function. Hypothermic patients require an average of 40 minutes longer of PACU care than normothermic patients to reach discharge criteria when temperature was used as part of the criteria (Panagiotis et al, 2005; AORN, 2009).

In a perioperative cost-finding analysis of the routine use of intraoperative active warming during general anesthesia, Fleisher et al (1998) conducted a prospective, randomized, and blinded study with 100 patients allocated to either active warming (normothermic group) or routine thermal care (hypothermic group). Researchers found that the time from completion of surgery until extubation was significantly less in the normothermic group versus the hypothermic group ($P = .01$), although PACU lengths of stay were similar. There were no demonstrable differences in attainment of PACU discharge criteria between the two groups; however, the normothermia group used fewer cotton blankets than the hypothermia group. The additional recovery time associated with hypothermia added up to $7000 to total hospitalization costs (Fleisher, 1998).

PREVENTION OF HYPOTHERMIA

Prevention of unplanned perioperative hypothermia is important for both patient comfort and prevention of the complications that result from hypothermia. A large body of research over several decades has demonstrated that the normalization of body temperature during the perioperative period significantly improves patient outcomes and patient satisfaction and dramatically reduces the cost of treating complications related to ineffective thermal management.

Evidence supports that general and regional anesthetic techniques produce intense heat loss during the surgical experience. The most significant change in temperature occurs during the first 60 minutes that the patient receives anesthesia agents. As a result, the patient's temperature should be monitored when the length of the procedure exceeds 30 minutes. Evidence suggests that patients should be assessed for risk for developing unplanned hypothermia in the preoperative stage and managed accordingly. The patient's temperature should be recorded before anesthesia is induced and then taken at least every 30 minutes until surgery is complete. If the patient's temperature is rapidly changing, more frequent assessments should be made. Whenever possible, a core temperature site should be used. There are four sites for reliable measurement of core temperature: tympanic membrane, distal esophagus, nasopharynx, and pulmonary artery. Table 15-1 displays the advantages and disadvantages of reliable temperature sites for measurement of core temperatures. Axillary, bladder, oral, rectal, temporal artery, infrared tympanic, and skin sites provide less reliable means to assess a patient's temperature (Hooper and Andrew, 2006; Sessler, 2008).

The selection of the best device for monitoring patient temperatures should be dependent

TABLE 15-1 Temperature Sites for Reliable Measurement of Core Temperature

Site for Measurement	Advantages	Disadvantages
Tympanic Membrane	• Non-invasive approach of measurement by thermocouple • Preferred method in many pre and postoperative areas	• Not always a readily available measurement site for intraoperative measurements
Distal Esophagus	• Less prone to artifact • Desirable site intraoperatively	• Not usually desirable site for pre and postoperative measurements
Nasopharynx	• Reliable monitoring site for intraoperative monitoring	• Not usually desirable site for pre and postoperative measurements • Measurements may be influenced by inspired gases and may be 0.5° C (0.9° F) lower than pulmonary artery temperatures
Pulmonary artery	• Most accurate measurement of core body temperature	• Invasive form of monitoring

From Association of periOperative Registered Nurses: Recommended practices for the prevention of unplanned perioperative hypothermia. In Association of periOperative Registered Nurses: *2009 standards and recommended practices*, Denver, 2009, The Association.

upon accuracy of measuring core temperature, device reliability, accessibility of monitoring site, patient safety, and ease of use. Use of one device for continuous patient monitoring is ideal, but not always realistic in the perioperative setting. The use of one reliable monitoring site is considered important for continuity of data gathering and aids in obtaining consistent data.

Prevention of hypothermia should begin in the preoperative phase and continue into the postoperative and recovery phases of care. Thermal management should be consistently undertaken throughout perioperative care and encompasses both temperature monitoring and thermal care measures. Any abnormal patient temperatures should be communicated and managed as a coordinated effort among members of the perioperative team. All temperature measurements and interventions should be documented on the perioperative record (AORN, 2009).

Preoperative Phase

Temperature is generally recognized as a fundamental component of a patient's perception of well-being during the perioperative experience. Beginning in the preoperative phase of care, patients often complain about feeling cold. One of the most common nursing approaches for addressing this complaint is to cover the patient with warmed cotton blankets.

A preoperative temperature should be monitored and documented to provide baseline data for development of a thermal management plan. The patient's risk factors for unplanned perioperative hypothermia should be assessed. Thermal care should be focused on the prevention of unplanned hypothermia, and it may include warming a cold, stressed patient before transferring the patient to the operating room. The patient's subjective thermal comfort status should be assessed as well. Determining the best thermal management approach is the nurse's responsibility and it may include active warming techniques.

Treatment of redistribution hypothermia is easier said than done, both because the internal heat flow is large and because heat applied to the skin surface requires considerable time to reach the core thermal compartment. One way to minimize this substantial core-to-peripheral temperature gradient is to actively warm patients before anesthesia induction with an approach called prewarming. Prewarming, either preoperative or preinduction warming, can be completed either in the preoperative area or in the operating room before induction of anesthesia. Prewarming can be achieved only with the use of active warming techniques.

Examples of active warming techniques include the use of convective (warmed air) warming blankets and fluid warming to maintain and/or increase a patient's temperature, whereas passive warming methods include the use of insulation type of coverings such as reflective or conventional cotton blankets and head coverings (Figure 15-3). Active warming to the overall body and to localized areas has been found to be an effective intervention for reducing anxiety and complaints of pain during the preoperative phase of care (Wagner, 2006).

Prewarming of the skin before induction of anesthesia has little effect on core temperature, but it does increase the peripheral skin temperature and reduce the core-to-peripheral temperature gradient. Prewarming is important because induction of anesthesia would then produce little redistribution hypothermia because heat can only flow down a temperature gradient (Keikkas and Karga, 2005; AORN, 2009). Several factors may affect this gradient, including ambient temperature, degree of adipose tissue, and concurrent medications. Therefore the degree to which redistribution will decrease the core temperature in individual patients is difficult to predict. For example, an obese patient essentially is prewarmed by self-predilation. Both the first-rate insulation provided by fat and the increased heat production mean that obese patients are usually in a vasodilated state and usually have a reduced gradient for hypothermia redistribution if undergoing surgery (Sessler, 2008).

If the patient is undergoing a procedure that is expected to take at least 1 hour, prewarming should be considered to ensure the normalization of temperature during the intraoperative care (AORN, 2009). Evidence demonstrates prewarming for 30 minutes with a forced-air warming system provides sufficient heat to ensure the normalization of temperature for 1 hour. However, even 15 minutes of prewarming before induction of anesthesia results in higher core body temperatures upon arrival in the PACU (Kim et al, 2006; Wagner, 2006; Andrzejowski et al, 2008).

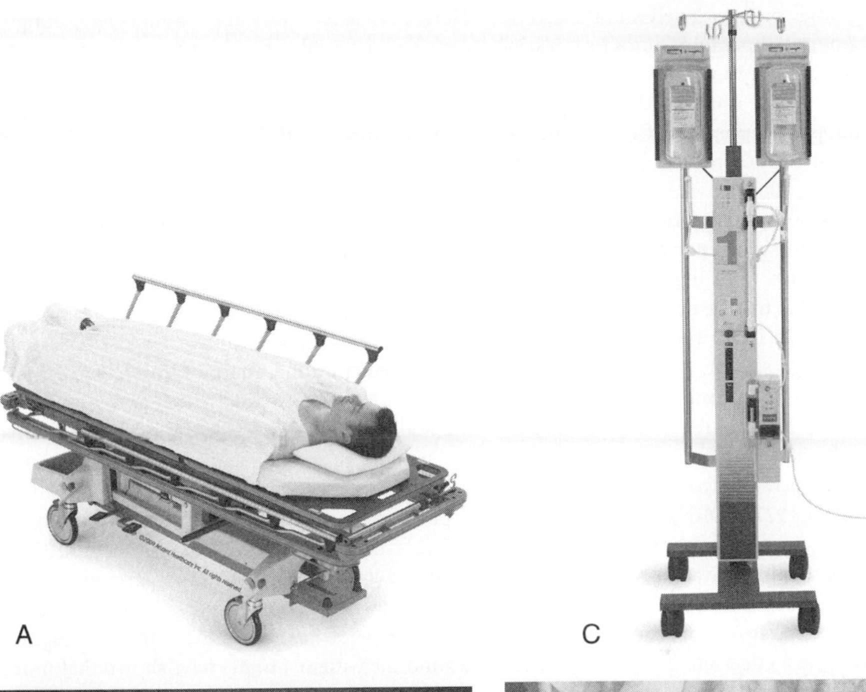

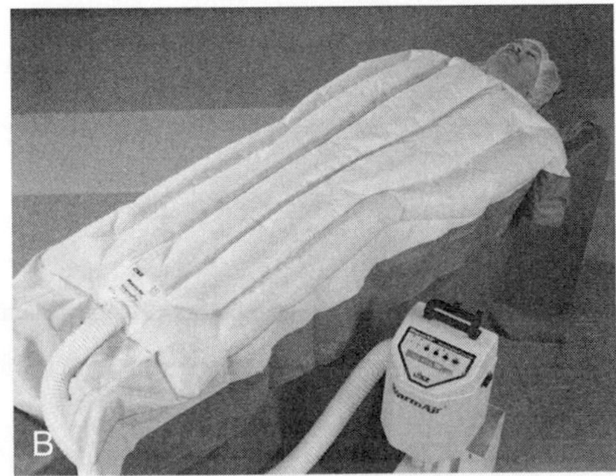

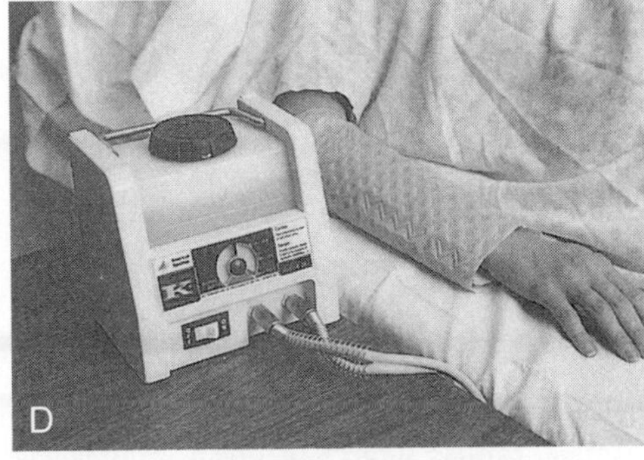

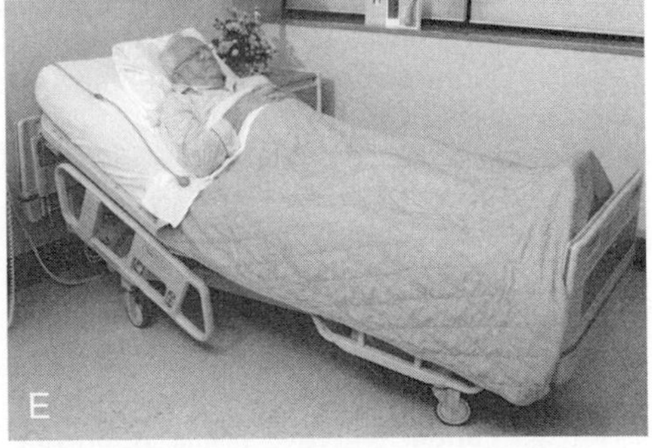

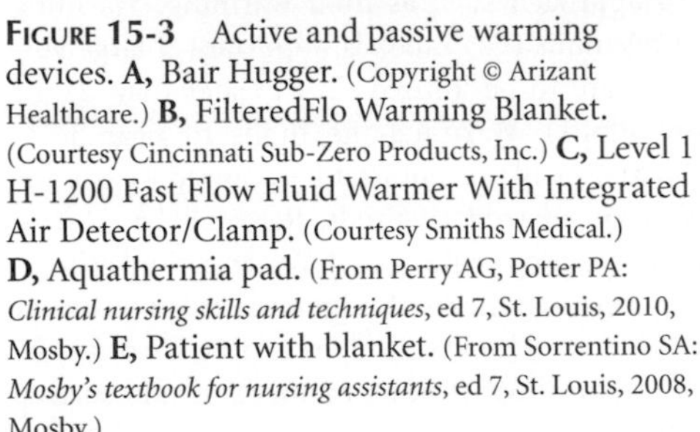

Figure 15-3 Active and passive warming devices. **A,** Bair Hugger. (Copyright © Arizant Healthcare.) **B,** FilteredFlo Warming Blanket. (Courtesy Cincinnati Sub-Zero Products, Inc.) **C,** Level 1 H-1200 Fast Flow Fluid Warmer With Integrated Air Detector/Clamp. (Courtesy Smiths Medical.) **D,** Aquathermia pad. (From Perry AG, Potter PA: *Clinical nursing skills and techniques*, ed 7, St. Louis, 2010, Mosby.) **E,** Patient with blanket. (From Sorrentino SA: *Mosby's textbook for nursing assistants*, ed 7, St. Louis, 2008, Mosby.)

Warming fluids preoperatively should also be considered. Room-temperature fluids or refrigerated blood products are included as risk factors for the development of unplanned hypothermia. Fluid warming is recommended if 2 L or more of fluids is administered preoperatively (Hasankhani et al, 2007; AORN, 2009).

Increasing the room temperature may be feasible if active warming is not available for use or in addition to active warming when additional warming approaches may be needed (e.g., trauma patient, burn patient). It may be considered appropriate when a large surface area is exposed for surgery and forced-air warming (FAW) may not be a sufficient warming approach. The severity or level of hypothermia may be reduced by raising the ambient temperature to more than 23 °C (73.4° F) (Morris, 1971; AORN, 2009).

The use of equipment to humidify and warm anesthetic gases should be available, especially for the pediatric population. Less than 10% of heat is lost through the respiratory tract and has not been found to have much effect on core temperatures. However, use of warmed gases during anesthesia has been found effective in infants and children (Bissonnette et al, 1989; AORN 2009). This warming method should not be used in place of skin surface warming because it transfers much less heat.

Intraoperative Phase

During surgery the patient's temperature should be normalized unless therapeutic hypothermia is indicated for tissue and organ preservation, for example, cardiac surgery or organ transplantation. When a hypothermic technique is required, the temperature should be normalized as soon as medically appropriate to minimize the untoward side effects of heat loss (AORN, 2009).

Patients who maintain normothermia intraoperatively experience fewer adverse outcomes. The use of passive insulation will usually be adequate to normalize body temperature during local anesthesia, moderate/procedural sedation, and monitored anesthesia care cases, because a body cavity is not opened. Passive warming blankets (e.g., cotton, reflective blankets) provide a level of thermal comfort and reduce heat loss by approximately 30%, but are not sufficient to prevent hypothermia in anesthetized patients (Sessler and Schroeder, 1993; Bujdoso, 2009). However, active warming should be strongly considered for all general and regional anesthetics, because these techniques produce profound heat loss and typically attend more invasive surgical procedures (AORN, 2009). See Figure 15-3 for several types of passive and active approaches to patient warming.

Effective methods of active warming that prevent hypothermia during the intraoperative phase involve continuing or beginning skin surface warming. There are several types of devices available for skin surface warming: FAW; circulating-water garments, and energy transfer pads. FAW devices are the most widely used active warming method. The method is effective in all age groups and types of surgical patients. The efficacy of FAW in the prevention and correction of unplanned hypothermia has been demonstrated in many clinical trials (Wong et al, 2007; Wagner et al, 2008; AORN, 2009). Circulating-water garments circulate warm water through a special segmented, conductive type of heating garment that is wrapped around the patient. Studies have shown that more heat is transferred to the patient by a circulating-water garment than a FAW upper body blanket when undergoing abdominal surgery and also during rewarming after cardiopulmonary bypass (Hofer et al, 2005; Nesher et al, 2005). Energy-transfer pads, which circulate water through heat exchange pads that adhere to the patient's skin, are relatively new warming devices and have been found to be an effective approach during off-pump cardiac surgery (Grocott et al, 2004).

One of the most efficient techniques to actively warm patients is to combine body surface warming by a FAW system with another active warming approach such as fluid warming. Warming intravenous (IV) fluids is important if large volumes are to be infused (i.e., greater than 2 L/hr for adults). Warming the fluids to near 37 °C (98.6° F) will prevent heat loss caused by administration of cold IV fluids. Research has shown that the combination of FAW and fluid warming decreased the risk for hypothermia more than FAW alone. However, fluid warming is not a substitute for FAW or other methods of skin surface warming. Studies show that warmed fluids alone will not usually keep patients normothermic (AORN, 2009).

Where significant volumes of irrigation solution are used, warming of solutions should be considered. Procedures that routinely use a large volume of irrigation include transurethral resection of the prostate, knee arthroscopy, hysteroscopy, and percutaneous nephrolithotomy. Warming irrigation solutions for use inside the abdomen, the pelvis, or the thorax should also be considered important. Again, warming the fluids to near 37° C (98.6° F) will prevent heat loss caused by administration of cold fluids, but is not sufficient alone to prevent hypothermia. When using warmed irrigation solutions, the measurement of the solution should be taken with a thermometer at time of use. Irrigation with hot solutions can lead to patient burn injuries (AORN, 2009).

Postoperative Phase

The evidence supports that normothermic patients experience less shivering, recover from anesthesia more quickly, and report higher satisfaction with their care than hypothermic patients. The patient should not be transferred back to the unit or home until the temperature is within the normal range. The normalization of temperature should be incorporated into discharge criteria (AORN, 2009).

Assess the patient's temperature on admission to the PACU. If the core temperature is less than 36° C (96.8° F), active warming is warranted. If the patient is shivering, the nurse should consider active warming measures. If the patient is receiving volume resuscitation, warm the intravenous fluids before infusion. Discharge from the PACU should be considered only when the patient's core temperature is normalized at or above 36° C (96.8° F) (AORN, 2009).

Effectiveness of Warming Devices

Numerous warming approaches are available, including increasing room temperature, humidification of anesthetic gases, warmed cotton blankets, thermal drapes, fluid warmers, circulating-water garments, energy transfer pads, and FAW systems. However, a meta-analysis of studies regarding these different warming methods showed FAW systems to be the most effective method to prevent and treat perioperative hypothermia (Mahoney and Odom, 1999). Additional precautions, such as increased temperature monitoring and increasing the room temperature to minimize heat loss, should be undertaken to prevent unplanned hypothermia in infants/neonates, patients with severe trauma, and patients with extensive burns (AORN, 2009).

PRINCIPLES OF WARMING SAFELY

Thermal management activities should be carried out using U.S. Food and Drug Administration (FDA)–approved devices. Because all warming devices have the potential to cause a patient burn when misused, the devices must be used in accordance with the manufacturer's instructions and in a way that minimizes the potential for injury. One of the most serious misuses is applying active heating devices to ischemic limbs. A health care facility's policies and procedures for warming device use must comply with the Safe Medical Devices Act. Any injury related to the use of a warming device should be reported to the FDA as mandated by this act.

Serious burn injuries have occurred in operating rooms because of "hosing," the misuse of a FAW system by failing to attach a blanket to the end of the hose and thereby blowing heated air directly onto the patient (ECRI, 1999). The FAW system is designed for use with the blanket and hose attached to distribute warm air safely and evenly across a large portion of the patient's body. Blanket air temperature is typically 2.5° C to 5.6° C (3.6° F to 10° F) lower than the temperature of the hose air. Therefore failure to use the warming blanket decreases the efficiency of the FAW system while significantly increasing the probability of thermal injury caused by concentrated hot air, contact between skin and the hose surface, and elevated air temperature at the hose nozzle (ECRI, 1999). Legal implications when using medical devices/equipment are listed in Box 15-4.

Nurses should receive initial education, as well as continuing education, regarding maintenance of competency in the use of warming devices and the prevention of unplanned hypothermia. Planning, using thermal protection modalities, and understanding patient safety issues should be part of any learning program related to warming competencies (AORN, 2009). Box 15-5 provides recommendations for safe warming system use.

BOX 15-4 Legal Implications When Using Medical Devices/Equipment

- Consider membership on policy and procedure committees to ensure clear policies and procedures concerning product identification, evaluation, and repair.
- Learn policies and procedures concerning actions to be taken when an injury or death occurs with equipment, including whom to contact and preservation of the product.
- Obtain adequate orientation and continuing education in-service on patient care equipment to ensure competency.
- Use equipment according to manufacturer's directions.
- Document all instances of patient injury accurately and completely in the patient's medical record and other required forms.

Data from Brent NJ, editor: *Concepts of negligence, professional negligence and liability in nurses and the law: a guide to principles and applications*, ed 2, Philadelphia, 2001, Saunders.

BOX 15-5 Recommendations for Reducing Burn Risk with Forced Air Hyperthermia Units

- Never depart from the unit's operating instructions without first checking with the supplier to learn about potential problems. The rationale for any alternate approach should be documented.
- Never treat patients using the unit's hose alone. Hyperthermia units and blankets are designed to be used as a system, not as independent components.
- If there is a reasonable chance that the patient will need to be warmed during surgery, apply the warming blanket before draping. The cost of using a disposable blanket unnecessarily is small compared to the cost of treating a patient for burns.
- Monitor the patient's body temperature and vital signs throughout treatment. Periodically check the appearance of the patient's skin under the blanket. Air temperature should be reduced or the unit turned off if vital signs become unstable or if redness of the skin is observed.
- Do not use the maximum temperature setting for patients with compromised circulation or patients who require warming for an extended period of time. Also, monitor such patients even more closely than patients without these conditions.

From ECRI: Hazard report: misusing forced-air hyperthermia units can burn patients, *Health Devices* 28(5–6):229–230, 1999. ECRI Institute publishes a variety of resources on perioperative safety, including additional information on forced air hyperthermia units. For more information on these resources contact ECRI Institute at (610) 825-6000.

CONCLUSION

Perioperative nurses should approach the prevention of unplanned hypothermia as a major patient safety initiative to focus on prevention of harm. Prevention measures are cost-effective, at low risk for injury, and may not be a major change in practice for many. Avoiding unplanned hypothermia is an obvious clinical goal for patient safety. Box 15-6 lists some of the initiatives and recommendations related to perioperative thermal management in the United States.

Nurses have an important role in the prevention and treatment of unplanned perioperative hypothermia and should advocate thermal management for every patient cared for by the perioperative health care team. Hypothermia is nurse controlled, and normothermia can be easily managed without a physician's order. Temperature management during the perioperative experience can decrease costs for both the hospital and, more importantly, the patient. The proactive practice of preventing unplanned perioperative hypothermia prevents patient harm and can have a profound impact on patient outcomes and safety.

BOX 15-6 Initiatives and Recommendations Related to Perioperative Thermal Management

ASSOCIATION OF PERIOPERATIVE REGISTERED NURSES (AORN)—RECOMMENDED PRACTICES FOR THE PREVENTION OF UNPLANNED HYPOTHERMIA

- Designed to provide recommended practices to implement to prevent unplanned hypothermia.
- Includes prewarming of patients for 15 minutes immediately before anesthesia induction and intraoperative warming to keep patients normothermic perioperatively.
- Web site: http://www.aorn.org

AMERICAN SOCIETY OF PERIANESTHESIA NURSES (ASPAN)—CLINICAL GUIDELINE FOR THE PREVENTION OF UNPLANNED PERIOPERATIVE HYPOTHERMIA

- Designed to provide guidance for instituting active warming measures for patients who are hypothermic.
- Website: http://www.aspan.org

INSTITUTE FOR HEALTHCARE IMPROVEMENT (IHI)—INITIATIVE: 5 MILLION LIVES CAMPAIGN

- Designed to protect patients from 5 million incidents of medical harm over a 2-year period (2006–2008).
- Initiative targeted SSIs and advised facilities to use warmed forced-air blankets perioperatively.
- Web site: http://www.IHI.org

SURGICAL CARE IMPROVEMENT PROJECT (SCIP)

- Multiyear national campaign aimed at decreasing surgical complications.
- Initiative recommended immediate postoperative normothermia for colorectal surgery patients to reduce the incidence of surgical infection.
- SCIP Infection 10—*Surgical Normothermia* will measure the proportion of patients undergoing any anesthesia-provided procedure of more than 1 hour who have active warming provided or achieve normothermia within 15 minutes before or after the end of anesthesia. Measure to be aligned with the Physician Quality Reporting Initiative (PQRI) measure and excludes intentional hypothermia cases.
- Web site: http://www.qualitynet.org

THE JOINT COMMISSION (TJC)

- In the *Specifications Manual for National Hospital Quality Measures,* TJC supports implementation of SCIP –Inf-7: *Colorectal Surgery Patients With Immediate Postoperative Normothermia.*
- Web site: http://www.jointcommission.org

CENTERS FOR DISEASE CONTROL AND PREVENTION (CDC)

- The CDC *Guideline for the Prevention of Surgical Site Infection* (1999) posits that excellent surgical technique is widely believed to reduce the risk for SSI. Among the techniques included was the prevention of hypothermia.
- Web site: http://www.cdc.gov

SSI, Surgical site infection.

REFERENCES

Akata T, et al: Changes in body temperature following deflation of limb pneumatic tourniquet, *J Clin Anesth* 10:17–22, 1998.

Andrzejowski J, et al: Effect of prewarming on post-induction core temperature and the incidence of inadvertent perioperative hypothermia in patients undergoing general anaesthesia, *Br J Anaesth* 101(5):627–631, 2008.

Association of periOperative Registered Nurses: Recommended practices for the prevention of unplanned perioperative hypothermia. In Association of periOperative Registered Nurses: *Standards and recommended practices*, Denver, 2009, The Association.

Ayres U: Older people and hypothermia: the role of the anesthetic nurse, *Br J Nurs* 13(7):396–403, 2004.

Bay J, et al: Factors influencing arterial PO_2 during recovery from anaesthesia, *Br J Anesth* 188(6):685–696, 1986.

Beilin B, et al: Effects of mild perioperative hypothermia on cellular immune responses, *Anesthesiology* 89(5):1133–1140, 1998.

Bissonnette B, et al: Passive or active inspired gas humidification increases thermal steady-state temperatures in anesthetized infants, *Anesthes Analg* 69:783–787, 1989.

Bujdoso P: Blanket warming: comfort and safety, *AORN J* 89(4):717–722, 2009.

Camus Y, et al: The effects of warming intravenous fluids on intraoperative hypothermia and postoperative shivering during prolonged abdominal surgery, *Acta Anaesthesiol Scand* 40:779–782, 1996.

Corallo JP, et al: Core warming of a burn patient during excision to prevent hypothermia, *Burns* 34(3):418–420, 2008.

ECRI: Hazard report: misusing forced air hyperthermia units can burn patients, *Health Devices* 28(5–6):229–230, 1999.

Fleisher LA, et al: Perioperative cost-finding analysis of the routine use of intraoperative forced-air warming during general anesthesia, *Anesthesiology* 88(5):1357–1364, 1998.

Frank SM, et al: Relative contribution of core and cutaneous temperatures to thermal comfort and autonomic responses in humans, *J Appl Physiol* 86(5):1588–1593, 1999.

Frank SM, et al: The catecholamine, cortisol, and hemodynamic responses to mild perioperative hypothermia. A randomized clinical trial, *Anesthesiology* 82(1):83–93, 1995.

Grocott HP, et al: A randomized controlled trial of the Arctic Sun temperature management system versus conventional methods for preventing hypothermia during off-pump cardiac surgery, *Anesth Analg* 98:298–302, 2004.

Hasankhani H, et al: The effects of intravenous fluids temperature on perioperative hemodynamic situation, postoperative shivering, and recovery in orthopedic surgery, *Can Oper Room Nurs J* 25(1):20–24, 26–27, 2007.

Heier T, Caldwell J: Impact of hypothermia on the response to neuromuscular blocking drugs, *Anesthesiology* 104:1070–1080, 2006.

Hofer C, et al: Influence of body core temperature on blood loss and transfusion requirements during off-pump coronary artery bypass grafting: a comparison of 3 warming systems, *Thorac Cardiovasc Surg* 129:838–843, 2005.

Hooper VD, Andrew JO: Accuracy of noninvasive core temperature measurement in acutely ill adults: the state of the science, *Biol Res Nurse* 8:24–34, 2006.

Kiekkas P, Karga M: Prewarming: preventing intraoperative hypothermia, *Br J Perioper Nurs* 15(10):444–451, 2005.

Kim JY, et al: The effect of skin surface warming during anesthesia preparation on preventing redistribution hypothermia in the early operative period of off-pump coronary artery bypass surgery, *Eur J Cardiothorac Surg* 29(3):343–347, 2006.

Kumar S, et al: Effects of perioperative hypothermia and warming in surgical practice, *Int Wound J* 2(3):193–204, 2005.

Kurz A, et al: Heat balance and distribution during the core-temperature plateau in anesthetized humans, *Anesthesiology* 83(3):491–499, 1995.

Kurz A, et al: Perioperative normothermia to reduce the incidence of surgical-wound infection and shorten hospitalization, Study of Wound Infection and Temperature Group, *N Engl J Med* 334(19):1209–1215, 1996.

Leslie K, Sessler DI: Perioperative hypothermia in the high-risk surgical patient, *Best Pract Res Clin Anaesthesiol* 17(4): 485–498, 2003.

MacFie CC, et al: Effects of warming on healing, *J Wound Care* 14(3):133–136, 2005.

Mahoney CB, Odom J: Maintaining intraoperative normothermia: a meta-analysis of outcomes with costs, *AANA J* 67(2):155–163, 1999.

Matsukawa T, et al: Heat flow and distribution during induction of general anesthesia, *Anesthesiology* 82(3):662–673, 1995.

Mestyan J, et al: The significance of facial skin temperature in the chemical heat regulation of premature infants, *Biol Neonate* 7:243–254, 1964.

Moore K: Hypothermia in trauma, *J Trauma Nurs* 15(2): 62–64, 2008.

Moore S, et al: The role of irrigation in the development of hypothermia during laparoscopic surgery, *Am J Obstetric Gynecol* 176:598–602, 1997.

Morris RH: Influence of ambient temperature on patient temperature during intraabdominal surgery, *Ann Surg* 173(2):230–233, 1971.

Nesher N, et al: Thermowrap technology preserves normothermia better than routine thermal care in patients undergoing off pump coronary artery bypass and is associated with lower immune response and lesser myocardial damage, *J Thorac Cardiovasc Surg* 129:1371–1378, 2005.

Panagiotis K, et al: Is postanesthesia care unit length of stay increased in hypothermic patients? *AORN J* 81(2):379–392, 2005.

Rajagopalan S, et al: The effects of mild perioperative hypothermia on blood loss and transfusion requirement, *Anesthesiology* 108(1):71–77, 2008.

Roe CF: Effect of bowel exposure on body temperature during surgical operations, *Am J Surg* 122:13–15, 1971.

Rutherford, et al: Hypothermia in critically ill trauma patients, *Injury* 29:605–608, 1998.

Sanders B, et al: Intraoperative hypothermia associated with lower extremity tourniquet deflation, *J Clin Anesth* 8:504–507, 1996.

Sato, et al: Forced-air warming effectively prevents midazolam-induced core hypothermia in volunteers, *Eur J Anaesthesiol* 26(7):566–571, 2009.

Schmied H, et al: Mild hypothermia increases blood loss and transfusion requirements during total hip arthroplasty, *Lancet* 347:289–292, 1996.

Scott EM, Buckland R: A systematic review of intraoperative warming to prevent postoperative complications, *AORN J* 83(5):1090–1113, 2006.

Sessler D: Temperature monitoring and perioperative thermoregulation, *Anesthesiology* 109(2):318–338, 2008.

Sessler D, Schroeder M: Heat loss in humans covered with cotton hospital blankets, *Anesth Analg* 77:73–77, 1993.

Sessler D, et al: Heat loss during surgical skin preparation, *Anesthesiology* 78:1055–1064, 1993.

Silva JE: Thyroid hormone and the energetic cost of keeping body temperature, *Biosci Rep* 25(3–4):129–148, 2005.

Tayefeh F, et al: Circadian changes in the sweating-to-vasoconstriction interthreshold range, *Pflugers Arch* 435:402–440, 1998.

Wagner D: Unplanned perioperative hypothermia and surgical complications: evidence for prevention, *Perioperative Nurs Clin* 1(3):267–281, 2006.

Wagner D, et al: Effects of comfort warming on preoperative patients, *AORN J* 84(3):427–448, 1996.

Wagner K, et al: Comparison of two convective warming systems during major abdominal and orthopedic surgery, *Can J Anesth* 55(6):358–363, 2008.

Wenisch C, et al: Mild intraoperative hypothermia reduces production of reactive oxygen intermediates by polymorphonuclear leukocytes, *Anesth Analg* 82(4):810–816, 1996.

Wong PF, et al: Randomized clinical trial of perioperative systemic warming in major elective abdominal surgery, *Br J Surg* 94(4):421–426, 2007.

ELECTROSURGERY

Chapter 16

Brenda C. Ulmer MN, RN, CNOR

The use of electrosurgery generators (ESUs) have become commonplace throughout the world wherever surgical and invasive procedures are performed. The caustic "cautery" and "clamp, cut, and tie," which was the gold standard for hemostasis for centuries, has been transformed by today's surgeons to electrosurgery coagulation, vaporization, and vessel fusion.

HISTORICAL BACKGROUND

Papyrus documents from Egypt dated about 3000 BC are among the earliest records of surgery and the use of cauterization to control bleeding. Further examples of cautery use can be found in early manuscripts throughout the Middle Ages. Many researchers and physicians contributed to the body of knowledge of electrosurgery throughout the past two centuries.

In the 1800s researchers around the world were independently conducting experiments with electricity. In both England and America Michael Faraday (1791–1867) and Joseph Henry (1797–1878) were conducting experiments on the relationship between magnetism and electricity. They discovered that a moving magnet could induce an electrical current in a conductive wire. Electromagnetism was a very important principle that led to improved electromedical devices (Goldwyn, 1979).

The research conducted in the years between 1881 and 1900 saw electrical current moved into the higher-frequency ranges. In 1881 William J. Morton reported that current in the 100-kHz range did not produce the painful tissue effects of current in the lower-frequency ranges. By 1891 Arsenne d'Arsonval of France had documented that the alternating current frequency could safely be lowered to 100 kHz (Pearce, 1986).

An early use of electrosurgery clinically was by Joseph A. Riviere. While treating a musician with electricity for insomnia, Riviere accidentally touched one of the wires on a device he was using and produced a spark. This incident prompted Riviere to use the spark on an ulcer on the musician's hand. Repeated treatments resulted in healing of the ulcer. Riviere reported his results at the First International Congress of Medical Electrology and Radiology in Paris in 1900. This is said to be the first surgical use of high-frequency current to treat a human condition (Kelly and Ward, 1932).

The first patent for an electrosurgical high-frequency generator was filed by Lee DeForest on February 10, 1907. The DeForest electrosurgery unit was not the device that came into general use in operating rooms. That distinction goes to the man whose name has become synonymous with electrosurgery—William T. Bovie—and his work with Harvey Cushing, MD. They are the two men whose names are most closely associated with electrosurgery. The Bovie and Cushing partnership yielded successful contributions to the field of electrosurgery that have stood the test of time.

Bovie's interest in electrosurgery came about because of his work with radium at the Harvard Cancer Commission. He believed that the cautery effect achieved from radium emanation could be achieved more easily with electrocoagulation. Bovie's work with high-frequency generators continued, and his machine developed into one that was better suited for the operating room.

The advances Cushing made in surgical care and specifically neurosurgery are legendary. He was one of the first proponents of blood pressure monitoring during surgery and used primarily local anesthesia. There were also great advances made in controlling blood loss during surgery through the methods that Cushing used. There were, however, still patients that were considered inoperable due to the concern of uncontrolled bleeding. Cushing's first true consideration of the use of electrosurgery seems to have occurred at a medical conference in the summer of 1925. Samuel Harvey and John Morton, both residents of Cushing's, were watching an electrosurgery demonstration when Cushing joined them. One of them jokingly suggested that Cushing use the machine on the brain. Instead of discounting the possibility, Cushing stopped and looked thoughtfully at the demonstration (Voorhees et al, 2005). Cushing later visited Bovie's laboratory at Harvard to inquire further about his electrical machine.

By the fall of 1926 Cushing had arranged to use Bovie's device during a surgical procedure. Over the next two years the two worked together to use and make refinements to the electrosurgical generator. Cushing's adoption of the use of electrosurgery changed the landscape of surgery throughout the world. Both Cushing and Bovie gave credit to the work done by other researchers in the field of electrosurgery, but it is the work that the two of them accomplished together that contributed to the advancement of Bovie's device. The combination of Cushing's skill as a surgeon and Bovie's genius made the difference. They worked with Liebel-Flarsheim to develop a commercial unit, which also contributed to the success of the "Bovie." The continued refinement and evolution of electrosurgery devices did not end with Bovie and Cushing, but have continued throughout the twentieth and twenty-first centuries. Electrosurgery is one of the most common devices used in surgical and invasive procedures around the world.

ELECTROSURGERY

Basic Principles of Electricity

Electricity is the power behind radio-frequency electrosurgery generators; therefore it is useful to understand how electricity works. Electricity is a naturally occurring phenomenon arising from the existence of atoms. Atoms consist of negatively charged electrons, positively charged protons, and neutral particles called neutrons. Atoms that contain equal numbers of electrons and protons are charge neutral. Movement of electrons can change the charge of the atom. Atoms that lose electrons and gain protons have a positive electrical charge; atoms that gain electrons and lose protons have a negative electrical charge. During atom movement, like charges repel and unlike charges attract. Electron movement is termed electricity, and it can move at nearly the speed of light. The following two constant properties of electricity can have an impact on patient care in the operating room:

1. Electricity always follows the path of least resistance.
2. Electricity always seeks to return to ground (Columbia Encyclopedia, 2001).

Electrical current—electricity—is produced as electrons flow through a conductor. The pathway of the electrical current as it flows through the conductor is called the electrical circuit. There must be a complete circuit before the device will function. The two types of electrical current in use today are direct current (DC) and alternating current (AC). Direct current is a simple circuit, and the electricity flows in only one direction. All types of batteries employ a simple DC circuit. Energy flows from one terminal on the battery and returns to the other terminal to complete the circuit.

AC changes, or alternates, direction of the electrical flow. The frequency of these alterations is measured in cycles per second or Hertz (Hz), with 1 Hz being equal to one cycle per second. Household current alternates at 60 cycles per second, as does much of the electrical equipment used in operating rooms. Alternating current at 60 Hz can cause tissue injury. As early researchers discovered, neuromuscular stimulation ceases at about 100,000 Hz as the alternating current moves into the radio-frequency range. Electrosurgery generators take 60-cycle household current and raise it to the radio-frequency range of 200,000 Hz to 3.3 MHz (Figure 16-1). As electrons flow through a conductor, that flow is measured in amperes, or amps (Hutchisson et al, 1998).

Additional factors that affect current flow and electrosurgery generator performance include resistance, voltage, and power.

Resistance is the opposition to the flow of the electrical current. Resistance or impedance is measured in ohms. In the operating room one source of resistance or impedance is the patient. All patient tissues have different ohms of resistance—muscle and blood have the lowest resistance and easily allow for the flow of electrons.

Voltage is the force that will cause 1 amp to flow through 1 ohm of resistance. It is measured in volts. The voltage in an electrosurgical generator provides the force that pushes electrons through the circuit. Electrosurgery generator voltages can range from about 2000 to as much as 10,000 volts of electricity, depending on the type of generator and how the generator is used.

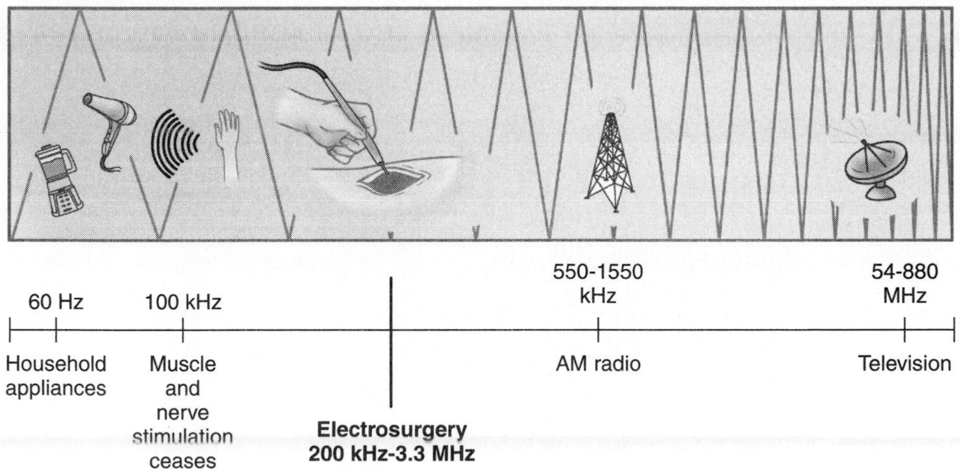

FIGURE 16-1 Electrosurgery frequency spectrum. (Courtesy Covidien, Inc.)

Power is the energy produced. The energy is measured in watts. A watt is the amount of energy produced by 1 volt times 1 amp of current. Electrosurgical generator power settings are either printed on a light-emitting diode (LED) screen in watts, or a percentage of the wattage is demonstrated on a numerical dial setting. Most electrosurgical generators have a maximum coagulation output of 120 watts, and a maximum vaporization or cut output of 300 watts.

Current flow through a completed circuit, impedance/resistance, and voltage are all components that must be present for the electrosurgical generator to function. Knowing the role that each one plays during use of the generator will help to ensure safe use of the electrosurgery generator.

Electrosurgery Waveforms

One of the important discoveries during the early development of the electrosurgery generator was that the electrical output from the generators could be manipulated to produce different waveforms, or electrosurgical modes. There are three basic waveforms that have distinct tissue effects. The modes or waveforms are cut, fulguration, and blend (Figure 16-2).

Vaporization (Cutting)

The cutting current produced by an electrosurgical generator is a continuous waveform. Because the delivery of current is continuous, much lower voltages are required to achieve tissue vaporization. To produce a cutting effect the active electrode tip is held just over the tissue. The current vaporizes cell walls and divides the tissue. The cut mode can also be used for coagulation of tissue through desiccation. In this application the active electrode is in direct contact with tissue.

Fulguration

Tissue fulguration is produced with the coagulation (coag) mode on the generator. The coagulation current is an interrupted or dampened waveform with a duty cycle that is on only about 6% of the time. The tissue is heated when the waveform spikes and then cools down during the 94% off-time of the duty cycle, thus producing coagulation of the cell. The proper method for achieving hemostasis when using coagulation is to hold the active electrode tip slightly above the target tissue and let the spark from the tip do the work.

Blend

The blend mode on a generator is a function of the cut waveform, typically indicated by the yellow section on most generators. When "blend" is selected, the cut current is modified to a dampened waveform that produces some hemostasis. The voltage is increased, and the off-time of the generator is

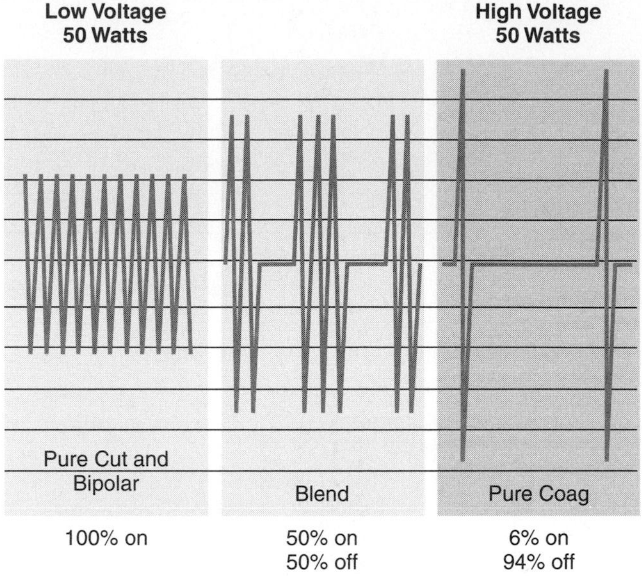

FIGURE 16-2 Typical electrosurgery waveforms. (Courtesy Covidien, Inc.)

adjusted, depending on the blend setting selected. There are several blend settings that provide different ratios of coagulation to cutting current. The ratios and number of blend settings vary depending on the manufacturer of the generator.

Desiccation

Electrosurgical desiccation can be produced using either the cut or the coagulation mode on the generator. The difference is that the active electrode tip must contact the tissue to achieve desiccation. The desired mode to achieve tissue desiccation through direct contact is the cut waveform because of the lower cut voltage (Ulmer, 2007b).

Electrosurgical Tissue Effect

The electrosurgery waveform the surgeon selects affects patient tissue. Other variables can also alter the outcome of the electrosurgical tissue effect. The time that the surgeon activates the active electrode determines the degree of tissue effect. Activations that are too long produce wider and deeper tissue damage. Activations that are not long enough will not produce the desired tissue effect. The power setting the surgeon selects alters tissue effect. The surgeon should always use the lowest possible power setting to achieve the desired tissue effect, which will vary with the patient. The size of the active electrode influences the tissue effect of the generator. A large electrode will require a higher power setting than a small electrode. It is also important to note that a clean electrode will conduct current more effectively than a dirty electrode, thereby requiring lower power settings. Patient tissue can determine the effectiveness of the generator. A lean, muscular patient will conduct the electrosurgical current better than an obese or emaciated patient. The physical condition of the patient determines the amount of impedance encountered by the current as it attempts to return to the generator to complete the circuit.

Electrosurgical Technologies

The history of electrosurgery demonstrates a surgical tool that has evolved over time. Since Cushing's early use of the technology, electrosurgery has developed from nondifferentiating electrical current to computer-controlled systems that adjust output according to the demands of patient tissue (Table 16-1). The role of the perioperative professional is to be familiar with old and new technology and to understand how technology improvements benefit both the patient and perioperative practitioners.

TABLE 16-1 Evolution of Electrosurgery Technology in the Twentieth and Twenty-First Centuries

Year	Development
1926	Cushing uses Bovie's ground-referenced device
1968	Solid-state circuit
1981	Quality contact monitoring
1995	Tissue-density feedback control
1999	Tissue fusion
2006	Closed-loop coagulation

Electrocautery

The electrocautery device is the simplest electrical system used in the operating room today. It uses a simple DC generated from a battery within the system. The small handheld eye cautery is an example of this device. The battery heats up a wire loop at the end of the device. The current never leaves the instrument to travel through the patient's tissue. A cautery device is useful in minor procedures where very little bleeding is expected. It cannot cut tissue or coagulate large bleeders, and tissue has a tendency to stick to the heated wire.

Bipolar

Bipolar electrosurgery is the use of electrical current in which the circuit is completed by using two parallel poles located in close proximity to one another such as bipolar forceps. One pole is positive, and the other is negative. The flow of current is restricted between the two poles. Because the poles are close together, low voltages are required. Many bipolar units use the cut waveform. A patient return electrode is not needed because the current never flows through the patient's body. This also makes bipolar very safe. Bipolar, however, cannot spark to tissue, and the low voltage makes it less effective on large bleeders.

Monopolar Electrosurgery

When monopolar electrosurgery is used, the electrical current originates in the generator and is delivered to patient tissues by an electrosurgery active electrode tip. The current travels through patient tissue to and is collected by the patient return electrode and returned to the generator. This is the intended pathway for the electrical current. Monopolar electrosurgery should be used in a way that restricts current flow to the intended pathway and reduces the likelihood of producing stray electrical current.

Ground-Referenced Generators

The first generation of electrosurgery generators, such as the original Bovie unit, were ground referenced. During operation the ground completed the electrosurgical circuit. The units were spark-gap systems that were high output and high performance (Massarweh et al, 2006). This made them a favorite with surgeons. One major hazard of a grounded system is that current division can occur. If the electrical current finds an easier and quicker way to return to ground, the patient could be burned at any point where the current exits the patient's body. That could be where the patient's hand touches the side of the bed, a knee touches a stirrup, or any number of alternate exit sites. Patient burns could occur. Later models offered a cord fault alarm that alerted the perioperative staff if the patient return electrode was not plugged into the generator. The disadvantage was that electrosurgery could still be used even if the return electrode was not on the patient.

Solid-State Generators

Solid-state generators were introduced in 1968. The inventor of the solid-state generator was a National Aeronautics and Space Administration (NASA) scientist who realized it was possible to replace the large ground-referenced generators with smaller machines. Isolated generators reference the electrical current between the unit and the patient, and, even if the patient touches another grounded object, the current will ignore that contact. Current division does not occur with isolated generators, which eliminates the possibility of alternate site burns. During the use of an isolated generator, the unit will not work if the patient return electrode is not on the patient. The generator, however, is not capable of determining the quality of the contact between the patient and the patient return electrode. Should the patient return electrode become compromised during surgery, a return electrode burn could occur.

Quality Contact Monitoring

In 1981 a technology was introduced to address patient return electrode burns. Quality contact monitoring or return electrode monitoring is a split pad system that allows the generator to continuously monitor the quality of the contact between the pad and the patient. An interrogation circuit from the generator constantly monitors impedance or resistance at the pad site. If a condition develops at the return electrode site that could result in a patient burn, the quality contact monitoring system will inactivate the generator (Phippen et al, 2009). Return electrode monitoring was a major breakthrough in the advancement of patient safety. For the first time in generator history, a technology could take into consideration the real-time condition of the patient's own tissues. This computer-controlled system heralded a new generation of electrosurgery technology innovation.

Tissue Density Feedback Electrosurgery

Progression of computer capabilities further advanced patient safety in 1995 when computer-controlled feedback generators were developed. The technology uses a computer-controlled, instant response system that senses tissue density. The feedback system provides consistent clinical effect through all tissue types. The generator rapidly senses tissue resistance and automatically adjusts the output voltage to maintain consistent tissue effect. This is called an adjustment mode, or effect mode. The feedback mode reduces the need to adjust power settings for different types of tissue. It also gives improved generator performance at lower voltages, which reduces the risk for patient injury. Instant response to changing patient conditions represents improved performance over conventional generators, and, just as with quality contact monitoring, was a tremendous advance in patient safety. This safety system, however, was only available in the cut or vaporization mode, and coagulation continued to be the primary mode used in the operating room (Eggleston et al, 1997).

Tissue Fusion

The progression of the computer technology quickened the pace of new developments in electrosurgery. Following on the heels of tissue response technology came tissue fusion capabilities in 1999. Tissue fusion was revolutionary in the world of electrosurgery. Using a combination of pressure and bipolar type of energy, the surgeon could fuse or seal vessel walls and tissue bundles. The pressure and energy change the nature of the collagen of the tissue between the forceps, creating a permanent tissue weld. The seal is strong and withstands three times normal systolic blood pressure. Use of the vessel fusion system reduced and/or eliminated the need for sutures, clips, and staples. Throughout the history of hemostasis the surgeon had never before had the ability to seal vessels and tissue bundles up to (and including) 7 mm in size. A tremendous added benefit to patient safety was that the bipolar-like design of the system did not require a patient return electrode. Pacemakers, implants, scar tissue, and jewelry were not affected by the vessel fusion current (Propkopakis et al, 2005).

Closed-Loop Coagulation

The most recent engineering breakthrough in electrosurgery occurred in 2006 with the introduction of increased tissue-sensing generator capabilities employing a closed-loop coagulation mode. The technology builds on, and then improves, the best tissue-sensing engineering developments of the past 25 years, beginning with quality contact monitoring. Closed-loop coagulation is a computer-controlled system that senses tissue resistance and adjusts output voltage, current, and generator power over 3000 times per second. This provides consistent electrosurgical effect across different patient tissues. This technology is the first time tissue sensing has been available to the surgeon in the coagulation mode. The differences between conventional coagulation and closed-loop coagulation can be seen by comparing waveform printouts of the generator output (Figure 16-3). The tissue-sensing technology communicates information about the patient's tissues back to the generator, making each surgical procedure customized and specific to each patient (Ulmer, 2007a).

Electrosurgical Accessories

Accessories used during electrosurgery procedures are an integral part of the system.

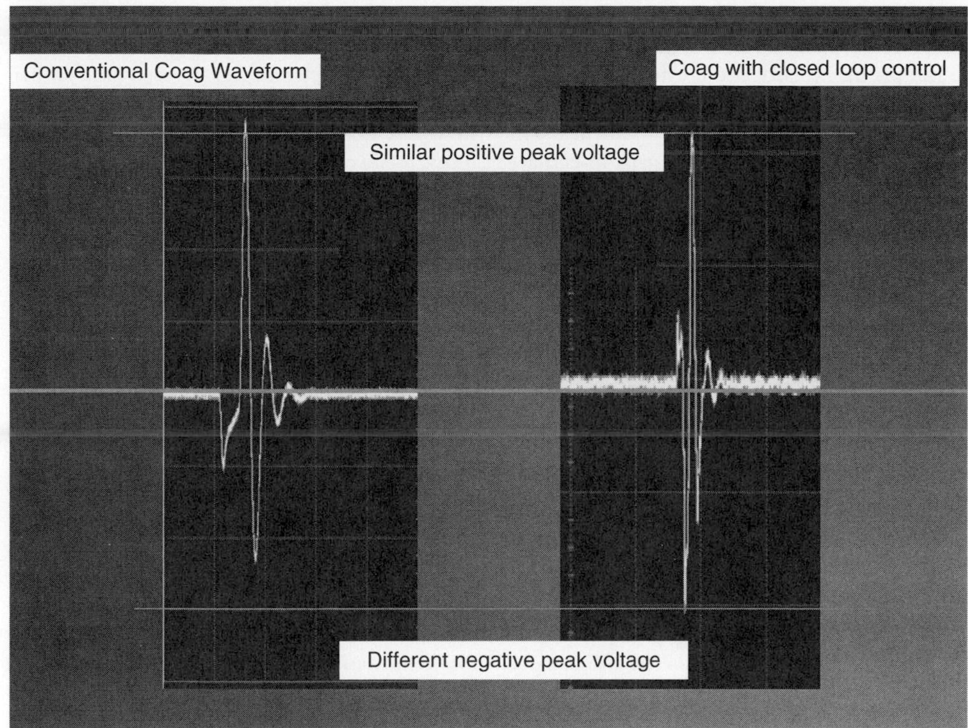

FIGURE 16-3 Closed-loop coagulation waveform compared with conventional coagulation waveform. (Courtesy Covidien, Inc.)

These include many types of active electrodes, holsters, and patient return electrodes.

Active Electrodes

The active electrodes deliver concentrated current to the surgical site. A wide assortment of active electrodes is available for both bipolar and monopolar units. Active electrode pencils or forceps may be hand controlled or controlled by a foot pedal. Pencil tips are available in needles, blades, balls, and loops. Some active electrodes contain a combined suction and coagulation instrument. Active electrode tips are available with an insulated area of the tip to further protect the patient. Coated tips are increasing in use because of the ease of cleaning eschar off the tip with a wet sponge. The advantage of being able to keep the active electrode tip clean is that it will also keep the voltages required to push the electricity out of the tip as low as possible, and lower voltages are always a good idea.

Holsters

Holsters are a vital part of the electrosurgical system. Active electrodes should be placed in holsters that are recommended by the manufacturer when not in use. They should be easily accessible and visible to the surgical team. Holsters are an essential part of the safe operation of the electrosurgical system and one of the least expensive safety mechanisms a hospital can provide. Holsters should meet standards for heat and fire resistance. Pouches and other makeshift holsters that are not intended for use with electrosurgery active electrodes could pose a threat to patient safety because such items will not protect the patient from the inadvertent activation of the active electrode.

Patient Return Electrodes

Patient return electrodes, or grounding pads, remove monopolar current from the patient and return it to the generator. There are many types of return electrodes used, ranging from metal plates to dual section pads. Reusable metal plates—which are not primarily used in the United States—are made of stainless steel and fit under the patient. A gel must be used to make the patient's skin more conductive and to fill any gaps in contact between the plate and the patient's skin. The quality of contact depends on gravity and the amount of gel used. A disposable version of this plate was also developed. It was made of cardboard and covered with foil. Neither plate conforms to body contours, so effectiveness may vary. More importantly, metal/cardboard plates do not have quality contact–monitoring capabilities.

Pregelled water-based foam pads, which are disposable, come in many sizes and shapes. They adhere well to body contours, and an adhesive edge helps hold the pad on the patient. When using gelled water-based pads, care must be taken to store cartons flat to prevent the gel from accumulating on one side of the pad. During use, the dryer side of an improperly stored pad could contribute to an electrosurgical burn. Gelled pads can also dry out during long storage periods, thereby compromising conductivity. When using gelled pads, care must be taken to rotate stock and store cartons properly.

Conductive adhesive pads were developed to replace gel with a layer of adhesive over the pad surface. The adhesive promotes conductivity and good contact with the patient's skin. These pads may be a dry conductive adhesive or a high-moisture conductive adhesive. Both conform well to body contours. This type of pad is also available in the split dual-section design. The split pad design denotes a quality contact–monitoring system.

Placement of the patient return electrode is an important consideration. The pad should be as close to the surgical site as possible, over a large muscle mass. Muscle is a better conductor of electrical current than fatty tissue. By placing the patient return electrode as described, lower power settings can be used on the generator to achieve the desired tissue effect. Scar tissue and any bony structures should also be avoided, because they are more resistant to current flow, and impedance can increase at these sites (Fairchild, 1996).

Manufacturer's Recommendations

It is also important to read and follow manufacturer's recommendations for any device, but particularly when using electrosurgery equipment and accessories. The patient injury that can occur when electrosurgery is used inappropriately makes following prescribed recommendations essential. User's guides and manufacturer's recommendations are legal, binding instructions. Failure to follow recommended uses could constitute negligence should an incident occur.

CONCLUSION

The concept of using heat to stop bleeding goes back thousands of years. Throughout the centuries researchers have constructed a variety of devices that use electricity as a means to heat tissue and control bleeding. Electrosurgery became more widely used in the late 1920s because of the urgent need to safely control bleeding in operative and invasive procedures. The evolution of the equipment has continued throughout its history to the devices of today that take the patient tissues into consideration during energy delivery for hemostasis. Application of safe practices in electrosurgery promote patient safety and minimize potential for untoward patient outcomes (Box 16-1).

BOX 16-1 Electrosurgery Clinical Recommendations

1. Be familiar with technology and patient safety implications.
2. Read and follow manufacturer's directions.
3. Always use the lowest power setting to achieve the desired tissue effect.
4. Apply short activations of power for the desired tissue effect.
5. Keep the electrosurgery active electrode tip clean; this will allow current to be conducted more effectively.
6. Always place the electrosurgery active electrode in nonconductive holster when not in use.
7. Apply patient return electrode appropriately and according to manufacturer's directions.
8. Place patient return electrode as close to surgery site as possible.
9. Avoid placement of the patient return electrode over scar tissue or bony structures.

REFERENCES

Columbia Encyclopedia, ed 6, 2001, Electricity, available at http://www.bartleby.com/65/el/electricity.html. Accessed April 24, 2009.

Eggleston JL, et al: Instant response electrosurgery generator for laparoscopy and endoscopy, *Minim Invasive Ther Allied Technol* 5(6):491–495, 1997.

Fairchild SS: Electrosurgery units. In Fairchild SS, editor: *Perioperative nursing principles and practice*, Boston, 1996, Little Brown.

Goldwyn RM: Bovie: the man and his machine, *Ann Plast Surg* 2(2):135–153, 1979.

Hutchisson B, et al: Electrosurgery safety, *AORN J* 68(5): 830–837, 1998.

Kelly HA, Ward GE: History. In Kelly HA, Ward GE, editors: *Electrosurgery*, Philadelphia, 1932, Saunders.

Massarweh NN, et al: Electrosurgery: history, principles, and current and future uses, *J Am Coll Surg* 202(3):520–530, 2006.

Pearce J: Early experiments with high frequency current. In *Electrosurgery*, London, 1986, Chapman & Hall.

Phippen ML, et al: Provide instruments, equipment and supplies. In *Competency for safe patient care during operative and invasive procedures*, Denver, 2009, CCI.

Propkopakis EP, et al: Tonsillectomy using the ligature vessel sealing system, a preliminary report, *Int J Pediatr Otorhinolaryngol* 69:1183–1186, 2005.

Ulmer BC: Electrosurgery: history and fundamentals, *Perioper Nurs Clin* 2:89–101, 2007a.

Ulmer BC: Electrosurgery mode differentiation. In Ulmer BD, editor: *Electrosurgery self study guide*, Boulder, 2007b, Covidien Energy-based Devices.

Voorhees JR, et al: Battling blood loss in neurosurgery: Harvey Cushing's embrace of electrosurgery, *J Neurosurg* 102:745–752, 2005.

UNIT III • Workplace Safety

WORKPLACE SAFETY ISSUES AND TRENDS

Donna S. Watson, MSN, RN, CNOR, ARNP-BC

Promoting patient safety has always been a fundamental philosophy for the profession of nursing. However, it has not been until the past decade that nurses have voiced their concerns related to issues affecting nurses—specifically, workplace safety issues. Many workplace safety issues that directly affect the nurse also have an indirect effect on patient safety, and the two should never be addressed in isolation from one another (Aiken et al, 2002; Needleman et al, 2002). Nurses today routinely deal with critical issues related to the provision of safe patient care; however, they often do not pay attention to their own workplace safety issues (Foley, 2004).

WORKPLACE SAFETY ISSUES

As a professional group, nurses are extremely dedicated, and most will always place patient needs first. As an example, nurses often volunteer to work extra shifts to provide adequate coverage for patients. The perioperative nurse will decline break and lunch relief when it is not in the best interest of the patient to depart from the case (e.g., critical time of cross clamping of the aorta). Perioperative nurses are required to stand for prolonged periods of time and may put their bodies in awkward positions when retracting with instruments during a surgical case. Daily, perioperative nurses are required to lift heavy equipment and transfer patients, frequently with minimal assistance. Although this list of nursing actions is not intended to be exhaustive, the list demonstrates that the patient's welfare is always placed first. Unfortunately, some of these nursing actions that are required for patient care place the nurse at an increased risk for injury (ANA, 2001b). As previously stated, it is common for nurses to overlook issues of their own well-being and safety to provide patient care. Many people may question the wisdom and the end result of this dedication.

Aging Workforce

It is projected that in 2010 40% of nurses in the United States will be older than 50 years of age (U.S. General Accounting Office, 2001). Research supports that one out of every five nurses will leave nursing prematurely for reasons other than retirement (Federation of Nurses and Health Professionals, 2001). Reasons for leaving the profession prematurely include factors such as fatigue, long work hours, stressors associated with the physical demands of the work, chronic lumbar pain, and personal injury (ANA, 2001b; Federation of Nurses and Health Professionals, 2001; U.S. General Accounting Office, 2001; Foley, 2004). Nurses who are now entering the profession appear less inclined to accept the status quo and expect that workplace issues will be addressed to adequately protect the nurse, which in return better protects the patient.

Nursing Shortage

How the recession will alter the nursing shortage remains unclear. Recent reports suggest that the nursing shortage appears to have decreased related to current economics. Many nurses have elected to delay retirement, resulting in fewer hospital vacancies for the registered nurse (RN) (Calvan, 2009). Despite the fact that there a fewer nursing vacancies, Buerhaus et al (2009) project a shortage of 260,000 RNs by 2025. This is attributed to the aging workforce.

The nursing shortage is not limited to the United States. The International Council of Nurses (ICN) (2006) recognizes a worldwide nursing shortage affecting developing and developed countries. Action plans are similar to those of the United States, with recommendations to address the practice environment for nursing (ICN, 2006).

In 2009 the Canadian Nursing Association recommended addressing environmental issues to decrease absenteeism for Canadian nurses, which is likely an outcome attributed to fatigue and workplace issues (Kyle, 2009). It is also being realized in the United States that workplace issues must be addressed to effectively recruit and retain nurses (Foley, 2004).

Work-Related Injuries

Nursing ranks among one of the highest professions for work-related injuries. Data on nonfatal occupational injuries and illnesses requiring days away from work collected by the U.S. Bureau of Labor Statistics (2008) from 2006 to 2007 identifies the occupation group of RNs as the tenth-highest occupation for work-related injuries. A subset of the nursing group identified as nursing aides, orderlies, and attendants is the third-highest injured group, falling just below the occupations of truck drivers (heavy and tractor-trailer), laborers, and material movers. Data collected from 2006 to 2007 reported a total of 64,950 work days for nursing personnel that were lost because of work-related injuries. The total for nursing aides, orderlies, and attendants was 44,930 days and for RNs, 20,020 days. The highest rate of injuries and illness in nursing occurs with the subset of nursing aides, orderlies, and attendants. The most frequent work-related injury is a musculoskeletal disorder, which occurs more frequently for this subset than for laborers, freight handlers, and delivery truck drivers (Figure 17-1).

Any work-related injury resulting in a day away from work has the potential to negatively affect patient care. When a nurse is off because of a work-related injury, this generally results in decreased staff. In the perioperative area that may result in

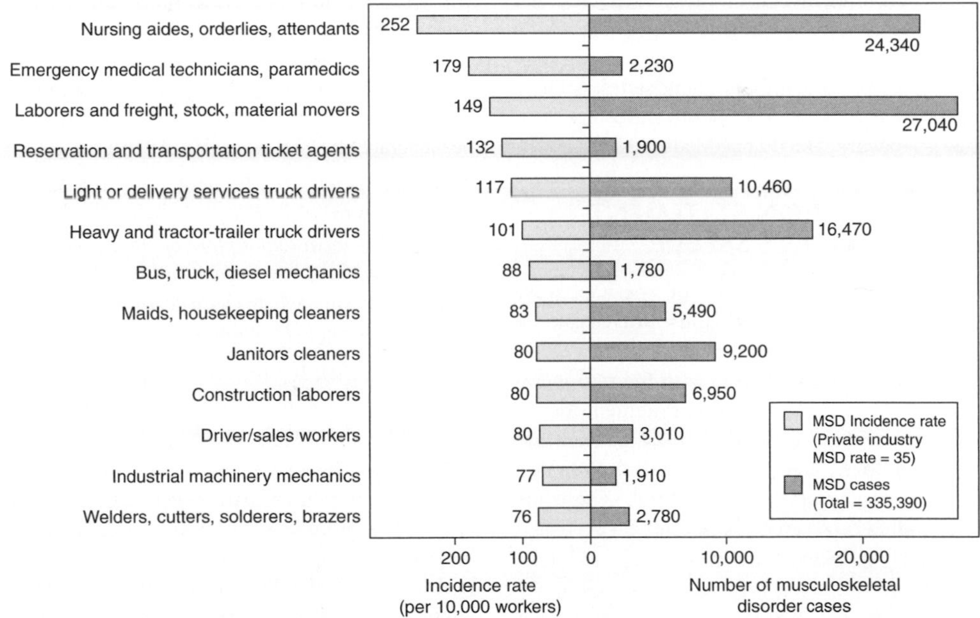

FIGURE 17-1 Incidence rate and number of injuries and illnesses due to musculoskeletal disorders by selected occupations, 2007. (Modified from Bureau of Labor Statistics: *Nonfatal occupational injuries and illness requiring days away from work,* Washington, DC, November, 20, 2008, U.S. Department of Labor Bureau of Labor Statistics, available at http://www.bls.gov/news.release/pdf/osh2.pdf. Accessed July 3, 2009.)

cancellation of cases because of lack of adequate staff, which can negatively affect patient care.

Personal Health and Safety

Today more nurses are cognizant of their personal health risk and are no longer "accepting" the idea of taking risks for personal injury or untoward health effects when there are preventive measures such as equipment that will minimize the risk for the nurse (e.g., smoke evacuation). In 2001 the American Nurses Association (ANA) (2001a) conducted a Health and Safety Survey to evaluate exposure to hazards in the workplace for registered nurses. Across the United States 4826 nurses participated in the survey to report health and safety concerns. Of these nurses, 60% expressed concern related to on-the-job disability resulting from a back injury, 45% were concerned about needlestick injuries and contracting a bloodborne pathogen, and 21% were concerned about developing latex allergies. Health care facilities are becoming more aware of the importance of addressing nursing issues, ensuring that every nurse feels safe, and supplying the necessary equipment and staffing to provide safe patient care. Nursing professionals are becoming more astute and understand that patient safety advocacy begins with advocacy for a safe workplace environment for the nursing staff. Mary Foley, past ANA president, states, "Nurses shouldn't fear for their own health and safety when they go to work" (Medscape Medical News, 2001).

AORN POSITION STATEMENT ON WORKPLACE SAFETY

In 2003 the Association of periOperative Registered Nurses (AORN) House of Delegates in the *AORN Position Statement on Workplace Safety* addressed safety issues specific to the perioperative environment. The position statement identified six categories of workplace safety exposure issues: biologic, ergonomic, chemicals, physical hazards, psychosocial, and cultural. These are detailed here, and several have chapters dedicated to discussing the issues in depth.

Biologic Risk

The first category of workplace exposure is biologic risk, which includes exposure to bloodborne pathogens, infectious agents, biologic components of surgical smoke, and allergens contained in latex products such as surgical gloves. The bloodborne pathogens' risks to health care workers were known for decades. However, no risk-reduction efforts or concerns were set forth until the human immunodeficiency virus (HIV) was described in 1981 (Berguer and Heller, 2004). Currently the pathogens of greatest concern are HIV, hepatitis B virus (HBV), and hepatitis C virus (HCV) (Centers for Disease Control and Prevention [CDC], 2003). In 1987 the Centers for Disease Control and Prevention (CDC, 1987) released the universal precautions for use on every patient, by all persons, all of the time.

The complex issues related to bloodborne pathogen exposures, especially in the operating room environment with needlestick injuries and other sharps-related injuries, continue to be a potential hazard. In 1991 the Occupational Safety and Health Administration (OSHA) issued the bloodborne pathogens standard (29 CFR 1910.1030) designed to protect health care workers at risk. The bloodborne pathogens standard has undergone revision based on new evidence for prevention and is expected to be implemented by each facility. The bloodborne pathogens standard required facilities to implement an exposure-control plan, compliance with the universal precautions, engineering controls, barrier protection, free HBV vaccinations, education and training programs, and postexposure evaluation (OSHA, 1991). This is enforced through the OSH Act of 1970, often referred to as the General Duty Clause (OSHA, 1970):

> *Section 5(a)(1) of the OSH Act, requires the employers to "furnish to each of his employees employment and a place of employment which are free from recognized hazards that are causing or likely to cause death or serious physical harm to his employees."*
>
> *Section 5(a)(2) requires employers to "comply with occupational safety and health standards promulgated under this Act."*

Even with the CDC's recommended standard precautions and the regulation behind the OSHA's bloodborne pathogens standard to decrease risk, the risk in the operating room remains evident. Quebbeman et al (1991) report that untoward outcomes for staff include cuts or needlestick injuries in approximately 15% of operations studied. Gerberding et al (1990) report accidental exposure (parenteral or cutaneous) of 6.4%. If study results are applied across the more than 50 million surgical procedures performed annually in the

United States, the adequacy of protection for health care personnel in the operating room environment must be questioned. Many suggest that even with the application of standard precautions and the OSHA bloodborne pathogens standard there remains the inability to fully understand and address the many issues surrounding bloodborne pathogen exposure in the complex operating room environment (Berguer and Heller, 2004). Chapter 19 reviews the issues and recommendations for prevention of sharps injuries in the operating room.

Ergonomics

The second category of workplace safety exposure is ergonomics. This includes static or awkward positions, standing for prolonged periods of time, back injuries, repetitive motion, lifting of heavy patients, and transportation of heavy equipment (AORN, 2006). Perioperative scrub persons and first assistants are frequently required to stand in awkward positions at the surgical field. It is not unusual to remain in an awkward position (e.g., holding instruments) for prolonged periods of time. Staff members who are "scrubbed in" on long cases and relieved by someone else only for mandatory breaks and lunch may complain of lumbar strain, aches, discomfort, and extreme muscle fatigue.

In addition to the above workplace ergonomics, there are issues related to patient transfer, patient positioning, holding extremities for the surgical preparation, and transferring the patient following surgery. The trend of implementing lift teams and using special equipment for moving and positioning patients has been minimally implemented in the surgical services area. Chapter 21 reviews the issues and challenges of preventing back injuries in the perioperative staff, with emphasis on the unique job requirements of the operating room.

Chemical Exposure

The third category of workplace safety exposure is chemical and associated with anesthesia gases, disinfecting/sterilizing agents, cleaning agents, and specimen preservatives (AORN, 2003). There is long-standing concern related to exposure to waste anesthetic gases and the potential for negative effects on health care workers. Waste anesthetic gases expose health care workers to volatile gases, generally in small amounts, as a result of leakage from the anesthesia breathing circuit into the operating room air (National Institute for Occupational Safety and Health [NIOSH], 2007). Waste anesthetic gas exposure may include exposure to halothane, enflurane, isoflurane, desflurane, sevoflurane, and nitrous oxide. There are studies that demonstrate adverse health effects from chronic exposure. Some studies link exposure to the occurrence of miscarriages, genetic disorders, and cancer (NIOSH, 2007).

The National Institute for Occupational Safety and Health (NIOSH) (2007) recommends that health care facilities develop a hazard communication program that includes a safety plan related to exposure, methods to minimize and control exposure, labeling of cylinders with anesthetic agents, availability of material safety data sheets (MSDSs), provision of training and education for health care workers as required by the OSHA hazard communication standard (20 CFR 1910.1200), and installation of a waste scavenging system to remove anesthetic gases in the perioperative area.

NIOSH recommends specific ventilation exchanges to minimize exposure to waste anesthetic gases that are routinely exhaled by the patient. NIOSH (2007) recommendations include a facility ventilation system for the operating room that should provide 15 air exchanges per hour, with a minimum of 3 air changes of fresh air hourly. The ventilation system for the postanesthesia recovery area should provide at least 6 air changes per hour, with at least 2 air changes of fresh air hourly (NIOSH, 2007).

The anesthetic equipment should be maintained, including the breathing circuits and the waste-gas scavenging systems. Staff should be educated and trained in awareness, prevention, and control recommendations related to minimizing exposure to waste anesthetic gases. Recommendations from NIOSH (2007) for operating room personnel and anesthesia providers include the following:

- Periodically monitor staff liver and kidney function.
- Monitor pregnancy outcomes for female workers and wives of male workers.
- Inspect anesthesia delivery system for any interruptions.
- Confirm that the ventilation system is working properly.
- Confirm that the waste scavenging system has been properly applied and is working correctly.

- Gas flow should be activated after the delivery system is connected to the laryngeal mask or endotracheal tube.
- Vaporizers should be filled using a ceiling-mounted hood with working evacuation system.
- Vaporizers should not be filled during delivery of anesthesia.
- Uncuffed endotracheal tube should have a completely sealed airway.
- Administer the lowest possible anesthetic gas flow rate.
- Avoid high anesthetic gas flow rates.
- Avoid anesthesia delivery via open drop methods.
- If a mask is applied, it should fit correctly.
- Apply waste scavenging system to eliminate residual gases before disconnecting from the breathing circuit.
- Stop gases by turning the valve off before disconnecting the patient's breathing system.

Concern about health care worker exposure to disinfecting/sterilizing agents, cleaning agents, and specimen preservatives requires the facility to provide a safe working environment for the health care worker. The OSHA hazard communication standard [20 CFR 1910.1200] not only applies to anesthetic agents, it also applies to any hazardous material (e.g., disinfecting/sterilizing agents, cleaning agents, and specimen preservatives). The standard requires that a facility develop and train on the hazard communication program, which includes a safety plan related to exposure, methods to minimize and control exposure, safety requirements, labeling instruction, availability of material safety data sheets, and provision of training and education to health care workers. The facility is required to supply the employee with the appropriate protective apparel based on the respective agent (e.g., goggles, face shields, specific gloves, mask, gown, jumpsuit, apron) (NIOSH, 2007). In addition, manufacturer's directions should be reviewed and followed for storage, transportation, staff safety precautions, and disposal.

Physical Hazards

The fourth category, physical hazards, addresses workplace risks associated with fire, electricity, radiation, lasers, smoke plume, and compressed gases (AORN, 2003). Surgical fires, although preventable, continue to occur at an alarming rate of 550 to 660 per year. In the event of a surgical fire, the surgical team is at risk and should be knowledgeable about the components of the fire triangle and preventive measures to ensure both patient and staff safety. Fire prevention and safety is discussed in Chapter 6. Electrosurgery safety precautions are discussed in Chapter 16. The issue of chronic exposure to surgical smoke has been ongoing for the past three decades. Unfortunately, there are many facilities that do not implement practices of smoke evacuation to protect staff from chronic exposure. Perioperative nurses are concerned about the health effects of chronic exposure and are the strongest advocates for the use of smoke evacuators. Chapter 18 reviews current evidence with recommendations for surgical smoke evacuation. Radiation safety is an area that is an important workplace safety concern. Chapter 23 provides education and preventive measures specific for the perioperative team. The remaining item in this fourth category, which is included in Chapter 20, involves laser risk and safety measures for the perioperative team.

Psychosocial Risks

The fifth category of workplace risks is the psychosocial. The psychosocial aspects for the perioperative team members include long hours, mandatory overtime, demographic diversity, nursing shortage, on-call requirements, trauma, burnout, verbal and physical abuse, and violence from staff, patients, patients' families, or nurses' families (AORN, 2003). Each issue is complex and can directly affect the quality of patient care delivered. For example, one solution facilities have implemented to provide adequate patient care coverage is mandatory overtime. Perioperative nurses and their colleagues on other units may be required to work more than 12-hour shifts and may work more than 60 hours per week. The outcome is an extremely fatigued nurse or perioperative team member providing care to a patient. Because of fatigue, the nurse can make poor patient care decisions that may negatively affect the patient (Study shows 12-hour shifts increase errors, 2004).

Symptoms of fatigue are described as "increased anxiety, decreased short term memory, slowed reaction time, decreased work efficiency, reduced motivational drive, decreased vigilance, increased variability in work performance, [and] increased errors of omission which increase to commission when time pressure is added to the task" (Battelle Memorial Institute, 1998). The symptoms of fatigue have been identified as being equivalent to or even greater than impairment from alcohol intoxication. Dawson and Reid (1997) studied performance impairment as a result of fatigue compared with performance impairment resulting from alcohol intoxication. Results revealed that following 17 hours of wakefulness the performance level decreased to a level of performance equal to a blood alcohol concentration (BAC) of 0.05%. Performance after sustained wakefulness at 24 hours was equal to a BAC of 0.10%. The mean relative performance between the tenth and twenty-sixth hours decreased on average by 0.74% per hour.

As a result of increasing awareness of fatigue and the implications for impairment of performance, the AORN House of Delegates in 2005 passed the *Guidance Statement on Safe/On-Call Practices*. The strategies are listed in Box 17-1. Most facilities recognize that fatigue related to

BOX 17-1 AORN Position Statement on Safe Work/On-Call Recommended Strategies

Recognizing the potential negative consequences of sleep deprivation and sustained work hours and further recognizing that adequate rest and recuperation periods are essential to patient and perioperative personnel safety, AORN suggests the following strategies.

- Perioperative registered nurses should not be required to work in direct patient care for more than 12 consecutive hours in a 24-hour period and not more than 60 hours in a seven-day period. Sufficient transition time is required for appropriate patient handoff and staff relief. Under extreme conditions exceptions to the 12-hour limit may be required (e.g., disasters). Organization policy should outline exceptions to the 12-hour limitation. All worked hours (i.e., regular hours and call hours worked) should be included in calculating total hours worked (Rosekind et al, 1997; Gaba and Howard, 2002; Page, 2004a).
- Off-duty periods should be inclusive of an uninterrupted eight-hour sleep cycle, a break from continuous professional responsibilities, and time to perform individual activities of daily living (Dinges et al, 1996; Page, 2004b; Rogers et al, 2004).
- Arrangements should be made, in relation to the hours worked, to relieve a perioperative registered nurse who has worked on-call during his or her off shift and who is scheduled to work the following shift to accommodate an adequate off-duty recuperation period.
- The number of on-call shifts assigned in a seven-day period depends on the type of facility and should be coordinated with the number of sustained work hours and adequate recuperation periods mentioned above.
- An individual's ability to meet the anticipated work demand should be considered for on-call requirements. Limited research indicates older people are more likely than younger people to be adversely affected by sleep deprivation; however, there is no research specific to the effects of on-call assignment and a person's age.
- Orientation to on-call should be included in the orientation process and should be accomplished using the preceptor system (i.e., having an experienced nurse serve as an immediate resource for the orientee). The time frame depends on the type of procedures and the scope of services.
- Perioperative registered nurses should uphold their ethical responsibility to patients and themselves to arrive at work adequately rested and prepared for duty (Gaba and Howard, 2002; AORN, 2004).
- Health care organizations should support perioperative RNs in changing cultural attitudes so that fatigue is recognized as an unacceptable risk to patient and worker safety rather than a sign of a worker's dedication to the job (Gaba and Howard, 2002).

AORN, Association of periOperative Registered Nurses; *RN*, registered nurse.

From Association of periOperative Registered Nurses: AORN position statement on safe work/on-call practices, April 2005, available at http://www.aorn.org/PracticeResources/AORNPositionStatements/Position_SafeWork OnCallPractices/. Accessed July 11, 2009.

sleep deprivation impairs performance with the potential negative effect on patient safety. As a result, creative solutions to staffing patterns have been developed that include splitting of weekend call, providing time off when staff approach a 60-hour work week, and providing a second call team as back-up (Kenyon et al, 2007).

Cultural Issues

The sixth category in workplace safety is that of cultural issues. These include the ongoing issue of nursing staff tolerance of abusive behavior from physician and nursing colleagues; poor management support for an optimal workplace safety program; lack or absence of respect from colleagues, including members of the perioperative team and other associated health care professionals; and lack of a code of conduct endorsed by all team members (AORN, 2003). Chapter 25 discusses strategies for dealing with disruptive behavior, and Chapter 27 discusses recommendations for implementing and establishing a culture of safety.

STRATEGY TO IMPROVE SAFETY

Hierarchy of Controls

The challenge for health care facilities is to acknowledge the many issues related to workplace safety and implement strategies that address and minimize workplace hazards. One strategy that has been successfully implemented is the "hierarchy of controls." Colleagues such as occupational health nurses, occupational physicians, industrial hygienists, and safety engineers have applied the framework referred to as the hierarchy of controls as a means of addressing and attempting to solve hazards in the workplace. De Castro (2003) and Foley (2004) have reviewed application of the hierarchy of controls as a methodology to reduce workplace safety risk. De Castro (2003) identifies the control measures in decreasing order of effectiveness: elimination of hazards, substitution controls, engineering controls, administrative controls, work practice controls, and personal protective equipment (Figure 17-2).

Elimination and Substitution Controls

Elimination and substitution are considered to be the most effective approach for intervention and risk reduction. Elimination involves "complete removal of a hazard from the work area" (de Castro, 2003). One example is the removal of latex products from the facility in an effort to go "latex-free." This method is highly effective because, in the case of removing all latex products from a facility, it removes the risk from the practice setting. Substitution is "replacing a conventional material or process with a less harmful alternative" (de Castro, 2003). An example is substituting a product that may cause dermatitis to the staff for an equally effective product that is less likely to result in dermatitis (e.g., surgical gloves).

Engineering Controls

Engineering controls "remove or isolate a hazard through technology" (de Castro, 2003). The goal

Most Effective

Elimination of Hazards: Remove all unnecessary needles, scalpels, sharps, and sharp instrumentation from the surgical field.

Substitution Controls: Remove latex products and replace with latex-free products in an effort to go latex free.

Engineering Controls: Examples include double-glove technique, blunt-tip suture needles, and safety scalpels.

Administrative Controls: Develop policies for reducing risk to perioperative team members.

Work Practice Controls: Use hands-free technique, neutral zone, and double-glove technique.

Personal Protection Equipment: Wear goggles, eye shields, mask, and gloves.

Least Effective

FIGURE 17-2 Reducing hazards in the workplace according to the hierarchy of controls.

of engineering controls is that, if the risk cannot be removed, some form of protection through the use of technology should be used to decrease the risk to the health care worker. An example is the use of puncture-resistant containers in the operating room environment. In surgery it is not feasible to remove all needles, sutures, scalpels, sharps, and sharp invasive medical devices. Therefore it is recommended that these be passed in a "safe zone" and then disposed of in a puncture-resistant container that should be used by the perioperative staff.

Administrative Controls

Administrative controls involve development and implementation of policies and procedures. The policies are aimed at "limiting worker exposure to a hazard, typically accomplished through work assignment" (de Castro, 2003). For example, to prevent excessive radiation exposure, staff are required to wear appropriate attire, use shielding, and maintain distance from the source.

Work Practice Controls

Work practice controls "reduce exposure to occupational hazards through the behavior of workers" (de Castro, 2003). Policies and procedures should be developed to protect the health care worker, such as mandating gloves when working with body fluids or blood or banning recapping of contaminated needles. However, in the operating room banning recapping of needles can be difficult to enforce, especially with anesthesia providers. In this situation education is essential.

Personal Protective Equipment

Personal protective equipment (PPE) is considered to be the least effective measure and is implemented provided the risk cannot be decreased by the other controls. PPE includes the use of barrier type of protections such as goggles, eye shields, gowns, gloves, and mask. The effectiveness of PPE depends on its quality, the application of each item, and whether it is user efficient. For example, a regular surgical mask will offer little protection to the health care worker against surgical smoke exposure.

The use and implementation of the hierarchy of controls is one method of reducing risk of workplace safety hazards. The perioperative team should be knowledgeable of these risk-reduction strategies and take appropriate measures for prevention of injuries.

CONCLUSION

In the United States there are approximately 2.9 million licensed RNs, representing the largest group of health care professionals (Health Resources and Services Administration [HRSA], 2004). It is estimated that over 83% are employed in nursing (HRSA, 2004). Despite a recession, employment and career opportunities in health care have continued to increase, with gains of approximately 21,000 new job opportunities per month for 2009 (BLS, 2009). The prospects of a nursing career are excellent. It is anticipated that the nursing shortage will intensify because fewer are entering into nursing and many nurses are baby boomers and will likely retire in the near future (Buerhaus et al, 2009). This makes it imperative that these issues of workplace safety be addressed both for nurses currently in practice and for future nurses.

Focusing on a healthy workplace environment is the responsibility of every perioperative nurse. The promotion and development of a culture that addresses workplace safety is most effective when it is multidisciplinary. The multidisciplinary team should address each workplace safety issue with the premise of patient safety and the implication of care provided. If nurses do not push the agenda of workplace safety for nursing and our perioperative team, no one else will do this for us. To achieve this goal, the culture of many facilities will need to change to recruit and retain nursing professionals. One example is the use of lift teams and equipment in the operating room for patient transfer and positioning. The use of lift teams and special lift equipment may be the normal standard for many institutions, with housewide implementation. However, implementation is often forgotten or ignored in the operating room. The perioperative staff is at very high risk for injuries and must not be forgotten when workplace issues are addressed.

The average age of the registered nurse is 46.8 years, and it is well known that the nursing shortage is anticipated to intensify (HRSA, 2004). Mentoring new nurses and listening to their suggestions will enhance the workplace environment for improved retention and recruitment efforts.

To improve the workplace environment, old attitudes must change, including those such as "that's the way it is always done." Nurses and managers need to look at new and better ways to deliver care that promote safety for the patient as well as for the nurse.

The profession of nursing has the largest representation for a medical group of professionals in the United States. Collectively that makes for one strong voice to influence the political process, the legislative process at state and national levels, and the regulatory agencies. Nurses should voice their concerns and bring issues to the attention of administrations, managers, and those in public office. Lastly, every nurse must work on his or her personal health, well-being, and safety. Nursing is a highly stressful environment, and nurses must learn to provide to themselves the same preventive care and measures provided to their patients.

REFERENCES

Aiken LH, et al: Hospital nurse staffing and patient mortality, nurse burnout and job dissatisfaction, *JAMA* 288(16): 1987–1993, 2002.

American Nurses Association: Health and safety survey, *Nurs World*, September 2001a, available at http://www.nursingworld.org/MainMenuCategories/OccupationalandEnvironmental/occupationalhealth/HealthSafetySurvey.aspx. Accessed July 19, 2009.

American Nurses Association: Hearing on ergonomic safety in the workplace, *Nurs World*, July 20, 2001b, available at http://www.nursingworld.org/MainMenuCategories/OccupationalandEnvironmental/occupationalhealth/handlewithcare/Resources/HearingonErgonomicsSafety.aspx. Accessed August 18, 2009.

Association of periOperative Registered Nurses: AORN Position Statement: Ergonomically Healthy Workplace Practices, *AORN J* 83(1):119–122, 2006.

Association of periOperative Registered Nurses: Explications for perioperative nursing. In *Standards, recommended practices, and guidelines*, Denver, 2004, The Association.

Association of periOperative Registered Nurses: AORN position statement on safe/on-call practices, *AORN J* 81(5):1054–1057, 2005.

Association of periOperative Registered Nurses: Delegates try new key pad voting system, listen to task force reports, and vote on workplace safety statement, *AORN J* 77(6): 1108–1109, 2003.

Battelle Memorial Institute: *An overview of the scientific literature concerning fatigue, sleep, and the circadian cycle*, Federal Aviation Administration,January 1998, available at http://cf.alpa.org/internet/projects/ftdt/backgr/batelle.htm Accessed July 12, 2009.

Berguer R, Heller PJ: Preventing sharps injuries in the operating room, *J Am Coll Surg* 199(3):462–467, 2004.

Buerhaus P, et al: The recent surge in nurse employment: causes and implications, *Health Aff* 20(1):s657–w668, 2009, available at http://content.healthaffairs.org/cgi/content/abstract/hlthaff.28.4.w657. Accessed August 18, 2009.

Bureau of Labor Statistics: *Nonfatal occupational injuries and illness requiring days away from work*, U.S. Department of Labor Bureau of Labor Statistics, November 20 2008, available at http://www.bls.gov/news.release/pdf/osh2.pdf. Accessed July 3, 2009.

Bureau of Labor Statistics: *The employment situation: June 2009*, U.S. Department of Labor Bureau of Labor Statistics. July 2 2009, available at http://www.bls.gov/news.release/empsit.nr0.htm. Accessed July 3, 2009.

Calvan B: Recession forestalls anticipated nursing shortage, *Miami Herald*, August 17 2009, available at http://www.miamiherald.com/business/story/1188410.html. Accessed August 18, 2009.

Centers for Disease Control and Prevention: Recommendations for prevention of HIV transmission in health-care settings, *MMWR* 36(Suppl 2S):1, 1987.

Centers for Disease Control and Prevention: *Exposure to blood: what healthcare personnel need to know*, July 2003, available at http://www.cdc.gov/ncidod/dhqp/pdf/bbp/Exp_to_Blood.pdf. Accessed July 4, 2009.

Dawson D, Reid K: Fatigue, alcohol and performance impairment, *Nature* 388(6639):235, 1997.

de Castro AB: "Hierarchy of controls" providing a framework for addressing workplace hazards, *Am J Nurs* 103(12):104, 2003, available at http://www.nursingworld.org/DocumentVault/AJN/2003/AJNWorkplaceHazards.aspx. Accessed July 12, 2009.

Dinges DF, et al: *Principles and guidelines for duty and rest scheduling in commercial aviation*, (NASA Technical Memorandum 110404).Moffett Field, California, 1996, NASA Ames Research Center.

Federation of Nurses and Health Professionals: *The nurse shortage: perspectives from current direct care nurses and former direct care nurses*, April 2001, available at http://www.aft.org/pubs-reports/healthcare/Hart_Report.pdf. Accessed August 18, 2009.

Foley M: Caring for those who care: a tribute to nurses and their safety, *Online J Issues Nurs* 9(3):September 30, 2004. Manuscript 1, available at http://www.nursingworld.org/MainMenuCategories/ANAMarketplace/ANAPeriodicals/OJIN/JournalTopics/NurseSafety.aspx. Accessed July 12, 2009.

Gaba DM, Howard SK: Patient safety: fatigue among clinicians and the safety of patients, *N Engl J Med* 347(16):1249–1255, 2002.

Gerberding JL, et al: Risk of exposure of surgical personnel to patients' blood during surgery at San Francisco General Hospital, *N Engl J Med* 322:1788–1793, 1990.

Health Resources and Services Administration: *The registered nurse population: findings from the 2004 national sample survey of registered nurses*, U.S. Department of Health and Human Services, 2004, Washington, DC, available at http://bhpr.hrsa.gov/healthworkforce/rnsurvey04/. Accessed July 3, 2009.

International Council of Nurses: *Priorities to address global nursing shortages*, March 29 2006, available at http://www.icn.ch/PR04_06.htm. Accessed August 18, 2009.

Kenyon TG, et al: On call: alert or unsafe? On-call electronic task force, *AORN J* 86(4):630–639, 2007.

Kyle A: Report predicts nursing shortage will continue to grow, *Leader-Post* May 11, 2009, available at http://www.leaderpost.com/health/Report+predicts+nursing+shortage+will+continue+grow/1585852/story.html. Accessed July 2, 2009.

Medscape Medical News: Nurses say health and safety concerns play major role in employment decision, *Medscape Medical News* 2001, available at http://www.medscape.com/viewarticle/411358. Accessed August 18, 2009.

National Institute for Occupational Safety and Health: *Waste anesthetic gases—occupational hazards in hospitals*, Washington, 2007, The Institute, available at http://www.cdc.gov/niosh/docs/2007-151/. Accessed July 11, 2009.

Needleman J, et al: Nurse staffing levels and quality of care in hospitals, *N Engl J Med* 346(22):1715–1722, 2002.

Occupational Safety and Health Administration: OSH Act of 1970, available at http://www.osha.gov/pls/oshaweb/owadisp.show_document?p_table=OSHACT&p_id=3359December 29 1970. Accessed August 18, 2009.

Occupational Safety and Health Administration: *Bloodborne pathogens*, December 6 1991. Standard number 1910.1030, available at http://www.osha.gov/pls/oshaweb/owadisp.show_document?p_table=STANDARDS&p_id=10051. Accessed August 18, 2009.

Page A: Work and workspace design to prevent and mitigate errors. In *Keeping patients safe: transforming the work environment of nurses*, Washington, 2004a, Academies Press.

Page A: Work hour regulation in safety-sensitive industries. In *Keeping patients safe: transforming the work environment of nurses*, Washington, 2004b, National Academies Press.

Quebbeman EJ, et al: Risk of blood contamination and injury to operating room personnel, *Ann Surg* 214(5):614–620, 1991.

Rogers AE, et al: The working hours of hospital staff nurses and patient safety, *Health Aff (Millwood)* 23(4):202–212, 2004.

Rosekind MR, et al: Managing fatigue in operational settings 2: an integrated approach, *Hosp Top* 75(3):31–35, 1997.

Study shows 12-hour shifts increase errors, *Healthc Benchmarks Qual Improv* 11:105–106, 2004.

U.S. General Accounting Office: In *Nursing workforce: emerging nurse shortages due to multiple factors*, Report to the Chairman, Subcommittee on Health, Committee on Ways and Means, House of Representatives, July 2001 No. GAO-01-944.

HAZARDS FROM SURGICAL SMOKE

Decreasing Your Risk

Kay A. Ball, PhD, RN, CNOR, FAAN

The general population has been concerned about the inhalation of contaminated air for years. The harmful toxins from tobacco smoke, the toxic gases from artificial turf, the air pollution in confined areas such as airplane cabins, and the airborne debris from fires have all made the headlines in local and national newspapers and reports. Clean air is necessary for good health and longer lives (Maugh, 2009), but attention has not been focused on the air quality behind the closed doors of surgery. Erin Anderson (2005) once stated, "In hindsight, will health care professionals be embarrassed about their cavalier attitudes toward surgical smoke as they once were with cigarette smoke?"

Research has demonstrated that over 500,000 health care workers are exposed to the hazards of surgical smoke (Barrett and Garber, 2004). Even though evidence-based smoke evacuation recommendations have been widely publicized, compliance by perioperative nurses and other surgical team members is still not consistent (Edwards and Reiman, 2008; Ball, 2009). Perioperative nurses have reported an increased incidence of respiratory problems when compared with the general population (Ball, 2009). This alarming information could be the result of breathing in surgical smoke for years in the operating room. Some of the health conditions associated with surgical smoke include those listed in Box 18-1 (Alp et al, 2006).

This chapter will review the hazards of surgical smoke, discuss the recommendations for smoke evacuation practices, describe different smoke evacuation methods, and provide information about compliance in the elimination of all surgical smoke.

HAZARDS OF SURGICAL SMOKE

When hot tools, such as electrosurgical energy or laser beams, impact tissue, heat is created that causes the cells to explode and cellular contents to be released into the air. This debris, consisting of water and particles, is known as surgical smoke or plume. There are few differences between electrosurgery and laser-generated plume. A classic study published in 1989 by Tomita et al compared the hazards of surgical smoke to those of cigarette smoke. When they used a CO_2 laser to vaporize 1 g of tissue, the effect of breathing in the resultant plume was compared with the hazard potential of smoking three unfiltered cigarettes. When electrosurgery was used to vaporize tissue, the results compared the smoke inhalation hazards with those of smoking six unfiltered cigarettes (Tomita et al, 1989). This research demonstrates that electrosurgery plume may be more hazardous than laser smoke, but actually both types of smoke are very similar and can cause identical inhalation hazards (Tomita et al, 1989).

Even though research findings suggest that there may be differences between laser plume and electrosurgery smoke, both types of surgical smoke should be treated the same and properly evacuated (Bigony, 2007). Reports show that plume is more consistently evacuated during laser surgery (Edwards and Reiman, 2008). The appropriate evacuation of plume generated during electrosurgery procedures continues to be inconsistent and lacking (Ball, 2009).

The hazards of surgical smoke can be grouped into four categories: the odor, the particulate matter size, the potential for transmission of viable organisms, and the challenges with laparoscopic plume.

Odor of Surgical Smoke

When surgical smoke is generated, an awful, offensive odor is produced by the inorganic and organic compounds that are created. Inorganic compounds, such as carbon monoxide, carbon dioxide,

BOX 18-1 Conditions Caused by Surgical Smoke

Acute and chronic inflammatory respiratory problems
- Emphysema
- Asthma
- Chronic bronchitis

Anemia
Anxiety
Cancer
Cardiovascular problems
Dermatitis
Eye irritation, lacrimation
Headaches, light-headedness
Hypoxia, dizziness
Nasopharyngeal lesions
Nausea, vomiting
Sneezing
Throat irritation
Weakness
Fatigue

sulfur, and nitrogen, can lead to hypoxia if inhaled. Organic compounds, such as acrolein, benzene, and polycyclic and aromatic hydrocarbons, can lead to nausea, headaches, and fatigue. The odor is from the combination of these toxic gases that are found in trace amounts in the plume; however, the cumulative effect makes surgical smoke an inhalation hazard. Some of these toxic gases, such as benzene and formaldehyde, are also known carcinogens, so continual inhalation of these gases must be avoided (Ball, 2007; Ulmer, 2008).

The Centers for Disease Control and Prevention (CDC) (2006) has warned health care professionals that the toxic gases produced within surgical smoke can cause eye irritation. Providers wearing contact lenses may have difficulty if exposed to a lot of surgical smoke; therefore adequate smoke evacuation practices must be in place.

Size of Particulate Matter

The size of the particles within surgical smoke has been shown to be extremely small. Mihashi et al (1981) found that 77% of the particles in smoke are less than 1.1 μm in size. If inhaled, these particles can be carried to the bronchioles and alveoli of the lungs, where they can cause respiratory problems (Taravella et al, 2001). The mean particle size of smoke particulate produced by electrosurgical energy is approximately 0.07 μm in size, whereas laser plume particulate is approximately 0.31 μm in size (Bigony, 2007; Ulmer, 2008).

Baggish et al (1988) conducted research involving laboratory rats inhaling surgical smoke with and without the use of a smoke evacuator to filter the plume. The rats breathing in filtered plume had no lung changes, whereas the rats inhaling surgical smoke that was not filtered by a smoke evacuator developed hypoxia and other respiratory problems. This research demonstrated that smoke evacuation systems are effective if used properly.

Many surgical team members today have reported respiratory problems that may be connected to the inhalation of surgical smoke (Ball, 2009). Latex allergies and sensitivities have often been associated with repeated exposure to latex. In much the same way, allergies or respiratory conditions may be attributed to the continual exposure to surgical smoke.

Potential Viability

Of great concern is the potential for the transmission of viable organisms within surgical smoke. Garden et al (2002) conducted a classic research study on the probability of transmission of viable particulate during laser surgery. Laser energy was used to vaporize lesions on a cow. In the surgical smoke, intact DNA for bovine papilloma virus was identified. This intact DNA was then injected into another area of the cow, which led to the growth of more viral lesions. The cow was injected with the infective particulate; the cow did not inhale it. Results note that there is a high potential for the transmission of viable organisms within surgical smoke. Other studies have been conducted that have demonstrated similar results (Sawchuck et al, 1989; Bigony, 2007).

There are many anecdotal stories related today about health care professionals contracting a disease similar to that of their patients. Surgical smoke has been implicated as the carrier that can potentially transmit disease from the patient to the provider. Hallmo and Naess (1991) reported that a 44-year-old surgeon in Norway became hoarse after years of inhaling surgical smoke from the vaporization of condyloma. When biopsies of the surgeon's lesions were performed, examination revealed the presence of the same DNA strain as is found in anogenital warts, not normally found in the throat. The theory is that surgical smoke that is not evacuated can spread disease to another host.

Laparoscopic Plume

When a laparoscopic procedure is performed using a hot tool, such as the laser or electrosurgery device, surgical smoke is created within the abdominal cavity. Visibility is obscured, making the surgery difficult and sometimes unsafe to perform. When the smoke is directly evacuated, the CO_2 gas pressure is decreased and the pneumoperitoneum that is needed for proper visualization is compromised. Performing a laparoscopic procedure requires the delicate balance between smoke evacuation and insufflation to maintain the pneumoperitoneum.

Ott et al (1997) performed a research study to determine the reason for postoperative laparoscopic patients' complaints of headaches, nausea, or vision problems. When surgical smoke was not evacuated during the laparoscopy, the patients with untoward symptoms also had an increase in blood methemoglobin and carboxyhemoglobin. When these elements increase, the oxygen-carrying capabilities of the patient's red blood cells decrease, leading to symptoms of nausea, headaches, and visual problems. When the surgical smoke is properly evacuated during laparoscopy, the patient does not complain of these symptoms postoperatively and an increase in methemoglobin or carboxyhemoglobin is not detected. Therefore, to prevent the patient from absorbing the byproducts of combustion during laser or electrosurgery, proper smoke evacuation methods must be employed.

SMOKE EVACUATION RECOMMENDATIONS

Many research studies and papers have been published about the hazards of surgical smoke. Because of this increased attention, standards and recommendations have been written to provide guidelines on proper smoke evacuation practices. In existing policies, verbiage has been changed from "should" (meaning smoke evacuation is recommended) to "shall" (meaning that smoke evacuation is more highly recommended) to "must" (meaning that smoke evacuation is required or consequences may be employed). Many organizations and agencies have addressed the hazards of surgical smoke and have written recommendations that can be referenced to provide appropriate smoke evacuation practices.

The Association of periOperative Registered Nurses (AORN) (2009) has addressed the need for smoke evacuation in four different recommended practices: the recommended practices on laser, electrosurgery, endoscopic minimally invasive surgery, and safe environment of care. The recommendations are easy to read, understand, and follow and offer guidance and reference for the creation of hospital or surgery center policies and procedures. A sample smoke evacuation policy is provided in Box 18-2.

In March 2008 the AORN House of Delegates ratified the *AORN Position Statement on Surgical Smoke and Bio-aerosols.* This statement acknowledges the documented hazards of surgical smoke and describes acceptable smoke evacuation practices. In 2009 the AORN *Surgical Smoke Evacuation Tool Kit* was introduced. This unique tool kit can be downloaded for free by AORN members at http://www.aorn.org/PracticeResources/ToolKits/SurgicalSmokeEvacuationToolKit. This tool kit provides a PowerPoint presentation, practice reminder signs for the evacuation of all surgical smoke, a sample policy, a sample skills checklist, a comprehensive bibliography, and links to vendors selling smoke evacuation equipment and supplies.

The Occupational and Safety Health Administration (OSHA) mandates under the General Duty Clause that an employer must provide a safe workplace environment for all workers. Therefore, if an employee is forced to work in an environment contaminated with surgical smoke because smoke evacuation equipment and supplies are not available, an employee can report his or her own facility anonymously to OSHA. OSHA can then perform a surprise inspection and cite the facility for not providing a safe workplace environment. The Joint Commission is also beginning to ask what practices are being performed to evacuate surgical smoke so that a safe surgical environment is maintained. Standards passed in January 2009 by the Canadian Standards Association entitled *Surgical Plume Scavenging for Health Care* (CSA Standards, 2009) address the requirement that surgical smoke must be evacuated appropriately. This is the first dedicated worldwide standard on smoke evacuation. Many other countries will use this standard in formulating their own recommendations and requirements.

BOX 18-2 Sample Policy for the Evacuation of Surgical Smoke

1. Use the appropriate smoke evacuation system depending on the amount of plume generated. If small amounts of plume are generated and room suction is to be used, an in-line suction filter is positioned between the suction canister and the wall outlet to capture the surgical smoke particulate. An individual smoke evacuation system is used if larger amounts of plume are generated.
2. Change the smoke evacuation filter or filters according to the manufacturer's written instructions.
3. Hold the smoke evacuation suction tube close (<1 inch away) to the tissue interaction site to remove as much plume (odor and particulate matter) as possible. If possible use a special electrosurgery device that also provides smoke evacuation through the tube surrounding the electrosurgical pencil blade.
4. Smoke evacuation tubing should have a smooth inner lumen to eliminate any whistling noise.
5. Use a reducer fitting to adapt a large smoke evacuation tube to a smaller suction or evacuation tube.
6. The scrub person or first assistant can operate the smoke evacuation foot pedal (if available) to minimize the wear and tear on the smoke evacuator motor and to decrease noise. Ideally a sensing system should be used on the laser or electrosurgery device that automatically activates and shuts off the smoke evacuator whenever plume is created.
7. Evacuate surgical smoke generated during endoscopic or laparoscopic procedures. Endoscopic smoke evacuation instruments help decrease the presence and retention of plume inside a body cavity or organ. During laparoscopic procedures, a delicate balance between smoke evacuation and insufflation is needed to maintain the pneumoperitoneum. A low-pressure suction valve or other smoke evacuation device can be attached to the trocar system sleeve to remove plume gently during a laparoscopic procedure without destroying the pneumoperitoneum. A special smoke evacuator that provides automatic plume removal also can be used to evacuate the intraabdominal smoke without destroying the pneumoperitoneum. A high-flow insufflator is recommended to replace any lost insufflation gas quickly.
8. Wear a surgical mask that provides adequate filtration (0.1 μm filtration) to protect against any residual smoke particulate matter that has not been evacuated. The high-filtration mask must fit snugly around the face. Wearing a high-filtration mask does not replace the need to use a smoke evacuation system to remove the surgical smoke from the environment.
9. Continuing education helps health care personnel understand the hazards of surgical smoke and encourages the use of appropriate methods for evacuation.

Modified from Association of periOperative Registered Nurses: *Perioperative standards and recommended practices,* Denver, 2009, The Association; Ball K: *Lasers: the perioperative challenge,* ed 3, Denver, 2004, Association of periOperative Registered Nurses.

SMOKE EVACUATION PRACTICES

There are many devices and pieces of equipment available today that provide adequate smoke evacuation. The amount of plume produced will determine which method is appropriate for smoke evacuation.

In-Line Filter

For years the most common method to evacuate surgical smoke is to merely use the suction device without a filter (Ball, 2009). This practice allows the particulate within the surgical smoke to coat the inside lumen of the suction system. An in-line filter is needed to protect the wall suction from contamination by surgical smoke. The filter is placed between the wall outlet and the suction canister (Figure 18-1). If the filter is placed between the patient and the suction canister, then fluids can invade the filter and decrease its efficiency. The filter is changed according to the manufacturer's recommendations.

The suction line is engineered to evacuate fluids from the surgical site, not air contaminants. Therefore the suction ability or air movement of the wall suction may not be forceful enough to provide adequate collection of all of the particulate matter and odor within surgical smoke. The suction line should only be used when very small amounts of plume are expected.

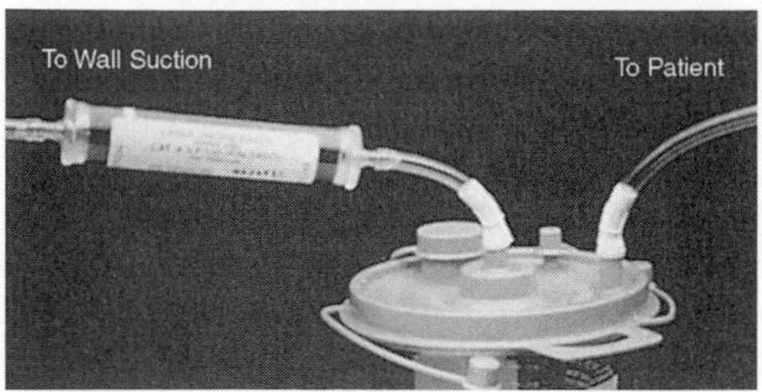

FIGURE 18-1 An in-line filter is placed between the wall outlet and the suction canister and is used to evacuate small amounts of surgical smoke. (From Ball KA: *Endoscopic surgery*, St. Louis, 1997, Mosby.)

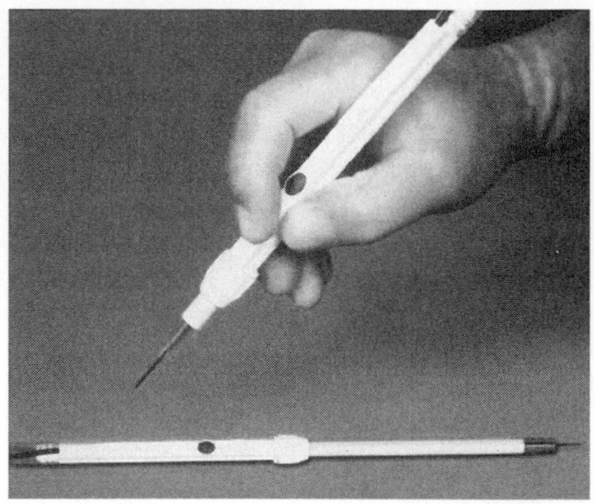

FIGURE 18-2 An electrosurgical pencil with the smoke tube built into the pencil design. (From Rothrock JC: *Alexander's care of the patient in surgery*, ed 13, St. Louis, 2007, Mosby.)

Smoke Evacuator

The most appropriate method of evacuation is using an individual smoke evacuator that has been designed to remove surgical smoke from the surgical site (Figure 18-2). Smoke evacuation involves the processes of collection and filtration. The smoke evacuator provides enough air movement to collect and then filter the particulate matter and odor.

Collection of the surgical smoke involves a high velocity of air movement at the suction tip to gather all of the plume. The National Institute of Occupational Safety and Health (NIOSH) publication entitled *Hazard Controls: Control of Smoke From Laser/Electric Surgical Procedures (HC11)* (2009) states that the smoke evacuator should have the capability of producing a capture velocity of about 100 to 150 ft/min at the inlet nozzle. Therefore a smoke evacuator must have high suction power to create this type of velocity.

For proper filtration, most smoke evacuators have a triple filtration system. The first part of the filtration system is a moisture filter that collects any moisture and removes large particulate matter. The next type of filtration involves an ultra-low penetration air (ULPA) filter that removes particulate of 0.12 μm in size at 99.9999% efficiency (Ball, 2004). This means that only one particle in a million will escape capture.

High-efficiency particulate air (HEPA) filtration is not appropriate for smoke evacuation because it filters 0.3-μm particles at only 99.97% efficiency. The activated charcoal filter neutralizes the odor from the surgical smoke. Coconut-based charcoal is more absorptive than wood-based charcoal.

The smoke evacuation filters should be changed as recommended by the manufacturer. Many smoke evacuation systems have an indicator light that illuminates when the filter needs to be changed. Some indicators are activated using a timed method—when a certain amount of time has passed while the smoke evacuator is on, the indicator light will illuminate. In other, more trustworthy indicator systems, when the air movement through the filter is diminished, the indicator light will glow, meaning that the filter has become occluded and is no longer effective.

When a smoke evacuator filter is changed, gloves should be worn because this practice is listed as an occupational hazard. When disposing of the contaminated filter, the manufacturer's recommendations and hospital policy should be followed. Many times the contaminated filter is disposed of as biohazardous waste even though disease has never been transmitted by a contaminated smoke evacuator filter in a landfill.

When purchasing a smoke evacuator, different characteristics need to be considered. Smoke evacuators should not be noisy. A documented barrier to the use of smoke evacuators has been the amount of noise the unit produces (Ball, 2009). Many surgical team members and surgeons refuse to use the older smoke evacuation systems because they produce too much noise and are distracting during the procedure. These older systems may be able to be refurbished to minimize the noise. Another characteristic of a smoke evacuator may be portability if the unit is to be moved from room to room. The smoke evacuator should be easy to use with a filter that is easy to change. Foot pedal of automatic activation systems are available today so that the smoke evacuator is operating only when plume is created. The cost of the equipment and the supplies is also considered when smoke evacuation devices are being evaluated.

The most critical features of a smoke evacuator continue to be the effectiveness of plume capture and the filtration system. The type of motor in the smoke evacuator will determine the velocity of capture. Turbine motors often take time to "ramp up" before the smoke is actually being evacuated. In comparison, a rotary vein pump will provide an instant negative static pressure needed to capture the plume particulate as it is first being generated.

Many times when a smoke evacuation program is being introduced, standardized products and devices are easier to incorporate into a surgical suite. When evaluating smoke evacuation devices and supplies, a side-by-side assessment can often determine which devices are most acceptable to the surgical team.

Smoke evacuators need little maintenance but should be checked from time to time to keep them in good working order. Ideally there should be a smoke evacuator system positioned in every surgical suite, just as suction for fluids is available in every operating room.

Laparoscopic Smoke Evacuation

Smoke left in the abdomen during a laparoscopic procedure will obstruct the surgeon's view and can also be absorbed by the patient, which in turn will create unwanted symptoms during the postoperative recovery phase. Evacuation of surgical smoke during laparoscopy requires the delicate balance between smoke evacuation and carbon dioxide insufflation to maintain the pneumoperitoneum.

Various devices are on the market to provide this balance. A low-pressure suction valve is available that provides a gentle movement of the abdominal air to decrease the smoke. Other devices that connect to the trocar system sleeve provide a mild movement of the insufflation gas to remove the smoke. A recirculator is also available that removes the plume, filters it, and then directs it back into the insufflated cavity to reduce the need for as much CO_2 gas for insufflation. A special smoke evacuator has been designed to evacuate surgical smoke during the laparoscopic procedure while monitoring and maintaining the pneumoperitoneum. This unit can also be used to remove the insufflation at the end of the procedure by using a closed system that minimizes exposure by the surgical team to the contaminated insufflation gas. This provides a much safer environment for the surgical team.

Face Mask Protection

A surgical face mask should never be worn as the first line of defense to protect against surgical smoke inhalation. A surgical face mask is worn only to protect the user from any residual plume that may have escaped capture by smoke evacuation practices. A regular surgical face mask usually filters 5-µm particulate. Surgical smoke particulate flows right through this type of mask. A high-filtration mask providing 0.1-µm filtration is appropriate for use in conjunction with smoke evacuation practices. The mask must be worn appropriately and disposed of when the procedure is complete. Again, the face mask when used alone does not offer adequate protection from surgical smoke inhalation.

COMPLIANCE WITH SMOKE EVACUATION RECOMMENDATIONS

Research has demonstrated that surgical smoke evacuation recommendations are not being consistently followed (Edwards and Reiman, 2008; Ball, 2009). As previously stated, the most common method for evacuation of surgical smoke is to use the suction provided in each surgical room. Increased education on surgical smoke hazards and smoke evacuation methods leads to increased compliance with smoke evacuation recommendations (Ball, 2009). Reviewing and posting articles, information pieces, AORN's recommended practices, or AORN's *Position Statement on Surgical Smoke and Bio-aerosols* helps to increase awareness and also leads to greater compliance with guidelines.

The documented barriers to compliance must be discussed when a smoke evacuation program is being implemented. The most common barriers to compliance are not having a smoke evacuator available, physicians prohibiting smoke evacuation practices during their procedures, the loud noise of some smoke evacuators, and complacency often exhibited by the surgical staff (Ball, 2009). How to overcome these barriers must be openly discussed and solutions suggested.

Reminder signs posted throughout the surgical department are an easy way to continually remind the surgical team members of the importance of evacuating all surgical smoke. AORN has created unique and powerful reminder signs that are offered with the AORN *Surgical Smoke Evacuation Tool Kit.* These signs can be downloaded, printed, and laminated for hanging in highly visible areas to remind everyone about the hazards of surgical smoke and the need to evacuate it.

A policy that addresses all of the aspects of surgical smoke evacuation is needed to ensure practice changes. Any updated or revised policy should be posted so everyone in the operating room can review it. The Joint Commission may ask to see a department's policy on surgical smoke evacuation and then may determine if the policy is being followed. A smoke evacuation competency checklist can be incorporated into the annual skills review to ensure smoke evacuation is being employed appropriately.

The smoke collection tube must be held as close to the tissue-impact site as possible (less than 1 inch away from the site). The further the collection tube is held away from site, the more particulate matter and toxic gases will escape. Devices have been introduced that provide the suction collection tubing around the electrosurgical pencil. As surgical smoke is created by the electrosurgical energy, the smoke tube captures the plume by creating a whirlwind motion (Figure 18-3). This vortex provides a powerful movement to capture all of the plume. There are shrouds available that can be positioned over the electrosurgical pencil, and there are also electrosurgical pencils with the smoke tube incorporated within the pencil design. This technology is able to capture more plume than using a suction tubing that pulls the plume in a unidirectional motion.

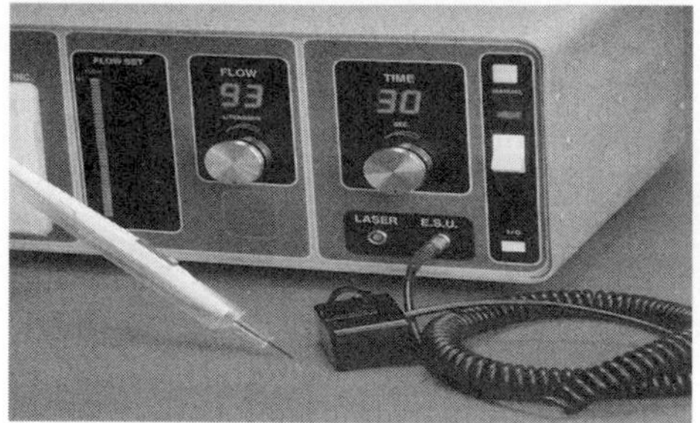

FIGURE 18-3 Individual smoke evacuator. (From Rothrock JC: *Alexander's care of the patient in surgery*, ed 13, St. Louis, 2007, Mosby.)

CONCLUSION

Implementing a comprehensive smoke evacuation program depends on the passion and dedication of many surgical team members. The program should be transparent to the surgeon. Each specialty should review smoke evacuation needs and recommend practices that will ensure clean air is provided during all procedures. Physician preference cards should always list smoke evacuation practices if any plume is generated during the procedure. If a surgeon insists that smoke evacuation is not needed, then the perioperative nurse needs to intervene and communicate that this is a workplace issue, not a patient issue. Maintaining a safe workplace is a huge responsibility of the perioperative nurse, and he or she must be dedicated to ensuring workplace safety is always followed.

On the front door of the hospital a "no smoking" sign is usually prominently displayed. Yet in the surgical department, smoking is still permitted. It is not tobacco that is burning, but human flesh and tissue that are producing the smoke. However, smoke is smoke, and it all contains contaminants that pollute the air, leading to inhalation hazards. In the past, miners would take canaries into the mines to ensure they were breathing clean air. If the canary would become unconscious, then the miner would exit the mine because the air was contaminated. The surgical team today is serving as the canary. Surgical team members are presenting with more respiratory problems, indicating that clean air is not always available in operating rooms. We must quit killing the canaries by starting to evacuate all surgical smoke (IC Medical, 2009)!

REFERENCES

Alp E, et al: Surgical smoke and infection control, *J Hosp Infect* 62(1):1–5, 2006.

Andersen E: Surgical smoke—is there a fire? *AAOHN J* 53(3):103–104, 2005.

Association of periOperative Registered Nurses: *Perioperative standards and recommended practices*, Denver, 2009, The Association.

Baggish MS, et al: Protection of the rat lung from the harmful effects of laser smoke, *Lasers Surg Med* 8(3):248–253, 1988.

Ball K: *Lasers: the perioperative challenge*, ed 3, Denver, 2004, The Association.

Ball K: Making the case for smoke evacuation, *Outpatient Surg* 6(8):53–57, 2007.

Ball K: *Surgical smoke evacuation guidelines: assessing compliance among perioperative nurses,* unpublished doctoral dissertation, 2009, Virginia Commonwealth University.

Barrett W, Garber S: Surgical smoke—a review of the literature, *Business Briefing: Global Surgery* 1–7, 2004, available at: http://www.touchbriefings.com/cdps/cditem.cfm?nid=952#Contents. Accessed, November 26, 2007.

Bigony L: Risks associated with exposure to surgical smoke plume: a review of the literature, *AORN J* 86(6):1013–1020, 2007.

Centers for Disease Control and Prevention: *NIOSH health hazard evaluation report,* HETA #2001-0066-3019, Dunedin, Fla, 2006, Centers for Disease Control and Prevention.

CSA Standards: CSA Standard help clear toxic smoke form operating rooms, March 18, 2009, available at: http://www.csa.ca/cm?c=CSA_Content&childpagename=CSA%2FLayout&cid=1238189000724&p=1239124789907&pagename=CSA%2FRenderPage. Accessed October 24, 2009.

Edwards BE, Reiman RE: Results of survey on current surgical smoke control practices, *AORN J* 87(4):739–749, 2008.

Garden JM, et al: Viral disease transmitted by laser-generated plume (aerosol), *Arch Dermatol* 38:1303–1307, 2002.

Hallmo P, Naess O: Laryngeal papillomatosis with human papillomavirus DNA contracted by a laser surgeon, *Eur Arch Otorhinolaryngol* 248(7):425–427, 1991.

Hazard controls: control of smoke from laser/electric surgical procedures (HC11), March 2, 1998, National Institute for Occupational Safety and Health, available at http://www.cdc.gov/niosh/hc11.html. Accessed May 11, 2009.

IC Medical, Inc.: Marketing slogan, 2009.

Maugh TH: Cleaner air linked to longer lives, *Columbus Dispatch* 2009.

Medscape: *Secondhand smoke damages lungs,* 2007, available at http://www.medscape.com/viewarticle/566487?sssdmh=dm1.320965&src=nlpatient. Accessed November 27, 2007.

Mihashi S, et al: *Some problems about condensates induced by CO_2 laser irradiation,* Fourth Congress of the International Society for Laser Surgery, Tokyo, 1981, Japan Society for Laser Medicine.

Ott DE: Smoke and particulate hazards during laparoscopic procedures, *Surg Serv Manage* 3(3):11–13, 1997.

Sawchuck WS, et al: Infectious papillomavirus in the vapor of warts treated with carbon dioxide laser or electrocoagulation: detection and protection, *J Am Acad Dermatol* 21:41–49, 1989.

Taravella MJ, et al: Respirable particles in the excimer laser plume, *J Cataract Refract Surg* 27(4):604–607, 2001.

Tomita Y, et al: Mutagenicity of smoke condensates induced by CO_2-laser irradiation and electrocauterization, *Mutat Res* 89(2):145–149, 1989.

Ulmer BC: The hazards of surgical smoke, *AORN J* 87(4):721–734, 2008.

Chapter 19

BLOODBORNE PATHOGENS

Lieutenant Colonel Laura D. Desnoo, MSN, RN, CNOR

It has long been understood that blood from infected patients can transmit viral disease through percutaneous inoculation or blood contact with nonintact skin. In the past, exposure to blood was considered to be a hazard of the position. The perioperative nurse and members of the surgical team recognized that the exposure risk to blood and body fluids in surgery is arguably greater than in other departments such as the emergency department or laboratory department (Jagger, 1994). It was not until the human immunodeficiency virus (HIV) was described in 1981 that greater attention was given to health care worker (HCW) safety and implementation of safe practices intended to protect the health care worker (Berguer and Heller, 2004).

Contracting a disease from a bloodborne pathogen infectious agent has been identified as an occupational hazard for HCWs and specifically for the perioperative team members in the operating room (OR) and procedural areas. These areas of practice are complex and consist of dynamic events for the perioperative teams that result in a challenging environment to control.

Makaray et al (2007) surveyed 699 surgical residents in 17 U.S. medical centers with the shocking results that 51% of needlestick injuries in this group were not reported. Of needlestick injuries not reported, 16% involved a high-risk patient whose blood tested positive for HIV, hepatitis B virus (HBV), or hepatitis C virus (HCV) (Makaray et al, 2007). Ninety-nine percent of the surgical residents reported an average of eight needlestick injuries during their first 5 years.

Needlestick and sharps injuries continue to occur even with best practices and recommendations in place. This chapter will explore the history of needlestick safety and prevention, pathogen prevalence, pathogen transmission, injury pattern, OR-specific engineering controls and work practices, and recommendations for management of occupational exposure to needlestick or sharps injuries.

HISTORY

During the early to mid-1980s, transmissible, potentially fatal diseases became of great concern to HCWs. In response the Occupational Safety and Health Administration (OSHA) developed standards addressing workplace safety and bloodborne pathogens (Cuming et al, 2008). In 1991 OSHA (2008) issued the bloodborne pathogens standard (29 CFR 1910.1030) to protect workers from this risk. Beginning in 1996, nursing organizations along with grassroots groups lobbied for legislation at the federal level to mandate safer needlestick devices and improve HCW education (Peterson, 1997). It was not until November 6, 2000, that President Clinton signed the Needlestick Safety and Prevention Act (Murphy, 2001). In 2001, as a response to the Needlestick Safety and Prevention Act, OSHA revised the bloodborne pathogens standard.

OSHA requires that employers reduce and eliminate employee risk through the use of engineering and work practice controls. The revised standard clarifies the need for employers to select safer needle devices and to involve employees in identifying and choosing these devices, to annually review advances in technology to reduce risk or injury, and to maintain a log of injuries from contaminated sharps (OSHA, 2009).

PATHOGEN PREVALENCE

Bloodborne pathogens are pathogenic microorganisms that are present in human blood,

The opinions or assertions contained in this chapter are the private views of the author and are not to be construed as official or as reflecting the views of the U.S. Army Medical Department or the Department of Defense.

or blood components, that can cause disease in humans. There are more than 20 pathogens that can be transmitted with occupational exposure. The pathogens that are of greatest concern are HBV, HCV, and HIV. They are the most commonly transmitted pathogens during patient care (Centers for Disease Control and Prevention [CDC], 2008b) (Table 19-1). The operating room and perioperative services are areas of high risk for exposure, and the risk for becoming infected is a concern for all perioperative team members. Other bloodborne diseases that pose sporadic but infrequent occupational infection risks include syphilis, malaria, babesiosis, brucellosis, relapsing fever, human T-lymphotropic viruses, viral hemorrhagic fever agents, and arboviruses.

TABLE 19-1 Infections Transmitted via Sharps Injuries During Patient Care (PC) and/or Laboratory/Autopsy (L/A)

Infection	PC	L/A
Blastomycosis		+
Cryptococcosis		+
Diphtheria		+
Ebola	+	+
Gonorrhea		+
Hepatitis B	+	+
Hepatitis C	+	+
HIV	+	+
Herpes	+	
Leptospirosis		+
Malaria	+	
M. tuberculosis	+	+
Rocky Mountain spotted fever		+
Scrub typhus		+
Strep pyogenes		+
Syphilis		+
Viral hemorrhagic fever	+	+

From Centers for Disease Control and Prevention: *Workbook for designing, implementing, and evaluating a sharps injury prevention program*, 2008, available at http://www.cdc.gov/sharpssafety/pdf/sharpsworkbook_2008.pdf. Accessed September 6, 2009.
HIV, Human immunodeficiency virus.

Hepatitis

Six different hepatitis viruses have now been characterized, and other hepatitis viruses are likely to be identified in the future. Hepatitis B and C are the two hepatitis infections that are of greatest concern for the perioperative team because of several features that they share: (1) both are bloodborne infections; (2) both are associated with chronic infection ultimately leading to cirrhosis, portal hypertension, and hepatocellular carcinoma; and (3) both can be occupational infections for the HCW after percutaneous injury associated with infected blood.

HBV is an inflammation of the liver that can lead to liver damage and death. Approximately 1.2 million persons in the United States have chronic HBV infection, and an estimated 4000 to 5000 persons die each year from HBV-related liver diseases (CDC, 2002). HBV constitutes the primary infection hazard to HCWs; however, hepatitis B vaccine immunizations and compliance with other provisions of OSHA's bloodborne pathogens standard have been effective in reducing HBV infections. Since the hepatitis B vaccine became available in 1982, the number of occupational infections has decreased significantly, from over 10,000 in 1982 to fewer than 400 in 2001 (CDC, 2003).

For a susceptible person (a person who has not received the vaccination), the risk from a single needlestick or cut exposure to HBV-infected blood ranges from 6% to 30% and depends on the hepatitis B e antigen (HBeAg) status of the source individual. Hepatitis B surface antigen (HBsAg)-positive individuals who are HBeAg positive have more virus in their blood and are more likely to transmit HBV than those who are HBeAg negative. Although there is a risk for HBV infection from exposure to mucous membranes or nonintact skin, there is no known risk for HBV infection from exposure to intact skin.

HCV infection is present in nearly 4 million people in the United States and is the most common chronic bloodborne infection in the United States. Hepatitis C infection is caused most commonly by needlestick injuries. It has a lower rate of transmission than hepatitis B following needlestick injury and often occurs with no symptoms; however, it has a 50% to 80% rate of chronic disease after acute infections. There is no vaccine for hepatitis C, and only prevention of blood exposure will avoid the risks of this occupational infection. No data are available related to the risk for occupation exposure and infection following a needlestick or sharps injury contaminated with hepatitis C blood. Studies indicate that the percentage of HCWs with confirmed HCV infection is 1%, compared with confirmed cases in 3% of the U.S. general population (CDC, 2003).

Human Immunodeficiency Virus

The Centers for Disease Control and Prevention (CDC) (2008a) estimated that 1,106,400 U.S. adults and adolescents were living with HIV infection at the end of 2006 (95% confidence interval). HIV infection has been reported following occupational exposures to HIV-infected blood by needlesticks or cuts; splashes in the eyes, nose, or mouth; and skin contact. Most often, however, infection occurs from needlestick injury or cut injury (e.g., sharps). The overall risk for seroconversion has been estimated at close to 0.3% after percutaneous injury (i.e., needlestick injury, cut) with an HIV-contaminated instrument (Stringer et al, 2001). No vaccine can currently prevent HIV infection, and no treatment exists to cure it.

BLOODBORNE PATHOGEN TRANSMISSION

To develop strategies for reduction of occupational exposures to bloodborne pathogens it is important to examine the types of exposures: cutaneous contact, mucous membrane contact, percutaneous penetration, and aerosolization of blood.

The first means of transmission is through cutaneous contact, and the intact skin is the first line of defense for the body to help prevent contamination. Most cutaneous exposures are breaks in the skin and remain unnoticed by the HCW (Stringer et al, 2001). Many HCWs, especially OR personnel, develop these breaks in their skin. Breaks in the skin also are thought to be caused by repeated scrubbing, hand washing, and dermatitis linked to latex allergy (Stringer et al, 2001). The prevalence of latex sensitivity is reported to be 3% in hospital workers as a whole and 6% in OR personnel (Stringer et al, 2001).

The second means of transmission is through mucous membrane (i.e., the lining of the mouth, eyes, and nostrils), which are more vulnerable to disease organisms than intact skin. The risk for HIV transmission from mucous membrane contamination has been estimated to be 0.09% (Stringer et al, 2001). There have been at least four documented cases of U.S. workers who seroconverted after being exposed to HIV-infected blood through contact with mucous membranes (Stringer et al, 2001). There are many cases of both HBV and HCV that were transmitted via contaminated blood contact through the mucous membrane.

The third means of transmission is percutaneous contamination; it may also be referred to as transcutaneous or parenteral route. This type of transmission occurs when a sharp instrument such as a scalpel, bone hooks, needles, or bone penetrates the skin.

The fourth means of exposure is aerosol. As technology has advanced, high-speed cutting devices produce an aerosol that may be contaminated with pathogens from an infected or colonized patient (Taylor, 2006). This method of transmission has not been well studied and requires further research.

Prevention of blood exposure—by implementing the use of barriers in the operating room and modification of surgical techniques—is recommended to minimize risk for needlestick or sharps injury to prevent occupational infection from both known and unknown bloodborne viruses from the surgical patient.

INJURY PATTERN

To understand the mechanism of injury and implement best practices to prevent exposure to bloodborne pathogens, the perioperative nurse must be aware of the contributing factors for exposure. One recognized factor is related to the invasive nature of surgical procedures, which places the perioperative team in a highly vulnerable position for percutaneous exposure. Taylor (2006) identifies contributing factors related to occupational needlestick or sharps injury: (1) extended contact with open surgical sites, (2) manipulation of equipment and sharp instruments, and (3) exposure to large quantities of blood and body fluids and other types of tissue.

Wright et al (1991) investigated the mechanisms of glove tears and injuries resulting from sharp objects in the operating room. Each person who experienced a glove tear or sharps injury was interviewed immediately after the incident. During 2292 operations, 249 glove tears and 70 injuries from sharp objects were documented.

In 63% of the glove tears, there was visible contact with the patient's blood. The cause of the glove tear could be identified in only 81 incidents (33%). Ninety-two percent of the glove tears occurred when personnel were wearing one glove. These findings suggest that most glove tears are the result of unknown causes; however, changes in the number of gloves worn was suggested to reduce risk. Sixty-seven percent of the sharps injuries were caused by needlesticks, usually during suture placement. The majority of the sharps injuries (57%) occurred with the injured hand stationary or holding an object (16%), while the hand was retracting tissue (17%), and by instruments not in use (24%) (Wright et al, 1991).

Tanner and Parkinson (2006) conducted a systematic review to include 31 randomized controlled trials investigating various parameters, which included glove perforations, double-gloving practices, and effectiveness of indicator gloves. Tanner and Parkinson (2006) concluded that the practice of double gloving is effective in significantly decreasing exposure to bloodborne pathogens. The recommendation for double gloving has since become endorsed as a best practice by the Association of periOperative Registered Nurses (2009), American College of Surgeons (2007), and American Academy of Orthopedic Surgeons (2008).

Berguer and Heller (2004) state that needlestick injuries may occur in as many as 15% of operations. Scrub nurses and scrub technicians sustain the second-highest frequency of injuries in the OR at 19%; surgeons and first assistants are the highest at 59% (Berguer and Heller, 2004). Suture needles are the main source of needlesticks to OR personnel, causing 51% of all sharps injuries in surgical settings. Scalpel blades cause 12% of injuries (Jagger et al, 1998). The most common body part injured is the nondominant hand, usually suturing the fascia. Surgeons also fail to report as many as 70% of their injuries and do not participate in recommended postexposure strategies (Patterson et al, 1998). Knowing the mechanism of sharps injuries should lead to the development of effective preventive strategies aimed at protecting operating room personal from exposure to bloodborne pathogens.

The Exposure Information Network (EPINet) is a voluntary surveillance program to report needlestick and sharp-object injury and blood and body fluid exposure. The database is managed by the International Healthcare Worker Safety Center at the University of Virginia. Data are reported by hospitals voluntarily. Using EPINet data from 2007, there were 29 health care facilities that participated from the United States. The total cases of percutaneous injuries in 2007 were 951 (Perry et al, 2009). The majority of percutaneous injuries, 35.9% (341), occurred in the operating room. Suture needles were involved in 23.9% of all reported percutaneous injuries. Data were then pulled out as to when the injury occurred; 47.5% of the percutaneous injuries occurred during use of the device. Ninety-two percent of the sharps injuries were contaminated. If the injury that occurred was by needle, the data were then broken down by whether the needle was a "safety design." Injuries continue at a high rate, but there is still a high rate of use of items that are not "safety devices." It is not known if injury by an item occurred because no safety device has been developed or because the institution had not implemented available safety-engineered devices. Of the injuries that occurred with a safety needle, the safety mechanism was activated in only 11.9% of the cases. The data suggest that there needs to be more training and education on safety devices to determine that the devices are used correctly. Training and education should include information on the device's intended use. The issues of why HCWs chose not to use safety devices when available also demands further research.

ENGINEERING CONTROLS AND WORK PRACTICES

Engineering Controls

Engineering controls are defined in OSHA's bloodborne pathogens standard as controls that isolate or remove the bloodborne pathogens hazard from the workplace (29 CFR 1910.1030[b]) (National Institute for Occupational Safety and Health [NIOSH], 2008). The standard states, "Engineering and work practice controls shall be used to eliminate or minimize employee exposure" (29 CFR 1910.1030[d][2][i]). This means that if an effective and clinically appropriate safety-engineered sharp exists, an employer must evaluate and implement it. However, if using a safer device compromises either patient safety or medical integrity, its use would not be required (NIOSH, 2008).

There are both general and specific engineering controls, as well as work practices, that can occur and be modified to allow for the reduction of exposure to bloodborne pathogens in the perioperative arena. The work that is necessary to redesign surgical sharps and procedures to reduce exposure to blood and body fluids may not be easy because change in culture is hard to produce and sustain. Surgeons are more likely to adopt strategies to prevent the transmission of bloodborne diseases if they do not have to make frequent or extensive behavioral changes (Wright et al, 1995).

Some of the suggested engineering controls include double gloving, blunt suture needles, safety scalpels, needleless fascia closing device, use of needleless skin closures, and use of robotics. Work practice controls suggested are use of hands-free technique, neutral zone, double gloving, and removing all unnecessary sharps from the surgical field and all unnecessary instrumentation from the procedure sets. The perioperative team should use personal protective equipment (PPE) with application of goggles, eye shields, mask, and gloves as appropriate.

Double Gloving

Many, if not all, perioperative team members who have scrubbed in on cases have encountered blood on their fingers or hands at the conclusion of the case without ever realizing that there had been a break in the glove barrier (e.g., failure, tear, or puncture) or that an injury had occurred. Glove failure is not an uncommon occurrence; in fact the U.S. Food and Drug Administration (FDA) permits 2.5% of new unused sterile gloves to fail standardized quality control testing (Berguer and Heller, 2004). The practice of double gloving affords a high degree of protection from this common event. Perforation rates as high as 61% for thoracic surgeons and 40% for scrub nurses have been reported (Berguer and Heller, 2004).

Blunt Suture Needles

Blunt-tip suture needles are identified by OSHA as an example of an engineering control to reduce percutaneous injuries (NIOSH, 2008). As an alternative to sharp-tip suture needles, blunt-tip suture needles can be used to suture less-dense tissue such as muscle and fascia. As many as 59% of suture needle injuries occur during suturing of muscle and fascia (Stringer et al, 2001). The replacement of conventional sharp-tip suture needles with blunt-tip suture needles for these surgical tasks will reduce injury rates to surgical personnel. Conventional sharp-tip suture needles may be needed to suture skin, bowel, and blood vessels, although suture-less techniques for these procedures are available for use at the discretion of the surgeon. Alternate skin closure devices should also be considered. These include 3M Steri-Strip Adhesive Skin Closures, 3M Steri-Strip Wound Closure System, Dermabond Topical Skin Adhesive, Indermil Tissue Adhesive, INSORB Subcuticular Skin Stapler, and SuturTek 360° Fascia Closure Device.

Other considerations to minimize risk include use of technology such as robotics, needleless medical devices, and safety scalpels. The use of the robotic hands can help to reduce the number of hands in the surgical field, also reducing the potential for exposure of the team members to the bloodborne pathogen. In addition, several companies produce safety scalpels that are both disposable and reusable (Figure 19-1). There are retractable blades, blade shields, and both passive and active systems. The use of vessel ligation and sealing devices eliminates the risk for needlestick or sharps injury to the perioperative team members (e.g., LigaSure system [Covidien, Boulder, Colo.]; Gyrus PK Tissue Management System [Gyrus Medical, Minneapolis, Minn.], Harmonic Scalpel [Ethicon Endo-Surgery, Cincinnati, Ohio], and EnSeal PTC tissue sealing and hemostasis system [SurgRx, Redwood City, Calif.]).

Work Practice Controls

Several work practice controls (i.e., changing the way in which the work is performed) exist. The following are some work practice controls that are used in organizations and meet OSHA's requirements:

- Hands-free technique
- Neutral zone
- Substituting staples for sutures
- Announcing that a sharp will be passed
- Removing all unnecessary sharps from the surgical field

The hands-free technique (i.e., the indirect transfer of instruments between surgeons and other scrub people so that only one person touches the same sharp item at any time) is a work practice recommended to decrease risk for percutaneous

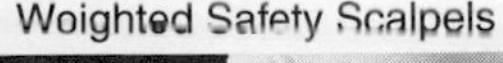

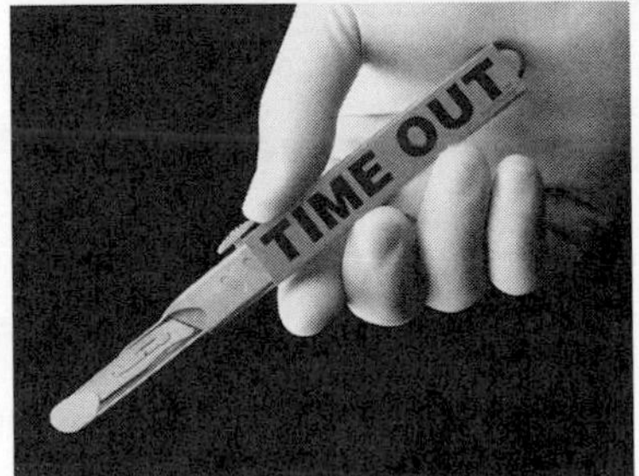
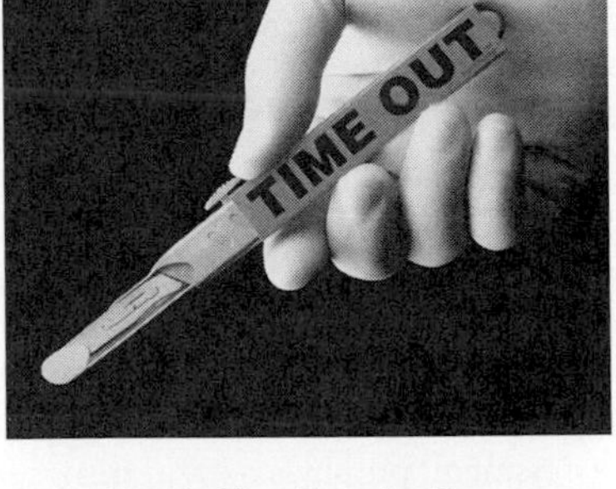

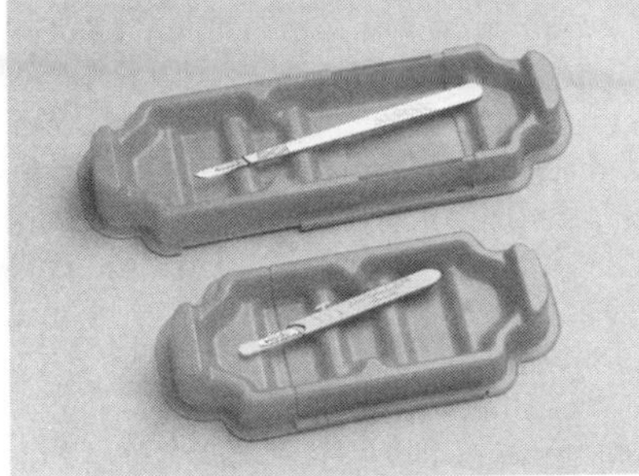

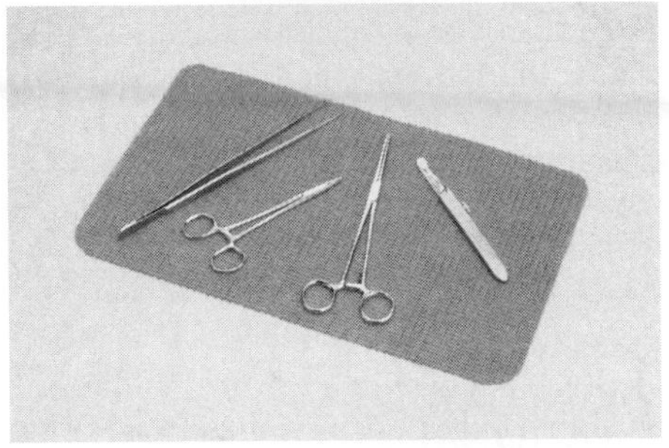

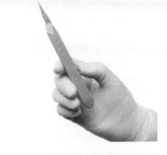

FIGURE 19-1 Examples of safety scalpels, hands-free transfer trays, and neutral zone products. (Courtesy of Sandel Medical Industries, LLC, Chatsworth, Calif.)

injury during surgery. A neutral zone should be used during all surgical procedures to prevent two individuals from simultaneously handling a contaminated sharp, including scalpel blades, suture needles, hypodermic needles, and sharp surgical instruments. The neutral zone may be established by using an emesis basin, instrument mat, or magnetic pad (see Figure 19-1).

Each time a sharp is placed in the neutral zone, the user (i.e., surgeon, physician assistant, registered nurse first assistant, scrub person) indicates placement of the sharp verbally and completely withdraws his or her hand from the neutral zone until the sharp is retrieved. The scrub person should allow only one sharp at a time in the neutral zone. When loading the needle holder, the scrub person should avoid manually positioning the suture needle. Instead the suture pack, a needle holder, forceps, or hemostat may be used to aid in positioning the suture needle onto the suture driver. Perioperative team members should avoid placing hands in the direct area that is being sutured.

When the sharps are organized in the work area, Mayo stand, or back table, the sharps should be pointed away from the handler and receiving personnel. With procedural custom packs, extra blades and hypodermic needles that are not required for the procedure should be passed off before count to minimize sharps on the field. All of these solutions require team commitment. All members of the perioperative team, including surgeons, must be included in the search for solutions; without their participation, implementation of the change and sustaining it will most likely fail (Stringer et al, 2001).

Personal Protective Equipment

PPE is designed to supplement both engineering controls and work practices. Perioperative service leaders should ensure that eye shields, goggles, reinforced gowns, other liquid-repelling garments, and sufficient gloves to allow for double gloving are readily available (Cuming et al, 2008). Standard precautions require that gloves be worn whenever there may be contact with blood and body fluids, when touching mucous membranes and nonintact skin, when handling contaminated instruments, and when performing venipuncture or other vascular and arterial access procedures (Stringer et al, 2001). Gloves are worn to protect the HCW and maintain sterility of the surgical wound, and they are an extension of standard precautions. Gowns, like gloves, are worn during a surgical procedure to protect the HCW, maintain asepsis, and to reduce exposure to blood and body fluid. The composition of a surgical gown allows for variation in the ability of a liquid to penetrate the material. Stringer et al (2001) attributed this variation to the material used, if the gown is reinforced or coated, length of time the gown may be in contact with fluids, and, if reusable gowns, the number of launderings. For selection of appropriate gown material, the product evaluation team should determine the type of procedures, the length of cases, and the material permeability based on these factors.

RECOMMENDATION FOR MANAGEMENT OF OCCUPATIONAL EXPOSURE

Bloodborne pathogens continue to be a source of occupational infection for health care workers, but particularly for the perioperative team. Over 1% of the U.S. population has one or more chronic viral infections. Hepatitis B is the infection that has the longest known role as an occupational pathogen, but infection with this virus is largely preventable with the use of the effective hepatitis B vaccine. Hepatitis C affects the largest number of people in the United States, and there is no vaccine available for the prevention of this infection. HIV infection still has not been associated with a documented transmission in the operating room environment, but six cases of probable occupational transmission have been reported. A total of 57 health care workers have had documented occupational infection since the epidemic of HIV infection began.

Infection of patients by bloodborne pathogens from infected surgeons remains a concern. Surgeons who are e antigen positive for hepatitis B have been well documented to be an infection risk to patients in the operating room. Only four surgeons have been documented to transmit hepatitis C, although other transmissions have occurred in the care of patients when practices of infection control have been violated (Fry, 2007). No surgical transmission of HIV to a patient has been identified at this time.

To improve compliance with the exposure plan, the reporting process of the injury needs to be easy and streamlined. The perioperative team member should be well informed of the expected process should he or she experience a needlestick or sharps injury. Figure 19-2 is a sample survey to evaluate personnel on occupational exposure to blood and body fluids. The OSHA bloodborne pathogens standard requires employers to evaluate and provide treatment based on the most recent data from postexposure assessment, prophylaxis, and treatment recommendations by the CDC.

Recommendations from OSHA (2008) for a needlestick or sharps injury include the following:

1. Immediately flood the exposed area with water, and clean any wound with soap and water or a skin disinfectant if available.
2. Report this immediately to your employer.
3. Seek immediate medical attention.

Hazards associated with working in the OR will always be present and may never be totally mitigated, but behaviors associated with protection can be modified to decrease the potential for exposure. Institute appropriate policies and procedures, jointly evaluating products with staff to ensure that the front-line team members have a voice in product selection (Figure 19-3). When this is implemented, compliance is more likely to occur.

The members of the perioperative team should have appropriate training and education, which includes identifying and using safety-engineered needlestick-avoidance devices and maintaining an injury log to collect data regarding the nature of the injuries and potential preventive methods. Maintaining a sharps-injury log will help to identify the number of employees injured, as well as annotating the products and circumstances involved in the injury. This information will allow accurate tracking of injuries, looking for trends based on data collected, and encourage employees to report injury. The goal is to work toward prevention of a single injury from a needlestick or sharp.

Many costs are associated with contracting a bloodborne illness from an occupational source, including human costs, medical expenses, and organizational losses (Taylor, 2006). Human costs include not only physical pain from the injury and discomfort from the treatment, but also psychologic and emotional trauma. Multiple personal consequences may occur for an HCW after a needlestick injury involving patients who

SAMPLE Survey of Healthcare Personnel on Occupational Exposure to Blood and Body Fluids

If you have questions or problems completing this form, please ask for help.

1. Which of the following best describes your occupation/work area? *(Check one.)*

- ☐ Nursing staff
- ☐ Nonsurgical medical staff
- ☐ Surgical medical staff
- ☐ Laboratory staff
- ☐ Dental staff
- ☐ Phlebotomy team
- ☐ V team
- ☐ Technician
- ☐ Clerical/administrative staff
- ☐ Transport service
- ☐ Central supply staff
- ☐ Maintenance/engineering staff
- ☐ Housekeeping/laundry services
- ☐ Other staff
- ☐ Security
- ☐ Medical student
- ☐ Other student

2. Which shift do you usually work? ☐ 1st ☐ 2nd ☐ 3rd

Part A. Reporting Occupational Exposures

The following questions are about exposures to blood or body fluids, including injuries from sharp objects such as needles, or blood or body fluid contact to the eyes, mouth, or skin.

3. Does our organization have a procedure/protocol for reporting exposures to blood and body fluids?

☐ No ☐ Yes ☐ Don't know

If yes, are you familiar with how to report these exposures?

☐ No ☐ Yes

4. Who would you contact first if you were injured by a needle or sharp object, or if you were exposed to blood or body fluid?

- ☐ Supervisor
- ☐ Occupational/employee health
- ☐ Infection control
- ☐ Emergency room
- ☐ Personal physician
- ☐ Don't know
- ☐ Would not contact anyone
- ☐ Other (please explain) ______________________________

5. In the past 12 months, have you been injured by a sharp object, such as a needle or scalpel that was previously used on a patient?

☐ No ☐ Yes ☐ Don't know if the object was previously used on a patient

If yes, how many contaminated sharps injuries did you sustain during this time period? _______
For how many of these exposures did you complete/submit a blood/body fluid exposure report? _______

6. In the past 12 months, did blood or body fluids come in direct contact with your eyes, mouth, or skin?

☐ No ☐ Yes

If yes, how many blood/body fluid exposures did you sustain during this time period? _______
For how many of these exposures did you complete/submit a blood/body fluid exposure reports? _____

Please go to the next page

FIGURE 19-2 Sample Survey of Healthcare Personnel on Occupational Exposure to Blood and Body Fluids. (From Centers for Disease Control and Prevention: *Workbook for designing, implementing, and evaluating a sharps injury prevention program,* 2008, available at http://www.cdc.gov/sharpssafety/pdf/sharpsworkbook_2008.pdf. Accessed September 6, 2009.)

Continued

are HCV or HIV positive. These may include the following (Taylor, 2006):

- Altering of sexual practices
- Chronic disabilities
- Denial of worker compensation claims
- Postponement of childbearing
- Punitive disciplinary action
- Job discrimination
- Need for a liver transplant
- Loss of employment
- Side effects of prophylactic medications
- Premature death

7. If you had an exposure that you did not report, please indicate the reasons for not reporting: *(Check all that apply.)*

☐ I did not have time to report.
☐ I did not know the reporting procedure.
☐ I was concerned about confidentiality.
☐ I thought I might be blamed or get in trouble for having the exposure.
☐ I thought the source patient was low risk for HIV and/or hepatitis B or C.
☐ I thought the type of exposure was low risk for HIV and/or hepatitis B or C.
☐ I did not think it was important to report.
☐ Other (please explain) ____________________

Part B. Postexposure Experience

Please answer the following questions only if you had an exposure to blood or body fluids that you reported to a supervisor or health official.

8. Where did you go to receive care after you were injured by a needle or other sharp object or were exposed to blood or body fluid?

☐ Employee/occupational health service
☐ Infection control
☐ Emergency room
☐ Personal physician
☐ Outpatient clinic
☐ Other (please explain) ____________________
☐ Did not receive care

9. If you received treatment for your injury or splash, please circle the number that best describes your experience with the health service where you received care.

	Strongly Disagree	Disagree	Neither Agree nor Disagree	Agree	Strongly Agree
a. I was seen in a timely manner.	1	2	3	4	5
b. I was given sufficient information to make a decision about postexposure treatment.	1	2	3	4	5
c. My questions were answered to my satisfaction.	1	2	3	4	5
d. I was encouraged to call or come back if I had any concerns.	1	2	3	4	5
e. Staff made me feel that it was important to report my exposure.	1	2	3	4	5
f. I did not feel rushed during my visit.	1	2	3	4	5
g. The place where I received treatment was convenient for me.	1	2	3	4	5

10. Please add any additional comments below.

THANK YOU FOR COMPLETING THIS SURVEY.

FIGURE 19-2—cont'd

SAMPLE Device Evaluation Form

Product: *(Filled in by health care facility)* Date: ____________

Department/Unit: ____________ Position/Title: ____________

1. Number of times you used the device.

☐ 1-5 ☐ 6-10 ☐ 11-25 ☐ 26-50 ☐ More than 50

2. Please mark the box that best describes your experiences with the device. If a question is not applicable to this device, do not fill in an answer for that question.

	Strongly Disagree	Disagree	Neither Agree nor Disagree	Agree	Strongly Agree
Patient/Procedure Considerations					
a. Needle penetration is comparable with the standard device.	1	2	3	4	5
b. Patients/residents do not perceive more pain or discomfort with this device.	1	2	3	4	5
c. Use of the device does not increase the number of repeat sticks of patient.	1	2	3	4	5
d. The device does not increase the time it takes to perform the procedure.	1	2	3	4	5
e. Use of the device does not require a change in procedural technique.	1	2	3	4	5
f. The device is compatible with other equipment that must be used with it.	1	2	3	4	5
g. The device can be used for the same purposes as the standard device.	1	2	3	4	5
h. Use of the device is not affected by my hand size.	1	2	3	4	5
i. Age or size of patient/resident does not affect use of this device.	1	2	3	4	5
Experience With the Safety Feature					
j. The safety feature does not interfere with procedural technique.	1	2	3	4	5
k. The safety feature is easy to activate.	1	2	3	4	5
l. The safety feature does not activate before the procedure is completed.	1	2	3	4	5
m. Once activated, the safety feature remains engaged.	1	2	3	4	5
n. I did not experience any injury or *near miss* of injury with the device.	1	2	3	4	5

FIGURE 19-3 Sample Device Evaluation Form. (From Centers for Disease Control and Prevention: *Workbook for designing, implementing, and evaluating a sharps injury prevention program,* 2008, available at http://www.cdc.gov/sharpssafety/pdf/sharpsworkbook_2008.pdf. Accessed September 6, 2009.)

Continued

	Strongly Disagree	Disagree	Neither Agree nor Disagree	Agree	Strongly Agree
Special Questions About this Particular Device					
(To be added by health care facility)	1	2	3	4	5
	1	2	3	4	5
	1	2	3	4	5
Overall Rating					
Overall, this device is effective for both patient/ resident care and safety.	1	2	3	4	5

03. Did you participate in training on how to use this product?

☐ No *(Go to question 6.)* ☐ Yes *(Go to next question.)*

04. Who provided this instruction? *(Check all that apply.)*

☐ Product representative ☐ Staff development personnel

☐ Other ______________________________

05. Was the training you received adequate?

☐ No ☐ Yes

06. Was special training needed in order to use the product effectively?

☐ No ☐ Yes

07. Compared with others of your gender, how would you describe your hand size?

☐ Small ☐ Medium ☐ Large

08. What is your gender?

☐ Female ☐ Male

09. Which of the following do you consider yourself to be?

☐ Left-handed ☐ Right-handed

10. Please add any additional comments below.

____

____

THANK YOU FOR COMPLETING THIS SURVEY

Please return this form to: ______________________________________

Figure 19-3—cont'd

Follow-up for percutaneous injuries costs between $500 and $2500 (if no infection is contracted), with an average of $672 reported in one study; for the estimated 54,000 injuries caused by suture needles each year, this translates to a potential cost to U.S. hospitals of $36.3 million per year (U.S. General Accounting Office, 2000). This cost is for follow-up only; the costs of treatment for HCV conversion reached nearly $14,000 (Taylor, 2006). These costs do not consider the impact on the health care facility.

CONCLUSION

Prevention of the occupational hazard associated with needlestick and sharps injury requires use of protective barriers, avoidance of exposure risk by modification of techniques, and a constant awareness of sharp instruments in the operating room. The exposure risk will always be present in the OR, and there are certain aspects of the perioperative physical environment that are difficult to change. Perioperative staff and other team members can promote safe practices by modifying behaviors and attitudes toward implementation of standard precautions and compliance with reporting protocols.

REFERENCES

American Academy of Orthopedic Surgeons: *Information statement: preventing the transmission of bloodborne pathogens*, revised June. 2008, available at http://www.aaos.org/about/papers/advistmt/1018.asp. Accessed September 6, 2009.

American College of Surgeons: *Statement on sharps safety from the American College of Surgeons*, 2007, available at http://www.facs.org/fellows_info/statements/st-58.html. Accessed September 6, 2009.

Association of periOperative Registered Nurses: AORN recommended practices for prevention of transmissible infection in the perioperative practices setting. In Association of periOperative Registered Nurses, *2009 Standards, Recommended Practices, and Guidelines*, Denver, 2009, AORN, p. 477.

Berguer R, Heller P: Preventing sharps injuries in the operating room, *J Am Coll Surg* 199:462–467, 2004.

Centers for Disease Control and Prevention: Achievements in public health: hepatitis B vaccination—United States, 1982-2002, *MMWR* 51(25):549–522, 2002, available at http://www.cdc.gov/mmwr/preview/mmwrhtml/mm5125a3.htm. Accessed September 6, 2009.

Centers for Disease Control and Prevention: *Exposure to blood: what healthcare personnel need to know*, Washington, DC, 2003, Department of Health and Human Services, Centers for Disease Control and Prevention.

Centers for Disease Control and Prevention: *New estimates of U.S. HIV prevalence, 2006*, 2008a, available at http://www.cdc.gov/hiv/topics/surveillance/resources/factsheets/prevalence.htm. Accessed July 26, 2009.

Centers for Disease Control and Prevention: *Workbook for designing, implementing, and evaluating a sharps injury prevention program*, 2008b, available at http://www.cdc.gov/sharpssafety/pdf/sharpsworkbook_2008.pdf. Accessed September 6, 2009.

Cuming R, et al: Improving compliance with Occupational Safety and Health Administration standards, *AORN J* 87(2):347–356, 2008.

Fry D: Occupational risks of blood exposure in the operating room, *Am Surg* 73(7):637–646, 2007.

Jagger J: Comparative injury risk among operating room, emergency department and clinical laboratory personnel, *Infect Control Hosp Epidemiol* 15:345, 1994.

Jagger J, et al: A study of patterns and prevention of blood exposures in OR personnel, *AORN J* 67(5):979–996, 1998.

Makary M, et al: Needle-stick injuries are common but unreported by surgeons in training, *N Engl J Med* 356(26):2693–2699, 2007.

Murphy E: Needlestick Safety and Prevention Act, *AORN J* 73(2):458–461, 2001.

National Institute for Occupational Safety and Health: *Use of blunt-tip suture needles to decrease percutaneous injuries to surgical personnel*, Safety and health information bulletin, New York, 2008, U.S. Goverment Printing Office.

Occupational Safety and Health Administration: *Bloodborne pathogens*, 2008. Standard number 1910.1030, available at http://www.osha.gov/pls/oshaweb/owadisp.show_document?p_table=STANDARDS&p_id=10051. Accessed September 6, 2009.

Occupational Safety and Health Administration: *Bloodborne pathogens and needlestick prevention*, 2009, Washington, DC, available at http://www.osha.gov/SLTC/bloodbornepathogens/standards.html. Accessed December 11, 2009.

Patterson J, et al: Surgeons' concerns and practices of protection against blood borne pathogens, *Ann Surg* 228(2):266–272, 1998.

Perry J, et al: EPINet report: 2007 percutaneous injury rates, *International Healthcare Worker Safety Center* 1–3: August, 2009.

Peterson C: Health worker safety: ANA applauds safer needle device bill, *Am J Nurs* 97(12):16, 1997.

Stringer B, et al: Quantifying and reducing the risk of bloodborne pathogen exposure, *AORN J* 73(6):1132–1146, 2001.

Tanner J, Parkinson H: Double gloving to reduce surgical cross-infection, *Cochrane Database Syst Rev* 2002 (3): CD003087, 2006.

Taylor D: Bloodborne pathogen exposure in the OR—what research has taught us and where we need to go, *AORN J* 83(4):833–846, 2006.

U.S. General Accounting Office: *Occupational safety: selected cost and benefit implications of needlestick prevention devices for hospitals*, 2000, available at http://www.gao.gov/new.items/d0160r.pdf. Accessed July 27, 2009.

Wright J, et al: Mechanisms of glove tears and sharp injuries among surgical personnel, *JAMA* 266(12):1668–1671, 1991.

Wright J, et al: Reported use of strategies by surgeons to prevent tranmission of bloodborne diseases, *Can Med Assoc* 152(7):1089–1095, 1995.

LASER RISKS AND PREVENTIVE MEASURES FOR THE STAFF

Vangie Dennis, RN, CNOR, CMLSO

This is a remarkable age in which humanity rides the surging crest of a great wave of scientific and technologic achievement. Technologic advancements have fashioned an ingenious tool to develop a device that produces a type of light energy that has never been seen before—the laser. Light may come from a chemical reaction, light may come from energy conversions, but light from lasers is unique.

HISTORY OF LASERS

In the seventeenth century Sir Isaac Newton discovered that sunlight was composed of a rainbow of many colors. He believed that light was propagated by tiny particles, but could only speculate about the origins of this phenomenon. By the end of the nineteenth century it was known that light was a visible manifestation of a primary force of nature, electromagnetism. This also includes radio waves, microwaves, and x-rays. Light energy, like atoms, emits other waveforms of energy as it spontaneously changes from one energy state to another. By itself, a spontaneous process cannot produce light. It was in the twentieth century that Albert Einstein predicted that, under special circumstances, photons (particles of light) could bombard a substance and could stimulate the release of identical photons. This process is called stimulated emission. It had never been described before.

The word *LASER* is an acronym for ***L***ight ***A***mplification by ***S***timulated ***E***mission of ***R***adiation (Bertolotti, 2004). A laser beam is merely light; however, it is light that is amplified by stimulated emission, unlike normal light, which is produced by spontaneous emission. The differences between laser light and normal light are part of the reason that the laser has so rapidly assumed, and is continuing to assume, such a prominent position in science and medicine. Understanding the physics of the laser is necessary to understanding and optimizing safe practice within the perioperative setting.

The concept of a laser actually began in 1913 when Niels Bohr developed his theory of the atom (Carruth and McKenzie, 1986). This theory uses the model so familiar today of the atom consisting of a nucleus around which electrons circulate. Based on this model, Bohr was able to describe the atomic basis for the production of light energy by spontaneous emission. Using Bohr's model, in 1917 Albert Einstein speculated on the possibility of both spontaneous and stimulated emission. However, the existence of stimulated emission remained primarily a theory until 1954, when Charles H. Townes, Nikolay Basov, and Alexander Prokhorov were able to physically produce measurable stimulated emission with the MASER (***M***icrowave ***A***mplification by ***S***timulated ***E***mission of ***R***adiation) (Carruth and McKenzie, 1986).

Based on work with the maser, Charles H. Townes and Arthur L. Schawlow published a paper in 1958 discussing the possibility of extending the maser principles into the optical portion of the electromagnetic spectrum (Bertolotti, 2004). A year earlier, Gordon Gould, a graduate student at Columbia University, developed the principle of laser. He recognized that he had something great, so he had the notebook containing this theory notarized. He received bad legal advice, however, and did not pursue a patent until 9 months after Townes and Schawlow had submitted their patent. After many years of legal battles, Gould finally received credit and recognition for coining the word *laser* (Ball, 2004). However, it was not until 1960 that Theodore H. Maiman of Hughes Research Laboratories developed the first visible laser, a ruby laser (Maiman, 1960). Following this breakthrough, the entire area of visible and near-visible lasers grew rapidly. The development of other lasers quickly followed: the helium-neon (He-Ne) and neodymium:yttrium-aluminum-garnet (Nd:YAG) lasers were developed in 1961. The first semiconductor laser was developed in 1962, and 1963 brought the development of the carbon dioxide (CO_2) laser.

Laser technology continues to grow as physicists strive to develop laser in the ultraviolet spectrum and into the x-ray spectrum. Similar growth is seen in the clinical and commercial use of lasers. Nowhere is this growth more evident than in the medical applications of laser, not only in surgery, but also in diagnosis and treatment. The growing prominence of lasers in medicine is rapidly approaching the point where no physician's education will be considered complete until his or her training has included some knowledge of basic laser physics and experience with laser applications. Lasers today have a myriad of uses. They are used as target designators for DNA research, in magnetic resonance imaging (MRI) medical systems, and to create holograms.

LASER PHYSICS

Light Properties

In understanding the fundamentals of laser physics, it is essential to first have a basic understanding of the areas of science that deal with light properties and electromagnetic energy. Understanding the fundamentals of laser physics is directly proportional to understanding the safety practices of operating room personnel.

Light can be described as a beam or a ray. This beam or ray of light travels in a straight line until it encounters another object. Once surface contact is made, three things may occur: (1) the light can be absorbed by the surface, (2) it can be reflected back from this surface, or (3) it can penetrate and be transmitted beyond this surface.

When light is absorbed by a surface or material, the energy of the light beam is normally transformed into heat energy. This thermal effect of light energy absorption is the principle behind laser surgery. The laser light is absorbed by the tissue and transformed into thermal energy, causing the desired ablation or coagulation of tissue. Thus laser surgery is similar to many other means of delivering heat energy to the tissue. However, it is by far the most efficient and most precise means of delivering thermal energy to date. It is this efficiency and preciseness that makes the laser so valuable to all fields of surgery (Laserscope, 2002).

The reflection of a laser beam from a surface is primarily a safety hazard in laser surgery. All laser light can be reflected off any shiny surface, and the flatter and smoother the surface, the worse the safety hazard. Surgical tools with roughened or blackened surfaces have been developed to minimize the risk for inadvertent reflections. There are times, in procedures such as those in the upper airway, when reflection of the laser energy serves as a means of diverting the thermal energy away from the endotracheal tube.

The transmission of laser light through a surface is a factor that is very much dependent on the frequency or wavelength of the laser light and the properties of the tissue at that frequency. For example, glass transmits light in the visible spectrum almost completely, while completely blocking the transmission of the far-infrared energy produced by the holmium:yttrium-aluminum-garnet (Ho:YAG) or CO_2 laser. When light transmits into any solid surface, the light will interact. Each particle will then reflect, absorb, or transmit the light off or through the surface layer. This random reflection, absorption, and transmission scatters the light in all directions within the material. The deeper the light is able to transmit within the material, the more the scattering and spreading of the light energy. Laser energy at wavelengths that transmit deeply into biological tissue will cause thermal destruction at greater depths, but will also cause a subsurface area of thermal damage, the radius of which is larger than the radius of the laser beam spot size (Laserscope, 2002).

Laser Energy Generation

The physical basics of light energy are the foundation of the generation of laser light. Stimulated emission does not occur in nature. The environmental conditions must be very precisely controlled to make stimulated emission predominant over spontaneous emission. The key to laser energy generation lies within the laser tube, or optical resonator cavity. The laser tube is almost always cylindrical, designed so that laser propagation can occur in all directions. Within the laser tube is the active medium, which contains the atoms whose electrons undergo an energy-level transition to produce the laser light.

The name of a particular laser is derived from the active medium within the laser tube, which is responsible for the actual lasing. The medium can be a solid, a liquid, or a gas. A solid medium is usually in crystal form, although semiconductor lasers, so important in the communication industry, are also considered solid-state lasers. The potassium-titanyl-phosphate (KTP) laser and the Nd:YAG lasers are among the most common solid-state lasers. Liquid lasers are almost exclusively dye lasers. Dye lasers are very versatile, because, by changing the concentration or type of dye within the resonant chamber, the laser can actually be tuned to almost any desired frequency. However, a major drawback to dye lasers is a severe limitation in the amount of output power possible. Dye lasers are often used in ophthalmology and dermatology procedures. Gas lasers are by far the most common and popular types of lasers. Examples of gas lasers include the CO_2, the helium-neon, and the argon laser. Gas lasers are generally considered to be the most economical, efficient, and reliable type of laser (Carruth and McKenzie, 1986).

Characteristics of Laser Light

Laser light produced by stimulated emission possesses three properties that distinguish it from ordinary light produced by spontaneous emission. These three properties are monochromaticity, coherence, and collimation (Laserscope, 2002).

Monochromaticity means that all of the photons of light emitted by the laser are at one frequency and are moving in the same space and time. However, laser light is as close to being at one frequency as is physically possible. White light produced by spontaneous emission consists of light of all visible frequencies or all colors mixed together. Even visible light that might be considered a single color actually consists of a considerably wider spectrum of frequencies than light produced by stimulated emission. Therefore laser light is one color of light—monochromatic (Laserscope, 2002).

Coherence is a term referring to the wave nature of light and describes the fact that all of the peaks of the sine waves representing each photon are exactly in phase with each other, or both in the same space and time. In other words, all of the peaks of the waves exactly coincide, allowing all of the numerous small oscillations to accumulate. White light produced by spontaneous emission consists of all different frequencies. Therefore it is impossible for the waves of the white light to sum up consistently as does monochromatic light, because each frequency has its own wavelength, and the difference in wavelength will ensure that the photons of different frequencies will be out of phase the majority of the time. White light is composed of many colors of the light spectrum and will cancel each frequency out. With laser light, because of the coherency, the frequency will become in sync. This accounts for the brilliance so often seen with a laser beam (Laserscope, 2002).

Collimation describes the fact that all of the photons, or waves, produced by the stimulated emission process are going in exactly the same direction, parallel to each other. This property allows the stimulated emission photons to remain in phase while traveling for a long distance away from the laser source. Light produced by spontaneous emission tends to spread in all directions, as does the light produced by a light bulb. Although spontaneous emission light can be "collimated" using special optical lenses or mirrors to form a beam, it can never be as well collimated as light produced by stimulated emission (Laserscope, 2002).

Several characteristics of laser light result from these three properties. Although white light can be used to form images, laser light cannot form images, primarily because the laser light is collimated and coherent. Image formation requires light to travel in a wide range of directions from a given point. Because laser light photons all travel in the same direction, the light cannot be used to form an image. It can, however, be used to form holograms, but these are not "true" images (Bertolotti, 2004).

Laser light can be focused to an extremely sharp point using a lens. White light, however, can never be focused to a sharp point, because it consists of a mixture of light frequencies. Each frequency of light will have its own individual focal point after passing through a physical lens. Therefore, when the red portion of the spectrum is focused, the blue portion is not, and vice versa. Laser light can be focused to such a fine point that the molecules of air will literally explode if their breakdown voltage threshold is exceeded.

Operating Parameters

Three operating parameters determine precisely what the laser beam will do when exposed to tissue during surgery. These parameters are power, spot size, and exposure time. These parameters are used in combination to achieve the desired tissue effects.

Power

Power is an operating parameter expressed in watts. When the laser is turned on, the laser surgeon must decide what power setting will be used for the procedure. This parameter should be dictated by that surgeon's own experience and by consensus recommendations. The power setting usually is the highest recommended wattage with the shortest duration of exposure (time impacting tissue) so that thermal conductivity does not become a concern.

Spot Size

Spot size is the second operating parameter and describes the diameter of the minimum spot size achievable with a given lens. This parameter is typically given in millimeters. It is important to remember that spot size specifications are usually given for the spot size diameter, not the spot size radius, which is typically used in power density calculations. The spot size determines how concentrated the beam's power will be at the focal point of the laser beam. The minimum spot size is usually fixed by the focal length of the focusing lens. The spot size can be changed by using another lens with a different focal point (Laserscope, 2002).

Exposure Time

Time is the feedback parameter during laser use. Generally it is given in seconds, but it can be expressed in milliseconds (1 msec = 1×10^{-3} seconds). The longer the beam impacts tissue at a given power and spot size, the deeper that beam will penetrate. A surgeon uses time as the feedback mechanism in the same manner that a surgeon uses the feeling of pressure as feedback when cutting with a scalpel. There is also a similar learning curve that must be mastered when first using the laser. Learning to use the scalpel takes time and experience to master how much pressure is necessary to make a cut that is neither too shallow nor too deep. Learning to use the laser also necessitates the accumulation of experience to master how much time on tissue is required to cut or ablate tissue to the depth desired.

Power Density

Power density is a parameter that combines two of the three operating parameters to describe how concentrated the laser beam is on the surface of the tissue. Power density determines the effect of the laser beam when applied to the tissue. High power densities of the CO_2 laser correlate with vaporization of tissue, whereas lower power densities are associated with tissue coagulation. Power density is expressed in watts per square centimeter (W/cm^2), although occasionally this parameter is given in watts per square millimeter (Ball, 2004).

Increasing the power density will increase the laser beam's ability to vaporize as opposed to coagulate. The power density is directly proportional to the power setting. Therefore doubling the power will double the power density. However, the power density is inversely proportional to the square of the spot size diameter. Thus decreasing the spot size by half will quadruple the power density (Bertolotti, 2004).

The power density is influenced to a much greater extent by the beam spot size than it is by the power setting alone. Because of this relationship, a laser can be easily taken from full vaporization to full coagulation merely by focusing and then defocusing the laser beam. When the delivered laser light is at the focal point (which is determined by the focusing lens), the laser beam will have its maximum power density and will perform vaporization most efficiently. Backing away from the focal point, or defocusing, allows the laser beam to diverge and enlarge the spot size, thus decreasing the power density.

Radiant exposure is the true determinant of the amount of thermal damage caused by the laser. Radiation exposure takes into account all three of the operating parameters of the laser using the following equation:

$$\text{Radiant exposure (W sec/cm}^2\text{)} = \frac{\text{Power} \times \text{Time}}{\text{Spot size}}$$

Radiant exposure is directly proportional to the amount of thermal damage done to the tissue and is a better description of the tissue effect than is power density (Bertolotti, 2004). The actual time the laser impacts tissue is extremely difficult to estimate, particularly when the laser beam is in almost constant motion over the tissue surface as it is during most surgical procedures. Most descriptions of laser surgical procedures deal with the parameter of power density, leaving variations in the application of the time parameter to the discrimination of the individual laser surgeon.

EFFECTS ON BIOLOGICAL TISSUE

A laser beam's effect on tissue will vary with the frequency of the laser light and the type of tissue with which the laser interacts. Two properties of the tissue are often used to describe this interaction: the coefficient of absorption and the selective absorption (American National Standards Institute [ANSI], 2005)

Coefficient of Absorption

The coefficient of absorption describes how a particular substance absorbs a specific frequency of light. Because soft tissue is normally 70% to 90% water, water is used as the standard for biological tissues; it is also useful as a model for nonpigmented soft tissue. Water is a particularly good model for describing the interactions of different lasers with the clear structures of the eye.

The three major lasers used in medicine are the KTP, the Nd:YAG, and the CO_2. Because each laser operates at a fairly specific wavelength, each laser is associated with its own, individual coefficient of absorption.

The coefficient of absorption is a factor describing how rapidly the particular frequency of energy will be absorbed with depth. Low coefficients of absorption often correspond to very high percentages of scatter. If the energy is not well absorbed and is not highly reflected, it will attempt to transmit beyond the surface. As some laser energy penetrates, it allows for a large degree of scattering. Nd:YAG laser energy, in particular, scatters to a great degree, especially in tissue. In fact, scattering is the main factor that limits the penetration of the Nd:YAG laser in tissue. The absorption coefficient commonly given for 1064-nm wavelengths (Nd:YAG) in tissue are taking into account not only absorption but also scattering. Because "tissue" is not uniform in composition, these values will vary a great deal for different types of soft tissue and even for the same type of soft tissue from different locations (ANSI, 2005).

Selective Absorption

Selective absorption takes into account the absorption of laser energy by constituents of the medium other than water. Laser energy in and near the visible spectrum is readily absorbed by pigments and dyes.

Normal white light is composed of all of the frequencies or colors of electromagnetic energy in the visible spectrum (e.g., red, yellow, blue). Pigments absorb certain frequencies of the spectrum very well and other frequencies not as well. The color of an object determines how well those wavelengths are absorbed. In effect, the pigments take certain portions of the visible spectrum out of white light by absorption, allowing the portions that are perceived as the color to be transmitted, reflected, and scattered. For example, hemoglobin is a very good absorber of the blue and green portions of the visible spectrum, allowing the red portion to be perceived as the color of hemoglobin. Thus hemoglobin is a very good absorber of the blue-green argon and the green KTP laser energies, but not as good an absorber of the red ruby or helium-neon laser energies. Hemoglobin also absorbs the near-infrared energy from the Nd:YAG lasers fairly well, although not as well as blue and green light. Melanin tends to absorb all frequencies of visible light equally well.

The selective absorption by pigmented tissues is the principal reason why the argon laser was initially so popular in ophthalmic surgery. The blue-green light energy from the argon laser transmits easily through the clear structures of the eye with minimal absorption by the lens and aqueous humor while being readily absorbed by the pigmented retina. Thus the laser energy is preferentially absorbed in the retinal area of the eye as is desired for performing many retinal procedures. The argon laser is now being replaced by the KTP 532-nm wavelength and diode laser technology. Similarly, both the KTP and Nd:YAG laser are extremely useful for the treatment of surface pigmented lesions, allowing laser energy to be absorbed primarily in the pigmented areas while sparing (relatively) the nonpigmented areas (Dennis, 2008).

Wavelength Versus Transmission

The properties of soft tissue absorption and transmission are dependent upon the laser wavelength. The properties of soft tissue determine the amount of laser energy that will be reflected from, absorbed by, or transmitted between air and tissue. Transmission or penetration into soft tissues is very good for low-frequency electromagnetic energy.

Beginning in the very-low-frequency infrared (invisible) portion of the spectrum, transmission begins to increase with increasing frequency or decreasing wavelength. A high degree of transmission is seen in the x-ray spectrum, which makes these frequencies particularly good for medical imaging.

The far-infrared energy produced by the CO_2 laser (wavelength = 10,600 nm) has extremely low transmission in soft tissue. Thus the CO_2 laser energy is very well confined to the upper 0.1 mm of the tissue surface. The near-infrared energy produced by the Nd:YAG laser (wavelength = 1064 nm) penetrates deeper in nonpigmented soft tissue than the CO_2 laser energy and scatters significantly. In fact, it is primarily the scattering by the tissue rather than absorption that limits the depth of penetration of Nd:YAG energy. The visible blue-green energy of the argon laser (wavelength = 488 nm) or the KTP (wavelength = 532 nm) would penetrate the deepest of the three lasers if the tissue were completely devoid of pigment and hemoglobin. However, the presence of pigment and blood, even in relatively avascular tissues, changes the depth of penetration drastically as a result of selective absorption. Therefore the depth of penetration by the argon or KTP laser energy is less than that of the Nd:YAG laser energy, and in extremely pigmented tissues the penetration depth can closely approximate that of the CO_2 laser (ANSI, 2005).

Effects of Temperature on Tissue

Laser surgery is an accurate and efficient method of performing thermal surgery, in contrast to other modalities used in operating rooms. Of course, other considerations are the operator's experience and understanding of the tool. The actual surgery results from the conversion of the laser energy into heat. In tissue, protein denaturation occurs at and above 60° C (140° F), which results in irreversible tissue injury. At 100° C (212° F), water converts into steam. At some point between 300° and 400° C (572° and 752° F), tissue will begin to carbonize, resulting in surgical smoke or plume. At approximately 530° C (986° F) and in the presence of oxygen, tissue will burn and evaporate. Although these temperature-related effects are similar for all medical lasers once the energy is converted to heat, the differences in absorption of the various wavelengths by the various components of tissue make a great difference in the actual heat conversion during laser surgery (ANSI, 2005).

Heat coagulation of tissue is generally a slow process until carbonization begins. When carbonization occurs, energy absorption increases as does the rise in surface temperature. This is true for all types of medical laser energy because carbon is such a good absorber in the infrared and visible portion of the electromagnetic spectrum. A laser beam should be activated continuously on carbonized tissue. This is particularly true for the CO_2 laser, but also applies to the Nd:YAG, the diode 830 nm, the KTP, and the argon lasers. Carbon will absorb laser energy extremely well and will rapidly heat the surface of the tissue to 300° C to 500° C (572° to 932° F). Surface temperatures this high will significantly extend the zone of thermal necrosis underlying the tissue surface as thermal conductivity spreads to heat the adjacent structures (ANSI, 2005).

LASER SAFETY

When lasers are introduced into a health care environment, whether in a hospital, surgery center, or a physician's office, health care professionals must be prepared to address issues of safety for both the staff and the patient. All lasers present safety hazards and should be used in accordance with established regulations, standards and recommended practices, manufacturer's recommendations, and institutional policies. Laser safety is based on knowledge of the specific laser wavelength being used, its instrumentation and delivery systems, mode of operation, laser parameters, power densities, absorption in tissues, and associated risks specific to the wavelength.

Federal Regulatory Agencies and Nongovernmental Controls

Lasers are classified as medical devices and are subject to regulation. The Performance Standards for Light-Emitting Products (21 CFR 1040) provides specifications for manufacturers of medical laser systems. Becoming acquainted with the organizations, laws, and standards regulating or affecting the use of lasers in a medical setting familiarizes the health care professional with the information necessary to develop and implement an appropriate laser safety program.

The federal Performance Standards for Light-Emitting Products (21 CFR 1040.10) (U.S. Food and Drug Administration, U.S. Department of Health and Human Services, 2009) requires that the operating manuals from the manufacturers provide the following information: calibration, maintenance, warning signs, nominal hazard zone, specific laser eyewear, and safety instructions that the laser safety officer can incorporate into standard operating procedures.

FDA and the National Center for Devices and Radiological Health

All medical lasers are regulated by the U.S. Food and Drug Administration (FDA) under the Medical Device Amendments to the Food and Drug Act, which apply primarily to laser manufacturers. These regulations are enforced by the National Center for Devices and Radiological Health (NCDRH). The FDA regulates more than 250 types of lasers, including those intended for medical and surgical use. The federal guidelines require manufacturers to classify the medical laser systems based on the laser's ability to cause damage to the eye and skin. They are categorized under FDA classification of medical devices as class III, subdivision class 4, because of the potential hazards. Manufacturers must conform to all safety requirements of the federal standard. They must also be approved by the NCDRH before any marketing or testing of a laser for a particular clinical application or use and must comply with the labeling requirements (ANSI, 2005).

American National Standards Institute

The American National Standards Institute (ANSI) is a voluntary organization of experts, including manufacturers, consumers, and scientific technical and professional organizations and government agencies, that determines industry consensus standards in technical fields. ANSI's mission is to provide a guide for the safe use of lasers and laser systems for diagnostic and therapeutic use in health care facilities. The first cohesive blueprint for building safe clinical laser services was the "American National Standard for the Safe Use of Lasers in Health Care Facilities," or ANSI Z136.3. ANSI Z136.3 implies that an adequate program for control of laser hazards be established in every health care facility that uses surgical lasers. The program must include provisions for a laser safety officer, education of users, protective measures, and management of accidents. ANSI Z136.3 covers many areas of lasers and their safe use, including terminology, hazard evaluation, classification, control measures, and administrative controls. Federal legislation and state laser safety regulations, as well as professional and advisory standards, are based on the ANSI (2005) standard.

Occupational Safety and Health Administration

The Occupational Safety and Health Administration (OSHA) is concerned primarily with the safety of health care workers. OSHA is the agency that can enforce the ANSI standards despite the fact that it does not have specific legislated regulations governing laser safety in health care facilities. OSHA can cite violations under the General Duty Clause (mandating that employers provide a safe workplace environment) if the level of compliance is not satisfactory (ANSI, 2005).

Nongovernmental Agencies

American Society for Lasers in Medicine and Surgery

In 1989 the American Society for Lasers in Medicine and Surgery (ASLMS) issued reports that were adopted as recommendations by the society's members. In 1990 the board of directors released nine recommended perioperative practices relating to patients undergoing laser procedures. These recommendations address assessment, nursing diagnosis, planning, implementation, and evaluation of nursing care (ANSI, 2005).

Association of periOperative Registered Nurses

"Recommended Practices for Laser Safety in the Practice Setting" was first published by the Association of periOperative Registered Nurses (AORN) (2009b) in 1989 with scheduled periodic review and update. These broad recommended practices provide recommendations to support perioperative nurses in developing policies and procedures for the safe use of lasers in their practice setting. These recommended practices represent an optimal level of practice. The AORN (2008) published "Surgical Smoke and Bio-Aerosols," a position statement that recommends the control of surgical smoke in surgical and laser procedures. In 2009 the AORN (2009c) *Surgical Smoke Evacuation Took Kit* was released to assist nurses with strategies to implement a smoke-free surgical environment.

The Joint Commission

The Joint Commission does not currently recommend specific guidelines for laser use; however, it recently added a statement about the control of hazardous gases, which includes the proper evacuation of surgical smoke. The Joint Commission inspectors note if health care facilities enforce compliance with their own specific laser policies and procedures (ANSI, 2005).

State Regulations

State regulations, along with the FDA, are the only guidelines for laser safety that are backed by legislative action. All other guidelines are recommended practices or standards and are based on the ANSI Z136.3 guidelines (ANSI, 2005). The concern over laser safety is reflected in the increasing number of states that are enacting medical laser safety legislation. Regulations governing the safe use of lasers present health care personnel with a complex set of guidelines.

Medical Device Regulations and Recommendations

The hazard classification system is based on the accessible radiation as set by the FDA and ANSI (Box 20-1). Both the FDA and ANSI define the classification of laser energy. Medical lasers typically follow the ANSI Z136.3 classification, but either classification system is acceptable (ANSI, 2005).

BOX 20-1 American National Standards Institute Classification of Lasers*

Class 1 Laser: Considered to be incapable of producing damaging levels of laser emission.
Class 2 Laser (low power): Applies only to visible laser emissions which may be viewed directly for time periods less than or equal to 0.25 seconds, which is the aversion response time.
Class 1M and 2M Laser: Poses the same risk to the unaided eye as do the class 1 and class 2 lasers, but may pose an increased ocular hazard from intrabeam viewing with certain optical instruments.
Class 3 Laser: May be hazardous for direct exposure or exposure to specular reflection, and are divided into two subclasses, 3R and 3B. Class 3R is a transitional, lower-risk group of lasers with reduced requirements. (Class 3R was formerly Class 3A)
Class 4 Laser: Presents significant eye, skin, and fire hazards and may pose hazardous diffuse reflections.

* Lasers are classified according to potential hazard of exposure.
From American National Standards Institute: *Safe use of lasers in health care facilities Z136.3*, Orlando, Fla., 2005, American National Standard for Safe Use of Lasers in Health Care Facilities, Laser Institute of America.

STANDARDS OF PRACTICE

Control of potential health hazards associated with the use of surgical laser systems requires adoption of appropriate safety standards and policies. It is imperative that everyone involved with medical lasers understand how to safely manage each type of laser in a medical setting. Before a laser is used clinically, a laser program should be established with written policies and procedures to establish authority, responsibility, and accountability.

The laser safety officer (LSO) is a person who has been appointed by the administration and has attained the training and education to administer a laser safety program. This does not mean the LSO must be present during every laser procedure. The LSO is responsible for appropriate classification of lasers within the facility, hazard evaluation, control measures, procedural approval, protective equipment, maintenance of equipment, training of all personnel associated with lasers, and medical surveillance. Box 20-2 lists requirements of the LSO.

Hazard Evaluation and Control Measures

Hazard evaluation is influenced by various factors of the laser system being used. The classification of the laser and the wavelength of the laser may also assist in defining the necessary control measures

BOX 20-2 Laser Safety Officer Requirements

- Certification: CMLSO Certified Medical Laser Safety Officer.
- Validation of training to include procedures and equipment or a minimal of 10 years' experience with multiple laser wavelengths and delivery systems.
- Basic understanding of the federal regulations associated with lasers.
- Professional Organizations: Member of the Laser Institute of America and the American Society for Lasers in Medicine and Surgery
- Candidates must have a 4-year degree or an AS degree from an accredited institution.
- One (1) year of experience with laser safety or acting as LSO, having performed the specific responsibilities outlined in ANSI Z136.3 Safe Use of Lasers in Health Care Facilities Standard.

Courtesy Vangie Dennis, Gwinnett Hospital System, Lawrenceville, Ga.

to be incorporated into the safety program. These factors affect which control measures need to be incorporated into the laser safety program and implemented into practice. Control measures are those procedures or methods implemented to minimize hazards associated with a particular laser when it is in the operational mode. Control measures may be influenced by the ability of the laser energy to injure, the environment in which the laser will be activated, personnel that may use or be exposed within the nominal hazard zone, the delivery systems, and the nonbeam hazards associated with the specific laser. Ancillary hazards create the potential for significant injuries to occur. Injuries, including death, may occur during testing of laser equipment, during electrical servicing, and from fires, explosions, and even embolisms.

Administrative Controls

Administrative controls specify the criteria for implementation of engineering controls or work practices for personnel protection. Standard operating procedures (SOPs) are established from institutional policies and procedures. Safety controls, maintenance and service, and the function of the laser should be incorporated into the facility's SOPs. SOPs may also include documentation requirements for preprocedure safety checklists and intraprocedural laser operation and safety. The LSO is responsible for the execution of the SOPs. Box 20-3 is an example of a system laser safety program policy that should be implemented if lasers are present within your system. Figure 20-1 is an example of a laser log that can be part of the permanent record. This is a paper version, but it can be replicated electronically.

Procedural and Equipment Controls

Engineering and procedural controls are determined by the LSO and implemented when appropriate to circumvent potential hazards. Procedural controls require adherence to written SOPs to ensure the safety of all personnel working in the region of lasers. For example, SOPs should provide for operational guidelines, emergency shut-off mechanisms, standby functions, use of low-reflective materials near the laser beam path, and laser storage.

Operational guidelines should require laser switches, whether foot pedal or finger trigger (which control the laser energy), to be guarded to prevent accidental activation. This may necessitate one foot-pedal access for the individual controlling the delivery device to prevent inadvertent activation of the laser. Accessory attachments to lasers must comply with the laser safety guidelines. This includes ensuring that there are laser filters on operating microscopes that protect the operator at the binocular viewing tube and through the accessory viewing tubes.

Lasers should be placed in the "standby" mode when the laser is on but not being fired or when the user in no longer in control of the delivery device to prevent accidental discharge. When not in use, storage of the laser and/or disabling of the laser is necessary to prevent inadvertent activation of the laser by nonauthorized personnel.

Nonreflective instruments (dull, anodized, or matte finished) should be used in or near the laser beam to defocus or disperse the laser beam. Appropriate backstops or guards should be used to prevent the laser beam from striking normal tissue or nontargeted tissues (ANSI, 2005).

Laser Treatment Controlled Area

The nominal hazard zone (NHZ) is the space in which the level of the direct, reflected, or

BOX 20-3 Laser Safety Program Safety Manual

POLICY

The Laser Safety Program (LSP) is established to promote safety in the use of lasers and for laser users at the Hospital System, in particular Class 3b and 4 lasers. The LSP is developed and administered in collaboration with the HS Safety Committee, Campus Director of Surgical Services, Patient Safety Coordinator and the Campus Laser Safety Officer. The Laser Safety Program is set up to provide guidelines that protect hospital associates, physicians and patients against hazards associated with the operation of lasers.

PROCEDURE/GUIDELINES

A. Responsibilities

1. Safety Committee—The Safety Committee establishes laser safety guidelines based on OSHA and ANSI accepted standards for laser users and provides support to laser users in complying with safety guidelines.
2. Patient Safety Coordinator
   a. Provides system oversight of LSP.
   b. Provides indirect supervision of LSP and Laser Safety Officers (LSOs) as delegated by the Safety Committee.
   c. Coordinates system-wide compliance with external regulatory requirements and reporting to the Safety Committee.
3. Director, Surgical Services
   a. Responsible for safe use of lasers in accordance with LSP.
   b. Provide direct supervision of the LSO.
   c. Establish and maintain an environment for the safe use of lasers.
   d. Address issues concerning laser safety that cannot be resolved by LSO.
   e. Ensure annual safety surveys of class 3b and 4 lasers for compliance with laser safety guidelines.
   f. Ensure that all physicians are properly credentialed to utilize lasers prior to use for patient care and treatment.
   g. Ensure that all lasers are reviewed for safe operations prior to purchase by LSO prior to use for patient care and treatment.
   h. Ensure that associates, physicians and/or contractors that use or work in the proximity of lasers receive the proper safety training.
4. Laser Safety Officer (LSO)
   a. Establish and maintain adequate policies and procedures for the control of the laser hazards.
   b. Verify classifications of lasers.
   c. Conduct hazard evaluation of laser work areas.
   d. Ensure that prescribed control measures are implemented and maintained.
   e. Approve Class 3 and Class 4 standard operating procedures (SOPs).
   f. Recommend, approve and audit protective equipment required to assure personnel safety.
   g. Review signs and equipment labels.
   h. Review Class 3 and Class 4 laser installations, facilities and laser equipment prior to use. This also applies to modification of existing facilities or equipment.
   i. Coordinate safety education and training for laser personnel.
   j. Determine the personnel categories as part of the medical surveillance program.
   k. Maintain required records, such as government regulations, maintenance of the safety program, training records, audits, SOP approvals, medical staff credentialing records, etc.
   l. Conduct inspections for the presence and functioning of laser safety features and control measures required for Class 3 and Class 4 lasers.
   m. Accompany regulatory agency inspectors (such as OSHA, FDA/NCDRH, state or local agencies) reviewing the laser safety program or investigating an incident and document any discrepancies or issues noted. Coordinate completion of corrective actions.
   n. Develop a response plan for notifications of incidents of actual or suspected exposure to potentially harmful laser radiation. Conduct investigations of accidents involving lasers.
   o. Maintain inventory of lasers and laser systems, and assign a Controlled Laser Authorization (CLA) for each laser.
   p. Make recommendations to the Patient Safety Coordinator and the Safety Committee for any changes or controls necessary for regulatory enforcement, and educational requirements and records.
   q. Inform the appropriate Occupational Safety and Health and the Safety Committee and request their assistance to help implement necessary safety recommendations.

Continued

BOX 20-3 Laser Safety Program Safety Manual—cont'd

r. Provide an annual report on the status of the Laser Safety Program to the Patient Safety Coordinator.

5. Other Personnel Responsibilities:
   a. Know the hazards and the precautionary procedures for laser use in their work area.
   b. Attend required training.
   c. Plan and conduct operations in accordance with established procedures and laser safety practices.
   d. Use personal protective equipment in accordance with prescribed training and policy.
   e. Operate lasers in a manner consistent with the requirements of the safety review.

B. Laser Education
1. The LSO, in collaboration with the Department Director/Manager, will assess and coordinate all education and training of the personnel who will operate the laser.
2. The LSO is responsible for validating competency of the vendor representative and those who train the authorized laser operators.
3. The LSO will work with the Medical Staff Coordinator and provide all necessary in-service records and training for physicians who utilize the laser.
4. The LSO has the authority to validate physicians on specific wavelengths of laser systems, but this does not negate the credentialing requirements of the specific surgical applications.

C. Laser Protective Eyewear
Approved protective eyewear will be worn whenever hazardous conditions may result from laser operations. Assistance in selecting eyewear may be obtained from the Laser Safety Officer.

D. Visual Warnings
Appropriate warning labels will be conspicuously displayed on the laser system. Appropriate warning signs will be posted outside the operating area. The signal word "CAUTION" will be used on all signs and labels associated with Class 2 lasers. The signal word "DANGER" will be used on all signs and labels associated with Class 3 and Class 4 lasers.

Courtesy Vangie Dennis, Gwinnett Hospital System, Lawrenceville, Ga.
ANSI, American National Standards Institute; *FDA,* U.S. Food and Drug Administration; *NCDRH,* National Center for Devices and Radiological Health; *OSHA,* Occupational Safety and Health Administration.

scattered radiation used during the normal laser operation exceeds the applicable maximum permissible exposure (MPE). A NHZ should be identified by the LSO to prevent unintentional exposure to the laser beam. Determination of the NHZ should take into consideration information gathered from the manufacturer's labeling and by analysis, the radiation transmission of the beam, and the potential for equipment failure. The NHZ is usually contained within the room but may extend through open doors or transparent windows, depending on the type of laser used. It is the responsibility of the LSO to define the NHZ and ensure that the proper safety practices are adhered to in the NHZ (ANSI, 2005).

The appropriate warning signs should posted at every entryway into the laser treatment controlled area and should define the NHZ. The symbols and wording on the warning sign should be specific for the type of laser in use and designed according to the information described in ANSI Z136.3.

Windows and viewing areas should be limited because the NHZ may reach beyond the room in which the laser is in use. Additional safety controls, such as closing doors and covering windows with applicable filters or barriers or restricting traffic, depend on the laser used. Screens, curtains, or a blocking barrier may be placed near entryways to avert laser radiation.

Only authorized persons, approved by the LSO, should be in the vicinity of the NHZ. Only authorized laser operators that have been delegated specific responsibilities by the LSO may operate a laser. An authorized laser operator is a person trained in laser safety and approved by the facility to operate the laser. This person is

LASER PROCEDURE RECORD

PLACE LABEL HERE

Date: ________

Diagnosis: ________

Procedure: ________

SURGICAL TEAM

Physician: ________

Assistant: ________

Anesthesia: ________

CRNA: ________

Scrub: ________

Circulator: ________

Laser Personnel: ________

Comments: ________

LASER SAFETY PRECAUTIONS

	Yes	No	N/A
Electrical cords inspected			
Laser signs all entrances			
Appropriate eyewear on door			
Cover windows			
Laser mask			
Smoke evacuator			
Rectal pack			
Check fiber integrity			
Basin of water/saline			
Fire extinguisher			
Laser retardant drapes			
Nonflammable prep			
Nonreflective instruments			
Cover fiber tip/handpiece			
Wet towels/4 × 4s at surgical site			
One equipment foot pedal access			
Glasses inspected upon distribution			
PM verified per rental company			

EQUIPMENT/DELIVERY SYSTEMS

Laparoscope	____	Laryngoscope	____
Handpiece	____	Bronchoscope	____
Cystoscope	____	Scanner	____
Gastroscope	____	Disc Probe	____
Micromanipulator	____		

FIBERS

Size: ________

Type: ________

LASERS

Type: ________

Biomed #: ________

Assessment: ________

LASER ENERGY

Watts	____	Ultra/super pulse	____
Milliwatts	____	Pulses	____
Average watts	____	Spot size	____
Total energy	____	Mill joules	____
Joules	____		
Hertz	____		

HEAD, NECK, AND CHEST

Time on	____	Time off	____
Time on	____	Time off	____
Time on	____	Time off	____
Time on	____	Time off	____
Time on	____	Time off	____

EYE PROTECTION

Surgeon	____	Patient	____
Scrub	____	Taped	____
Circulator	____	Wet 4 × 4	____
Anesthesiologist	____	Eyewear	____
Anesthetist	____	Opaque block	____
Laser operator	____		

ANESTHESIA PRECAUTIONS

Endotracheal Tubes:		Gases:	
Mallinckrodt	____	Helium	____
Laser Shield II	____	Compress air	____
		Circuit lines protected	____
		O_2 sat. @ 30%	____
		Location of:	
		Trach tray	____
		Trachs	____
		Bronchoscopes	____

COMMENTS

____

____

Laser Personnel Signature: ________

FIGURE 20-1 Laser procedure record. (Courtesy Vangie Dennis, Gwinnett Hospital System, Lawrenceville, Ga.)

responsible for the safety of the equipment and the treatment environment in the NHZ. The person must remain at the laser control while the laser is in use. The operator's responsibilities include the following:

- Assessing the procedure needs, including anesthesia needs, type of laser, and accessory equipment
- Checking equipment before use, including accessories, operation, and safety equipment, to ensure safe working order

- Implementing safety controls for all personnel (including the patient) in the treatment area, such as wearing appropriate eyewear
- Displaying appropriate signage
- Setting the laser wattage and exposure as requested by the physician
- Monitoring activation of the laser and observation of team members for breaks in safety
- Completing a safety checklist and laser log

All health care personnel in the vicinity of the NHZ should be trained in implementation of all laser safety precautions to avoid inadvertent exposure to laser hazards. All personnel, including the patient, within the NHZ should use appropriate personal protective equipment (PPE) (ANSI, 2005).

Maintenance and Service of Lasers

Preventative maintenance should be performed every 6 months. Only properly educated, trained, and approved technicians should be allowed to work on the laser or handle the electrical components.

Protective Equipment

Eye Protection

The eye is the organ that is most susceptible to laser injury. Everyone in the NHZ, including the patient, should wear appropriate eyewear approved by the laser safety officer. The optics of the eye can concentrate and focus laser light, at wavelengths ranging from 400 to 1400 nm. This creates an optical concentration of 100,000 times on the retina, which increases the potential ocular hazard. Ultraviolet and far-infrared wavelength regions (outside 400 to 1400 nm) principally produce corneal effects. Also, laser radiation at certain wavelengths may cause damage to the lens of the eye. Appropriate laser safety eyewear filters out the hazardous wavelength of laser radiation. In addition to direct exposure from misdirected and damaged fibers, scattered, diffused, and reflected laser beams can cause eye injuries. Laser protective eyewear may include goggles, face shields, glasses, prescription glasses with special filters or coatings, and patient corneal shields (Laser Institute of America, 2007a).

The patient's eyes and eyelids should be protected from the laser beam by appropriate methods when the eyes are in the NHZ. Protective methods may include wet eye pads, laser protective eyewear, or laser-specific eye shields. Corneal eye shields may be necessary when goggles or glasses interfere with the laser treatment.

All personnel in the NHZ should wear protective eyewear that is labeled with the appropriate optical density and wavelength while the laser is in use. Ocular hazards may transpire during operational pretesting of the laser to confirm beam alignment and calibration. Potential for ocular hazards is also present during fiberoptic procedures as a result of the fiber becoming disconnected or breaking. Both instances also require protective eyewear to be used to prevent exposure of the eye. Protective eyewear should be available outside the room near the posted warning signs designating the specific type of laser in use. For optimal protection, inspect eyewear for pitting, cracking, discoloration, coating damage, frame condition, and light leaks. If any of these are present, the eyewear is considered inadequate for eye protection and should be discarded (ANSI, 2005).

Skin Protection

Whenever there is a potential hazard of thermal burns from high-powered lasers, all persons in the laser treatment area should be protected from laser beam exposure to their skin and other nontargeted tissues. Overexposure to ultraviolet radiation can lead to skin sensitivities or even burns from direct or reflected laser energy. Surgical gloves, tightly woven fabrics, and flame-retardant material, depending on the laser being used, may provide skin protection. Protection of exposed tissues around the operative site may be accomplished by covering the areas with saline-saturated or water-saturated, fire/flame-retardant materials (e.g., towels, sponges, drapes, fabrics). These materials must remain moist to absorb or disperse the energy of the laser beam. Polypropylene or plastic drapes can melt if a laser beam strikes them, and woven or nonwoven fabrics can be ignited. Laser handpieces or fiber tips should be placed on a moistened surface to prevent fire from the hot tip or shattering of the tip if placed on a cold surface (Laser Institute of America, 2007b).

LASER SAFETY AND TRAINING PROGRAMS

A laser safety program establishes and maintains policies and procedures to ensure control of laser hazards. The policies and procedures should include the following:

- LSO guidelines defining the authority and responsibility for evaluation and control of laser hazards. A laser committee may need to be developed when increased laser usage necessitates maintaining enforcement of SOPs.
- Criteria and education for procedures for all personnel working in an NHZ. All personnel working with lasers should attend laser safety education courses periodically.
- Credentialing and clinical practice privileges of the medical staff are the health care facility's responsibility. Credentialing should be for specific laser procedures with specific laser types.
- Implementation of laser hazard control measures.
- A continuous quality improvement program that includes appropriate use and maintenance of equipment, management and reporting of accidents, and prevention actions to minimize injuries.

A laser education program for personnel working with or around lasers, for the facility's specific laser(s) and specific to the procedures being performed in the facility, must be implemented. The program must comply with applicable standards and regulations covering all procedures necessary to provide a safe environment. Personnel should demonstrate and complete competency skills periodically (ANSI, 2005).

Medical Surveillance

Medical surveillance for all Class 3b and Class 4 laser users exposed to laser radiation in the NHZ should be performed as a preemployment examination and when abnormal exposures have occurred. Surveillance is specific to the personnel category and the known risks associated with the particular laser operated. Personnel categories are divided into laser personnel who routinely work in the NHZ and incidental personnel who are unlikely to be exposed to laser energy (e.g., custodial, supervisory, clerical). Surveillance may be required to assess a baseline level of visual performance to assist in the evaluation of laser damage in the case of inadvertent exposure to the eye. Surveillance can also identify those individuals who may be at risk from ultraviolet hazards, specifically to the skin. Laser accidents must be documented to define the need for further evaluation of the injured person (ANSI, 2005).

Laser Hazards

Nonbeam Hazards

Hazards other than those directly related to exposure to the laser (e.g., eye, skin, and other tissues) are known as nonbeam hazards. Potential hazards related to nonbeam hazards are diverse, and the LSO must determine the appropriate control methods to be implemented. Evaluations of the hazards may necessitate enlisting the assistance of safety and/or industrial hygiene personnel from OSHA.

Electrical Hazards

Lasers contain high-voltage electrical circuits that may lead to shock, electrocution, or fire. These types of hazards are some of the leading causes of laser-related accidents and deaths. Potential electrical hazards from damaged electrical cords, faulty grounding, lack of compliance with training programs, or inadequate or inappropriate use of lockout/tag out procedures can be prevented by adherence to SOPs of the facility. Visual inspection of the laser, including electrical, plumbing, accessory equipment, delivery systems, gas supply, and sterile draping, before use may prevent injuries from occurring. Observance of general electrical safety (e.g., no fluids placed on or near lasers, extension cords not used to power lasers) will also support the maintenance of safety.

Smoke Plume

Vaporization of tissues may release toxic substances (e.g., acetone, isopropanol, toluene, formaldehyde, metal fumes, and cyanide), as well as carcinogens and viruses, from the cells. This laser plume contains water, carbonized particles, mutated DNA, and intact cells. At certain concentrations, ocular and upper respiratory tract irritation and unpleasant odors may transpire. These substances should not be inhaled; this initiates the need for some type of smoke evacuation system to be used to prevent personnel and the patient from inhaling plume. Removal of plume will also enhance the visualization of the surgical/treatment site and may prevent the laser beam from potentially being reflected.

Smoke plume inhalation should be reduced to a minimum by using multiple controls. These controls may include the use of high-filtration masks, wall suction units with in-line filters, and smoke evacuators. High-filtration masks should be used in conjunction with other controls and not as a sole means for protection. These masks should be tight fitting and capable of filtering particles as small as 0.1 μm. Wall suction systems with an in-line filter may be used when the generation of a minimal amount of plume is expected, such as during laparoscopic cases. Wall suctions generate low suction rates and are designed for fluids; thus an in-line filter should be used to collect particulate matter. A mechanical smoke evacuator or suction with an ultra-low penetration air filter and activated charcoal filter should be used when a large amount of laser plume is expected. These systems should be turned on simultaneously with the activation of the laser energy and placed as close as possible to the laser site. Standard precautions (gloves and mask) should be taken when using lasers, as well as when handling contaminated filters, because of the amount of potential contaminants generated. Box 20-4 is an example of a surgical plume policy. Keep in mind that electrosurgical plume can be generated with all types of energy sources, such as electrosurgical units.

BOX 20-4 Methods of Removing Surgical Smoke Plume

Examples of procedures which require an in-line filter on the suction line which is positioned between the wall outlet and the suction canister:

Temporal artery biopsy
Hand procedures
Vocal cord polyps
Tonsillectomies
Laparoscopies
Ear procedures
Dermatological procedures
Nasal procedures
Thoracoscopy
Back procedures
Craniotomies
Breast biopsies

Examples of procedures which require a smoke evacuator with an evacuation hose:

Abdominal surgical procedures
Breast reduction procedures
Large extremity procedures
Vaporization of condyloma
Thoracic procedures
Excisional neck procedures
Spinal fusions

Courtesy Vangie Dennis, Gwinnett Hospital System, Lawrenceville, Ga.

Fire and Explosion Hazards

Fire is a potential hazard that can have devastating consequences. Laser energy can ignite flammable liquids, solids, and gases. Fire occurring with these types of materials most often materializes outside the patient, but fires can ignite with materials in the patient. The AORN (2009b) states that "all persons in the laser treatment area should be protected from flammability hazards associated with laser use." Becoming aware of the potential hazards and adherence to safeguards can protect the patient and health care personnel.

Personnel should be aware of the items that have a potential for causing fire, burns, or explosions. These may include surgical drapes, endotracheal tubes, paper or gauze materials, gases (e.g., oxygen, methane, anesthetic gases), and flammable liquids or ointments (e.g., skin preparation solutions, oil-based lubricants). Irrigation solution (e.g., water or saline) and CO_2 fire extinguishers should be readily available where lasers are used.

Methane gas from the anus or large bowel should be prevented from entering the area where laser energy is dispersed by covering the area with wet towels or packing the anus with wet gauze or packing. Preparation solutions should be nonflammable. Any compound or solution containing alcohol (e.g., alcohol-based preparation solutions, tape removers, degreasers, benzoin, and tinctures) can ignite from contact with laser energy. Alcohol vapors should not be allowed to accumulate under drapes. Overheating of iodoforms that tend to pool on or around the skin or aerosolized preparation solutions can lead to flash fires when laser energy is used.

Oxygen concentration in the room should be kept to a minimum. The anesthesia provider should be aware of the hazards of oxygen leaking from around a patient's face mask. The anesthesia provider should be prepared to turn off the free flow of oxygen immediately, if needed.

SPECIALTY PROCEDURES

Fiber Optic Delivery

When a fiber is used to deliver laser energy, whether through a flexible or rigid endoscope, the fiber should extend beyond the end of the endoscope. This will prevent laser beam exposure to the inside lumen or the end of the sheath. Endoscope lenses can easily be damaged, resulting in lens pitting or even shattering. The endoscope sheath may become overheated if the laser energy is activated while the fiber is still within the sheath, resulting in thermal damage not only to the scope but also potentially to the patient's adjacent or surrounding tissues.

Coupling Arm

There are automatic shut-off features incorporated into some laser equipment. There is no protection from inadvertent beam delivery if the arm becomes unattached; therefore the laser operator must make certain the coupled attachment is secured and must be at the laser panel in the event that the deactivation of the laser is required.

Bronchoscopic Couplers

Couplers used with the CO_2 laser with bronchoscopy must have an optical system that allows the visible helium-neon beam to pass coaxially with the invisible CO_2 laser beam. Burns to the patient's trachea, larynx, pharynx, and oral cavity have occurred as a direct result of a misaligned beam.

Airway Concerns

Guidelines to minimize the risks associated with lasers and other energy modalities should be incorporated into the OR team's practices. There are various types of laser-dedicated endotracheal tubes. The type of laser wavelength used dictates the specific type of endotracheal tube. Some tubes have FDA clearances for specific wavelengths of lasers. The red rubber reusable tube wrapped in aluminum foil tape is not an acceptable laser tube and is not approved by the FDA. This tube is an evolved practice for which there are articles published in the medical literature stating that this is an acceptable tube in the beginning of laser ear, nose, and throat (ENT) airway applications, but with the advent of new FDA-approved laser tubes for specific wavelengths, this wrapped tube should not be used. The polyvinylchloride (PVC) endotracheal tube is contraindicated with laser airway procedures when the tube is in direct contact with the laser beam. PVC material is very flammable, and the byproducts of combustion are hydrochloric gas and, in the presence of fluid, hydrochloric acid. All tubes under pressure are potentially explosive. Special endotracheal tubes designed for use during laser procedures should be used when surgery is being performed on the airway. The manufacturer's specific guidelines must be adhered to when these tubes are being used.

Considerations should be taken when choosing the appropriate anesthetic agent. No one anesthetic technique is used to the exclusion of others. Helium and compressed air are acceptable gases to use during laser procedures. Helium is a less-dense gas and has the ability to flow through compromised airways more easily than compressed air. Helium will also retard burning, but the risks of delivering hypoxic levels can be a problem. Pulse oximetry should always be used with helium delivery. Nitrous oxide is contraindicated in upper airway laser surgery. Nitrous oxide, in the presence of oxygen, will present as if 100% oxygen is being delivered. The fraction of inspired oxygen concentration (FiO_2) should be no higher than 30%. A value above the 30% range supports combustion.

The cuff of the endotracheal tube should be instilled with normal saline or water mixed with methylene blue dye. The saline or water will serve as an extinguisher and the methylene blue dye as an indicator that the cuff has been breached (ANSI, 2005).

Areas of the patient's face accessible to the laser should be protected from stray beams. The patient's eyes should be covered with wet sponges or laser conformers as indicated by the surgical procedure. Water-soluble lubricant is indicated if a laser is used. Petroleum-based lubricant is flammable and therefore contraindicated.

Before any laser airway procedure, staff should familiarize themselves with the procedural steps to managing an airway fire. The steps are as follows:

1. Immediately disconnect the breathing circuit and remove the endotracheal tube (ECRI Institute, 2009). Disconnection of the breathing circuit is the quickest method of stopping the gas flow.
2. Extinguish the fire with water/saline. This may be done by another member of the surgical team. The operating room staff and anesthesia provider should have water/saline readily available on the operating room back table and anesthesia cart.
3. Remove any remaining material in the airway that may be left smoldering. Irrigate airway tissue with sterile water/saline, allowing for cooling of tissue and to extinguish any remaining embers (ECRI Institute, 2009).
4. Access to the bronchoscopes and tracheotomy trays should be readily available. The location of the instruments should be established prior to any airway procedure. Failure to remove any pieces of the tube will allow the tube to continue to burn in the patient.

During head and neck surgeries the patient is mechanically ventilated in the majority of the procedures. If precautionary protocols are not followed and instantaneous action is not taken if an airway fire occurs, hot gases can be forced deep into the lungs, causing extensive injuries. Seconds of indecision or confusion can cause irreparable damage or death to the patient. The management of airway procedures, as well as the collaborative communication among the operating team members, is essential for patient safety and quality care. The development of airway safety protocols involving head, neck, and chest procedures should be a collaborative effort between the department of anesthesia and surgical services (Box 20-5) (ANSI, 2005).

LASER RENTALS

Health care costs are rising, and reimbursements are dwindling. Many hospitals are considering alternatives to bringing expensive technology into the operating rooms. Over the past decade, the use of laser rental companies has increased. Renting a laser system has proved to be a viable solution for providing laser services without incurring the costs of expensive capital acquisitions, service contracts, and personnel to operate the laser system. Health care facilities often have the misconception that when a laser is rented, the health care facility does not have the responsibility or accountability for the laser operator provided by the rental company or for actions of their own personnel. Laser rental companies and health care facilities need to consider and should understand the roles and responsibilities each has during the laser procedure.

Laser rental companies' competencies should be no less stringent than those required for health care facility personnel. The AORN (2009a) guidance statement "The Role of the Health Care Industry Representative in the Perioperative/Invasive Procedure Setting" states that the competency of an individual who provides direct or indirect patient care should be held to the same requirements as the hospital employee. AORN recognizes the need for a structured process for education, training, and introduction of procedures, techniques, technology, and equipment to health care professionals practicing within the perioperative/invasive procedure setting. Competencies are not and should not be limited to validation of a laser course as recommended by ANSI (2005), which includes laser physics, safety, and hands-on demonstration that is wavelength and specialty specific. Other requirements for credentialing may include Health Insurance Portability and Accountability Act regulations, health and safety protocols, age-specific competencies, immunizations, background checks, and operating room protocols. The laser company should appoint an LSO for the company to develop and monitor its own policies and procedures, as well as designing and monitoring its own laser log. Validation and competencies should be required yearly for the laser rental personnel just as a hospital or medical facility requires competencies to be assessed annually. Furthermore, when the laser rental company brings a laser into the health care facility, the employee of the company must understand the policies, procedures, and credentialing criteria specific to that health care facility (Dennis, 2008).

Laser companies have provided an alternative to the purchase of expensive laser systems, and many health care facilities rely heavily on these companies to provide the expertise in assisting with their laser services. Many health care facilities assume that the medical-legal responsibility and accountability is the liability of the company. Both the laser rental company and the health care facility must understand their own medical-legal responsibility and accountability.

CONCLUSION

Regardless of the clinical setting, the presence of laser equipment creates a need for unique control measures and work practice. Laser safety is the responsibility of both the company and the hospital, with a collaborative approach to patient and personnel safety. All personnel involved in the care of a patient during laser procedure and in the vicinity of the NHZ should be educated appropriately to maintain a safe environment for patient care. A well-developed laser safety program that is created and administrated according to the ANSI Z136 standards can minimize hazards and promote patient safety when implemented properly. When everyone understands and puts into practice the fundamentals of maintaining a laser-safe environment, the risk of accidents resulting from lack of education, training, or noncompliance with policy is greatly reduced (Dennis, 2008).

REFERENCES

American National Standards Institute: *Safe use of lasers in health care facilities Z136.3*, Orlando, Fla, 2005, Laser Institute of America.

Association of periOperative Registered Nurses: *Position statement on surgical smoke and bio-aerosols*, April 2008, available at http://www.aorn.org/PracticeResources/AORNPositionStatements/SurgicalSmokeAndBioAerosols/. Accessed August 21, 2009.

Association of periOperative Registered Nurses: Guidance statement: the role of the health care industry representative in the perioperative setting. In Association of periOperative Registered Nurses: *Perioperative standards and recommended practices*, 2009 ed, pp. 204–206, Denver, 2009a, The Association.

Association of periOperative Registered Nurses: Recommended practices for laser safety in practice settings. In Association of periOperative Registered Nurses, Denver, 2009b, The Association *Perioperative standards and recommended practices*, 2009 ed, pp. 367–372.

Association of periOperative Registered Nurses: *Surgical smoke evacuation tool kit*, 2009c, available at http://www.aorn.org/PracticeResources/ToolKits/SurgicalSmokeEvacuationToolKit/. Accessed August 21, 2009.

Ball K: *The perioperative challenge*, ed 3, Denver, Co, 2004, Association of periOperative Registered Nurses.

Bertolotti M: *The history of the laser*, Bristol, UK, 2004, (translation; originally published in1999), Institute of Physics.

Carruth J, McKenzie A: *Medical lasers—science and clinical practice*, Bristol, UK, 1986, A Hilger.

Dennis V: Play it safe with medical lasers, *Biophotonics International*. December 2008, available at http://www.photonics.com/Content/ReadArticle.aspx?ArticleID=36060. Accessed August 10, 2009.

ECRI Institute: New clinical guide to surgical fire prevention, *Health Devices* 38(19):314–332, October 2009.

Laser Institute of America: *Guide for the selection of laser eye protection*, ed 6, Orlando, 2007a, The Institute.

Laser Institute of America: *Laser safety guide*, ed 11, Orlando, 2007b, The Institute.

Laserscope Greenlight PV: *Physician training manual, revision F.0126-3230*, San Jose, Calif, 2002, Laserscope.

Maiman TH: *Nature*, 187, 493–494, 1960.

U.S. Food and Drug Administration, U.S. Department of Health and Human Services: *CFR—Code of Federal Regulations Title 21*, 2009. Silver Springs, Md., available at http://www.accessdata.fda.gov/scripts/cdrh/cfdocs/cfcfr/CFRSearch.cfm?FR=1040.10. Accessed November 9, 2009.

PREVENTING BACK INJURIES

Patient Transfer and Mobility

Reuben J. DeKastle, MSHA, BN, RN, CNOR

PERIOPERATIVE BACK INJURIES—PERSPECTIVES AND CHALLENGES

Nurses have traditionally been willing to sacrifice their own bodies for the sake of their patients. When a patient begins to slip, nurses are more inclined to seek to catch them rather than safely guide their fall. The urgency of setup and turnovers in the operating room (OR) may prompt a perioperative nurse to ignore assistive devices or not take the time to call for extra help. For many it is an expectation that they will have a back injury as an outcome of their career. Nurses will compromise their own well-being for the benefit of others. Although the intent of these actions is noble, the outcomes often leave nurses in physical states in which they can no longer care for anyone but themselves.

Back Injuries Statistics

Nurses are typically within the top ten categories of professions to suffer from work-related spine injuries. When combined with associated caregivers such as nursing aides, attendants, and orderlies, they make up the largest single number (de Castro, 2004). Nelson et al (2009) state, "Patient transfer tasks are high risk and occur in every clinical setting." Some studies indicate that annually 40,000 nurses report back-related injuries, and that 12% of nurses who leave the profession each year do so because of back injuries (O'Malley et al, 2006; American Nurses Association, 2009). Another 52% complain of back pain (Nelson and Baptiste, 2004). The nursing shortage could potentially be eliminated if qualified nurses were able to live out their careers rather than have their careers cut short by spine injuries. It stands to reason that if back injuries account for the highest percentages of nurses leaving the profession and are the largest factor contributing to the nursing shortage (O'Malley et al, 2006), then preventive programs should be at least as important as additional nursing programs. It is estimated that back injuries in the health care industry account for approximately $20 billion annually (Bell et al, 2008). In addition, there are indirect costs of "overtime, decreased morale, use of replacement workers, continual hiring and training cycles, and increased worker compensation and employee healthcare costs" (Spry, 2009).

Bariatrics

Another factor that has changed the nature of patient handling is the rise in obesity. The bariatric population of North America is growing and shows no signs of plateauing anytime soon (Hurd, 2009). In the United States alone, the bariatric population has soared to 38 million in the past decade. Muir et al (2007) define the obese patient as anyone over 350 lb or someone with a body mass index of greater than 49. They further estimate that about one quarter of the bariatric population is classified as severely obese. These patients arrive with increased morbidity and mobility issues. They are making up an increasing percentage of the surgical population, not just for bariatric-specific procedures, but often for the comorbidities that are associated with excessive weight. Michelle McCleery, RN, PHD, manager of safety programs for Hill-Rom, has said, "I've never talked with one hospital that did not see a relationship between the increase in the severely obese patient population and staff injuries" (Safety in mobility, 2004). No longer are perioperative staff safe to just count to three and then "heave-ho." To prevent spinal injury, it will take a team effort, using all available resources accompanied by a change in culture, emphasizing safety over expediency. If we do not initiate some of the back injury prevention measures from a nursing model, it will be done for us by a legislated mandate, as has already occurred in a number of states.

The Gender Factor

Further contributing to the high numbers of back injuries in the nursing profession is the well-known fact that it is a predominantly female profession. In a classic article published in the *Lancet* in 1965, the authors used scientific measures to indicate the physiologic differences between males and females in their oxygen consumption, lifting power, and degree of sustaining capabilities when lifting an object over a period of time. The evidence was clear that females in the nursing profession are at a distinct physical disadvantage while doing tasks that would not be tolerated in male-dominated professions (Tsolaki et al, 1965). Some studies have specifically focused weight-tolerance measurements on what is safe for females. The small percentage of men in the nursing profession might find it frustrating if they were to be considered the brawn of the unit. We may all agree that simply recruiting men into the profession will not likely solve the musculoskeletal injuries in the nursing profession and especially in the operating room. We will need to look to other more viable and sustainable solutions that work for both genders.

The Aging Workforce

As society and legislated expectations gradually raise the anticipated age of retirement, aging nurses will seek to remain employed longer into the years that traditionally have been considered the retirement years. Minimizing the risks of personal injury in the workplace may provide a safe place to live out those years, as well as serve as an enticement for novice nurses to seek employment in a distinctly safer environment. The discerning nurse may begin choosing a place of employment based not merely on money and geography, but rather on the safe work culture of the prospective employer.

BARRIERS AND HAZARDS

A multitude of factors may negatively influence back injuries. The aging workforce, staffing shortages, nurse's self-sacrificing ethic, obesity of both patient and staff, increasing acuity of the patient population accompanied by decreased patient mobility, and institutional cultural expectations are all factors that influence the prevalence of back injuries.

One of the largest barriers to eliminating back injuries in the perioperative setting is the nursing ethic of putting the patient's well-being ahead of one's own. There are numerous other barriers to safe back care within the perioperative setting. Most equipment and safe patient handling programs that are available in the hospital setting are designed for a medical/surgical floor and adapt very poorly to the OR. Lift teams are outlined in the literature but focus exclusively on non-OR environments. Many of the patient transfer devices are not designed to fit into the OR context. For example, the spread legs of a typical lift device will not go under a solid-based OR bed, yet to be stable, especially for bariatric patients, this would be required. Ceiling lifts are very difficult to retrofit into existing ORs because of the existence of booms, ceiling lights, and ventilation systems. Murphy (2009) states, "You wouldn't be able to use overhead lifts in the OR."

Defining the Limits

"No one can define a weight where it is safe to lift" (Safety in mobility, 2004). The National Institute for Occupational Safety and Health (NIOSH) had estimated that the average worker should limit his or her lifting to 51 lb (de Castro, 2004). Since then, further studies have lowered that number to 35 lb (Nelson et al, 2009; Waters et al, 2009). Measures that have sought to quantify how much weight an individual should be able to safely lift fail to factor in the fact that patients do not come with handles, do not have their weight evenly distributed, and can be either predictably or unexpectedly combative. Added to this is the fact that patients are often in positions that require flexion and awkward posture of the caregiver, combining for a less-than-ideal position or location for lifting, even if the patient is an appropriate weight. Waters et al (2009) indicate that a female should not lift more than 11.1 lb in a one-handed lift. In the OR this may exclude lifting limbs for preparation or even some pieces of equipment that exceed this weight. Table 21-1 shows the typical weights of various body parts.

TABLE 21-1 Lifting and Holding Legs, Arms, and Head for Prepping

Ergonomic Tool #3

Patient Weight lbs (kg)	Body Part	Body Part Weight lbs (kg)		Lift 1-hand	Lift 2-hand	Hold 2-hand <1 min	Hold 2-hand <2 min	Hold 2-hand <3 min
<120 lbs (< 54 kg)	Leg	< 19 lbs	(9 kg)					
	Arm	< 6 lbs	(3 kg)					
	Head	< 10 lbs	(5 kg)					
120–160 lbs (54–73 kg)	Leg	< 25 lbs	(11 kg)					
	Arm	< 8 lbs	(4 kg)					
	Head	< 13 lbs	(6 kg)					
160–200 lbs (73–91 kg)	Leg	< 31 lbs	(14 kg)					
	Arm	< 10 lbs	(5 kg)					
	Head	< 17 lbs	(8 kg)					
200–240 lbs (91–109 kg)	Leg	< 38 lbs	(17 kg)					
	Arm	< 12 lbs	(6 kg)					
	Head	< 20 lbs	(9 kg)					
240–280 lbs (109–127 kg)	Leg	< 44 lbs	(20 kg)					
	Arm	< 14 lbs	(6 kg)					
	Head	< 24 lbs	(11 kg)					
280–320 lbs (127–145 kg)	Leg	< 50 lbs	(23 kg)					
	Arm	< 16 lbs	(7 kg)					
	Head	< 27 lbs	(12 kg)					
>360 lbs (>163 kg)	Leg	> 57 lbs	(26 kg)					
	Arm	> 18 lbs	(8 kg)					
	Head	> 30 lbs	(14 kg)					

No shading: OK to lift and hold; use clinical judgment and do not hold longer than noted.

Heavy shading: Do not lift alone; use assistive device or more than one caregiver.

From Nelson A et al: Development of the AORN guidance statement: safe patient handling and movement in the perioperative setting. In Peterson C, editor: *AORN guidance statement: safe patient handling and movement in the perioperative setting*, Denver, 2007, Association of periOperative Registered Nurses.

Unique Operating Room Challenges

The challenges of the OR are unique to the OR. Positioning a patient into a prone position on a spine table, tower table, or Wilson frame would be impractical with lift equipment. Repositioning an intubated patient requires the gentle measures of the human touch. Adding an equipment component to this action should be as an adjunct to fine-tuning the personal element rather than the other way around.

Ergonomic Stressors

The *AORN Position Statement on Ergonomically Healthy Workplace Practices* (2006) identifies ergonomic stressors that are likely to contribute to back injuries during patient handling tasks. These include the following:

1. Forceful tasks—such as pushing a stretcher over carpeted floors
2. Repetitive motions—such as passing instruments
3. Awkward posture—such as holding a retractor in a vaginal hysterectomy (Figure 21-1)
4. Static posture—such as maintaining a position for a prolonged period while scrubbed in (Figure 21-2)
5. Moving or lifting patients and equipment—without adequate support or equipment
6. Carrying heavy instruments and equipment—such as hastily retrieving a tray of instruments from the supply room rather than finding a cart to wheel it with

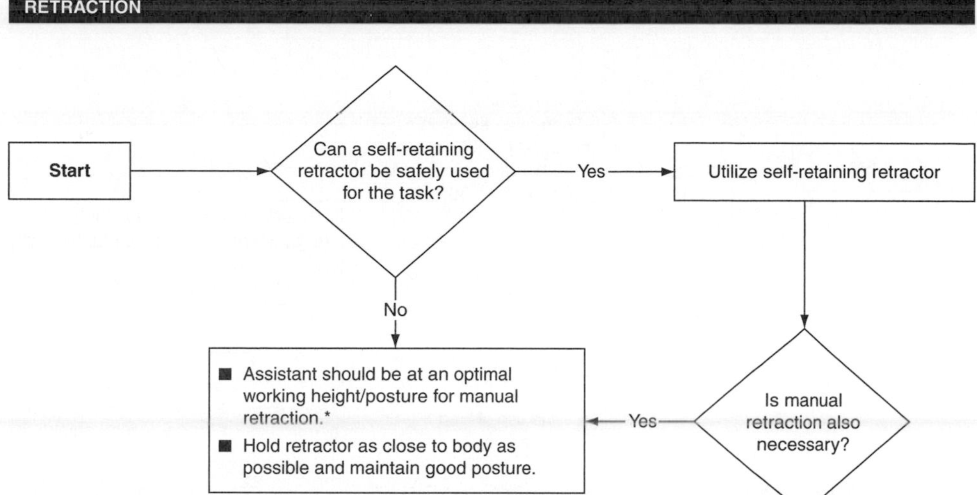

FIGURE 21-1 Ergonomic tool for retraction. (From Nelson A et al: Development of the AORN guidance statement: safe patient handling and movement in the perioperative setting. In Peterson C, editor: *AORN guidance statement: safe patient handling and movement in the perioperative setting*, Denver, 2007, Association of periOperative Registered Nurses.)

7. Overexertion—such as dealing with a combative patient

Other ergonomic stressors are listed in Box 21-1.

Expectations of Efficiency

Another barrier to eliminating back injuries is the inherent expectation of speed in the OR. When it is difficult to get the whole team to stop for a surgical time-out, who will have the patience required to wait for the OR team to appropriately position a patient for surgery with elaborate lift equipment? The culture of the OR may need to be confronted until safety outweighs expediency.

Ergonomic Hazards

Many additional hazards await the OR team member. Night shifts are noted to produce higher rates of injuries, because the lack of resources may lead one to take more risks. Working long shifts of greater than 12 hours or working over 40 hours per week is also "associated with a 50% to 170% age-adjusted rate of musculoskeletal disorders of the neck, shoulders and back" (Mathias and Patterson, 2005). In addition, mandatory overtime, increased work pace, and increased physical and psychologic demands are further hazards for back injury (*Safe patient handling*, 2006).

Musculoskeletal injuries increase in proportion to the frequency of actions such as forceful pushing and pulling, twisting, and assuming awkward positions for lifting or transferring (Nelson et al, 2009). The activity most likely to lead to back injury while lifting is the action of twisting while lifting a load (Lavender et al, 2007). The study also concluded that when proper body mechanics were employed, the injury rates were not affected significantly until a twisting motion was included in the activity (Lavender et al, 2007). Wardell (2007) stated that "Nurses spend between 20% and 30% of their work time bending

PROLONGED STANDING

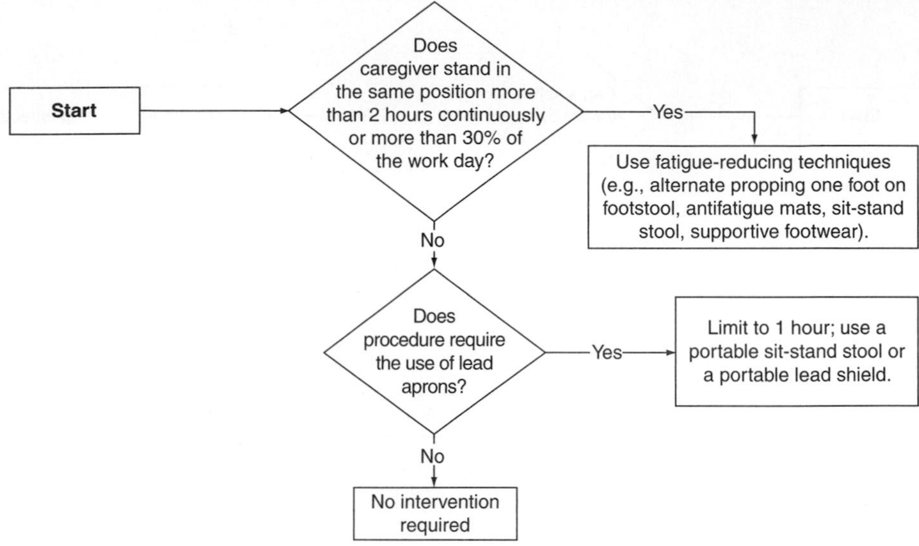

General recommendations

- ☐ Caregiver should wear supportive footwear that has the following properties:
  - Does not change the shape of the foot
  - Has enough space to move toes
  - Shock-absorbing, cushioned insoles
  - Closed toe
  - Height of heel in proportion to the shoe
- ☐ Caregivers may benefit from wearing support stockings/socks.
- ☐ Antifatigue mats should be on the floors.
- ☐ Antifatigue mats should be placed on standing stools.
- ☐ The sit-stand chair should be set to the correct height before setting the sterile field so caregivers will not be changing levels during the procedure.
- ☐ Be aware of infection control issues for nondisposable and antifatigue matting.
- ☐ Accommodations for pregnancy were considered, but the 2-hour limit on prolonged standing covers this condition.
- ☐ Scrubbed staff should not work with the neck flexed more than 30 degrees or rotated for more than 1 mintue uninterrupted.
- ☐ Two-piece, lightweight lead aprons are recommended.
- ☐ During the sit-to-stand break, staff should look straight ahead for a short while.

* "Recommended practices for maintaining a sterile field" in *Standards, Recommended Practices, and Guidelines* (Denver, Colo: AORN, Inc. 2007) 665-672.

FIGURE 21-2 Ergonomic tool for prolonged standing. (From Nelson A et al: Development of the AORN guidance statement: safe patient handling and movement in the perioperative setting. In Peterson C, editor: *AORN guidance statement: safe patient handling and movement in the perioperative setting*, Denver, 2007, Association of periOperative Registered Nurses.)

forward or with their bodies twisted." Figure 21-3 illustrates a common hazard of twisting. A draped microscope is often pushed all the way into a corner, leaving little choice for the nurse but to drag this cumbersome item from a sideways twisted position. Lifting or moving patients in beds does not lend itself to the classic lifting posture of keeping the weight close to your body and using your legs as the lifters. Often the smaller muscles of the arms and hands do much of the lifting because of the compromised positions in which nurses find themselves. Murphy (2009) reflected on the fact that an increasing number of caregivers now fall into the bariatric category. Thus, when the traditional body mechanics concept of keeping the weight close to your core is followed, the lifted weight may still be a long distance from the spinal cord, significantly increasing the mechanical stressors.

A joint project of the Association of PeriOperative Registered Nurses (AORN), NIOSH, the Patient Safety Center of Inquiry at the James A. Haley

BOX 21-1 CLINICAL POINTS

Operating Room Ergonomic Stressors

- Overexertion
- Forceful tasks
- Walking long distances in larger operating rooms
- Flooring not ergonomically designed
- Working in low light conditions
- Repetitive motions
- Lateral transfers of patients
- Static standing positions
- Moving heavy equipment
- Trip hazards
- Holding or carrying instruments
- Awkward posture
- Working in crowded environments
- Retrieving or storing items stored too high or too low
- Fast-paced work expectations
- Holding or moving patient extremities
- Pushing or pulling motions
- Wearing lead aprons
- Standing on tubes or cords
- Positioning patients
- Reaching for supplies above one's head
- Bending to retrieve items from low shelves or off the floor
- Manual handling of bariatric patients
- Wearing orthopedic helmets
- Wet flooring
- Fatigue
- Prolonged work hours
- Manual cranking of equipment
- Pushing wheeled equipment in the presence of tubes and cords

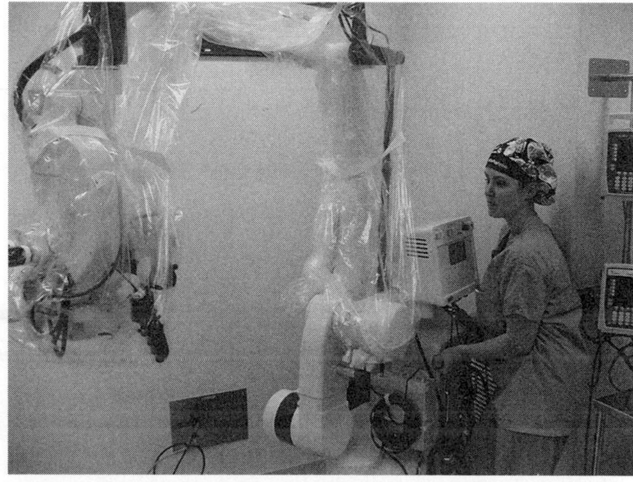

FIGURE 21-3 Twisting hazard. Moving heavy equipment from awkward positions is a critical hazard encountered in the operating room. In this staged photo the microscope is additionally difficult to move because of its position in the corner and the presence of a sterile drape.

Veterans Administration Medical Center (VMAC), and the American Nurses Association (ANA) determined seven "high-risk" activities within the OR that were most likely to lead to musculoskeletal injuries (Nelson et al, 2007). In this case the term "high-risk" referred to those activities "that push the limits of human capabilities—e.g., heavy loads, sustained awkward positions, bending and twisting, reaching, fatigue or stress, force, or standing for long periods of time. It is the combination of frequency, duration and stress of these tasks that predispose nurses to MSDs" (musculoskeletal disorders) (Nelson et al, 2007). More specifically, seven identified high-risk tasks are as follows (Nelson et al, 2007):

1. Lateral transfer from stretcher to OR bed
2. Repositioning patients on OR beds

TABLE 21-2 Recommendations for Pushing, Pulling, and Moving Equipment on Wheels

Ergonomic Tool #7

OR Equipment	Pushing		Max Push Distance ft/(m)		Ergonomic Recommendation
Electrosurgery unit	8.4 lbF	(3.8 kgF)	>200 ft	(60 m)	
Ultrasound	12.4 lbF	(5.6 kgF)	>200 ft	(60 m)	
X-ray equipment portable	12.9 lbF	(5.9 kgF)	>200 ft	(60 m)	
Video towers	14.1 lbF	(6.4 kgF)	>200 ft	(60 m)	
Linen cart	16.3 lbF	(7.4 kgF)	>200 ft	(60 m)	
X-ray equipment, C-arm	19.6 lbF	(8.9 kgF)	>200 ft	(60 m)	
Case carts, empty	24.2 lbF	(11.0 kgF)	>200 ft	(60 m)	
OR strecher, unoccupied	25.1 lbF	(11.4 kgF)	>200 ft	(60 m)	
Case carts, full	26.6 lbF	(12.1 kgF)	>200 ft	(60 m)	
Microscopes	27.5 lbF	(12.5 kgF)	>200 ft	(60 m)	
Hospital bed, unoccupied	29.8 lbF	(13.5 kgF)	>200 ft	(60 m)	
Specialty equipment carts	39.3 lbF	(17.9 kgF)	>200 ft	(60 m)	
OR strecher, occupied, 300 lbs	43.8 lbF	(19.9 kgF)	>200 ft	(60 m)	
Beds, occupied, 300 lbs	50.0 lbF	(22.7 kgF)	<200 ft	(30 m)	**Min two caregivers required**
Specialty OR beds, unoccupied	69.7 lbF	(31.7 kgF)	<100 ft	(30 m)	
OR beds, unoccupied	61.3 lbF	(27.9 kgF)	<25 ft	(7.5 m)	Recommend powered transport device
OR beds, occupied, 300 lbs	112.4 lbF	(51.1 kgF)	<25 ft	(7.5 m)	
Specialty OR beds, occupied, 300 lbs	124.2 lbF	(56.5 kgF)	<25 ft	(7.5 m)	

No shading Minimal risk—Safe to lift

Light shading Potential risk—Use assistive technology as available

Heavy shading Considerable risk—One person should not perform alone or weight should be reduced.

kgF, Kilogram force; *lbF*, pound force; *OR*, operating room.

From Nelson A et al: Development of the AORN guidance statement: safe patient handling and movement in the perioperative setting. In Peterson C, editor: *AORN guidance statement: safe patient handling and movement in the perioperative setting*, Denver, 2007, Association of periOperative Registered Nurses.

3. Lifting and holding legs, arms, head for preparation
4. Prolonged standing
5. Holding retractors for extended periods of time
6. Lifting and carrying supplies/equipment
7. Pushing, pulling, moving equipment on wheels

Any OR nurse looking at this list would agree that each task has strong potential for back injuries. The *AORN Guidance Statement: Safe Patient Handling and Movement in the Perioperative Setting* (Peterson, 2007) created a list of the degrees of stress involved with various movements in relation to equipment in the OR (Table 21-2). Mathias and Patterson (2005) identifies prolonged standing for the perioperative nurse as the number one hazard for back strain. Prolonged standing was placed ahead of patient movement and positioning, no matter what the age of the care provider.

ALGORITHMS

To deal with each of the seven high-risk tasks, the AORN task force developed algorithms, also referred to as "Ergonomic Tools" to provide guidance in the patient handling decision-making process. Many safe patient handling programs have instituted similar lift algorithms. Algorithms are visual maps that guide the caregiver very clearly through a decision-making pathway when considering patient handling. In a publication designed as a bariatric patient–handling toolkit, Baptiste (2007) developed algorithms specifically for the bariatric population.

Patient assessment is essential when considering how to approach mobilizing or transferring a patient. Assessment should include cognitive status, weight, ability to assist, potential for unexpected movements, and presence of tubes, drains and intravenous (IV) lines. In the OR some of these variables are commonly present. Even transferring the patient just from the OR bed to the stretcher will often involve most of them and often in multiples. Depending on such an assessment of the patient's ability to assist, the algorithm may direct whether additional care or equipment is needed (Figure 21-4). A patient's weight or level of consciousness may also lead to another level of equipment use or higher number of patient caregivers. It may seem embarrassing at first to ask for assistance to lift a leg into a stirrup. Nurses have always bravely done these tasks on their own. As the weight of legs has increased with the bariatric evolution, nurses' conditioning may have led them to continue to single-handedly lift increasingly heavy legs because that is what has always been done. It may take a shift in perspective to be willing to ask for additional help. At times it may be beneficial to use a lift device when positioning a very large leg. At other times, four people may coordinate their efforts to lift both legs simultaneously to accomplish the task in the manner recommended by the AORN (2009) *Recommended Practices for Positioning the Patient in the Perioperative Practice Setting.* Sufficient help and movement aids need to be employed to safely transfer the patient or even position a heavy limb. Manual lifting should never be attempted if it involves lifting most or all of the patient's weight. Transfer aids should be employed along with sufficient personnel to ensure safety of the patient and the care providers.

THREE REALMS OF PREVENTION

It is evident that prevention is vastly preferable to treating injuries. Traditionally there has been one predominant method of musculoskeletal injury prevention: expecting the caregiver to be more prepared for and more careful in performing patient handling tasks. The startling ineffectiveness of this approach has led to a broader approach that breaks the responsibilities of successful prevention into the three categories of engineering, administrative, and behavioral controls (Table 21-3).

Engineering Controls

Engineering controls are considered the most effective in prevention of work-related musculoskeletal injuries because of the relative permanency of the changes. These involve changing the work space, equipment, and tools used for patient handling; patient care environmental layout; and job flow alteration, resulting in a reduction of musculoskeletal hazards (Nelson and Baptiste, 2004). An example of a failed engineering control is the use of back belts. Research now shows no startling benefits from their use, although no one appears ready to say that it is inappropriate to use them (Nelson and Baptiste, 2004). Engineering controls that have been more successful recently have included height-adjustable beds and electrically driven beds. Ceiling-mounted lifts are useful in the preoperative area and recovery, but not as versatile within the OR. Sometimes it is a relatively simple and inexpensive device that can save a back. Wheel sleeves are a useful tool to push cords and hoses out of the way of wheeled equipment (Figure 21-5).

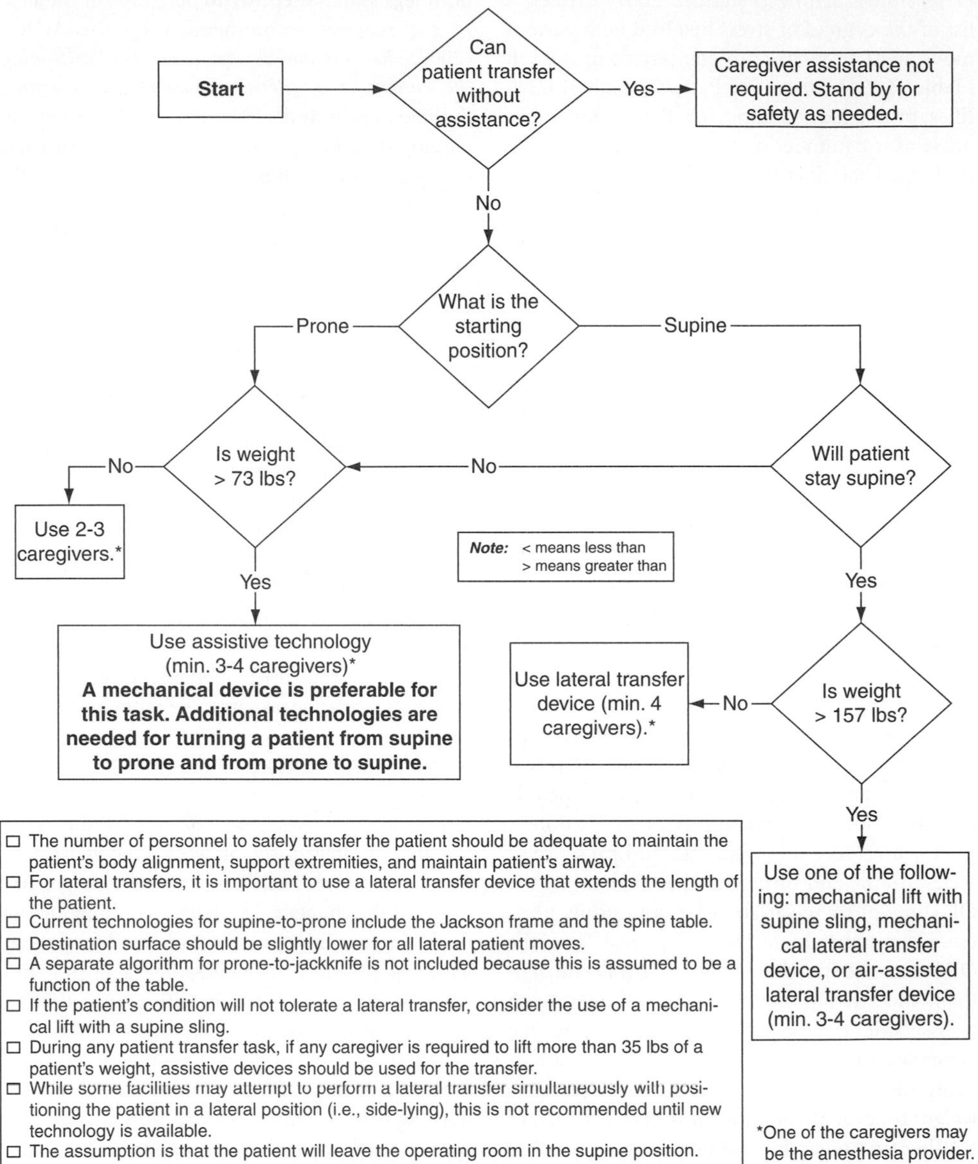

FIGURE 21-4 Ergonomic tool for lateral transfer from stretcher to and from the operating room bed. (From Nelson A et al: Development of the AORN guidance statement: safe patient handling and movement in the perioperative setting. In Peterson C, editor: *AORN guidance statement: safe patient handling and movement in the perioperative setting*, Denver, 2007, Association of periOperative Registered Nurses.)

Tools Available to Operating Room Staff

Although manual lifting and repositioning will always remain a part of positioning in the OR, it is increasingly necessary to identify the tools most beneficial to minimize the manual handling components. Convenience and accessibility are

TABLE 21-3 Control and Evidence

Type of Control	LEVEL OF EVIDENCE: Evidence That the Intervention Is Ineffective	Evidence That the Intervention Is Effective	Promising New Interventions Under Study
Engineering	Back belts	Use of patient handling equipment and devices	
Administrative		Patient care ergonomic assessment protocols No-lift policies Patient lift teams	Clinical tools, such as algorithms and patient assessment protocols
Behavioral	Training in safe lifting techniques Manual patient lifting Classes in body mechanics	Training in proper use of lifting equipment and devices	Unit-based peer leaders

Data from Nelson A, Baptiste A: Evidence-based practices for safe patient handling and movement, *Online J Issues Nurs* 9(3):Manuscript 3, September 30, 2004, available at http://www.nursingworld.org/MainMenuCategories/ANAMarketplace/ANAPeriodicals/OJIN/TableofContents/Volume92004/No3Sept04/EvidenceBasedPractices.aspx. Accessed May 22, 2009.

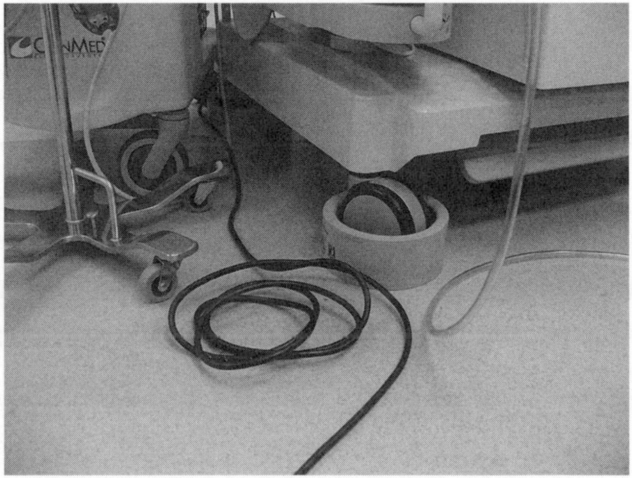

FIGURE 21-5 Wheel sleeves. Cords and hoses pose a trip and strain hazard. Wheel sleeves help slide these out of the way when moving equipment.

essential. If the device is too complicated or time consuming, nurses will likely revert to manual lifting to keep the expected pace going. Lateral-assist devices are designed to minimize friction and even weight, allowing for a safer transfer for both patient and caregiver while providing comfort to the patient as well. Following is a list of some of the assistive devices available to the OR team. Some may be new concepts, whereas others have been available for many years.

Inflatable lateral-assist devices. Several products on the market use a cushion of air to vastly reduce the weight and friction for transfers. In the appropriate size the devices are designed to lift patients of any size. It may be beneficial to place the device under the patient on the OR table so that when the procedure is completed, it can simply be inflated and the transfer completed with minimal effort. This may remain under the patient on the stretcher until the patient reaches the postsurgical floor and is positioned in his or her hospital bed. In some hospitals the device is assigned to the patient on admission and stays under the patient throughout the entire patient stay (Barry, 2006). The one caution that nursing staff have indicated is that in prolonged surgical procedures the texture of the device may have the potential for skin breakdown compared with placing the patient on the surface of the skin-friendly pads on most modern OR beds. When selecting this type of device, it is important to consider how it will be sanitized between patients. It requires a nonporous material that can be sanitized with usual hospital protocols. Another positive feature of these devices is the bridging factor. A small gap between the two beds may be easily bridged. The main safety feature for staff is that it takes minimal effort to transfer the patient from one bed to another. Although it would be physically possible to single-handedly move a bariatric patient on an inflatable lateral-assist device, it is recommended that nurses use the corresponding algorithm to determine the safe number of staff members to be involved in the patient transfer (Figure 21-6).

Friction-reducing lateral-assist devices. There are several devices available that use a two-layer vinyl sheet designed to minimize friction and aid in transferring laterally. This device does not have a bridging feature; thus the two bed surfaces must be in close proximity for the transfer. Some hospitals have even used large trash bags covered with a linen sheet to accomplish the same intent on a lower budget.

Powered full-body sling lift. This device may be operated by one or two caregivers, using a sling under the patient to transfer the patient. This equipment is available in a portable or ceiling-mounted application. The evident benefit of eliminating manual handling is countered by the more cumbersome and time-consuming nature of this equipment. Another drawback is the fact that there is still a requirement of manual handling to get the sling positioned appropriately under the patient before the lift can occur. Despite these drawbacks, there may be times when this is the best solution for positioning a bariatric patient even in the operative setting.

Roller board. This device has been the standard transfer device in ORs for many years. It is easily stored in most OR rooms, allowing for easy access. It has the feature of bridging over gaps between bed surfaces. The downside is the harsh surface that patients encounter in the transfer, along with the requirement for a significant amount of manual handling.

Sliding boards. Lighter than a roller board, this device uses the smooth surface of a vinyl board as a sliding surface through the use of drawsheets. Features also include convenient storage and the ability to bridge gaps between beds. The harder surface and the increased need for manual handling make it less desirable than the inflatable lateral-assist device.

Electric operating room tables. Larger operating rooms have enjoyed the convenience of electric beds for many years now. Where manual beds exist, it would be beneficial to replace them with electric beds, where the touch of a button provides bed positioning, rather than repetitive cranking in awkward positions.

Electric beds. Increasingly, hospitals with a bariatric population are acquiring postoperative beds that are self-propelled. Transferring a patient from the OR to recovery has usually been a job of the circulator and the anesthesia provider. This is awkward enough with a stretcher and normal-size patient. Add to this a bariatric-size bed with patient, and it far exceeds the limits of what two people should attempt to push or pull. A number of well-designed beds are available that will do this work for the team, thus reducing the risk for injury during transport.

Several of these tools may be enhanced by the use of proper transfer techniques. Phippen et al (2009) describe a bed tilt technique in which the bed from which the patient is being moved is tilted toward the receiving bed to use the advantage of gravity. Sometimes our best tools are not kept in closets or holders but rather in the thoughtful use of physics and gravity.

Administrative Controls

The second category of controls involves the use of policies and practices supported by management to ensure a reduction in ergonomic risk factors. It may include altering work expectations, such as providing for additional or prolonged breaks. It may also focus on suitability of shifts, such as the length of shifts depending on the rigors of a particular shift. It may be as simple as putting a limit on the maximum weight of an instrument tray. In addition, it may be beneficial

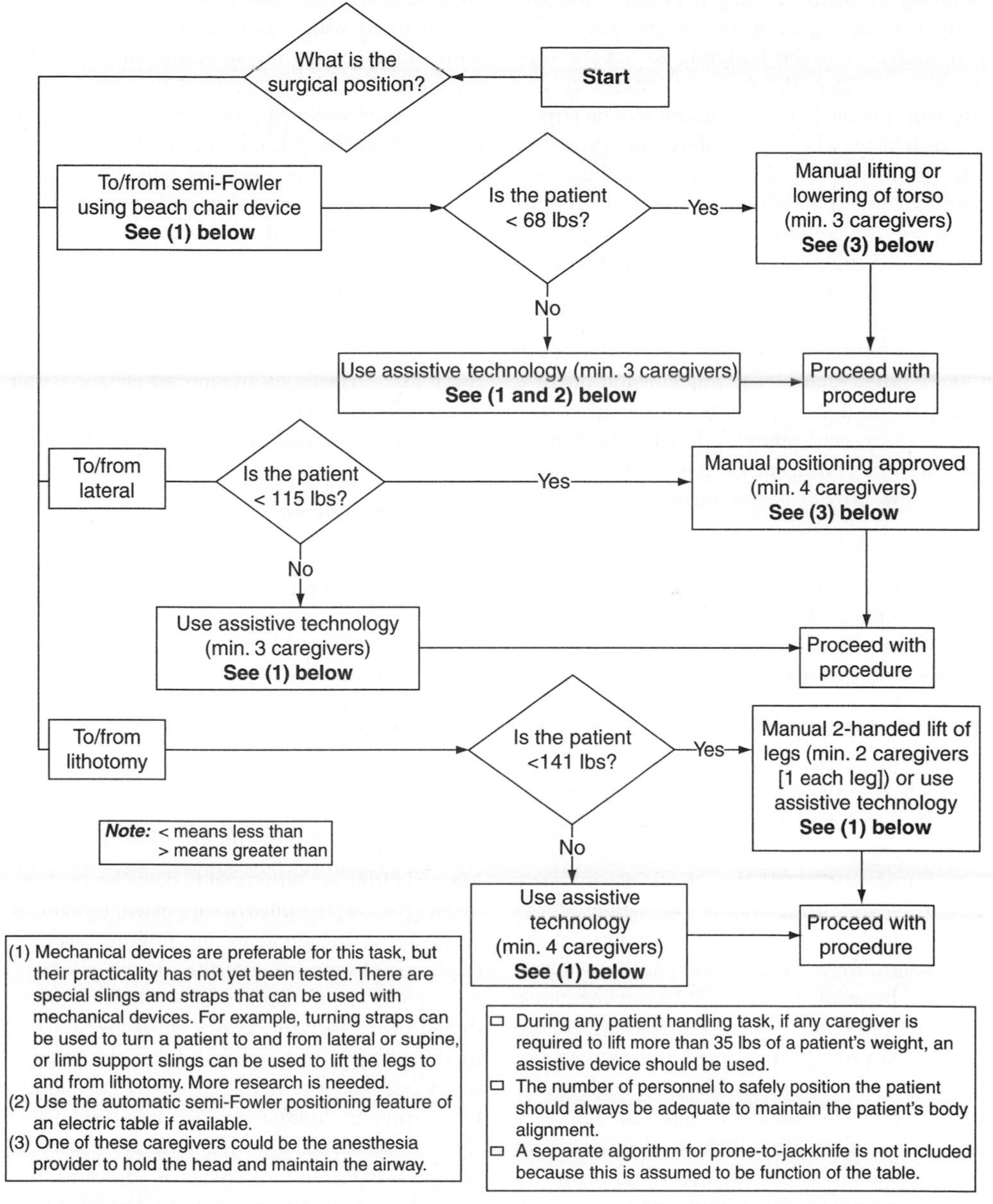

FIGURE 21-6 Ergonomic tool for positioning/repositioning the patient on the operating room bed into and from the supine position. (From Nelson A et al: Development of the AORN guidance statement: safe patient handling and movement in the perioperative setting. In Peterson C, editor: *AORN guidance statement: safe patient handling and movement in the perioperative setting,* Denver, 2007, Association of periOperative Registered Nurses.)

to teach stress-reduction techniques in response to personal awareness of risk factors (Nelson and Baptiste, 2004). An administrative control that is increasingly supported in the literature is the development of institutional "no-lift" policies and ergonomic assessment tools and algorithms.

Building a Culture of Spine Safety

Building a positive culture is essential for safe patient handling programs to be successful. Although it may be tempting to have a top-down approach in the context of administrative controls, the likelihood of success will be largely dependent on whether staff-level care providers have input into the development of their own culture. Muir et al (2007) defined the culture of safety as "the collective attitude of all care givers in assuming a shared responsibility for safety in the work environment which results in a safe, dignified, respectful and caring environment for both caregivers and patients." Wardell (2007) noted that in the implementation of a safe patient handling program, the investigators encountered some disheartening results. Seventy-one percent of the participants refused to use the provided equipment; of these, 64% felt that the equipment was not appropriate for their needs. In addition, the culture shifted away from teamwork because, after all, they now had equipment available.

In light of these findings, it is important to plan ahead sufficiently to predict barriers to success and address them with the intent of avoiding staff discouragement or disengagement. One strategy is to consider the model of crew resource management, in which all involved individuals have equal input. Many hospitals have spent considerable energy on the topic of scripting for targeted conversations. The Transformation of the OR (TOR) initiative within the Volunteer Hospital Association (VHA) is an example of restructuring the culture of the OR to allow for more open and positive communication between the varied OR team members, ranging from housekeepers to surgeons (DeKastle and Farnsworth, 2009). Some hospitals note significant improvements in communication and understanding between surgeons and staff with these types of initiatives. It may take these types of initiatives to allow for the needed time to safely position patients in the operating room.

Hospitals that incorporate a shared governance model of decision making are likely to accomplish such goals with minimal difficulty. According to the definition of Tim Porter-O'Grady, shared governance is an innovative organizational framework that affords nurses professional autonomy. It empowers the professional nursing staff and managers to contribute collectively to the decision-making process related to patient care, nursing practice, and the work environment (Shared governance, 2008). When frontline nurses are involved with exploring the barriers along with implementing the solutions, the initiatives are more likely to be successful. One OR using a broad model of shared governance commissioned one such staff-led team to explore movement devices. The staff-level research lent credibility to any forthcoming suggestions and changes. Team members coordinated the trials, as well as the staff education, leading to a comprehensive use of inflatable lateral-assist devices within their OR (DeKastle and Farnsworth, 2009).

A culture of safety within the perioperative setting is likely to foster positive morale, enhanced staff retention, and reduced loss of time as a result of injuries and potentially serves as a recruiting tool.

Policy Development

A significant component within administrative controls involves the research and development of policies pertaining to safe patient handling. Many hospitals address this topic in policy format without any regard to the unique implications for the operating room. It may require a separate policy specifically intended for the OR setting or at minimum, an addendum to a facility policy.

"No-Lift"—A Reasonable Philosophy?

Manual lifting is a term used to describe any time when a patient is handled or supported "by hand or bodily force, including pushing, pulling, carrying, holding and supporting of the patient or a body part" (Nelson and Baptiste, 2004). One common thread in the literature is that this type of activity should be at least minimized if not eliminated when possible. The ANA has described mandatory lifting as "'unsafe' and 'directly responsible for musculoskeletal disorders suffered by nurses'" (Hughes, 2006). In the context of administrative controls, it would be important to develop a hospital philosophy regarding the commonly used term *no-lift* and then include it within written policies and staff education.

The term *no-lift* has become more popular in the literature as well as in recent legislation. Although the term may be somewhat misleading by making people believe that they will no longer be required to lift anything at all, it actually refers to a more reasonable measure of lifting than what nurses would naturally allow themselves to lift on behalf of their patients. Other terms also associated with this concept include *safe patient handling and movement, lift-free, minimal lift,* and *zero lift* (Nelson and Baptiste, 2004). One study drew the differences between the perceptions of nurses and physiotherapists (PTs) in regards to zero lift. Nurses actively supported implementing zero-lift policies. The PTs were strong in their opinion that this would inhibit the rehabilitative progress of their patients (Trossman, 2007). Although some may assume that these strong terms absolve the nurse of any lifting at all, the concept actually is broadly defined as a commitment by health care leadership to provide proper equipment in sufficient quantity and quality to minimize manual lifting wherever and whenever possible. This commitment is formalized through appropriate policies and equipment training to guide the care providers.

Behavior Controls

Behavior controls may be less effective than the previous two controls, but are not without merit. This approach has been the main focus of prevention for a number of decades now without remarkable favorable statistics. The use of body mechanics training is the core of this focus, although now it also includes training for the equipment that is introduced as a result of engineering and administrative controls.

Basic Body Mechanics Principles

Behavioral controls may involve instruction in basic body mechanics. Some of the most pertinent components of this focus for the perioperative setting include the following:

- Make sure that you plan ahead when considering your patient-handling task.
- Lift with your legs rather than your back.
- Maintain the natural curvature of your spine.
- Determine your center of gravity, and then seek to keep it centered above your base of support.
- Preferentially use large muscles over the smaller ones. In doing so, remember to use your hands and arms as instruments of attachment rather than using them for lifting.
- Work from a position of balance by keeping your knees bent and feet apart at shoulder width with one foot leading slightly ahead of the other.
- Bend hips and knees at the same time.
- Use a pushing or pulling rather than a lifting motion when possible. Pushing is preferable to pulling. Push or pull from the center of gravity.
- When bearing weight, pivot on your feet rather than twisting your back.
- Use the mechanics of movement rather than strength alone.
- Allow your patient to assist in other ways than by holding on to your neck or arms.

In a 2008 conference in Washington State devoted to the topic of creating a culture of safe patient handling (Piazza, 2008), the lectures not only focused on zero-lift or no-lift topics, but also included a workshop on safe body mechanics. It appears that even in a state where "no lift" has been legislated, it is still reasonable to consider the need for personal physical preparation and education. The acronym LITE was used at this conference. It encourages the care provider to consider the ***L***oad, ***I***ndividual, ***T***ask, and ***E***nvironment (Table 21-4) (Murphy and Rickerson, 2008).

Some basic instruction on the topic of proper body mechanics must be provided in a chapter on prevention of back injury. Several approaches may need to be explored to ensure that all learning styles are accommodated.

Spine classes. Traditional methods of lift training have not had the dramatic impact on decreased back injuries that one would anticipate. One study showed that there was little difference between those who watched a video on body mechanics and those who went through prolonged classroom-based training (Lavender et al, 2007). A number of myths exist regarding back injuries in the health care setting (Box 21-2). Evidence based on two decades of research further indicates that other traditional preventive programs using administrative changes, engineering controls, and worker training in such skills as safe lifting and body mechanics classes along with the use of back belts have not had a positive impact on the musculoskeletal injury rates suffered by health care providers (Nelson and Baptiste, 2004; ANA, 2009). Despite these findings, many hospitals still choose to provide spine care classes to the staff who are at most risk for back injury. These are not necessarily irrelevant, just not the definitive means to reduce injuries. Eliminating these programs altogether would have a negative

TABLE 21-4 LITE Principles

Term	Meaning
Load	Load means patient characteristics that can affect the handling risk, such as age, gender, diagnosis, dependency, neurologic status, size, weight, ability to cooperate, and fall risk.
Individual	Individual means the capabilities of caregivers, such as language, education, training, physical limitations, stress and fatigue, which can affect their ability to do the job safely.
Task	Task means the nature of the task, what has to be done, how, and when. Different tasks have different requirements, each needing assessment and a unique approach.
Environment	Environment means the working environment and covers factors such as facilities, staffing levels, culture, and resources, which all impact on how the task is done.

Modified from *Introduction to the New Zealand patient handling guidelines*, available at http://www.acc.co.nz/PRD_EXT_CSMP/idcplg?IdcService=GET_FILE&dID=35375&dDocName=PI00287&allowInterrupt=1. Accessed September 29, 2009.

BOX 21-2 CLINICAL POINTS

Safe Patient Handling Myths

Myth #1: Nurses get hurt because they lift improperly.

Truth: Evidence indicates that most injuries relate to performing tasks beyond physiologic limits (Mathias and Patterson, 2005).

Myth #2: Education and training regarding body mechanics is an effective method of musculoskeletal injury prevention.

Truth: Evidence clearly shows that despite several decades of this approach, injury rates have not been positively affected.

Myth #3: Manual lifting provides increased dignity for patients.

Truth: Studies that capture patients' responses to lift devices show positive results (Mathias and Patterson, 2005).

Myth #4: The risks associated with patient handling are eliminated with mechanical lift devices.

Truth: Manual handling will always remain at least a minimal component of patient handling. Positioning the equipment or slings may involve some risk. The risks are minimized, but not eliminated.

Myth #5: If hospitals buy equipment, nurses will use it.

Truth: Obstacles to effective and consistent use may include lack of education, availability, confinement of work space, haste, and patient preference (O'Malley et al, 2006).

Myth #6: Workers sustain injuries because of nonwork activities such as hobbies.

Truth: These are not significant factors contributing to musculoskeletal injuries (Mathias and Patterson, 2005).

Myth #7: The use of back belts effectively protects the caregiver from spine injuries.

Truth: Statistical evidence has not shown these to be effective (Murphy and Rickerson, 2008).

Myth #8: Equipment is redundant when enough staff is available.

Truth: The more staff who help, the more staff are exposed to a potential injury.

Myth #9: Patient handling equipment is not worth the expense.

Truth: Numerous hospitals have been able to prove a financial saving in workers' compensation payments in addition to the decrease in lost productive time (Mathias and Patterson, 2005).

Myth #10: Mechanical lifts impede a patient's rehabilitation.

Truth: Rehabilitative progress has not been shown to be impeded when lift equipment is used appropriately (Murphy and Rickerson, 2008).

impact on spine injury statistics. According to one physical therapist involved with teaching basic principles of lifting, body mechanics, communication techniques, and the use of core body strength, this approach has been beneficial in preventing injuries (Craig, 2009).

Peer leaders. Another concept in some health care environments is the use of peer leaders or "train the trainer" programs. In this model, key individuals are given the essential training and then expected to return to their units to share their newly acquired skills and knowledge with their colleagues. For example, when introducing an inflatable lateral-assist device, rather than taking all staff through hospital-based training, it would be more efficient and effective to train peer leaders to take the training back to their colleagues. An increased benefit of this method is that the education is more respected when coming from peers than from someone who may be an unknown suspected of potentially having an agenda.

Personal preparedness. A previous proponent of personal preparedness, Murphy (2009) now admits to shifting further away from teaching personal preparedness in favor of simply teaching the use of equipment. Murphy does not state that it is unnecessary to teach body mechanics, just that it is important to ensure that all caregivers are operating safely. She has shifted her energies predominantly to the proper use of equipment. It may be necessary to balance training programs to include components of both approaches so as to maximize the safe patient handling preparedness of staff.

Murphy and Rickerson (2008) are clear in suggesting that if you have to choose between the use of strength or equipment, always defer to the use of equipment. Nurses are known for their critical thought. Employing this strength in the context of safe patient handling is preferential to shortcutting the processes, compromising their health for the sake of expediency. It is beneficial to use resources such as equipment, fellow workers, or even float pool staff as additional help when tired, sore, or not sure of one's abilities.

Equipment focus. Training in the use of equipment requires a two-pronged approach. First, the training may relate to the actual equipment and how to safely employ it. Second, it will require the critical thought processes that will lead to successful use of the items. Staff members need to be familiar with algorithms or ergonomic tools to include in their preparatory assessments (see Box 21-1 and Figure 21-4). The staff should know to prepare the work space by removing or minimizing obstacles. Next, equipment should be retrieved and used for the assessed task. Safety is paramount, including routine actions such as locking and leveling the transfer surfaces.

The Nurse's Personal Responsibility

The discussion up to this point has been strongly directed toward supporting and preparing the caregiver. Now the focus will shift, putting more responsibility upon the caregiver to take personal responsibility for his or her own back safety and use of provided resources.

Physical fitness. A number of strategies can be employed to support physical fitness even while performing the daily tasks of one's job. It would be good to start with becoming familiar with proper body mechanics and lifting techniques. When required to stand for prolonged periods, use good posture, put one foot up at a different elevation, change positions often, and use antifatigue mats when available. During long cases take short breaks by sitting on a draped stool (Mathias and Patterson, 2005). Practice good body posture during your off hours as well. Arrive to work early, and do some calisthenics or other physical preparation (Bissell, 2009). Communicate with a physiotherapist about stretching and relaxing techniques to employ at the beginning of and throughout the day. Persist in a personal exercise program. Murphy (2009) calls it "fit for duty," elaborating that "RNs as a group are terrible in their self-care habits." It stands to reason that if a large percentage of a nurse's job description consists of physically demanding activity, each individual has a vested interest in coming physically prepared and warmed up for the task.

Recognizing symptoms. A key to preventing exacerbated injuries is being able to recognize early symptoms when they arise. A sentinel back injury is not usually the result of an isolated incident. It most often occurs when an event pushes all previous negative encounters to a threshold leading to obvious injury (Craig, 2009). Some of the symptoms to be looking out for include numbness, tingling, pain, burning, stiffness, and cramping. Loss of strength and range of motion should also alert you to an underlying musculoskeletal dysfunction (Converso and Murphy, 2004). Early symptoms should serve as flags to the informed nurse to seek an evaluation before escalation toward injury or disability.

Communication. As with most encounters in life, communication is key to success. Team members may feel intimidated during a lift when looking around the table and recognizing a lot more credentials on other name badges than on their own. They may not be ready to lift or may be in an awkward position but unwilling to hold up the activity because of intimidation. In one case a certified assistive personnel (CAP) was new to her position. She was asked to assist in a lift that she was not familiar with. In her mind she knew that she should let the team know that she was not comfortable with participating but felt the urgency of the task and joined in regardless. Her injury from that lift caused prolonged unemployment and decreased confidence for future lifts (Craig, 2009). Craig strongly encourages communication in all lift endeavors. It should be a team approach where each one has an equal voice as to when he or she is ready to lift.

A common tactic that is used in the OR when lifting patients is to count to three and then all lift together. It is important to agree on whatever format is used to coordinate the team's efforts. Often it is the anesthesia provider who coordinates this, because that person is responsible for the airway and other vital monitoring systems. If at the last moment, someone is not ready or is unsure of his or her lift posture, it should be a group norm for that person to speak up and delay the lift or transfer. Communication is foundational to a successful handling event. When lifting tasks are attempted in an uncoordinated fashion, injuries are likely to occur.

LIFT TEAMS—COMBINING ALL PREVENTIVE CONTROLS INTO ONE PACKAGE

The aging nursing population is more likely to incur back injuries because of their age alone. The average age of nurses in the U.S. workforce is presently 46.8 years (Bell et al, 2008). By age 40, physical strength is measurably diminished in most people. By age 50 this diminished strength is accelerated (Wardell, 2007). Added to this is the significant diminished muscle strength with prolonged lifting. Muscle endurance is diminished by 48% after 1 minute of holding, 65% after 2 minutes and 71% after 3 minutes (Waters et al, 2009). Lifting is becoming an increasing challenge even as the patient population is becoming significantly heavier. This, along with the need to reduce injuries, has lead many hospitals to explore the concept of a dedicated lift team.

A lift team combines the three realms of prevention outlined previously when implemented successfully. A team typically consists of two physically fit, appropriately trained individuals who are dedicated to the task of patient lifting and transferring, following institutional safe patient handling policies and the appropriate lift equipment. Their primary task focuses on the high-risk patient-handling events (Nelson and Baptiste, 2004). Some hospitals have chosen to ensure that at least one of the two has sufficient credentials to be allowed to document the care that was given (Bissell, 2009). Some of the advantages of a lift team include eliminating "(1) lifts that are uncoordinated, (2) unprotected personnel, (3) lifting pairs with anthropometric disparities, (4) fatigue in nurses who lift, (5) injured nurses who lift, (6) lack of using mechanical lifting devices, and (7) lifters who are untrained" (Nelson and Baptiste, 2004) (Box 21-3). The concept of lift teams has been explored in hospitals around the nation over the past decade with a lot of satisfaction and support. Barry (2006) stated that institutions with lift teams reported half as many back injuries as those without lift teams. Some reports indicate that nursing injuries have diminished by about 70% since implementing an active lift program (O'Malley et al, 2006; Cantrell, 2009).

BOX 21-3 Advantages of Lift Teams

- Lifts are coordinated
- Personnel are more protected
- Pairing of lifting partners with anthropometric similarities
- Avoids dangerous lifts by fatigued nurses
- Injured nurses do not feel compelled to lift
- Use of mechanical lifting devices is the expectation
- The lift team members are specifically trained
- Significant decrease in nursing personnel injuries
- Safer transfer of patients
- Nurse retention

Data from Nelson A, Baptiste A: Evidence-based practices for safe patient handling and movement, *Online J Issues Nurs 2004*, 9(3): Manuscript 3, September 30, 2004, available at http://www.nursingworld.org/MainMenuCategories/ANAMarketplace/ANAPeriodicals/OJIN/TableofContents/Volume92004/No3Sept04/EvidenceBasedPractices.aspx. Accessed April 27, 2009.

One hospital requires all lift team members to go through a firefighter's fitness test and examination by a physician before initiating the training. This is repeated on an annual basis to establish continued suitability for the position (O'Malley et al, 2006). Some hospitals may choose to additionally substantiate the healthy spine through a radiograph and a history without spine injuries (Nelson and Baptiste, 2004). A Magnet hospital with a lift program noted that although the average age of all registered nurses (RNs) in their health care network was 41 years, the average age of the lift team was 23 years (Bissell, 2009). Bissell went on to state that her lift team had not had any injuries in the 3 years that the team had been in place, while reducing nursing back injuries by about 70%. She agreed that most of the lifting work was now being shifted to the typically younger and specifically trained lift team. For the lift team to have success it is essential that the nursing staff be educated in how to use the lift team, that the team be easily accessible through communication devices, and that nurses believe in the benefits of such lift teams. Where injuries persist when lift teams have been instituted, it is usually because nurses persist in owning patient handling and ignoring the availability of the supportive resource of a lift team. Other injuries have been noted to occur during urgent or emergent situations when waiting for a lift team was not reasonable (O'Malley et al, 2006).

The limitations in the literature regarding lift teams is that they stop at the red line of the OR. No studies researched by this author show lift teams supporting the patient transfer work within the OR. This may be an area for hospitals to explore. In some larger ORs some of the makeup of the staff includes unlicensed assistive personnel, also referred to as orderlies or OR aides. This group may present the opportunity to be developed as an OR-based lift team to work under the direction of the RN circulator. Job descriptions would need to be rewritten to reflect the physical demands of the position, as well as the necessary training. Ongoing competencies of these individuals may also need to be monitored. OR nurses on average are in their late 40s, well into the time of life when diminished physical strength is accelerating. Along with other OR-specific aids, it is increasingly necessary to explore the concept of an OR-dedicated lift team. As stated by O'Malley et al (2006), "Lift teams protect the most valuable resource of the healthcare organization—the nurse."

IMPLEMENTING SAFE PATIENT HANDLING PROGRAMS

Implementing a safe patient handling program may seem an arduous task at first. Nelson (2008) gives the disclaimer that development of such a program alone will not guarantee success of implementation. There are some logical steps that may assist in implementing such a program within the perioperative setting. Homsted (2004) outlined an eight-step approach that still has validity today. It will serve as the basis for the following suggested protocol.

1. **Organize an ergonomics team.** Using a shared-governance model would be ideal in assembling a variety of individuals to explore if, why, and when to implement a safe patient handling program. This team could include participants from purchasing, staff roles, management, industry, and risk management.
2. **Review the data, survey the staff, and conduct a departmental walk-through.** Occupational Safety and Health Administration (OSHA) 300 logs will give you a picture of the injuries that have occurred in your department. Risk management and human resources may also provide meaningful statistics.
3. **Assess patient dependency levels.** The OR may have a large range of dependency levels, from the patient with a local anesthetic to the intubated patient with multiple lines and tubes. It may be valuable to identify a number of levels of assistance that may be needed based on these criteria.
4. **Assess high-risk patient handling tasks.** This is discussed earlier.
5. **Determine the safest approaches to high-risk tasks.** Technology will need to be a big component of this approach. Input from staff-level caregivers is essential. Determine the types and numbers of equipment necessary to make equipment easily accessible.
6. **Research, pilot, select, and implement.** Again, staff-level caregivers are the ideal persons to make this a success. Without their buy-in, the whole process may fail.
7. **Plan detailed and interactive education for staff.** Providing an evidence-based practice approach is most likely to be received by the

adult learner. Hands-on training with return demonstration legitimizes the training and enhances retention of the skill and knowledge.

8. **Track injuries moving forward**. This step may cycle the process back to step 2, in which the evaluation of the data determines whether it was worth the effort. Post the results in visually understandable graphs where the staff can see the benefits of the program.

Nelson (2008) also favors a regimented process of implementation while discouraging general education classes and general reminders. In their place, energy should be given to developing unit peer leaders and an active method of receiving and responding to staff feedback. Nelson further promotes strategies that include involvement of frontline staff, financial incentives, marketing, and the use of champions. To strengthen the success of implementation, Nelson (2008) advocates a four-stage process of diffusion to include dissemination (awareness), adoption (commitment), implementation (delivery), and maintenance (continued use).

NEW INITIATIVES

Ergonomics

Health care ergonomics is a developing field. It is defined as "the science of adapting the work environment to the worker to improve safety" (Converso and Murphy, 2004). The influence of labor organizations along with professional nursing organizations, regulatory agencies, industry innovation, and scientific exploration have brought us to the point at which we now find ourselves (*Handle With Care backgrounder*, 2009). Research in ergonomics positively affects perioperative back injuries (Beck, 2008). Consultants are now available to come into most areas of a hospital and make recommendations for ergonomic adjustments to the workplace. It may be the mats on which scrubbed staff stand all day. It may be the weight of equipment or the height of the circulator's charting desk. All contribute to overall postural health. One long-awaited ergonomic change in patient care is the advent of motorized beds. A number of beds on the market will self-propel based on controls at the head of the bed. Too often the picture of the patient going from the OR to recovery shows a circulating nurse pulling the bed with one arm from a twisted posture while the anesthesia provider is juggling a piece of equipment and managing the airway (Figure 21-7). As noted previously, a twisting motion is responsible for more back injuries in health care than regular lifting postures. The self-propelled bed is a wonderful solution to this hazardous practice.

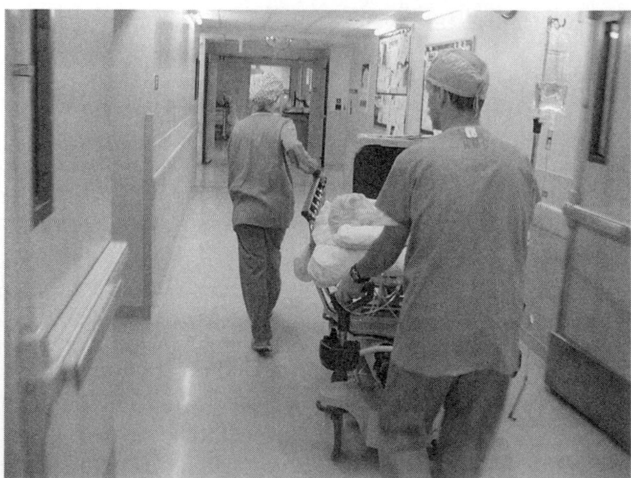

FIGURE 21-7 Twisting hazard. The RN circulator leading the gurney to recovery often pulls a lot of the weight from a twisted position, while the anesthesia provider tends to the airway and lines at the head of the bed.

Legislative Initiatives

Several states have legislated safe patient handling laws with the goal of protecting health care providers from work-related musculoskeletal injuries. This movement began when the ANA was granted funding by NIOSH in 2004 to launch "Safe Patient Handling and Movement Nursing School Curriculum." The overall goal of this program was to affect the next generation of nurses with the message of safe patient handling through nursing school curricula. As these nurses graduate, they will have the expectation of a safe environment, with the associated assistive devices already in place (*Handle With Care backgrounder*, 2009). Health care institutions need to be sure to be prepared for the arrival of this next generation of nurses.

Since the above-mentioned project in 2004, eight states have enacted legislation specifically targeted at safe patient handling. Seven other states are in the process of implementing safe patient handling and movement legislation (ANA, 2009). Washington State may be a model of this legislative initiative. Their model gives realistic timelines for compliance along with formulas and funding to purchase the necessary lift equipment.

Some political advocates come from the perspective that "Unless required by regulation, federal or state law, or collective bargaining agreements, hospitals are not likely to make safe working conditions a top priority" (Converso et al, 2004). Rather than having this despondent attitude, it is incumbent upon nurses to realize their collective backbones. They should advocate within their facilities and, from that vantage point, lead with safe practices that may be so much a part of their institutional culture that any ensuing legislation will only serve to validate the safe patient handling programs already in place. Safety is less likely to be accomplished by legislation than by nurses in a shared-governance model, owning their practice while holding leadership responsible for providing the necessary tools.

CONCLUSION

Perioperative nurses will need to be on the front lines in advocating for well-adapted safe patient handling programs, including the use of suitable mechanical devices and OR-specific lift teams. The research is clear as to the benefits of implementing appropriate safe patient handling programs. It is imperative that hospitals stop using outdated methods unsubstantiated by current evidence. It needs to be understood that, although advances in administrative and engineering controls have evolved, the caregiver mindset has not kept up. In many ways the challenges have grown all around nurses while the solutions and mindsets have remained unchanged. It will take changes in school curricula to prepare the next generation of safe patient handlers. It will also take policies, appropriate lift equipment, development of OR-based lift teams, algorithms, and ergonomic redesign, along with a change in the present way of looking at patient handling. It may also necessitate the broad use of the nursing-based concept of shared governance to propel the perioperative environment to a place of safety where aging nurses can finish out their careers and where novice nurses desire to work.

REFERENCES

American Nurses Association: *Safe patient handling and movement*, available at http://www.nursingworld.org/MainMenuCategories/ANAPoliticalPower/State/StateLegislativeAgenda/SPHM.aspx. Accessed April 27, 2009.

AORN position statement on ergonomically healthy workplace practices, 2006, available at http://www.aorn.org/PracticeResources/AORNPositionStatements/Position_Ergonomics/. Accessed June 24, 2009.

Association of periOperative Registered Nurses: Recommended practices for positioning the patient in the perioperative practice setting. In *Association of periOperative Registered Nurses: Perioperative standards and recommended practices*, Denver, 2009, The Association.

Baptiste A: Safe bariatric patient handling toolkit, *Bariatric Nursing and Surgical Patient Care* 2(1):17–46, 2007, available at http://www.liebertonline.com/doi/abs/10.1089/bar.2006.9996. Accessed April 27, 2009.

Barry J: Products to enhance productivity: the HoverMatt System for patient transfer: enhancing productivity, efficiency, and safety, *J Nurs Adm* 36(3):114–117, 2006, available at http://www.cinahl.com/cgi-bin/refsvc?jid=217&accno=2009139526. Accessed April 13, 2009.

Beck D: Ease that aching back, *OR Nurse* 2(5):47–49, 2008, available at http://www.ORNurseJournal.com. Accessed May 21, 2009.

Bell J, et al: Preventing back injuries in healthcare settings, 2008, available at http://www.cdc.gov/niosh/blog/nsb092208_lifting.html. Accessed May 21, 2009.

Bissell C: Personal communication, 2009.

Cantrell M: Personal communication, 2009.

Converso A, Murphy C: Winning the battle against back injuries, *RN* 67(2):52–58, 2004, available at http://web.ebscohost.com/ehost/pdf?vid=2&hid=115&sid=40d4a98e-9365-4e0f-ae64-f2dfd4f43ed5%40sessionmgr103. Accessed April 13, 2009.

Craig K: Personal communication, 2009.

de Castro A: Handle With Care: The American Nurses Association's campaign to address work-related musculoskeletal disorders, *Online J Issues Nurs* 9(3):2004. Manuscript 2, available at http://www.nursingworld.org/MainMenuCategories/ANAMarketplace/ANAPeriodicals/OJIN/TableofContents/Volume92004/No3Sept04/HandleWithCare.aspx?css=print. Accessed April 27, 2009.

DeKastle R, Farnsworth M: A shared governance model spawned by searing employee surveys, Paper presented at AORN fifty-sixth congress, Chicago, Ill, 2009.

Handle With Care backgrounder, *ANA Nursing World* 2009. available at http://www.nursingworld.org/MainMenuCategories/OccupationalandEnvironmental/occupational-health/handlewithcare/Backgrounder.aspx?css=print. Accessed April 27, 2009.

Homsted L: Preventing back injuries: safe patient handling and movement, *Fla Nurse* 52(3):3, 2004, available at http://web.ebscohost.com/ehost/pdf?vid=2&hid=120&sid=a0e6fe2f-7355-46cc-97dc-8ddba17ce6b1%40sessionmgr107. Accessed April 13, 2009.

Hughes K: Who's got your back? Reducing the incidence of on-the-job back injuries among nurses, *Am J Nurs* 106(7):2006. Hospital Extra):72A-B–72E-F, 2006, available at http://web.ebscohost.com/ehost/detail?sid=a9d04d35-5b25-4646-a578-ce183be61441@sessionmgr104&vid=1&hid=105&. Accessed April 13, 2009.

Hurd J: Personal communication, April 30, 2009.

Lavender SA, et al: Can a new behaviorally oriented training process to improve lifting technique prevent occupationally related back injuries due to lifting? *Spine* 32(4):487–494, 2007, available at http://journals.lww.com/spinejournal/pages/default.aspx. Accessed April 13, 2009.

Mathias J, Patterson P: New research looks at ergonomic stresses on operating room staff, *OR Manager* 21(7):1, 2005.

Muir M, et al: Handling of the bariatric patient in critical care: a case study of lessons learned, *Crit Care Nurs Clin North Am* 19(2):223–240, 2007, available at http://www.ccnursing.theclinics.com/article/abstracts?terms1=handling+of+bariatric+patient&terms2=&terms3=&terms4=. Accessed April 27, 2009.

Murphy J: Personal communication, 2009.

Murphy J, Rickerson N: *Tips and techniqes to ensure staff safety*, Paper presented at Creating a culture for safe patient handling, the Washington state law and beyond (conference), Tacoma, Wash, April 30, 2008.

Nelson A: *Implementing and sustaining successful SPH programs*, Paper presented at Creating a culture for safe patient handling: the Washington state law and beyond (conference), Tacoma, Wash, April 30, 2008 .

Nelson A, Baptiste A: Evidence-based practices for safe patient handling and movement, *Online J Issues Nurs* 9(3):2004, Manuscript 3 available at http://www.nursingworld.org/MainMenuCategories/ANAMarketplace/ANAPeriodicals/OJIN/TableofContents/Volume92004/No3Sept04/EvidenceBasedPractices.aspx. Accessed April 27, 2009.

Nelson A, et al: Development of the AORN guidance statement: safe patient handling and movement in the perioperative setting. In Peterson C, editor: *AORN guidance statement: safe patient handling and movement in the perioperative setting*, Denver, 2007, Association of periOperative Registered Nurses.

Nelson A, et al: *The illustrated guide to safe patient handling and movement*, New York, 2009, Springer.

O'Malley P, et al: No brawn needed: develop and implement a lift team policy to improve outcome, *Nurs Manage* 37(4):26–34, 2006.

Peterson C: *AORN guidance statement: safe patient handling and movement in the perioperative setting*, Denver, 2007, Association of periOperative Registered Nurses.

Phippen M, et al: *Competency for safe patient care during operative and invasive procedures*, Denver, 2009, Competency & Credentialing Institute.

Piazza A: *Safe patient handling legislative update*, Paper presented at Creating a culture for safe patient handling: the Washington state law and beyond (conference), Tacoma, Wash, April 30, 2008.

Safe patient handling: Washington gives nurses' backs a break, *Nursing* 36(6):33, 2006, available at http://web.ebscohost.com/ehost/pdf?vid=2&hid=120&sid=7057e0b3-43d5-432f-97e3-0d5093e654c2%40sessionmgr109. Accessed April 13, 2009.

Safety in mobility for patients and staff: *OR Manager* 20(5):12, 2004.

Shared governance, 2008, available at http://www1.wfubmc.edu/Nursing/Shared+Governance/index.htm. Accessed June 24, 2009.

Spry C: *Essentials of perioperative nursing*, ed 4, Sudbury, Mass, 2009, Jones & Bartlett.

Trossman S: Getting a lift: ANA, CMA and RN efforts continue to build momentum for safe patient handling movement, *Am Nurse (AM NURSE)* 39(4):1–11, 2007, available at http://web.ebscohost.com/ehost/pdf?vid=2&hid=113&sid=11881ae1-4a37-4ca6-ad84-a15a46ed85a0%40sessionmgr109. Accessed April 13, 2009.

Tsolaki T, et al: The nurse's load, *Lancet* 40:422–423, 1965.

Wardell H: Reduction of injuries associated with patient handling, *AAOHN J* 55(10):407–412, 2007, available at http://web.ebscohost.com/ehost/pdf?vid=2&hid=109&sid=85641cbe-adee-4733-95ae-818194cfd1e4%40sessionmgr104. Accessed April 13, 2009.

Waters T, et al: Recommended weight limits for lifting and holding limbs in the orthopaedic practice setting, *Orthop Nurs* 28(25):S28–S32, 2009.

LATEX ALLERGY

Anita Shoup, MSN, RN, CNOR

In the late 1980s allergy to natural rubber latex (NRL) became a concern for health care workers (HCWs) and patients. Although NRL allergy is rare, it can be career ending and/or life threatening with no current cure. NRL allergy affects people regardless of gender or racial or ethnic backgrounds. The Association of periOperative Registered Nurses (AORN) (2009) refers to NRL allergy as "a significant medical concern."

Various studies demonstrate prevalence rates for IgE-mediated latex allergy ranging from 0.8% to 6.5% of the general population. According to the American Academy of Allergy Asthma and Immunology (2009), in the population of normal adults the risk is up to 6%; in HCWs it is up to 10%; and in people with spina bifida/congenital defects it is nearly 50%. Latex protein allergy is believed to be responsible for 70% of anaphylactic reactions occurring in anesthetized children with myelodysplasia. NRL has been reported as the second most common cause of perioperative anaphylaxis with an incidence of 12% of all perioperative anaphylaxis (Hepner and Casstells, 2003).

Reports vary as to the exact number of people with an allergy to NRL. In general, the American Society of Anesthesiologists (ASA) (2005) identifies the following populations to be at an increased risk for NRL allergy:

- Patients with a history of multiple surgical procedures
- Health care personnel
- Other individuals with occupational exposure such as rubber industry workers and hairdressers
- Individuals with a history of atopy, hay fever, rhinitis, asthma, or eczema
- Individual with a history of food allergy to tropical fruits
- Individuals with severe hand dermatitis who wear latex gloves

Since the mid-1990s the sensitization rates have been declining steadily, attributed to the significant decrease in the use of higher-protein, powdered products. However, there are tens of thousands of products made of NRL and over 15,000 medical devices containing NRL. In addition, some products use NRL in their packaging. So there is still reason for caution.

To further complicate the issue, latex allergy reactions have been confused with two similar reactions that commonly occur with glove and other latex product use. These are an irritant dermatitis, which is non-allergenic in nature, and a delayed hypersensitivity reaction, which is allergenic, but not to the latex. These reactions have been noted in the literature for decades, while the true NRL allergy is relatively new.

WHAT IS NATURAL RUBBER LATEX?

Natural rubber is a milky fluid that is produced by the *Hevea brasiliensis* tree as a reaction to scoring or scarring of the tree. It is composed of water, natural rubber, and other nonrubber substances. In this mixture are many proteins, both water soluble and rubber bound. The proteins, specifically the water-soluble proteins, are the allergens responsible for NRL allergy. The rubber-bound proteins are responsible for making up the matrix, or film, that is the glove. These proteins are bound and therefore nonallergenic. The water-soluble proteins are free and can be leached, or washed, out of the gloves either intentionally during the manufacturing process or afterwards by other moisture such as perspiration (as when one's hands sweat while wearing gloves) or other source (such as blood and other moisture inside the body during surgery).

Latex is often referred to as the "sap" of the tree, but this is inaccurate. NRL is found in the latex ducts, which are closer to the surface of the tree trunk. A groove is cut in the trunk of the tree in a thin layer that causes the latex to start flowing, and it is then collected in a cup. Because latex is a natural product, it can spoil. Without the addition of a preservative, the latex will soon clump, or coagulate, hardening into a gumlike substance. To prevent this and keep the NRL in a liquid state, a stabilizing agent, or anticoagulant, is added to the cup. Ammonia is the most commonly used anticoagulant. If the product being made requires solid rubber for manufacture, the latex is allowed to coagulate in the cup. The process for solid production is different than that for liquid latex and destroys many of the proteins—or allergens—in the latex. As a result, products made from solid rubber tend to be less allergenic than products that are manufactured using liquid latex.

NRL is an elastic hydrocarbon polymer. The purified form is the chemical polyisoprene. Natural rubber latex can be cross-linked with sulfur, resulting in an elastomer that we know as rubber. Natural rubber latex is thus made stronger by cross-linking the *cis*-1,4-isoprene molecule with sulfur and heat.

This chemical, polyisoprene, can be synthetically produced. Synthetic production has allowed manufacturers of gloves and other products previously made with NRL to produce these items in a nonlatex version. Synthetic rubbers—nitrile rubber, polyisoprene rubber, and polychloroprene rubber (Neoprene)—all contain different basic molecules that can be cross-linked with sulfur and heat. Physical properties vary among the different rubber materials.

HISTORY OF GLOVES AND NRL

Surgical latex gloves have been worn for more than a century. Although numerous variations of the surgical glove were developed, Dr. William Halsted of Johns Hopkins Hospitals is often credited with their introduction. Before the adoption of routine surgical glove use, the surgical team members would disinfect their hands with carbolic acid, introduced by Dr. Joseph Lister, which is quite caustic. Dr. Halsted's scrub nurse, Carolyn Hampton, was on the verge of quitting her job because she could no longer tolerate the irritation to her skin. In trying to resolve this issue, Dr. Halsted contacted the Goodyear Rubber Company in Akron, Ohio, which had just refined the rubber vulcanization process. In response to Dr. Halsted's request, they manufactured rubber gloves for Ms. Hampton to wear, protecting her hands. Thus the first surgical gloves were developed to protect the hands of the worker, not to protect the patient.

When Goodyear made the first rubber surgical gloves, they probably contained only natural rubber cross-linked with a sulfur compound. In addition, they most likely took many hours to cure and probably were expensive compared with today's glove prices. For decades, medical gloves were so expensive that they were washed, checked for holes, powdered with talc, and sterilized repeatedly until they could no longer be used. Many nurses spent much of their time reprocessing surgical gloves.

As production methods improved, mass production of medical gloves reduced the costs of the gloves. In the 1960s single-use, disposable medical gloves were introduced. Low-cost medical gloves offered the convenience of throwing them away after use rather than rewashing and reprocessing them, which included steam sterilization. With the change to single-use gloves, the method for sterilization also changed to gamma irradiation. As a result, gloves were no longer washed or subjected to steam under pressure. The allergenic proteins in the gloves are water soluble. The proteins are denatured to some degree by steam under pressure. By removing both of these processes of steam and washing, the level of allergenic proteins in the gloves may have inadvertently increased, thus exposing wearers to greater levels of allergens. There is evidence of this in third world countries that still follow this practice. One study showed that in Venezuela, where gloves and catheters are reused, the incidence of latex allergy in the spina bifida population is not significantly higher than in the general population.

Allergic reaction to latex gloves was first reported in the literature by Downing in 1933. Reports of delayed allergic reactions appeared over the next several decades. NRL-induced anaphylaxis was first described in the literature in 1979, with a significant increase in the number of NRL-induced allergic reactions in the late 1980s. A number of events caused this rapid increase.

In the early 1980s the first cases of a new disease were being reported. We now know these were the first reports of human immunodeficiency virus (HIV) infection or acquired immunodeficiency syndrome (AIDS). The disease initially appeared to be found in the homosexual population but was soon found in persons with hemophilia and in infants whose mothers were infected with AIDS. In 1983 the Centers for Disease Control and Prevention (CDC) warned blood banks of a possible problem with the blood supply. Universal precautions were introduced in directives and guidelines issued by the CDC in 1987 and in standards published by the Occupational Safety and Health Administration (OSHA) in 1991 to protect HCWs and others from exposure to potentially contaminated blood and other bodily fluids. One of the key components of universal precautions is the use of gloves. One result of universal precautions was that HCWs who had historically not worn gloves (e.g., phlebotomists and dentists) began to wear gloves, and others who had sometimes previously worn gloves (e.g., nurses and physicians) began wearing them more frequently. It is estimated that glove use grew from 1.4 billion gloves in 1988 to 8.3 billion gloves in 1993. This resulted in increased exposure to both NRL and the chemicals used in the glove manufacturing process.

Universal precautions also resulted in the "Great Glove Shortage" of the 1980s, which had a significant impact on the manufacturing of latex gloves and other products. Scientists are not absolutely certain, however, whether changes in the manufacturing of latex gloves may have resulted in the increase in latex allergies. Manufacturers were having a difficult time keeping pace with the demand for surgical and examination gloves. In response to the demand for more raw latex to meet the shortage, plantation owners who grew and harvested the latex from their trees may have collected the latex before it had ripened. (Latex trees are not usually harvested until the plant is up to 7 years old, because the latex is considered immature.) This unripened or "green" latex contains proteins that are more allergenic or "potent." In addition, because of the increased demand for latex, the manufacturers, who had been harvesting and storing the raw latex until it was needed, were using it as quickly as possible to make gloves. This decreased the storage time of the raw materials, which previously had helped to destroy allergens. This action removed a natural ripening time in the latex manufacturing process, again allowing latex with more allergenic proteins to be used in glove manufacturing.

Up until this time a number of glove companies had manufacturing facilities located in North America. The raw latex was shipped in large tankers to plants for glove production. Some of these companies relocated their manufacturing plants to Southeast Asia, closer to the plantations where the latex is harvested. In doing so, once again a natural ripening time was removed from the process.

At the same time, new manufacturers were entering the market to fill the gap between supply and demand. The majority of latex in the world is produced in Malaysia. According to the Malaysian Industrial Development Association (MIDA), over 400 new licenses were issued to manufacturers between 1985 and 1990. Some of these new manufacturers may not have had the requisite knowledge, skill, or equipment to make a high-quality glove, thereby bringing potentially inferior products to the market. As health care workers from the time can attest, there were gloves coming into the hospitals that would tear apart on donning or completely stick together and be unwearable. In contrast, by 1995 MIDA reported the total number of glove manufacturers had fallen to approximately 100.

Another potential contributing factor worth considering is the weather. Some have speculated that variables such as hybridization and seasonal variation played a role. A drought occurred in areas where latex manufacturing facilities were located, which may have caused the manufacturers to reduce the amount of washing or "leaching" of the gloves and other latex products, resulting in more high-protein gloves entering the market.

The implementation of universal precautions coincided with another significant event. It was reported that over a dozen people in the United States were killed related to the use of barium enema tips (MedWatch, 1996). The latex cuff of the barium enema tips was suspected of containing an extraordinarily high level of latex proteins, which was attributed to a manufacturing anomaly. The fact that latex proteins could provoke anaphylactic responses, potentially injuring and killing people, stunned health care facilities and the medical latex glove industry. At the same time, because of the tremendous increase in medical glove use and the high latex protein content of some latex gloves, reported latex allergies among HCWs began increasing (MedWatch, 1996).

By 1992 the U.S. Food and Drug Administration (FDA) convened a meeting in Baltimore of government, academia, manufacturers, and scientists to discuss latex allergy. By this time it was well known that the allergenic proteins in the latex were the culprit. This meeting led to FDA selection of the Lowry testing method for total proteins in gloves and subsequent FDA labeling requirements for "low protein" claims.

From 1992 to the present, the levels of extractable latex proteins and antigens and powder and rubber chemicals have declined in most medical gloves. Most examination gloves used in the United States today are powder-free and nonlatex. Use of nonlatex gloves is growing quickly with the advent of better gloves made of chloroprene and polyisoprene. However, approximately 35% of surgical gloves used in the United States today are still powdered. Glove powder has been implicated in the transfer of latex proteins in the health care environment.

Today the number of new latex allergy cases appears to be declining, likely as a result of using fewer powdered, high-NRL antigen gloves (Early, 2005). However, type IV reactions to gloves (e.g., chemical reactions—primarily caused by accelerators) continue to occur. The chemical sensitivities may appear to be on the increase just because there are fewer new latex allergy cases.

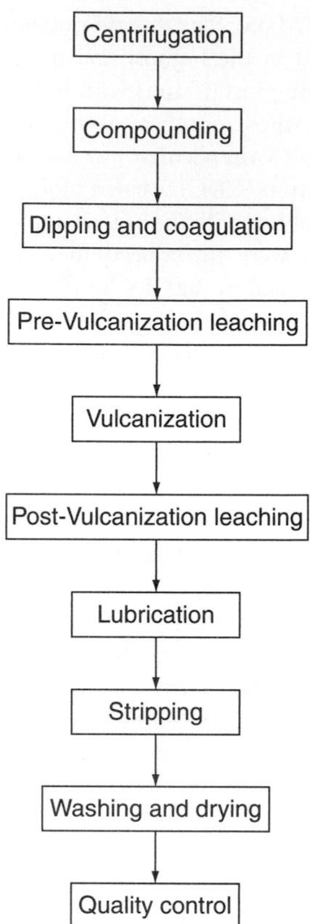

FIGURE 22-1 Glove manufacturing process.

MANUFACTURING PROCESS

Converting raw NRL into latex products is a complicated process, which actually consists of several separate processes. Because manufacturing plays an important role in the allergenicity of gloves and other products, a brief discussion of the latex manufacturing process is presented (Figure 22-1).

It is not uncommon for some glove factories to produce surgical gloves, examination gloves, industrial gloves, and even condoms. The primary differences in making these products are the level of quality and the formers used. The ASTM (originally known as the American Society for Testing and Materials) has developed Standard Specification for Rubber Surgical Gloves as well as Standard Specification for Rubber Examination Gloves. These cover certain requirements for the gloves used in conducting surgical procedures, medical examination, and diagnostic and therapeutic procedures.

Production of high-quality examination and surgical gloves includes ensuring that the environment throughout the glove factory and the quality of the latex are acceptable. The quality of the latex used has a direct effect on the quality of the glove produced. Therefore the manufacturing process starts with the preparation of the raw latex.

Ammonia is added to the latex as an anticoagulant. Ammoniation can, if performed at the right time, aid in the hydrolysis of the allergenic proteins in NRL. In addition, a small amount of chemicals may be added to stop microbiologic spoilage and curdling of the latex.

Centrifugation

Some manufacturers are experimenting with the addition of proteolytic enzymes before centrifugation to break down proteins in the mix and reduce the amount of available proteins in the final product. This development of deproteinized and purified NRL can significantly reduce protein levels. Some authors believe that these enzymes may also adversely affect the mechanical properties of the latex film.

Centrifuging the latex concentrates the rubber content and reduces the protein content. Double centrifuging can reduce protein content even further. In fact, many of the early cases of latex protein allergy might be traced to latex that had not been properly centrifuged (as well as to poor factory conditions). Today, improvements to latex quality such as pretreatment and additional centrifuging are performed to remove as many of the remaining impurities and proteins as possible, resulting in a better quality of latex for production.

Compounding

Compounding the raw latex (or nonlatex) material is mixing different chemicals such as accelerators, antioxidants, stabilizers, and colorants to a final solution suitable for the manufacturer's glove products and is a proprietary process. Manufacturers may add up to a dozen chemicals to the latex. Each manufacturer uses its own "recipe." Some manufacturers choose to control this compounding process themselves. Others may opt to purchase previously compounded NRL from other sources. Under the latter circumstances the amount and type of chemicals used from batch to batch may vary. Consequently, the number, type, and quantity of chemical allergens may also vary from batch to batch. Sulfur, one additive, is used to help form a product with superior stretch and recoil, adding strength to the glove, and to stabilize the latex for long-term storage.

Accelerator chemicals can cause type IV allergies in those individuals at risk. The chemicals most often implicated in type IV allergies are thiurams, mercaptobenzothiazoles (MBTs), and carbamates (dithiocarbamates).

- Thiurams are regarded as the most common cause of type IV delayed allergy. Thiurams are well known as sensitizing agents, and many manufacturers now replace thiurams with dithiocarbamates as the accelerators of choice.
- MBTs are used less frequently in glove production; thus the incidence of sensitization is lower than for other accelerator compounds.
- There are more than 34 types of carbamates (dithiocarbamates), and they are even less sensitizing than thiurams and MBTs.

Chemical accelerators are, for the most part, used up during curing and in the washing and leaching portions of the manufacturing process.

Dipping and Coagulation

Once compounding is complete, the latex mix is fed to the dipping tanks. In these tanks, hand-shaped formers are mounted on a continuous line that moves through the different steps of the manufacturing process. Glove formers are regularly inspected and cleaned before the molds are dipped into coagulant tanks. The formers are made of a material that can withstand high temperatures, usually porcelain. The hand-shaped formers must be smooth with no rough surface that could result in a pinhole or other imperfection in the glove. They are thoroughly cleaned so that the latex deposition can be even and continuous. Failure to clean the glove formers would cause the final product to possibly have defects such as holes. In the cleaning process the formers are dipped into an acid bath and rinsed with clean water. Then they are dipped into an alkaline bath to neutralize the acid and again rinsed in clean water. Afterward the formers are brushed to ensure that the surface of the formers is consistent. This is an important step to eliminate pinholes in the latex gloves.

The former is dipped into a coagulant (e.g., calcium nitrate), which assists in controlling the amount of latex that will be deposited on the glove (or how thick the glove is) and also ensures that the rubber will not adhere to the former. The thicker the requirements for the gloves, the longer the "dwell time" or the time the formers will travel in the coagulant tank. The clean and newly coated former then passes into a latex mixture. The solution may be an NRL or nonlatex compound, depending on what gloves are scheduled for manufacture on that particular run. The latex is allowed to build up some wet-gel strength before an initial leaching. The leaching is effective in removing residual calcium nitrate and soluble proteins. Hot water is used, and the tanks are continuously replenished with fresh water. It is here that the process deviates, depending on whether powder-free or powdered gloves are being manufactured.

Prevulcanization Leaching

Prevulcanization leaching, also known as wet-gel leaching, is the process of immersing the latex-coated formers into a bath or spray of water to wash out excess additives, such as coagulant, from previous stages. Chemical and protein content can be reduced at this stage. The effectiveness of the process depends on the temperature of the water, the duration of the leaching, and the rate of water exchange. Beading may be introduced at this stage to give each glove a rolled bead or rim at the open end.

Vulcanization

Vulcanization, or curing, was one of the key discoveries in the manufacture of rubber products. In this stage the latex film is heated, usually in hot-air ovens, initially at lower temperatures of 176° to 194° F (80° to 90° C) and then at higher temperatures of 212° to 284° F (100° to 140° C) where necessary. The combination of sulfur, accelerator, and heat causes cross-linking of the rubber, giving the film strength and elasticity .

Postvulcanization Leaching

Postvulcanization leaching, also called dry-film leaching, removes residual chemicals and proteins from the surface of the gloves. The effectiveness of this process is a function of time and temperature. This step is crucial to minimizing the occurrence of latex sensitivity. The key to making a good glove is to have a good leaching line. The glove leaching stage is one area in which factories will vary depending on the quality of gloves that are produced. Implementing a long leaching stage is more expensive and decreases the potential for profits as it relates to the reduced number of gloves produced. On-line washing is less expensive but tends to be less effective in removing the residual allergens. The best factories will constantly circulate fresh water, adding to the cost of making gloves. With on-line leaching the duration of leaching may be reduced to keep the lines moving at an acceptable rate. This may result in incomplete removal of water-soluble materials such as protein allergens. Off-line leaching does not pose this problem, because it is a separate operation that can last hours to days. Off-line leaching is used when complete removal of water-soluble materials is essential, but it involves more resources and therefore may be a more expensive process.

Lubrication

The next stage is one of a number of processes to aid in the ease of donning the gloves. A lubricant is added. Without this lubrication there is a high coefficient of friction between the glove surface and the hands of the wearer, which makes donning the glove more difficult, particularly if the hands are damp such as after performing surgical hand antisepsis. Historically a number of lubricants have been used, including, most commonly, talc powder and hydrolyzed corn starch. Unfortunately, much research over the past 60 years demonstrates numerous problems associated with cornstarch-powdered latex gloves, including postoperative adhesions and granulomas, peritonitis, aerosolization of protein allergens, and occupationally acquired asthma. Starch powder has been shown to bind the latex proteins and act as a vector for transfer of the protein to the skin and/or the lungs as an airborne dust. Research has shown that these latex protein allergens can sensitize individuals to NRL and/or exacerbate allergic reactions in the respiratory system of individuals already sensitive to latex. For this reason the health care community is shifting to the use of powder-free gloves.

Powder-Free Gloves

Latex gloves with very little or no powder lubricant can be prepared by either chlorination or addition of a polymer coating. Chlorination makes the glove surface slippery and allows the glove to slip on more easily without a powdered lubricant. Chlorination has been shown to substantially reduce protein levels in latex, but excessive chlorination can have a measurably detrimental effect on the aging and physical properties of the gloves.

A polymer coating replaces the powder with a suitable lubricating coat on the inner glove surface. Unlike chlorination, the addition of the polymer lining does not affect the physical properties of the latex. Both processes can be carried out on-line, without the powder-coating step, or off-line by first washing the finished powdered gloves, then subjecting them to the chlorination or polymer-coating treatment.

Powdered Gloves

If a powdered lubricant is used, the glove formers pass through a wet powder slurry to ensure even distribution over the glove surface. Interestingly, powder-free gloves may start out as powdered gloves. These gloves are rendered powder-free by thoroughly rinsing them in water.

With either powder-free or powdered gloves, in-line leaching, the use of the chlorination process, and high-temperature washing of gloves after they are removed from the formers are all highly effective methods to reduce the number of water-soluble latex allergenic proteins from the final latex glove. Issues surrounding the use of powdered gloves are discussed later in this chapter.

Stripping

This is the final operation on the production line. The latex gloves are stripped off the formers. This is often carried out manually, frequently with the assistance of compressed air, but an automatic stripping system is becoming more common. As the gloves are stripped, they are turned inside out so that what was the outer surface of the glove on the former is now the inner surface of the glove; the polymer lining that was on the outer surface is now inside the glove.

Washing and Drying

After the latex gloves are taken off the formers, they may be put into commercial washers and/or dryers to ensure that the powder is removed or, in the case of powdered gloves, more evenly distributed. A thorough washing can further reduce the number of latex proteins in the gloves. This process also makes the latex gloves more elastic.

Quality Control

A number of tests are required before receiving the gloves into the U.S. market. One of the quality tests is acceptable quality level (AQL). This is a standard for the number of holes allowed in the gloves. The FDA requires a 2.5 AQL or better for a shipment of medical-grade examination gloves and a 1.5 AQL or better for surgical gloves. The FDA requires the testing of medical gloves for pinholes by the water method. This is done by batches. In addition, in some plants the gloves undergo 100% testing by air inflation. These factories will inflate the latex gloves with air to visually detect any defects. Other tests will also be performed, such as tensile strength and elongation tests.

LATEX REACTIONS

As previously stated, there is more than one type of reaction to NRL products. The following are the three types of reactions that people may experience:

- Irritant contact dermatitis, which is nonallergic
- Type IV (delayed) hypersensitivity, also known as allergic contact dermatitis
- Type I (immediate) hypersensitivity

Understanding the difference between these three reactions is important in managing patients and workers with a suspected or documented latex allergy (Table 22-1). Exposure to NRL proteins occurs by several routes, including the following:

- Skin absorption when skin comes in contact with NRL products such as gloves
- Inhalation of aerosolized latex proteins bound to starch glove powder
- Ingestion by either failing to properly wash hands after contact with NRL proteins and before eating or eating food that has been handled with latex gloves
- Mucosal absorption when a mucous membrane such as the urethra, vagina, or rectum comes in contact with a latex product such as a catheter
- Intravenous (IV) absorption from syringes, tubing, Swan-Ganz catheters, and embolectomy catheters (although exposure via this route has decreased with the increase in use of nonlatex products such as syringes and IV lines)

Irritant Contact Dermatitis

The most common of the three glove reactions is a nonallergic, irritant dermatitis of the hand. Irritant contact dermatitis is a mechanical or thermal injury to the skin. Irritant dermatitis is NOT an allergic reaction. These reactions may appear similar to the type IV reactions, including dryness, redness, itching, peeling, and chapping, and if chronic they may cause cracking, fissures, and thickened skin, all of which end at the point of contact with the gloves (Figure 22-2). However, even though these may result from glove contact, they are not an allergic reaction. Irritant contact dermatitis can occur with either latex or nonlatex gloves. The condition may be caused and/or exacerbated by hand confinement in gloves, as well as frequent glove changes, frequent hand washing and wet working, exposure to chemicals, other

TABLE 22-1 Types of Natural Rubber Latex Reactions

	Irritant Contact Dermatitis	Type IV (Delayed) Hypersensitivity	Type I (Immediate) Hypersensitivity
Causes	Irritation to the outermost layers of the skin by chemical and/or mechanical irritants, including soaps and hand sanitizers, frequent hand washing, incomplete drying, friction from glove powder, chemicals.	Allergy to chemicals used in the manufacturing of both latex and nonlatex gloves.	Allergy to the natural rubber latex (*Hevea brasiliensis*) proteins found in such products as gloves (medical, household, and industrial), dental dams, condoms, balloons, and adhesives.
Prevalence	Common reaction. Is not an allergy.	Approximately 7%–18% of the population is affected.	The rarest of the three reactions. In normal adults the risk for sensitization to NRL may be as high as 6%. HCWs and others whose jobs require wearing latex gloves have a risk of about 10%. The estimated risk of individuals with spina bifida and people with congenital urinary tract defects is up to 50%.
Onset/reaction time	Can be hours to days.	Occurs 6–48 hours after exposure.	Immediate—within minutes and up to an hour after exposure.
Symptoms	Dryness, redness, cracking, peeling, chapping, fissures, thickened skin, ends at point of contact.	Skin may become fissured, thickened, and/or red. There may be a poison ivy–like rash, which can spread to areas above the level of the glove cuff, including the face, if touched.	Hives, runny/itchy nose, red/watery/itchy eyes, asthma and anaphylaxis (severe allergic reaction), nausea, and abdominal cramping. Severity depends upon the degree of sensitivity and amount of latex allergen to which the person is exposed.
Risk	Anyone who wears powdered gloves or gloves high in residual chemicals can develop this. In atopic individuals, contact dermatitis can be a sign of impending hypersensitivity if exposure to allergens continues.	If skin cracks, splits, or is bleeding from scratching, it is no longer considered intact. Intact skin is considered the primary barrier to pathogens. When skin is compromised, infection can occur more easily.	Emergency treatment for anaphylaxis may be required.
Treatment	Differential diagnosis must be conducted. Avoidance of substance(s) causing the reaction.	Differential diagnosis must be conducted. Avoidance of the chemical(s) causing the type IV hypersensitivity is the treatment of choice.	Avoid NRL allergen exposure. Anyone who has experienced a type I reaction, no matter the substance, should wear a medical ID bracelet and carry an EpiPen.

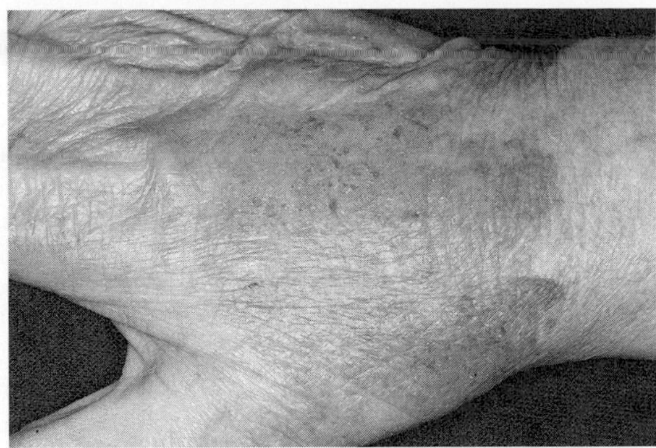

FIGURE 22-2 Irritant contact dermatitis. (From Habif T: *Color guide to diagnosis and therapy: clinical dermatology,* ed 4, St. Louis, 2004, Mosby.)

skin irritants such as soaps and lotions, and glove powder, which is a mechanical abrasive. Even the cold, dry air of winter can affect the skin.

There are risk groups for latex glove–induced occupational dermatitis. Occupational skin disease primarily affects workers younger than the age of 40. Contact dermatitis has a greater prevalence in workers 31 years of age or younger and in women. A risk factor for dermatitis may be the number of pairs of gloves used daily as opposed to the profession or degree of exposure to latex in the workplace. In one study, when workers wore 1 to 6 pairs of latex gloves per day, their risk for irritant dermatitis was 2.8%; with 7 to 30 pairs worn per day, the risk was 4.0%; and wearing more than 30 pairs carried a risk of 6.4% (Trape et al, 2000).

Diagnosis and Management

Because irritant contact dermatitis can mimic a type IV reaction, a differential diagnosis is performed. Because irritant dermatitis is the most prevalent of the three reactions, a reaction on the skin is initially presumed to be the cause. Treatment includes eliminating the irritant source to see if the skin improves. If using powdered gloves, switch to powder-free gloves. When washing hands, change the type of soap, decrease the amount of soap used, rinse hands thoroughly, and, when using hot water to wash, possibly switch to cool water at the end of the rinse. If stiff paper towels of low quality are used often, potentially switching to a softer, higher quality towel may have an effect. It is important not to change everything at once so as to be able to identify the culprit(s). If this does not resolve the issue, an occupational health practitioner, dermatologist, allergist, or immunologist may recommend the use of creams, lotions, or other similar agents on the hands. If the symptoms continue, a type IV reaction is suspected.

Caution must be used in selecting hand care products. Certain skin care products might increase the likelihood of antigen absorption by increasing protein extraction and protein transfer. Some agents that are petroleum based may cause breakdown of the latex product. Choose products that do not alter the physical characteristics of gloves or compromise barrier effectiveness. Only use water- or silicone-based products; no petroleum- or oil-based products. Remember to check ingredient labels carefully.

Type IV Delayed Hypersensitivity

Type IV delayed hypersensitivity, or allergic contact dermatitis, is a reaction to chemical additives in the gloves. To speed up the curing process, accelerators are added to the natural rubber latex. The following are the most commonly used glove accelerators:

- Thiurams (e.g., tetramethyl thiuram disulfide [TMTD], tetraethyl thiuram disulfide [TETD])
- Carbamates (e.g., dithiocarbamate [DTC], diethyl dithiocarbamate [DEC])
- Guanidines (e.g., diphenylguanidine [DPG])
- Thiazoles (e.g., 2-mercaptobenzothiazole [MBT] and zinc mercaptobenzothiazole [ZMBT])
- Thioureas (e.g., diphenylthiourea [DPTU], also known as: 1,3-diphenyl-2-thiourea or thiocarbanilide)

Because of sensitivity issues, the use of thiurams has been largely discontinued.

Although type IV allergy to glove chemicals is less common that irritant dermatitis, it is more common than type I allergy to NRL. Type IV symptoms appear as red (erythematous), irritated skin where the glove covers the skin, possibly extending slightly beyond the glove cuff. Pruritus, edema, eczema, blisters/pimples, and cracking of the skin are common (Figure 22-3). The skin can become inflamed and leather-like with time. Poison oak and poison ivy are other examples of type IV reactions and will have a similar appearance. Type IV reactions are usually localized and are mediated by T-lymphocyte cells in the skin. Type IV reactions are not usually life threatening.

Allergic contact dermatitis has an onset of 6 to 48 hours; thus reactions appear up to a day or two after wearing a glove. Persons with type IV reactions often report disappearance of symptoms when off work for a few days, such as over the weekend or while on vacation, with symptoms returning a day or two after reporting to work and reexposing the hands to the gloves. Allergic contact dermatitis can occur with either latex or nonlatex gloves because the same chemicals are used in the manufacture of nonlatex gloves as for NRL gloves. Consequently, persons who react to accelerators in NRL gloves might not find relief when switching to nonlatex gloves.

Diagnosis and Management

Chemical sensitivities can come from many sources—soaps, metals (such as nickel), gloves, and lotions, to name a few. Consequently, a diagnosis is made by testing for reactions to chemicals. This is usually done by an allergist using a patch test or sometimes a wear test. Treatment is the same as for irritant contact dermatitis—avoidance of the causative agent. For gloves this means identifying gloves that are not made with the offending chemical(s).

Manufacturers should make available a list of the chemicals used in their manufacturing process for appropriate glove selection. A potential cause for variation in allergens, both chemical and protein, is the fact that some companies do not make their own gloves. These companies buy gloves from different sources, called jobbers, and then attach their own label to them. This can result in gloves with the same brand varying greatly in the amount of allergens they contain.

People with type IV allergy may have to wear gloves made from a thermoplastic such as styrene-butadiene-styrene or a similar copolymer material that is manufactured without using the offending accelerators.

Type I Hypersensitivity

Type I reactions are the true allergy to NRL and the least common of the three reactions. Type I allergy is an IgE-mediated (or B-cell mediated) allergic response to water-soluble proteins in NRL. A type I allergic reaction is an immediate hypersensitivity reaction that usually occurs within minutes or even seconds of contact with the proteins. Allergic reactions to NRL proteins can range from skin redness and itching to rhinoconjunctivitis (Figure 22-4), difficulty breathing, hives, acute gastrointestinal distress, wheezing, hypotension, and, if untreated, anaphylaxis and death—though true

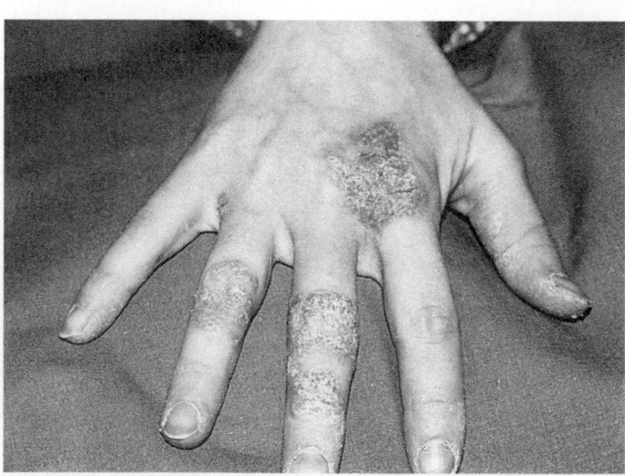

FIGURE 22-3 Type IV delayed hypersensitivity. (From Damjanov I, Linder J: *Anderson's pathology,* ed 10, St. Louis, 1996, Mosby.)

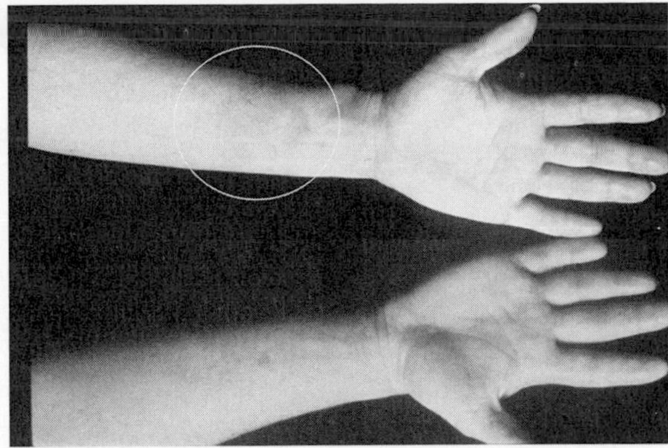

FIGURE 22-4 Type I (immediate) hypersensitivity. Allergic reaction on hands and arms. (Courtesy Mölnlycke Health Care, Norcross, Ga.)

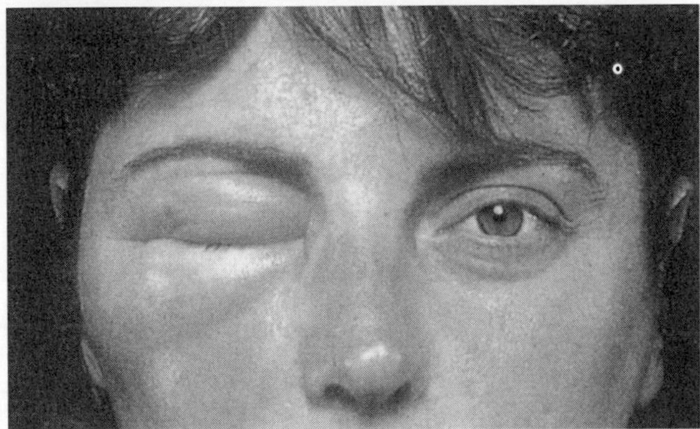

FIGURE 22-5 Type I (immediate) hypersensitivity. Allergic reaction on face. (From Male D et al: *Immunology,* ed 7, St. Louis, 2006, Mosby.)

allergic reactions to latex rarely progress to life-threatening patient conditions (Figure 22-5).

Diagnosis and Management

The gold standard for allergy testing is the skin prick test, because it has a sensitivity and specificity close to 100% (ASA, 2005). However, there is not currently an FDA-approved skin prick reagent for NRL. Practitioner-made preparations do exist. Because of the potential for severe allergic reaction, prick testing should be performed under controlled conditions with appropriate safeguards (e.g., emergency equipment and medication available) by medically qualified personnel.

Serum tests approved by the FDA are available in the United States. Unfortunately, these tests for specific proteins may not include the offending antigen for the individual being tested. There are over 240 proteins in NRL. So far, researchers have identified 13 proteins that can bind with IgE and therefore cause allergic reactions in humans (Table 22-2). Sensitivity appears to vary between groups, so false negatives (25% to 30%) are not uncommon. Cross-reactivity with certain pollens and plant food allergens may complicate the diagnosis. Unfortunately, no test can provide 100% confirmation of latex allergy. The ASA recommends a thorough history with the use of in vitro and/or in vivo tests.

Management of NRL-allergic individuals is dependent upon the type of reaction (i.e., irritant contact dermatitis, type IV [delayed] hypersensitivity, type I [immediate] hypersensitivity) and extent of symptomatology. The initial plan should begin with the implementation of removing sources of latex and promoting a latex safe environment for both the health care worker and patients to minimize exposure to materials that contain latex. This should include, but is not limited to, the development of an institution

TABLE 22-2 Registered Natural Rubber Latex Allergens

Name	Trivial Name	Molecular Weight*	Allergenicity
Hev b 1	Rubber elongation factor	14	SB 81%, HCW 52%
Hev b 2	Beta-1,3-glucanases	34	
Hev b 3	Small rubber-particle protein	24	SB 83%, HCW 24%
Hev b 4	Microhelix component	53–55	HCW 39%
Hev b 5	Acidic latex protein	16	SB 26%, HCW 65% and 92%
Hev b 6.01 Hev b 6.02 Hev b 6.03	Prohevein, Hevein preprotein Hevein Prohevein C-terminal fragment	20	HCW 63%
Hev b 7.01 = Hev b 13 (renamed) Hev b 7.02	Patatin homologue from B-serum Patatin homologue from C-serum	42	HCW 45%
Hev b 8	Latex profilin	15	
Hev b 9	Latex enolase	51	HCW 14.5%
Hev b 10	Mn-superoxide dismutase	26	
Hev b 11	Class I endochitinase	30	
Hev b 12	Lipid transfer protein	9	
Hev b 13 (= Hev b 7.01)	Latex esterase, early nodule-specific protein (ENSP)	42	HCW 63%

*SDS Page is a gel electrophoresis test.

HCW, Health care worker; *SB*, spina bifida.

From International Union of Immunological Societies Allergen Nomenclature Sub-Committee: *List of allergens*, 2009, available at http://dmd.nihs.go.jp/latex/allergen-e.html . Accessed July 21, 2009.

policy and procedure to address latex allergy and sensitivity management for HCWs and patients, availability of latex-free supplies and products, management expectations that address the care of a patient with latex allergies and the care of employees with latex allergies, and staff education to promote awareness of the issue.

Determining Latex Reaction

A final point to be made is that these three reactions—irritant dermatitis, type IV, and type I—are separate and distinct from one another. A common misperception is that a person will initially present with an irritant dermatitis reaction, progress to a type IV, and then develop a type I allergy to NRL. Although someone may progress through all three reactions, this is not necessarily—indeed not frequently—the case. A person may develop a type I systemic reaction, including symptoms such as hives and wheezing, without ever developing a rashlike symptom on the hands. Conversely, a person can be plagued by irritant dermatitis for years without ever developing an allergic reaction to either the chemicals or latex.

The relationship between the three is that if the skin becomes nonintact, such as through either the irritant dermatitis or type IV reaction, the absorption of allergens may occur at a more rapid rate. Therefore, if the patient is going to develop an allergy, this may occur more quickly than if the skin had remained intact.

Latex-Fruit Syndrome

There is a relationship between latex allergy and allergy to certain foods. Individuals with a history of NRL allergy seem to have a much higher rate of allergy to certain foods than the general public. In one study 70% of those who were allergic to latex reacted to one or more foods, compared with 15% of those who were nonallergic.

Foods implicated in the latex-fruit syndrome are classified as follows:

- Class I—clinical findings
- Class II—clinical findings and characterization of cross-reactive components (by extract inhibition assays)
- Class III—clinical findings and characterization of cross-reactive allergens.

Because of the close relationship between the reactive allergens, it is the class III foods that have the highest correlation with NRL allergy (Box 22-1).

Powder Issues

Originally, surgical gloves were disinfected by boiling in water and were then donned over the damp hands of the surgical team, who had just washed. The moistness of both hand and glove acted to reduce the amount of friction and allowed relatively easy donning. As the use of gloves expanded and the technology progressed, the gloves were sterilized using steam under pressure, which resulted in the surgical team members trying to don dry gloves over their wet hands—a very difficult proposition. To replace the moisture that had previously allowed the glove to slip easily over the skin, powder was added as the donning lubricant. Numerous powders were used over time, including lycopodium—the spores of a club moss—and talc—finely ground mica, a mineral substance. The dangers of these materials were clearly documented, and cornstarch powder was substituted as a safer alternative. Unfortunately, foreign-body reactions were also reported to cornstarch (Ellis, 2008).

BOX 22-1 Foods Implicated in the Latex-Fruit Syndrome by Class

CLASS I
Watermelon
Carrot
Apple
Cherry
Coconut
Apricot
Strawberry
Loquat
Spinach

CLASS II
Peach
Fig
Melon
Pineapple

CLASS III
Avocado
Banana
Chestnut
Cherimoya
Passion fruit
Kiwi
Papaya
Mango
Tomato
Bell pepper
Potato
Celery

It is not the purpose of this chapter to review in depth the issues related to the use of glove powder. However, because of the broad clinical impact powder has on the patient, a brief overview is required. Over the years there have been extensive reports of tissue reaction to these different lubricants, including the development of abdominal adhesions, granuloma formation, infection, poor healing, female reproductive sterility, and misdiagnosis of cancer. The effects of glove powder have long been reported in the peritoneum following abdominal surgery but have also been found in many types of tissue, including pericardium, pleura, meninges, retroperitoneum, testes and epididymis, inguinal and femoral regions, renal glomeruli, and synovial regions. Even the specialty of anesthesia has been shown to be affected with the demonstration that extradural catheters may be easily contaminated by starch powder from surgical gloves, which may then be deposited into the extradural space (Green et al, 1995).

With the appearance of latex allergy, the issues surrounding glove powder have increased. Glove powder has been clearly shown to bind to the NRL proteins and cause them to become aerosolized, thus increasing exposure to the allergens. As a result, numerous regulatory and professional organizations recommend that powdered gloves not be allowed around latex-allergic persons.

Occupational Asthma

The aerosolized powder may also contribute to the development of occupational asthma (FDA, 1999). Occupational asthma is asthma that is caused or worsened by breathing in a workplace irritant, such as chemical fumes, gases, or dust. Occupational asthma is caused by a response to specific allergens in the workplace. Examples of these are low-molecular-weight allergens such as glutaraldehyde, anhydrides, diisocyanates, varnishes, adhesives, laminates, and soldering resin, and high-molecular-weight allergens such as plant substances, including proteins found in natural rubber latex, flour, cereals, cotton, flax, hemp, rye, wheat, and papain. (Mayo Clinic, 2009)

The prevalence of latex protein–induced occupational asthma is estimated to be 2.5% to 6% among HCWs. Latex-induced asthma can lead to permanent respiratory disability, even after leaving the place of exposure. Once an individual becomes sensitized, exposure to even low doses will trigger asthma. "Patients with confirmed sensitizer-induced occupational asthma should have no further exposure to the causative agent, since the best outcome is achieved with early diagnosis and complete avoidance of exposure" (Tarlo and Liss, 2003).

According to the Mayo Clinic (2009), "When diagnosed and treated early, occupational asthma may be reversible. Long-term exposure to irritants can cause worsening symptoms and lifetime asthma. Treatment for occupational asthma is similar to treatment for other types of asthma, and it generally includes taking medications to reduce symptoms. But the only sure way eliminate your symptoms and prevent lung damage due to occupational asthma is to avoid whatever's triggering it."

In a 1999 report from the Rollins School of Public Health at Emory University, Phillips et al (1999) state that there are institutions that have gone powder-free and that it "significantly reduces the amount of latex allergen in the environment." In conclusion they stated, "Latex allergy appears to be a rare case in which primary prevention will likely prove to be a cost savings."

Investigators found that, following implementation of federal regulations that eliminated glove powder, the German health care system was able to significantly reduce occupationally acquired latex allergy disease on a national level when combined with increased awareness and depth of knowledge in facilities using powder-free, low-protein gloves. "These results show that primary prevention of occupational NRL allergies can be achieved if these straightforward and practical interventions are properly carried out and maintained" (Allmers et al, 2003).

PREVENTING LATEX REACTIONS

AORN (2009) states, "The goals of prevention are twofold: to prevent reactions in individuals who are latex-sensitized and to prevent initial sensitization of nonsensitized persons. The only effective preventive strategy at this time is latex avoidance. Working in an environment that is free of powdered, high-allergen latex gloves and products will help minimize sensitization of health care workers." Many professional and regulatory agencies, as well as health care providers, recommend and/or require the use of low-allergen, powder-free latex gloves because "the presence of even small amounts of residual aerosolized latex in the air or on surfaces can trigger a life-threatening reaction" (AORN, 2009).

PATIENT MANAGEMENT

Management of type I allergy includes strict avoidance of latex products for all NRL-allergic individuals and education for all HCWs, patients, and family members. When diagnosed as latex allergic, a patient needs to order and wear a medical alert tag to indicate his or her allergy. For type I allergic individuals, NRL protein avoidance through the use of synthetic gloves and products and the creation of a powder-free, latex-safe environment are important steps toward risk reduction. AORN (2009) states, "Although it is impossible to remove all latex from the environment (e.g., wheels on carts), all latex that may potentially contact the individual should be removed. Latex products selected for use should be low-allergen and powder-free."

According to the Mayo Clinic (2007), once a person is sensitized, the best way to prevent an allergic reaction is to avoid latex and take the following measures:

- Reduce your exposure.
- Talk to your employer about reducing the number of latex products you might come in contact with at work.
- Inform your health care professionals about your allergy.
- Choose alternative gloves.
- Avoid inhaling latex, and request that the people you work with use gloves that are not powdered.
- Wear a medical alert bracelet.
- Ask for advice. Talk to your doctor about your latex allergy. He or she might be able to suggest

other ways you can avoid latex in your daily life and reduce your chances of an allergic reaction. Your doctor might also suggest emergency medication to keep with you in case you have a severe reaction to latex.

Sensitized Versus Allergic Patients

The question has been asked, "What if the patient is only sensitive to latex, not allergic?" For management purposes, there is no distinction between the two. Sensitization is the development of an immunologic memory in response to exposure to an allergen (AORN, 2009). Although the patient may present as clinically asymptomatic, there is potential risk for severe reaction with additional exposure.

Persons allergic to NRL should wear only nonlatex gloves. Although there has been some recent discussion regarding hospitals changing to all nonlatex gloves, this may not be feasible and is not the most desirable approach for many facilities. The ECRI (2004) recommends the following:

1. Purchase gloves with protein levels that are as low as possible.
2. Purchase gloves that have protein levels printed on their labeling or that bear the Standard Malaysian Glove (SMG) label.
3. If possible, purchase gloves with 50 µg or less of protein per square decimeter of NRL.

Package Labeling and Protein Testing

As of September 30, 1998, manufacturers must display the following statement on all medical devices made from natural rubber latex that are designed for patient contact: "Caution: this product contains natural rubber latex which may cause allergic reactions" (U.S. Department of Health and Human Services, 1997). This ruling does not include pharmaceuticals or products that are not regulated by the FDA.

Knowing the levels of water-extractable proteins is important. The federal government has instituted guidelines regarding protein level claims. Using the modified Lowry assay (ASTM standard test method D 5712–99), a manufacturer may submit documentation requesting a low-protein claim. The documentation must show that the product consistently contains less than the claimed number of micrograms of total water-extractable protein per gram of latex. The lowest level claim that can be made is that the product contains 50 µg or less of total water-extractable protein per gram of latex by the modified Lowry assay.

The modified Lowry is not a perfect test. Some researchers and manufacturers believe that chemical substances can interfere with the results of the modified Lowry assay. In addition, the modified Lowry measures total protein, not just the 13 identified allergenic proteins, and the sensitivity of the test has been questioned because it cannot accurately measure below 50 µg. However, it is relatively inexpensive, rapid, and easily performed.

The ELISA (*E*nzyme-*L*inked *I*mmunosorbent *A*ssay) inhibition assay tests gloves for immunologically reactive latex protein. This method uses antibodies that specifically recognize latex antigens. According to manufacturers, it is more sensitive than the modified Lowry. It is sensitive to 15 ng/mL (1 ng = 10^{-9}g). When evaluating latex gloves, in addition to the required modified Lowry information, you may wish to consider asking manufacturers for the ELISA inhibition assay, which is very similar and is specified as an ASTM standard.

A word of caution: use of low-protein gloves is not the same as nonlatex gloves. The FDA requires that the following statement appear on the packaging whenever the low-protein claim is made: "Safe use of this product by or on latex sensitive individuals has not been established."

ENVIRONMENTAL MANAGEMENT

Hospitals and other health care facilities vary greatly in their size, structure, and function. Consequently, no one solution to the creation and maintenance of a latex-safe environment will apply to all circumstances. There are, however, guidelines that can be used to create a cost-effective, yet safe, latex allergy management program.

Creating a latex-safe environment does not mean eliminating latex products. Latex remains an extremely effective barrier against bloodborne pathogens and is cost-effective. Instead, the goal should be to provide a safe environment for persons who are already sensitized and reduce the sensitization of additional individuals. For sensitized patients or workers, the elimination of starch glove powder removes a source of airborne allergen.

Most departments have no control over the type of patients admitted to and treated on their unit. The arrival of a latex-sensitized patient may result in delay or cancellation of tests or procedures, waste of previously opened supplies, and inconvenience to patients. Latex exposure may place the patient at risk for an adverse reaction. These events are very costly to the institution or health care practice. Therefore maintaining the entire health care environment as latex-safe has proved to be an effective and cost-accountable method of environmental management.

Once latex products have been identified and synthetic substitutes found, the facility should develop specific guidelines, policies, and procedures. Latex use must be supervised to be certain the appropriate products are being used.

Workers with a confirmed latex protein allergy should use only synthetic gloves and should avoid all products containing NRL. Other persons in the same work environment should use only powder-free, low-allergen gloves, or, when appropriate, powder-free, synthetic gloves. Clinical units treating children with spina bifida or patients with medical conditions that require early and repeated surgical intervention and/or frequent mucosal contact with latex devices should consider these patients to be at high risk. Many hospitals treat such patients as though they are NRL allergic. Use of alternative products that do not contain natural rubber latex will help reduce the risk. Many resources are available on the Internet to assist in identification of products containing latex. However, the only sure mechanism is to contact the manufacturer directly.

An inventory or master list of all current products should be undertaken to determine products that contain NRL, and identification of appropriate latex-free substitutes is usually undertaken. Following this, whenever a new product is evaluated by the value analysis team or products committee, its allergenic content, barrier quality, and the presence of starch powder should be determined. Many institutions have a product screening questionnaire that is completed before a new product is considered. Adding these questions can assist in the latex-safe screening process.

AORN (2009) recommends having a latex-safe cart available for consolidating latex-free items in a single place for ease of location and use. This cart or bin contains commonly used patient care items. When a latex-allergic patient is admitted to the hospital, a staff member contacts materials management to obtain the cart. Critical areas such as the operating room or emergency department may choose to keep a latex-free cart permanently on the unit for use in emergency situations. After a cart is used, it may follow the patient to the next treatment area. If the cart is specific to a certain department such as the operating room, emergency department, or labor and delivery and differs from the general housewide cart, the department receiving the patient should be notified so they can order their own latex-free cart.

Some hospitals are actively replacing many latex products with latex-free items such as IV tubing, syringes, and tourniquets. As this shift occurs, some hospitals are deleting their latex cart and simply compiling a short list of the few products that contain latex and are to be avoided by latex-allergic patients. Emergency code carts should be completely latex-free.

An increasing number of facilities are banning latex balloons from the environment. Many facilities require that all balloons sold in the gift shop, delivered by florists, or brought in by visitors be made of Mylar. Posting a sign at all entrances will aid in public education and policy enforcement.

A couple of specific questions are often asked regarding the prophylactic treatment of surgical patients and the use of medications in multidose vials. Pretreating latex-allergic individuals before surgery or anesthesia remains controversial because it may mask the initial signs of an allergic reaction (ASA, 2005). Another controversial issue is the use of medication vials with rubber stoppers. AORN (2009) recommends that "Whenever possible, medications should be used from a latex-free vial. When this is not possible, arrangements with the pharmacy should be made in advance so medications can be drawn into a latex-free delivery device under aseptic conditions (e.g., inside the pharmacy's hood). If neither of these solutions is possible, the stopper should be removed and the medication withdrawn using a latex-free syringe. AORN does not recommend this practice unless all other options have been exhausted."

PATIENT ASSESSMENT FOR AN NRL ALLERGY

Because more facilities are implementing latex allergy protocols, and because latex-allergic surgery patients have become more common, managing patients with an allergy to NRL may be less stressful than in the past. The difficulty now may be determining which patients are at risk for a latex allergy, rather than actually providing a safe environment once it is determined that a patient is latex allergic.

A good screening questionnaire is an important first step and will screen out those who are obviously allergic to latex or obviously not allergic to latex. However, sometimes patients do not clearly fit into either category. People who have other hand problems, such as irritant dermatitis, may respond affirmatively to a latex screening questionnaire when indeed they do not have an NRL allergy. On the other hand, you may have patients who express some symptoms but are certain that latex allergy is not an issue with them. This is where patient assessment may become more of a challenge.

An initial assessment should identify risk factors and/or symptoms. It is important to elicit whether the patient is atopic, meaning they have either a personal or family history of hay fever, asthma, eczema, or multiple allergies. The patient may not express any of these; however, if a grandparent, parent, sibling, or other blood relative does, the patient is a greater risk. Consequently, asking about relatives is very important.

Another important risk factor to assess is NRL exposure. Occupational exposure is one source, which may include the following:

- Persons employed in health care occupations
- Persons employed in the NRL industry
- Food service workers
- Housekeepers
- Police, fire, and criminal justice workers
- Cosmetologists
- Day care workers
- Automobile mechanics

There is also an increase in the number of persons wearing gloves around the home. You may know of people who wear latex gloves to paint, work in their garden, or work on their car.

Other routes of exposure may be frequent surgeries or invasive medical procedures and extensive dental work, including orthodontia. Patients with congenital anomalies and infants who have been hospitalized for long periods may also have had increased exposure.

Assess for potential past reactions to the cross-reactive foods such as avocado, bananas, kiwi, chestnuts, and potatoes. In addition, when asking about reactions to potatoes, it is important to ask about peeling and slicing raw potatoes. When potatoes are cooked, the proteins in them tend to break down (as they are when gloves are steam sterilized) so a person may not react to them. However, there may be a response when handling raw potatoes.

The nurse should inquire about food avoidance or dislikes, which can lead to questions about specific reactions when these foods are eaten, such as tingly lips, tightness in the throat, or headaches. These are symptoms the patient typically may not associate with an allergy.

Once it has been determined that a person is at risk, it is important to assess for symptoms and/or specific reactions to products containing NRL. Some questions and rationales for their inclusion are the following:

- Do you have problems with adhesive bandages or tape? Many adhesives contain NRL.
- What happened the last time you went to the dentist? A common response is that the patient always gets "cold sores" following a dentist appointment. Or that his or her lips get tingly or swell, or the patient's throat gets tight. Leaving the question open-ended will allow the person to express any kind of symptoms from localized to systemic reactions. This question can also be asked about trips to the gynecologist and other health care providers.
- What happens when you blow up a rubber balloon? An interesting observation is that many times patients say, "I don't know. I don't blow up balloons." It is appropriate to follow up with "Why don't you blow up balloons? Are you never around them, or have you had problems in the past?" It may be that they simply are not around balloons. However, some patients respond, "Well, they just bother me so I don't blow them up." When asked about specific symptoms—"What 'bothered' you in the past?" —patients have reported a range of symptoms from tingly, swelling lips, to headaches, to wheezing.
- Do you ever have problems with condoms? Again, the response you receive may be, "I don't know, we don't use condoms." So asking the next assessment question is essential. "This is very important. May I please ask why you don't use a condom? Is it because you don't need birth control, you use another form of birth control, or you had problems with condoms in the past?"

Asking specific questions may assist patients with recalling past reactions they have had that could be latex related, but they did not realize the source of the reaction at the time. Many organizations, such as AORN and ASA, have sample screening questionnaires.

These guidelines are intended to assist the nurse in assessing a patient's reactions to NRL products. However, nothing replaces a complete workup with a knowledgeable allergist or other qualified health care provider. Any person who suspects he or she has a latex allergy should avoid contact with latex gloves and products until evaluated by a physician experienced in treating latex allergy.

CONCLUSION

Latex gloves have been used by HCWs for nearly a century. Their function is to prevent cross infection, for both the patient and the worker. Latex is the best, least expensive barrier we currently have at our disposal. It is nonporous, flexible, and relatively inexpensive compared with synthetic alternatives. It is derived from a natural renewable resource and is biodegradable, unlike the synthetic gloves, which are produced from oil.

Even if manufacturers solve the issues discussed, when a glove fails as a barrier, it ceases to fulfill its intended purpose. Glove failures result in exposures to HCWs and patients, putting them both at risk from bloodborne pathogens and pathogenic organisms (see Chapter 19).

Today, more than ever, health care decision makers must look at all factors to analyze outcomes for patients, HCWs, and the institution. For patients, positive outcomes mean successful procedures allowing quick recovery and maximum quality of life. For HCWs, positive outcomes depend on their being able to perform duties without undue personal risk. For the institution, it is important to ensure economic viability. A glove that has a low failure rate, is low in allergenic latex proteins, is low in residual chemical accelerators, and is powder-free greatly reduces risk and leads to desired outcomes for the patient, employee, and institution.

REFERENCES

Allmers H, et al: Primary prevention of natural rubber latex allergy in the German health care system through education and intervention, *J Allergy Clin Immunol* 110:318–323, 2002.

American Academy of Allergy, Asthma and Immunology: *Allergy statistics, 2009*, available at http://www.aaaai.org/media/statistics/allergy-statistics.asp. Accessed July 20.

American Society of Anesthesiologists: *Natural rubber latex allergy: considerations for anesthesiologists, 2005*, available at http://www.asahq.org/publicationsAndServices/latexallergy.pdf. Accessed July 20, 2009.

Association of periOperative Registered Nurses: Latex guideline. In *Association of periOperative Registered Nurses: Perioperative standards and recommended practices*, Denver, 2009, The Association.

Downing J: Dermatitis from rubber gloves, *N Engl J Med* 208:196–198, 1933.

Early PJ: Good news for people with latex allergies. In *HealthLink*, Milwaukee, Wis., 2005, Medical College of Wisconsin.

ECRI: Guidance article: lower-protein latex gloves, *Health Devices* 33:172, 2004.

Ellis H: Evolution of the surgical glove, *J Am Coll Surg* 207:948–950, 2008.

Green MA, et al: Starch, gloves and extradural catheters, *Br J Anaesth* 75(6):768–770, 1995.

Hepner DL, Castells MC: Anaphylaxis during the perioperative period, *Anesth Analg* 97:1381–1395, 2003.

International Union of Immunological Societies Allergen Nomenclature Sub-Committee: *List of allergens*, 2009, available at http://dmd.nihs.go.jp/latex/allergen-e.html. Accessed July 21, 2009.

Mayo Clinic: *Latex allergy: prevention, 2007*, available at http://www.mayoclinic.com/health/latex-allergy/DS00621/DSECTION=prevention. Accessed on July 20, 2009.

Mayo Clinic: *Occupational asthma, 2009*, available at http://www.mayoclinic.com/health/occupational-asthma/DS00591. Accessed on July 21, 2009.

MedWatch: *The clinical impact of adverse event reporting, 1996*, available at http://www.fda.gov/downloads/Safety/MedWatch/UCM168505.pdf. Accessed November 30, 2009.

Phillips VL, et al: Health care worker disability due to latex allergy and asthma: a cost analysis, *Am J Public Health* 89(7):1024–1028, 1999.

Tarlo SM, Liss GM: Occupational asthma: an approach to diagnosis and management, *CMAJ* 168:867–871, 2003.

Trape M, et al: Latex gloves use and symptoms in health care workers 1 year after implementation of a policy restricting the use of powdered gloves, *Am J Infect Control* 28:352–358, 2000.

U.S. Department of Health and Human Services: *FDATALK PAPER: latex labeling required for medical devices*, Rockville, Md, 1997, Food and Drug Administration, Public Health Service, available at http://www.fda.gov/bbs/topics/ANSWERS/ANS00826.html. Accessed on July 20, 2009.

U.S. Food and Drug Administration: Surgeon's and patient examination gloves, reclassification and medical glove guidance manual availability, proposed rule and notice, 21 CFR parts 801, 878, 880, *Fed Regist* 64(146):41710, 1999, available at http://www.fda.gov/OHRMS/DOCKETS/98fr/073099a.txt. Accessed July 22, 2009.

MINIMIZING RADIATION EXPOSURE

Kelly H. Austin, MS

Many perioperative nurses are involved with diagnostic, interventional, and therapeutic procedures in medical facilities that use ionizing radiation. Medical facilities that use ionizing radiation must have an established radiation safety program (RSP) with policies and procedures designed to protect the patient, health care workers, nurses, and physicians. The goal of the program is to ensure safety in these environments and minimize exposure to ionizing radiation. In order to use radioactive materials the facility must have a radioactive material license or permit with a state or the U.S. Nuclear Regulatory Commission (NRC). Facilities using radiation-producing machines for diagnostic x-ray examination and fluoroscopy must register each machine with the state. In each situation a radiation safety officer is designated as the individual responsible for managing the RSP. A successful RSP protects patients, radiation health care workers, members of the public, and the environment from ionizing radiation used in the facility.

Perioperative nurses are a critical component to successfully implementing the RSP because they are the "end user," the person who works directly with the patients undergoing procedures involving ionizing radiation. It is the goal of this chapter to provide perioperative nurses with practical information pertaining to the safe use of ionizing radiation, facilitating care and answering patients' questions regarding care specifics, and enhancing awareness of best practices when working around ionizing radiation.

TYPES OF IONIZING RADIATION

The term *radiation* is very broad; this discussion will focus on radiation that has the ability to cause ionization. Ionization is the process of removing or converting electrons from atoms. Ionizing radiation can be created from radiation-producing machines such as diagnostic x-ray units. Another source of ionizing radiation comes from radionuclides. A radionuclide is an atom with an unstable nucleus. The unstable nucleus is characterized as having excess energy, which is available to be imparted either to a newly created radiation particle within the nucleus or to an atomic electron. The radionuclide in this process undergoes radioactive decay and emits gamma ray(s) and/or particles. These rays and particles constitute ionizing radiation. Radionuclides may occur naturally but can also be artificially produced.

There are many types of ionizing radiation such as beta particles, gamma radiation, x-rays, positrons, alpha particles, and neutrons. The primary types of radiation used in the diagnosis and treatment of disease are gamma radiation, x-rays, and positrons. Occasionally beta radiation is used. Each of these types of radiation will be reviewed.

Gamma Radiation

Gamma radiation is electromagnetic radiation that has no mass and no electrical charge. Gamma radiation is emitted from the nucleus of a radioactive atom. Gamma radiation travels at the speed of light and is often referred to as a photon. Gamma rays are similar to visible light, but they have higher levels of energy. Gamma radiation is used most often in nuclear medicine procedures and in inpatient/outpatient thyroid therapy procedures.

X-rays

X-rays are very similar to gamma rays and have the same characteristics. Most x-ray photons used in medical facilities are created when electrons are accelerated to a high velocity within an x-ray tube and collide with a metal target. X-rays are predominantly used in diagnostic radiology, fluoroscopy, computed tomography (CT), and therapeutic x-ray procedures. X-rays typically provide information regarding anatomic structure.

Beta Particles

Beta particles are negatively charged particles that are emitted from an unstable nucleus. A beta particle is identical to an electron. One current medical use of beta particles involves yttrium-90, a radioactive material that emits a high-energy beta particle and is used in permanent brachytherapy procedures involving the liver.

Positrons

Positrons are positively charged beta particles emitted from the nucleus of some radionuclides. Similar to other types of radiation, positrons cause ionization as well. However, once a positron has lost most of its energy, it is annihilated when it interacts with an electron. As a result of this interaction, both particles are converted to photons. Positron-emitting radionuclides are used in positron emission tomography (PET) scans. PET scans are a newer modality that evaluates metabolic activity. PET can be used in combination with CT for more clinical information.

With each procedure using ionizing radiation there is the potential for health care worker and public exposure to radiation. Although the patient is intended to receive the radiation exposure for a medical benefit, individuals working with these patients in close proximity to the ionizing radiation sources may also be exposed to the ionizing radiation. The topics of radiation exposure and biological effects from radiation will be discussed. Methods of minimizing external exposure to radiation and preventing internal radiation exposure for the perioperative nurse will also be covered.

RADIATION EXPOSURE

Radiation exposure is defined as the transfer of energy in air from gamma or x-ray radiation. Radiation exposure is measured in roentgen (R), and exposure rate is quantified as roentgen/hour (R/hr) or, in smaller terms, as milliroentgen/hour (mR/hr). In the International System of Units (SI), the measure of radiation exposure is expressed in units of coulomb/kilogram. Another radiation dose unit is the roentgen absorbed dose (rad). This is the measure of the absorption of energy per unit mass by an object as a result of radiation interactions. In SI units the unit for radiation dose is the gray (Gy), where 1 Gy = 100 rad. Because different types of radiation cause varying degrees of damage to biological tissue, a system of estimating the potential harm was developed. The term *rem* is used to report the "equivalent dose" from exposure to different types of radiation. The rem is related to the rad by use of a radiation quality factor to account for the differences in damage done to tissues. In the SI system the unit of equivalent dose is sievert (Sv), where 1 Sv = 100 rem. The equivalent dose is the term used by the regulators to describe the radiation exposure that individuals may receive while working with or around ionizing radiation. These terms are often used interchangeably, which is incorrect. Simply stated, the roentgen refers to ionization of air, the rad refers to ionizing radiation energy deposited in matter, and the rem refers to the ability or tendency of ionizing radiation to cause harm to tissues.

BIOLOGICAL EFFECTS OF IONIZING RADIATION

The use of x-ray, gamma, and positron ionizing radiation for patient diagnosis and treatment can be quite disconcerting to the patient, as well as the perioperative nurse responsible for the care of the patient. It is not uncommon for staff and patients to raise questions regarding the safety of procedures involving ionizing radiation. Radiation health effects have been studied extensively. Evidence of human radiation health effects comes from many sources, but primarily from the studies of the survivors of the atomic bombings in Japan, uranium miners, radium dial painters, and medical studies. The Japanese Life Span Study was designed to evaluate the late mortality effects of the radiation and other trauma received by the survivors of the Hiroshima and Nagasaki A-19 atomic bombs. The sample population consisted of approximately 100,000 persons, including those exposed near to ground zero, persons exposed at such distances from ground zero as to guarantee that little radiation was received, and nonexposed immigrants to the cities (Beebe et al, 1961). The information obtained from these studies indicates a linear increase in adverse health effects from relatively large doses of radiation. There is minimal evidence to support increased risk to people at lower levels of radiation.

High levels of radiation are known to have an adverse effect on cells. Cells that are rapidly dividing, such as reproductive cells, blood-forming tissues, skin, and the gastrointestinal tract, are more sensitive to ionizing radiation. If a cell is exposed to ionizing radiation, several outcomes are possible. The cell can have no observed damage and continue to thrive; the cell may be damaged and die following division; it can become damaged but repair itself; or it can become damaged and misrepair itself, resulting in a change in cellular function, with the damage passing onto the next generation of cells. In the last scenario the formation of cancer results from changes in the cell's reproductive structure such that the cells can replicate into precancerous cells, which may eventually become cancerous. If the cells can be affected by ionizing radiation, then one must consider the result of ionizing radiation on living organisms. To better understand the effect that ionizing radiation has on living organisms, two types of health effects must be defined: deterministic health effects and stochastic health effects.

Deterministic Health Effects

When a tissue or an organism is exposed to very high doses of radiation (hundreds of rad) in a short period of time, the primary effect is cellular death. This is a deterministic health effect. As a result, the organ or system loses its ability to function or dies. The severity of the effect is directly related to the dose; the greater the dose, the more damage occurs. Deterministic effects exhibit a threshold radiation dose. Doses received below the threshold are not associated with adverse health effects. For example, cataract formation is evident when the lens of the eye receives a dose of approximately 200 to 300 rad (2 to 3 Gy) of gamma radiation. Note that "no radiogenic cataracts resulting from occupational exposure to x-rays have been reported. From patients who suffered irradiation of the eyes in the course of x-ray therapy and developed cataracts as a consequence, the cataractogenic threshold dose is estimated at about 200 rads" (Cember and Johnson, 2009).

Stochastic Health Effects

Stochastic health effects are health effects that occur by chance. Stochastic health effects are based on the probability of a health effect occurring and not on the severity of the effect. Regardless of a person's exposure to ionizing radiation, there is the random chance that the individual may or may not develop cancer in his or her lifetime. The conservative assumption is, if one is exposed to radiation, there is a future, random chance of developing an adverse health effect such as cancer. Therefore the probability of a health effect occurring is proportional to the radiation dose. However, there are no early observable effects from exposure to low levels of ionizing radiation, but adverse health effects such as cancer may occur many years later. The challenge is that radiation-induced cancer is not distinguishable from cancer caused by other factors. The other factors that can contribute to a cancer are inherited traits, age, sex, physical condition, diet, cigarette smoking, and exposure to other agents.

To further understand the difference between deterministic and stochastic health effects, the terms *acute dose* and *chronic dose* will be used, respectively. With an acute dose the individual receives a radiation dose in a very short time period. If the radiation dose is large enough, adverse health effects such as reddening of the skin, loss of hair, damage to the gastrointestinal tract, and damage to the central nervous system may occur within hours or a few days after exposure. If the acute radiation levels are high enough, death may occur.

On the other hand, with chronic dose, the individual may be exposed to low levels (a few millirem [mrem] each week) of ionizing radiation over their working lifetime. These chronic doses are unlikely to cause deterministic health effects, as a result of repair of damaged cells, but may cause a delayed health effect. Exposure to large amounts of sunshine is a good analogy for explaining acute and chronic doses. If an individual were to receive an acute exposure to the sun, a severe sunburn such as skin blistering and peeling may develop. If another individual were to receive chronic, low doses of sun, it may result in a golden tan year after year. Now assume that both the sunburned individual and the tanned individual reach the age of 75 and both are diagnosed with skin cancer. The sunburned individual may develop skin cancer as a result of the one-time acute sunburn, or the sun-tanned individual may develop skin cancer as a result of the chronic, low levels of exposure to the sun over many years. Both scenarios may lead to skin cancer, and yet there are so many other factors that have not been accounted for, such as inherited traits, age, and sex, that it is almost impossible to differentiate between the skin cancers that were a result of either acute or chronic exposure to the sun.

In a medical facility the possibility of a radiation health care worker receiving a high acute dose of ionizing radiation is extremely unlikely because of the presence of a RSP involving dose monitoring, education, and dose-reduction strategies. The main concern is for those health care workers who receive chronic, low levels of radiation exposure over their working lifetime. There are many dose-response models that describe the relationship between radiation dose and health effects. For doses greater than 50 rem (500 mSv), there is a definite linear relationship between dose and additional cancer risk (NRC, 1996). Fifty rem (500 mSv) is 10 times higher than the current annual limit of 5 rem (50 mSv). Below 50 rem (500 mSv), there is no definitive relationship between dose and additional cancer risk. Because of the uncertainty in the dose-response relationship at doses below 50 rem (500 mSv), it is assumed that there is a linear zero threshold-dose response at the lower levels of radiation dose. This means that all radiation doses are assumed to have some adverse effect. This is a conservative assumption that serves as the basis for our radiation protection programs throughout the world. By incorporating the philosophy of maintaining exposures from levels of ionizing radiation as low as reasonably achievable, additional effort is made to minimize radiation doses to health care workers and members of the public.

Another category of stochastic health effects that warrants attention is the perception that radiation and birth defects are directly linked. This is often referred to as hereditary effects. If a woman is exposed to ionizing radiation and later has children, there is the misperception that the offspring will exhibit birth defects or an increased risk for cancer. This has not been observed in studies of exposed humans, and the possibility of hereditary effects exists only from studies performed on animals. For this reason, additional precautions are recommended to continuously minimize exposure to ionizing radiation. To protect against deterministic and stochastic health effects, RSPs at medical facilities incorporate procedures and policies to protect radiation workers, patients, and the public from external and internal exposure to ionizing radiation.

Finally, teratogenic effects are developmental effects caused by intrauterine exposure to ionizing radiation. Irradiation of the developing fetus is a concern because of the rapidly dividing and developing cells. The risk to the fetus is a function of gestational age at the time of radiation exposure and the radiation dose. Based on this information, the risk from ionizing radiation to the fetus and children is higher than that for adults. The data to support a teratogenic effect come from experiments using animal models and from human populations exposed to very high doses of radiation such as the atomic bomb survivors. For humans the significant teratogenic effects observed included mental retardation, intrauterine growth retardation, and cancer development such as childhood leukemia. However, not all exposures to ionizing radiation cause these effects. For most diagnostic procedures involving ionizing radiation in which the fetal dose is less than 10 rem (100 mSv), very little data exist to support teratogenic effects in humans (Duke University, 2009; Edwards, n.d.). Even though there is very little evidence of teratogenic health effects below 10 rem (100 mSv), there is enough cause for concern that RSPs have established additional policies for the declared pregnant health care worker and the pregnant patient intended to further reduce the radiation dose to the fetus. The focus of this chapter is on the health care worker, and radiation safety policies for the declared pregnant health care worker will be discussed in greater detail later in this chapter.

RADIATION DOSE LIMITS

Based on the discussion regarding biological effects from exposure to ionizing radiation, it is prudent to explain radiation dose limits and how they are applied to protect individuals. Regulatory agencies have established specific limits of radiation dose for those working with ionizing radiation and for those considered members of the general public. Those individuals working with or around ionizing radiation that have been trained are considered occupational radiation workers. Individuals who work in or near areas where ionizing radiation is used, but are not directly involved in its use, are frequently referred to as ancillary personnel. Administrative staff, housekeeping, and maintenance staff may be considered ancillary personnel. These individuals may receive minimal training on radiation safety awareness. The term *general public* is applied to those individuals who are not directly working with ionizing radiation and who do not receive radiation safety training. Occupational radiation workers are limited to 5 rem (50 mSv) per year. Ancillary personnel and the general public are limited to 0.1 rem (1 mSv) in a year and less than 0.002 rem (0.02 mSv) in any hour. Annual dose limits in the United States are listed in Table 23-1 (NRC, 2009).

Maintaining Radiation Doses as Low as Reasonably Achievable

Because high doses of ionizing radiation have the potential to cause adverse health effects, the goal of a radiation protection program is to keep radiation doses below the annual limits. In addition, there is also a requirement that doses to health care workers and the general public will be maintained as low as is reasonably achievable (ALARA). RSP policies and procedures must be designed to minimize exposure to radiation as far below the limit as practical, taking into account economic and social factors. A facility cannot guarantee that its employees will receive no radiation exposure from their work with ionizing radiation, but, with implementation of policies and procedures that reduce external radiation exposure and prevent internal radiation exposure, exposure can be kept to a minimum.

TABLE 23-1 Annual Dose Limits in the United States

Total whole body dose (occupational)	5 rem/year (50 mSv/year)
Lens of the eye (occupational)	15 rem/year (150 mSv/year)
Skin (occupational)	50 rem/year (500 mSv/year)
Extremities (occupational)	50 rem/year (500 mSv/year)
Members of the general public and ancillary personnel	0.1 rem/year (1.0 mSv/year) not to exceed 0.002 rem (0.02 mSv) in any hour

From U.S. Nuclear Regulatory Commission: *Occupational dose limits for adults,* 10 CFR 20.1201, April 2009; U.S. Nuclear Regulatory Commission: Dose limits for individual members of the public, 10 CFR 20.1301, April 2009.

Declared Pregnancy Policy

A declared pregnancy policy applies to pregnant women whose assigned duties involve exposure to ionizing radiation. Exposure to any amount of radiation is assumed to carry some amount of risk. The conservative assumption is that as the dose increases, the likelihood of biological effects from the radiation increases as well. The annual limit of radiation exposure for an occupationally exposed worker is 5 rem (50 mSv). Although this limit is designed to protect the adult radiation worker, there is also another recommended limit for the embryo/fetus of declared pregnant radiation workers. The embryo/fetus of a declared pregnant worker is limited to 0.5 rem (5 mSv) over the gestation period. A declared pregnancy policy is designed to protect the fetus of an occupationally exposed health care worker. The staff working with and around ionizing radiation have the option to declare their pregnancy in writing to their employer. This is a voluntary decision. A woman may choose to make a formal declaration at any point in her pregnancy, or she may choose not to make a formal declaration at all. In the latter case the dose to the embryo/fetus would not be evaluated or limited by the facility. However, the woman's dose would still be subject to the limit for occupational radiation workers, typically 5 rem (50 mSv) per year.

Work restrictions for the declared pregnant health care worker are required if there is a significant potential for the embryo/fetus to receive a dose in excess of the 0.5 rem (5 mSv) limit as a result of the external exposure of its mother and/or from intakes of radioactive material by its mother. The expectation is that the radiation dose would be received at an even rate over the entire gestation period. To accurately assess the fetal dose, it is recommended that the declared pregnant health care worker receive a fetal dosimeter, which should be worn at the abdomen at about waist level (Figure 23-1). If the worker wears an

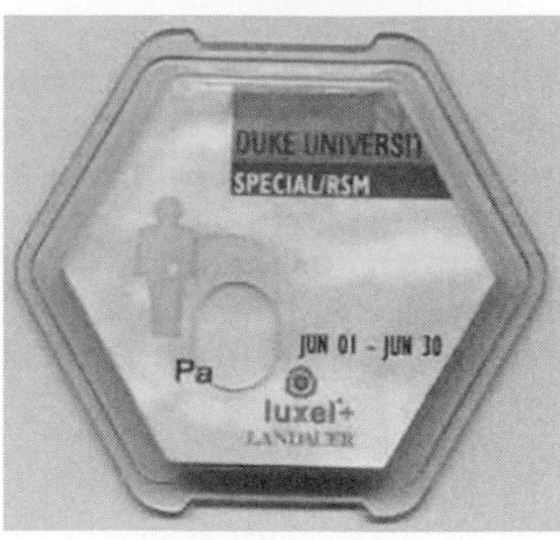

FIGURE 23-1 Fetal dosimeter. (From Duke University and Duke Medicine Radiation Safety Division: *Wearing your radiation dosimeter*, n.d., available at: http://www.safety.duke.edu/RadSafety/dosim/badge_tutorial.htm. Accessed November 12, 2009.)

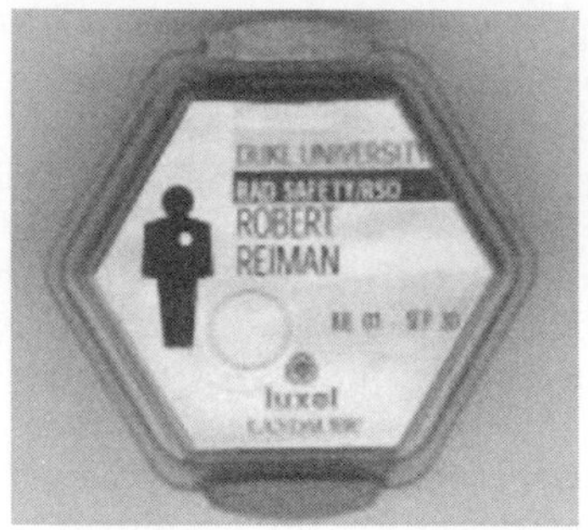

FIGURE 23-2 Body dosimeter. (From Duke University and Duke Medicine Radiation Safety Division: *Wearing your radiation dosimeter*, n.d., available at: http://www.safety.duke.edu/RadSafety/dosim/badge_tutorial.htm. Accessed November 12, 2009.)

x-ray–shielding apron, the fetal dosimeter must be worn *under* the apron. The fetal dosimeter should be exchanged monthly for analysis. A facility may elect to purchase maternity lead aprons designed specifically for use by the pregnant health care worker. Most maternity lead aprons increase lead shielding from 0.5 mm to 1.0 mm in areas to protect the fetus.

MONITORING RADIATION DOSE

Monitoring for radiation dose is required if the health care worker has the potential or is likely to receive 0.5 rem (5 mSv) in a year. Some facilities choose to monitor workers that may receive doses below 0.5 rem/yr. Employers use dosimeters, commonly referred to as badges, to monitor the radiation dose to radiation workers (Figure 23-2). Facilities are required to use a vendor that is certified by the National Voluntary Laboratory Accreditation Program (NVLAP). The NVLAP program provides a third-party accreditation to analytical laboratories that process and analyze dosimeters. Film badges, thermoluminescent dosimeters (TLD), and optically stimulated luminescent (OSL) dosimeters are examples of dosimeters that meet this accreditation criteria and are typically used in medical facilities. The purpose of these dosimeters is to detect and quantify the amount of radiation dose received while working with radioactive materials and/or radiation-producing machines. Film badges are limited in that their useful dose range is 0.01 rem to 500 rads (0.10 mSv to 5.0 Gy). In addition, film is quite sensitive to the effects of heat and humidity. TLDs have a useful dose range between 0.01 rem and 1000 rads (0.10 mSv to 10 Gy) and can withstand more rugged environments. OSL dosimeters have a useful dose range between 0.001 rem and 1000 rad (0.01 mSv to 10 Gy) and can also withstand rugged environments.

Dosimeters may be exchanged monthly, bimonthly, quarterly, or at other frequencies depending upon the needs of the facility. It is imperative that dosimeters be exchanged and replaced at the predetermined frequency to promptly and accurately assess the radiation dose to the individual. Dosimeters should be worn only while at work. Staff should be advised not to take the dosimeters home with them or to share them with co-workers. Placement of the dosimeter depends on how the wearer is exposed to radiation. For most perioperative nurses the dosimeter should be worn on the trunk of the body between the hip and the neck region under the lead apron. Typically those working in radiology and interventional radiology departments are issued two dosimeters. This can give a more realistic view of exposure than one dosimeter worn at the collar. One is worn under the lead apron and the other is worn at the collar outside of the shielded area to accurately assess the radiation dose received while working with radiation-producing machines. Dosimeters are a permanent personal record of occupational radiation dose. The radiation safety officer for the facility is typically responsible for monitoring the dosimeter results and investigating excessive or unusual doses.

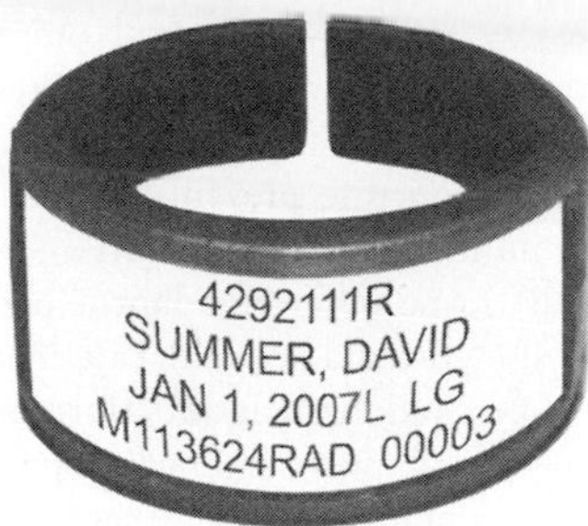

FIGURE 23-3 Ring dosimeter. (From Duke University and Duke Medicine Radiation Safety Division: *Wearing your radiation dosimeter*, n.d., available at: http://www.safety.duke.edu/RadSafety/dosim/badge_tutorial.htm. Accessed November 12, 2009.)

Ring dosimeters are used to assess the radiation dose to the extremities of radiation workers (Figure 23-3). The annual limit for extremities of radiation workers is 50 rem (500 mSv). Those individuals likely to receive 5 rem (50 mSv) to the extremities are required to wear ring dosimeters. The ring dosimeters currently on the market are TLD rings that are NVLAP certified. The health care worker may be issued one ring, which is typically worn on the dominant hand. Staff should wear the ring so that the label is on the palmar (inside) surface of the finger, *toward* the radiation source and *opposite* from the side one would normally wear the "stone" of a ring. In some situations the health care worker may be issued two TLD ring dosimeters so that one is worn on each hand to assess the extremity dose. Typically TLD ring dosimeters are exchanged at the same frequency as the whole body dosimeter. Some facilities sterilize the rings using gas sterilization procedures without rendering the dosimeter ineffective; however, it is suggested that each vendor be contacted for the best method for sterilizing ring dosimeters.

EXTERNAL RADIATION PROTECTION

An external hazard is a source of ionizing radiation that remains outside the body, but that emits radiation capable of penetrating the body. Certain types of radiation have the ability to penetrate skin and tissues and therefore present an external hazard. Sources of radiation that present external hazards are x-ray machines, various radionuclides used in diagnostic nuclear medicine procedures, and other sources used in radiation therapy. The three methods of reducing radiation doses from external sources are (1) reducing the time spent near the source, (2) increasing the distance from the source, and (3) shielding the source. Perioperative nurses are advised to minimize their time by working quickly and efficiently around radiation sources. The perioperative nurses should always maximize their distance from radiation sources. This may simply mean stepping away a few feet from the radiation source. The intensity of the radiation source decreases as the distance from the source increases. For example, if the distance between an individual and the radiation source is doubled, the intensity of the radiation is reduced by a factor of four.

Protective shielding is recommended for perioperative nurses working near radiation-producing machines such as fluoroscopy units. Lead aprons attenuate the radiation exposure in the diagnostic x-ray energy range and in fluoroscopy. Thyroid shields are also recommended for any exposures that place the perioperative nurse at a high risk for exposure because the thyroid is a radiosensitive organ (Association of periOperative Registered Nurses [AORN], 2008).

Leaded gloves are indicated when an individual's hands are frequently placed in the primary radiation beam during fluoroscopy procedures. Newer lead-equivalent protective gloves are available that help minimize exposure to the hands and allow for improved dexterity during fluoroscopy procedures. However, the health care provider should minimize direct exposure to the hands from the x-ray beam if possible.

For interventional radiologists, surgeons, nurses, and health care workers in this area, leaded eye protection is recommended to limit dose to the lens of the eye. The recommendation for leaded eye protection is applicable to radiologists, surgeons, and health care workers who are exposed to levels above 15,000 mrem annually (AORN, 2008). Lead aprons are not as efficient for attenuating radiation from gamma sources used in nuclear medicine or higher-energy x-rays used in radiation therapy and are not recommended for procedures using gamma radiation.

Proper Handling of Leaded Protective Equipment

The lead aprons, thyroid shields, and leaded gloves must be maintained to prevent anomalies in the lead that may render the protective equipment ineffective. Shielding devices when initially purchased should be tested to verify the integrity (AORN, 2008). Lead that is frequently folded over on itself can exhibit cracks, which allow for radiation to permeate the apron and expose the health care worker to unrecognized radiation exposure. Manufacturers of lead aprons recommend that aprons be hung vertically to prevent folding of the lead. Medical facilities that provide protective equipment should evaluate the integrity of the lead equipment (Michel and Zorn, 2002). The AORN (2008) recommends that shielding devices should undergo x-ray examination at least annually. Leaded protective equipment that does not meet the integrity standard must be removed from general use and replaced with new equipment. Shielding devices are cleaned with an Environmental Protection Agency (EPA)-registered hospital disinfectant following use (AORN, 2008).

INTERNAL RADIATION PROTECTION

Internal radiation doses result when the body is internally contaminated with radioactive material by inhalation, absorption, ingestion, and puncture. It is a concern for perioperative nurses who provide care for a patient undergoing a procedure that results in radioactive materials circulating in the patient's body. Examples may include nuclear medicine procedures, inpatient iodine thyroid therapy treatment, and sentinel lymph node biopsies. Occasionally, nuclear medicine patients may stay in the hospital for additional care after a nuclear medicine scan.

Internal radiation protection for perioperative nurses is necessary because of the potential for radioactive material contained in body fluids to splash and spill on their hands or skin. Ingestion of radioactive material may then occur from nurses eating with contaminated hands. Punctures to the skin from radioactively contaminated sharp objects such as needles or broken glass may result in absorption of radioactive material. To protect against internal radioactive hazards, it is necessary to follow universal precautions. The Centers for Disease Control and Prevention (CDC) defined universal precautions as a set of precautions designed to prevent transmission of human immunodeficiency virus (HIV), hepatitis B virus (HBV), and other bloodborne pathogens when providing first aid or health care. The basics of universal precautions include performing hand hygiene before and after each medical procedure. Staff must wear gloves whenever there is the possibility of coming into contact with blood or other potentially infectious materials such as body fluids and tissues. Staff must wear full-body gowns, face masks, and eye protection whenever there is the possibility of blood splashing onto the individual. Potentially contaminated sharp objects (sharps) must be properly disposed of in designated sharps containers to prevent needlesticks (CDC, 1996; Brouhard, 2007).

When working around radioactive materials, staff are encouraged to wear a double pair of gloves and to change gloves frequently. Staff should perform hand hygiene after contact with patients or radioactive specimens, especially before activities such as eating, drinking, smoking, and taking medications. Perioperative nurses should not eat, drink, take medications, use cosmetics, or handle contact lenses in areas where radionuclides are used (e.g., operating room and patient dosing, patient scanning, and specimen processing areas). When handling objects such as syringes, urine cups, and catheters, which may be contaminated with radioactive materials, the perioperative nurse is advised to wear protective clothing and plastic gloves. In the event of a suspected uncontrolled contamination incident involving radioactive materials, the perioperative nurse should contact the radiation safety officer for additional guidance.

Managing Contamination and/or Spills of Radioactive Materials

The following general recommendations are offered for managing spills of radioactive materials; however, each facility should have site-specific policies and procedures per state and federal regulations. For skin contamination involving radioactive materials, perioperative nurses should wash the affected area gently and thoroughly with soap and water. Slightly abrasive agents, such as brushes, scrub pads, or powders, may be used if skin contamination is not removed after repeated washings with soap and water. Attempts should be made not to abrade the skin. Resume washing with soap and water if contamination persists. A final survey should be completed by the radiation safety staff to ensure that contamination has been successfully removed.

For radioactive contamination of personal clothing, perioperative nurses should remove the contaminated clothing, check the skin underneath the clothing for possible skin contamination, and follow the recommended steps for decontamination of contaminated skin. Contaminated clothing or shoes should be placed inside a plastic bag labeled with "Caution Radioactive Material" tape or tags. Most radioactive materials used in the medical setting have relatively short half-lives, and clothes should be stored until the radioactive material has decayed to an acceptable level. The radiation safety officer should ensure that contaminated clothing and items do not leave the facility, are safely stored for decay, and are returned to the individual once they have decayed to lower levels.

For spills of radioactive urine or body fluids, it is helpful to define large-volume spills and small-volume spills. A large-volume spill typically consists of a large volume of liquid greater than the amount that may be absorbed by one large blue disposable underpad. For large-volume spills, staff should cover the contaminated area with absorbent material and guard the area to prevent others from stepping into the contamination. Staff should request assistance from the radiation safety office for decontamination procedures and verification that the area has been adequately decontaminated.

A small-volume spill may be defined as a spill involving an amount of liquid that may be absorbed by one large blue underpad. Staff should immediately isolate the area to prevent the spread of contamination and follow universal precautions. They should wipe up the spill with pads or paper towels and then clean the area with disinfectant. All material should be disposed of per decontamination protocol and procedure. Using an appropriate radiation instrument, the radiation safety officer or designated person should monitor the area with a survey meter to verify that no contamination remains. If contamination remains, rewipe the area until all contamination is removed. Additional follow-up by the radiation safety officer may be warranted. As a reminder, it is appropriate to check with facility policies and procedures regarding these types of incidents.

For situations that involve radioactive contamination with physical injury or illness, such as a heart attack, it is imperative to first address the injury or life-threatening medical issue. Lifesaving measures take priority over contamination concerns for the patient and the radiation worker. Remember that universal precautions will protect the perioperative nurse from potential internal contamination. To protect against external exposure to ionizing radiation, the nurse should minimize time, maximize distance, and use shielding when appropriate, provided this does not negatively affect the handling of the patient's injury. Radioactive contamination is not life threatening to the perioperative nurse or attending medical staff.

RADIATION SAFETY PRECAUTIONS FOR MODALITIES USING IONIZING RADIATION

Diagnostic X-ray

Radiographic procedures involve the use of x-rays to gain structural information about the body. The radiation output from the x-ray machine is based on two factors: the kilovoltage (kVp) and the milliamperes (mA). Kilovoltage indicates the energy of the radiation. The higher the kVp, the higher the energy, and therefore the radiation is more penetrating. Milliamperes refer to the current produced by the machine. The higher the current, the higher the number of x-rays produced. The radiation exposure produced by the x-ray tube is also determined by the time of the exposure, which is typically in seconds. In the diagnostic range the x-ray tube current is high, but the exposure time is quite short. Although the parameters can be manually adjusted by the operator, most modern x-ray units have an automatic adjustment capability to accurately and effectively image the patient and adjust the output depending on the size of the patient. Because of the automatic adjustment, the levels of radiation exposure are usually quite low for the patient, as well as other individuals in the immediate vicinity.

The highest area of exposure is in the primary beam directed at the patient. The major source of exposure for others in the room is from scattered radiation from the point where the primary beam enters the patient. If the perioperative nurse does not need to be in the room, it is recommended that the nurse stay out of the room until the x-ray procedure is completed. The perioperative nurse should not be directly involved in the positioning and holding of the patient during these diagnostic procedures. If the perioperative nurse must be in the room, he or she should keep as much distance as possible from the x-ray tube. Those who must be within 6 feet of the x-ray device are advised to wear a lead apron to minimize the dose from the radiation output near the x-ray tube. Individuals who are routinely in an x-ray room during diagnostic procedures should be issued a dosimeter to wear at the collar. Those who are infrequently assigned and exposed to x-rays are typically not issued a dosimeter because it is not likely that the individual would receive a dose in excess of 10% of the annual limit.

Fluoroscopy and Interventional Fluoroscopy

With fluoroscopic procedures the x-ray tube that produces the ionizing radiation is opposite an image intensifier that captures the x-ray image. Image intensifiers are capable of amplifying low-intensity x-rays to view the anatomic structure while minimizing radiation doses to the patient. Unlike diagnostic radiology, where the x-ray on-time is extremely short, in fluoroscopy the x-ray on-time can be quite long, on the order of minutes as opposed to a fraction of a second of exposure. There are two categories of fluoroscopic procedures. The first is used for simple procedures such as barium x-ray examinations and enemas, catheter insertion (to direct the placement of a catheter during angioplasty or angiography), cardiac catheterization, and orthopedic surgery (to view fracture and fracture treatments) (U.S. Food and Drug Administration [FDA], 2008). The second category is interventional fluoroscopy, which involves more complex surgical procedures such as endografts for the treatment of abdominal aortic aneurysms, the development of vertebroplasty, kyphoplasty, uterine artery embolization, and the use of fluoroscopic guidance during complex endoscopic biliary and upper urinary tract procedures (National Cancer Institute, 2005).

Typically the radiation output from a fluoroscopic procedure can be on the order of 2 to 10 R/min. In the high-level dose rate mode the output from the fluoroscopy unit can be as high as 20 R/min (FDA, 2005). A high kVp and low mA keep entrance skin dose rates at a minimum. With fluoroscopy units the highest radiation dose occurs in the primary radiation beam directed at the patient. Scattered radiation is a concern for health care workers. The recommendations for minimizing radiation doses from fluoroscopy units are (1) minimize time near the fluoroscopy unit, (2) maintain the maximum distance from the unit, and (3) use protective shielding where appropriate. By following proper radiologic techniques, radiation exposure to the patient and the staff can be minimized. For example, careful positioning of the tube is important for minimizing radiation doses. The x-ray tube should be under the patient and not above the patient because the largest amount of scattered radiation is produced where the x-ray beam enters the patient. By positioning the x-ray tube below the patient, the amount of scattered radiation that reaches the operator and those standing nearby is decreased. It is also suggested that the distance between the x-ray tube and the patient be maximized while minimizing the distance between the patient and the image intensifier.

Radiation dose to the patient and those nearby can be minimized by controlling the amount of fluoroscopic on-time to that which is essential for diagnostic and documentation purposes. It is prudent to keep the beam on-time ALARA. To further minimize the on-time, practice foot-pedal tapping. The operator should not abuse the pedal and leave the beam on if it is not needed to obtain the image. Employ last-image-hold to review findings instead of repeating the portion of the study. Collimation of the primary beam can also help minimize exposures. Collimate tightly to the area of interest, because this reduces the patient's total entrance skin exposure and improves image contrast. In addition, the scattered radiation to the operator and those nearby will decrease.

Perioperative nurses are advised to maintain their distance from the primary beam of radiation. With C-arm fluoroscopy units, those nearby should maintain awareness of their body position relative to the primary x-ray beam. For example, in a horizontal beam position, staff should stand on the side of the image intensifier. The intensity of the scattered radiation is less on the image intensifier side than on the x-ray tube side. For lateral and oblique projections, position the x-ray tube on the opposite side of the patient. The perioperative nurse should move to provide himself or herself with additional protection as indicated. The individual operating the fluoroscopy tube and those in the immediate vicinity should wear lead aprons, thyroid shields, and protective leaded glasses. Leaded gloves are also recommended if the operator's hands are in the primary beam of radiation.

Computed Tomography

CT is a special radiographic procedure in which an x-ray beam is rotated around the patient to take multiple cross-sectional images ("slices") of the area of interest. As the slices are taken, the examination table is moving through the scanner. The x-ray beam actually follows a spiral path. This is often called helical or spiral CT scan. A computer then creates a composite image of the area of interest based on information from these cross-sectional x-ray scans. CT imaging provides great anatomic detail. Modern CT scanners are extremely fast, and they can scan through large sections of the body in just a few seconds. The quick scan time is beneficial for all patients, but especially for children, older adults, and those who are critically ill.

Physicians use CT examinations to quickly identify injuries to the lungs, heart and vessels, liver, spleen, kidneys, or other internal organs in cases of trauma. Physicians also use CT examination for procedures such as abscess drainages and minimally invasive tumor treatments, to plan for and assess the results of surgery, and to plan and properly administer radiation treatments for tumors (Radiological Society of North America [RSNA], 2009a). The radiation safety aspects of CT imaging are quite basic—when the CT scan is in process, extraneous staff should not be permitted in the scanning room

Positron Emission Tomography

PET is a nuclear medicine procedure that uses high-energy positron-emitting radionuclides with very short half-lives. For example, fluorine-18 is a positron emitter that is labeled to a glucose (sugar) molecule and injected into patients as fluorodeoxyglucose (FDG). Those patients undergoing PET scans for cancer are void of sugar for a period of time before the procedure. The radioactive form of glucose (FDG) is injected and metabolized by the body; metabolism by cancer cells is especially rapid. As the positrons from the FDG interact with the electrons in the tissue, they are annihilated, resulting in photons that are emitted and analyzed by radiation detectors surrounding the patient. The location of increased metabolic activity, such as in malignant tumors, is then detected based upon the location of the photon emissions. PET scans are also used to evaluate decreased metabolic activity, as in the case of patients with Alzheimer's disease (Cember and Johnson, 2009). The use of PET is favored in the medical field because the half-life of the radioactive material is very short. Patients can be injected, scanned, and sent home the same day with very little residual radioactive material in their bodies.

Because of the emission of positrons and high-energy photons, the dose rates observed during these procedures are higher than those for the more routine nuclear medicine procedures. Staff directly involved with injecting the radioactive material and working closely with the patients during the procedure are usually issued whole-body dosimeters and ring dosimeters. Minimizing time around these patients and maximizing distance from the patient are the recommendations for those rendering care. Shielding the injection syringe is recommended to minimize radiation dose to the hands. Lead aprons are not efficient for minimizing exposure because of the higher-energy photons associated with PET. The short half-life of PET radionuclides means that radiation doses to perioperative nurses is low when the patient remains in the facility for other procedures. Once the scan is completed and the patient is elsewhere in the facility, no additional radiation safety precautions are necessary.

Manufacturers of imaging devices are now offering combined PET/CT scanners, which are a combination of both individual procedures previously described. In a PET/CT scan, both procedures can be performed with the patient in the scanner, which allows the structural information from the CT to be correlated with the physiologic function identified by the PET scan. The recommended safety precautions for minimizing radiation dose remain the same as described for each individual modality.

Nuclear Medicine

During a nuclear medicine procedure, radioactive material is injected into a patient's body and the body is scanned with a camera to generate an image showing the location of the radioactive material. Unusual uptake and retention of the radioactive material is used to diagnose or treat a variety of diseases, including cancers, heart disease, and other abnormalities. Typically the amounts of radioactive material administered for a diagnostic nuclear medicine scan are below 33 millicuries. A millicurie is a term used to describe an amount of radioactive material administered to a patient. Activity describes the rate at which a radionuclide undergoes nuclear transformations. As a result of the low activity administered to the patient, the radiation dose is usually very low to the patient, who may be released from the facility and sent home immediately following the scan. Nuclear medicine patients in the care of a perioperative nurse present a potential contamination problem because the patient's body fluids are radioactive. Gloves should be used when handling the patient's body fluids (universal precautions).

The external dose from a patient undergoing most routine diagnostic nuclear medicine procedures is small. Minimizing time and maximizing distance are very effective in minimizing the dose to the perioperative nurse from diagnostic nuclear medicine patients. Lead aprons are not beneficial for those assisting nuclear medicine patients because of the higher-energy gamma rays emitted from the radioactive materials used in the procedures.

Sentinel Lymph Node Biopsy

A sentinel lymph node biopsy is typically performed to assist in staging breast cancer and malignant melanoma. These procedures take place in the operating room. A trace amount of Tc-99m sulfur colloid is injected into the patient. A physician uses a radiation detector to determine if the radioactive material travels to the lymph nodes. The radioactive material has a 6-hour half-life and decays away within a few days. The trace amount (approximately 1 millicurie) that is initially injected does not pose a significant external hazard to those working near the patient, but the patient's body fluids or any removed lymph nodes may be contaminated, and the specimen should be labeled as radioactive as appropriate before transfer to the pathology department. Therefore universal precautions are recommended for handling patient specimens. There is very little concern with regard to external radiation safety because of the low level of radioactive material administered to the patient. As a general safety precaution, minimize time around the radioactive materials and maximize distance from the patient. Because of the low level of radioactive material, shielding is usually not necessary.

RADIATION THERAPY

Radiation therapy consists of two types: external beam therapy and brachytherapy. External beam therapy is a medical procedure that involves delivering ionizing radiation from sources outside the body to cancer cells in the body with the intent of destroying the cancer cells. The ionizing radiation is delivered from a machine (linear accelerator, cobalt machine, or orthovoltage x-ray machine) directed to the site of the cancer inside the patient. These procedures take place in an oncology department in specially shielded therapy rooms. Perioperative nurses are usually not involved with the therapy. Because the radiation source is outside the body, the patient's body fluids and tissues do not become contaminated with radioactive materials.

The term *brachytherapy* is derived from ancient Greek words for short distance (*brachy*) and treatment (*therapy*). Brachytherapy is sometimes called "seed implantation" and may be performed as an outpatient or inpatient procedure. These procedures are used in the treatment of different types of cancer. Radioactive "seeds" are carefully placed inside the cancerous tissue and positioned in a manner to maximize the lethal effect on the caner cells. Brachytherapy is used in the treatment of prostate cancer, cervical cancer, endometrial cancer, and coronary artery disease (American Brachytherapy Society, n.d.). It can be categorized as temporary brachytherapy and permanent brachytherapy.

Brachytherapy involves the temporary placement of a catheter, needle, or applicator into a tumor using fluoroscopy, ultrasonography, or CT to help position the radiation sources. The delivery device may be inserted into a body cavity such as the vagina or uterus (intracavitary brachytherapy), or applicators (usually needles or catheters) may be inserted into body tissues (interstitial brachytherapy) (RSNA, 2009b). In the event that these patients require surgery, the temporary implant would be removed before surgery to avoid exposing the surgical team to radiation. Body fluids do not contain radioactive material.

The perioperative nurse will be involved in permanent brachytherapy procedures because these procedures take place in the operating room. Currently, permanent brachytherapy involves seed implantation for early-stage cancer treatment involving radionuclides such as iridium Ir-192, iodine I-125, palladium Pd-153, and cesium Cs-131. With permanent brachytherapy, tumor sites are implanted with the radioactive seeds; tumor sites may include the brain, lung, recurrent head and neck cancers, retroperitoneal lymph nodes, and the prostate (National Council on Radiation Protection and Measurements [NCRP], 2007). The seeds are sealed sources containing radioactive material. The physician and medical physicist are responsible for seed placement and seed accountability. These patients contain sealed sources of radioactive material, and therefore the patient's body fluids are not contaminated. The most common location for permanent sealed-source implants is the prostate. When seeded, the prostate is the only source of ionizing radiation and poses an external hazard to the perioperative nurse. By minimizing time, maximizing distance, and using shielding where appropriate, the external exposure to the perioperative nurse can be significantly reduced. Typically, once these patients recover from the surgical procedure, they are sent home the same day and do not pose a serious hazard to those nearby.

Therapeutic Radionuclide Procedures

Inpatient Iodine-131 Thyroid Therapy

The use of radioactive iodine to treat thyroid cancer is common in the United States. Patients are administered a large dose of iodine-131, which is absorbed in thyroid cells, including cancerous cells. Radiation emitted from the iodine-131 kills the cancer cells. In some facilities, patients may remain in the facility until the levels of radiation have decreased as a result of biological elimination of the material and radioactive decay. These patients are typically quite healthy and do not require additional nursing care; however, on rare occasions these individuals may require surgery. The surgical patient who has received radioactive iodine in the immediate preoperative period is a source of external radiation exposure for the individuals caring for them in the perioperative period. The patient's body fluids are also contaminated with iodine-131 and are a potential source of internal radiation exposure. Universal precautions should be followed to prevent internal contamination, and using the principles of time, distance, and shielding will reduce external radiation doses.

Selective Internal Radiation Therapy

A relatively new permanent brachytherapy procedure involves the implantation of radioactive material in the form of micropolymer beads, also referred to as microspheres, for the treatment of liver cancer. The radioactive material used is yttrium-90, a beta emitter. The radioactive microbeads are infused into a catheter and travel in an artery until they lodge in the capillary bed of the liver. This procedure is typically performed in an operating room and involves the use of fluoroscopy. An interventional radiologist places the catheter in the appropriate location before infusing the radioactive microspheres. The syringe containing the radioactive microspheres must be shielded to reduce external exposure from the radioactive material. Precautions should be taken to prevent a potential spill of the microspheres. The patient does not present a potential threat for internal exposure to the perioperative nurse because the material is contained in the liver and is not likely to circulate throughout the patient's body. Universal precautions will adequately protect the staff from internal exposure concerns.

From an external radiation perspective the radiation emitted by yttrium-90 is very well shielded by the patient's body and does not present an external radiation hazard to the perioperative nurse. However, it is prudent to follow the principles of time and distance when working directly with these patients in the operating room and recovery area. The patient is discharged from the hospital within 24 hours of the procedure, and these patients do not pose an external hazard to others. No additional radiation safety precautions are warranted.

Radioactive Monoclonal Antibody Therapy

The use of monoclonal antibodies labeled with radioactive materials has increased in recent years. A monoclonal antibody is a protein created in a laboratory that is able to locate and bind to substances in the body such as tumor cells. The common radioactive materials used in monoclonal antibody therapy include the radioiodine I-131, indium In-111, yttrium Y-90, and technetium Tc-99m. The antibody can be paired with radioactive material so that when the antibody reaches the tumor cells, it also delivers the radioactive material to the tumor cells. The presence of the radioactive material assists in further localization of the suspect tumor and delivers a higher, more-specific radiation dose to the tumor. This procedure is currently used to diagnose and treat cancers of the colon, ovaries, breasts, lungs, and pancreas, as well as treating lymphoma and leukemia.

The patient undergoing this procedure presents an external source of radiation to the perioperative nurse and can also pose an internal contamination concern. Although the amount of radioactive material used in these procedures is low, on the order of a few millicuries, those caring for these patients must minimize time close to the patient and maximize distance from the patient when possible. The use of shielding such as lead aprons may not be beneficial because of the higher energy emitted from the radioactive materials used. Dosimeters may be issued to the operating room staff at the discretion of the radiation safety officer. Ring dosimeters may be issued to those preparing the dose and performing the infusion. The radioactive material injected into the patient circulates in the body fluids, and therefore patient specimens and body fluids are considered contaminated. The use of protective clothing and following universal precautions will adequately protect those working closely with this patient in the operating room. Additional procedures such as properly labeling specimens and handling radioactive waste generated from monoclonal antibody therapy must be addressed by the radiation safety officer.

CONCLUSION

Many of the concepts and terms described associated with ionizing radiation in this chapter have not changed over the years. However, the use of ionizing radiation in patient diagnosis and treatment is continuously evolving with new methods to detect, analyze, and treat certain diseases. Perioperative nursing staff must receive training on a regular basis to ensure that they are current on recommended practices and procedures. Although the basics of protection from internal radioactive material and external radiation protection have been explained, it is prudent to discuss new procedures with the hospital radiation safety staff and the radiation safety officer. Site-specific procedures such as proper handling and labeling of patient specimens, patient trash, operating room trash, and equipment used in these procedures involving radioactive material must be addressed. Frequent training sessions provide an opportunity to ask questions and ensure that policies and procedures are followed to minimize doses from ionizing radiation.

REFERENCES

American Brachytherapy Society: *What is brachytherapy?*, n.d., available at http://www.americanbrachytherapy.org/aboutBrachytherapy/brachy.cfm. Accessed May 5 2009.

Association of periOperative Registered Nurses: Recommended practices for reducing radiological exposure in the perioperative practice setting. In *Association of periOperative Registered Nurses: Perioperative standards and recommended practices*, Denver, 2008, The Association.

Beebe GW, et al: *Life span study Report 1: Description of study mortality in the medical subsample October 1950-June 1958*, Hiroshima, Japan, 1961, Atomic Bomb Casualty Commission, available at http://www.rerf.or.jp/library/scidata/lssrepor_e/tr05-61.htm. Accessed May 11 2009.

Brouhard R: *Universal precautions body substance isolation for everyone*, updated 2007, available at http://firstaid.about.com/od/ppe/qt/06_universal.htm. Accessed May 17, 2009.

Cember H, Johnson TE: *Introduction to health physics*, ed 4, New York, 2009, McGraw-Hill.

Centers for Disease Control and Prevention: *Universal precautions for prevention of transmission of HIV and other bloodborne infections, fact sheet*, updated 1996, available at http://www.cdc.gov/ncidod/dhqp/bp_universal_precautions.html. Accessed May 11, 2009.

Duke University and Duke Medicine Radiation Safety Division: *Fetal radiation dose estimates*, 2009, available at http://www.safety.duke.edu/radsafety/fdose/fdrisk.asp. Accessed May 12, 2009.

Edwards G: *Health and environmental issues linked to the nuclear fuel chain, section B: health effects*, n.d., available at http://www.ccnr.org/ceac_B.html#b.17. Accessed May 12, 2009.

Michel R, Zorn M: Implementation of an x-ray radiation protective equipment inspection program, *Health Phys* 82 (2, Suppl):S51–S53, 2002.

National Cancer Institute: *Interventional fluoroscopy: reducing radiation risks for patients and staff*, 2005, available at http://www.cancer.gov/cancertopics/interventionalfluoroscopy/allpages. Accessed April 29, 2009.

NCRP Report No. 155, *Management of radionuclide therapy patients*, Bethesda, Md, 2006, National Council on Radiation Protection and Measurements 2007.

Radiological Society of North America: *Radiology information*, 2009a, available at http://www.radiologyinfo.org/en/info.cfm?PG=bodyct. Accessed April 30, 2009.

Radiological Society of North America: *Radiology information on brachytherapy*, 2009b, available at http://www.radiologyinfo.org/en/info.cfm?PG=brachy. Accessed May 16, 2009.

U.S. Food and Drug Administration: *Performance standards for ionizing radiation emitting products, 2005*, 21 CFR 1020.32.

U.S. Food and Drug Administration: *FDA radiological health program, fluoroscopy*, 2008, Center for Devices and Radiological Health, available at http://www.fda.gov/cdrh/radhealth/products/fluoroscopy.html. Accessed April 29, 2009.

U.S. Nuclear Regulatory Commission: *Instruction concerning risks from occupational radiation exposure*, regulatory guide 8.29, revision 1 Washington, DC, 1996, U.S. Nuclear Regulatory Commission.

U.S. Nuclear Regulatory Commission: *Occupational dose limits for adults*, 2009 10 CFR 20.1201.

Chapter 24 INFECTIOUS DISEASE EXPOSURE

Elbridge A. Merritt, BSN, CNOR, CRCST, CHL

Infectious disease exposure in the operating room (OR) and sterile processing department (SPD) environments is a complex, multifaceted, and ever-changing challenge. Developing a comprehensive understanding of these evolving occupational risks within the OR and SPD environments requires dedication and a commitment to ongoing learning. Advancements in infection control and prevention (IPC) activities within the OR and SPD can be attributed to the involvement and collaboration of many governmental and professional organizations, dedicated professionals, and the patients who provide the impetus for our practices. Preventing infectious disease exposure should always be a primary consideration during the provision of patient care, but prevention must be viewed as a two-way street: the patient on one side and the health care provider on the other. In particular, everyone should strive to make personal hand hygiene the basis for providing quality health care for both the patient and oneself. Although the rationale for performing hand hygiene (HH) may not be ideal, the most recent release of the standard precautions guidelines provides the health care worker with a direction: "Standard precautions are intended to protect patients by ensuring that health care personnel do not carry infectious agents to patients on their hands or via equipment used during patient care" (Siegel et al, 2007). Standard precautions protect not only the patient, but the staff as well. Standard precautions and many other infection prevention and control principles assist with guiding our efforts to mitigate risk for and prevent infectious disease exposure in the OR and SPD.

This chapter will offer insight into a wide variety of topics related to infectious disease exposure in the OR, SPD, and IPC nursing practices. These three areas of the nursing profession overlap, providing many opportunities for collaboration, cooperation, and teamwork. These partnerships can make great leaps in the prevention of infectious disease exposures. The efforts ultimately will enhance and improve patient care, as well as the safety of health care personnel. The future challenges in preventing infectious disease exposure will require teamwork and collaboration like never before. Knowing, appreciating, and assisting in each other's work are essential components to establishing a culture of cooperation in preventing infectious disease exposure.

HISTORICAL BACKGROUND

Harvey Cushing (1869–1939) stated, "Certainly infections cannot be attributed to the intervention of the devil but must be laid at the surgeon's door" (Miller et al, 2005). This quotation provides a sample of the varying opinions of the time regarding infections. With the advancement and controversy regarding germ theory in the late 1800s one can understand the reasoning behind the thought process. Knowing what we know today regarding germ theory and the complexity of preventing infectious disease exposure, we must recognize how far the efforts have progressed.

Modern IPC as we know it now began to make solid progress during the mid-nineteenth century. As early as 1842 Oliver Wendell Holmes (1809–1894) of Harvard was recommending a hand wash of calcium chloride to prevent the spread of infection from the autopsy room to the ward (Miller et al, 2005). Similarly, Ignaz Philipp Semmelweis (1818–1865) provided a 2-year study demonstrating that a hand wash with a chloride of lime solution reduced puerperal sepsis mortality from 9.92% to 1.27% (Miller et al, 2005). Louis Pasteur (1822–1912) made additional advancements in the IPC world, most notably in germ theory. The germ theory postulated that most infectious diseases are caused by living organisms or germs. Pasteur is also well known for his work in the fermentation and pasteurization processes (Bellis, 2009). Joseph Lister (1827–1912) further advanced the work of Pasteur, applying it to surgical practice. Lister began applying carbolic acid to compound fracture wounds and documented a significant decrease in mortality rate from 45% to 15% (Miller et al, 2005). Upon hearing a lecture by Lister, U.S. neurosurgeon William W. Keen (1837–1932) began pioneering many of Lister's recommendations to neurosurgical practice with marked success (Miller et al, 2005).

The invention, development, and use of antiseptic solutions and supplies, aseptic technique, and sterilization of surgical instruments further improved the care and prevention of infection in surgical patients. In 1889, following a request by William Stewart Halsted (1852–1922) to Goodyear Rubber Company to develop rubber gloves for his scrub nurse because of an allergy to an instrument disinfectant, wearing of surgical gloves to protect the patient and staff members eventually emerged as common practice (Miller et al, 2005; Rothrock, 2007).

The first IPC efforts in the United States began in the 1950s concurrent with the growth of the intensive care unit and subsequent increases in staphylococcal infections (Friedman and Petersen, 2004). Formal IPC programs became common in hospitals in the 1970s, but it was not until 1976 that standards were established and an IPC program became a requirement for health care organizations (Friedman and Petersen, 2004).

The contributions of all the aforementioned professionals and countless others, as well as governmental and professional entities, have shaped and organized the current IPC programs, regulations, and requirements. Among the most influential in the modern IPC realm is the introduction by the Occupational Safety and Health Administration (OSHA) (2008) of universal precautions in 1991. Universal precautions, in addition to the standard and transmission precautions recommended by the Centers for Disease Control and Prevention (CDC), provided a solid foundation on which to build the modern IPC program. Without these modern-day IPC guidelines the number of infectious disease exposures in the OR and SPD would be astounding. These developments highlight only a few efforts in the development of a professional infection control program and provide a brief history in the evolution and development of modern IPC practices. Implementation of modern practices has been of great benefit to our patients, as well as preventing infectious disease exposure of staff members.

CHAIN OF INFECTION

The human body is resilient and has redundant but necessary and complementary layers in its defense against infectious disease. The body's defensive measures include external barriers, the inflammatory response, and the immune response (Rothrock, 2007). External barriers include healthy intact skin and mucous membranes. An inflammatory response can occur systemically or locally in tissue following injury in an attempt to isolate the offensive foreign object or pathogen (Phillips, 2004). The final defense measure, the immune response, may be passive or active immunity and is triggered by the inflammatory response (Phillips, 2004; Rothrock, 2007).

Essential to preventing disease exposure and subsequent infections is an understanding of the infectious process. The infectious process is often described as a chain of infection (Figure 24-1). Each link in the chain of infection has categories essential to understanding how to break, prevent, or interrupt the link in the infectious disease process.

The first link in the chain is the causative agent or the infectious agent. The causative agent may be bacterial, viral, fungal, protozoan, helminthic, or prionic in nature (Association for Professionals in Infection Control and Epidemiology [APIC], 2005). Activities that will break this link in the chain include early, accurate identification of signs and symptoms of illness and prompt identification of the causative agent. The occupational health screenings and policies must be clear, easy to understand, and available to staff members (APIC, 2005).

The second link in the chain is the reservoir or carrier. Reservoirs are a place for the infectious

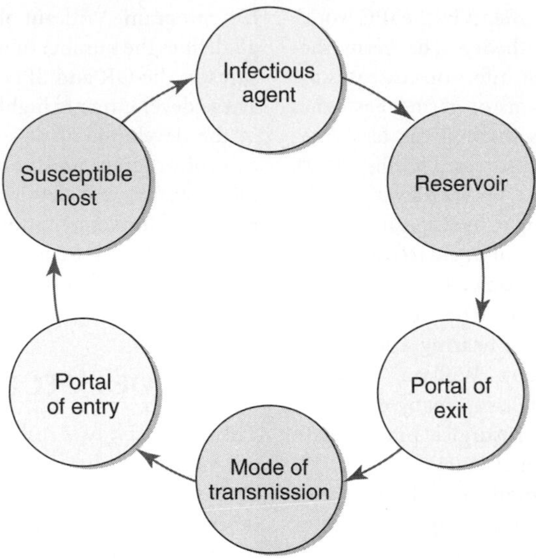

FIGURE 24-1 Example of chain of infection/infectious disease process. (From Potter PA, Perry AG: *Basic nursing,* ed 6, St. Louis, 2007, Mosby.)

agent to survive. The most common reservoirs are environmental, human, and animal (APIC, 2005). An infinite number of examples of environmental reservoirs are possible given an improperly cleaned OR or SPD environment. Activities that break this link in the chain related to the OR and SPD start at the point of use, either the OR or clinics. All instruments need to be cleaned of gross debris and sprayed with an enzymatic cleaner before being sent to the SPD department. Implemented processes include stringent monitoring, maintenance, and cleaning of the environment, as well as proper cleaning, disinfection, and sterilization of instruments and equipment. An example of a human reservoir is a health care worker who had a previous multidrug-resistant organism (MDRO) skin infection but now has MDRO skin flora or is colonized with the MDRO. Activities in the OR that can break this link in the chain related to the human reservoir include frequent personal hygiene (hand washing), effective occupational health screenings, and use of standard precautions. For personal safety and the safety of their patients, employees must be aware of and comply with occupational health screenings and policies.

The next three links are very closely related. The portal of exit, mode of transmission, and portal of entry links happen almost simultaneously. The portal of exit is the method by which the infectious agent leaves the reservoir. Portals of exit include respiratory, genitourinary, and gastrointestinal tracts; intact and nonintact skin; mucous membrane; placenta; and blood (APIC, 2005). The mode of transmission is the method by which the infection is passed on to a susceptible host (APIC, 2005). The mode of transmission may be by direct contact between the reservoir and susceptible host or between the environment and a susceptible host. Depending on the organism, the mode of transmission may also be by droplet or airborne transmission. The best opportunity to break the chain during these three links is with the mode of transmission link. This is accomplished in the OR by using appropriate contact, droplet, and airborne precautions based on the infectious illness, an action that may mitigate much of the risk for employee infectious disease exposure (see Appendix B). Portals of entry include the respiratory tract, genitourinary tract, gastrointestinal tract, intact and nonintact skin, mucous membrane, placenta, and parenteral (APIC, 2005).

The final link, the susceptible host, completes the chain of infection. A susceptible host is essential in contracting an infectious agent. The susceptibility of a host is influenced by many factors including age, sex, ethnicity, socioeconomic status, marital status, medical history, lifestyle, heredity, nutritional status, occupation, immunization status, diagnostic/therapeutic procedures, medications, pregnancy, underlying disease, and trauma (APIC, 2005; Otaiza and Pessoa Da Silva, 2008).

The chain of infection provides a good depiction of the infectious disease process. Typically staff members think the infectious disease process centers on mitigating exposure to the infectious patient. However infectious diseases do not discriminate. A susceptible host may come in the form of a patient or a staff member. The staff member who has an infection or is colonized can easily spread an infectious agent to a patient during the provision of health care. Staff members providing direct patient care must be aware of occupational health policies, and if they have an infection or are colonized, they must receive the appropriate treatment and evaluations before returning to their direct patient care job (Otaiza and Pessoa Da Silva, 2008). In addition, staff members must receive periodic occupational health screenings to ensure that they are healthy, are using personal protective equipment appropriately, and understand the postexposure protocols of their institution (Otaiza and Pessoa Da Silva, 2008).

BASIC COMPONENTS OF AN INFECTION PREVENTION AND CONTROL PROGRAM

Surveillance

Surveillance is the systematic, active, ongoing method of collecting, consolidating, and analyzing data concerning the distribution and determinants of a given disease or event, followed by the dissemination of that information to those who can improve the outcomes (APIC, 2005). IPC practitioners obtain, analyze, report, and distribute critical data and information related to the prevention and control of infections within their organization. Surveillance activities include collecting data that enable epidemiologic studies and illness tracking to be performed. The OR and SPD sections provide the IPC practitioner with an immense amount of surveillance data and have a profound influence on the effectiveness of any IPC program. Examples of surveillance activities in an OR include surgical site infection (SSI) rates; compliance with actions to prevent SSIs; monitoring and recording of the environmental parameters; environmental cleaning policies and procedures; flash sterilization rates and quality assurance monitoring, which includes biological and decontamination testing; and environment of care surveys. Examples of surveillance activities in the SPD include quality assurance testing, monitoring and recording environmental parameters and cleaning records, and environment of care surveys. The basic components of the IPC program can provide reciprocating data and information to the OR and SPD departments, including occupational health data, trending of SSIs, enhancing quality assurance activities, and assistance with education and training of OR, SPD, and environmental cleaning staff.

Intervention and Investigation

Following the analysis of the collected data, it is imperative to appropriately intervene to prevent infection. Surveillance may reveal an outbreak of infection. An outbreak is a cluster of infections greater than expected or the occurrence of an unusual infection (Friedman and Petersen, 2004). The source of an outbreak might be a patient, but it might also be a staff member stemming from an infectious disease exposure. Similar infection types of SSIs may indicate an outbreak and warrant an investigation. The goal of an investigation is to control and prevent further infections and to identify contributing factors so that prevention measures can be implemented (Friedman and Petersen, 2004).

Policy and Procedure Development

Developing policies and procedures that combine the efforts of leadership and staff members within the OR and SPD departments is imperative to subsequent compliance with those policies. Collaboration in developing the IPC policies enhances staff knowledge and compliance. Working with the laboratory and the licensed practitioners within the facility will assist in developing an appropriate antibiotic stewardship plan. Ultimately the collaboration in developing IPC policies with the OR, SPD, and the laboratory grows an effective IPC program that has been vetted by many organizational leaders and increases the overall commitment.

Competent Practitioners

One of the most critical effects an IPC practitioner has is that of an educator. The IPC practitioner provides education to both patients and staff members. The IPC practitioner teaches the staff the scientific rationale for the precautions that allow health care workers to apply procedures safely and correctly. IPC practitioners can also teach safely modified precautions based on changing requirements, resources, or health care settings (Siegel et al, 2007). Education requirements for newcomers and annual training, educational refreshers, and in-service programs for staff based on surveillance activities are just a few of the educational offerings an IPC practitioner provides to staff. In a recent study the likelihood of a health care worker's developing sudden acute respiratory syndrome (SARS) was strongly associated with less than 2 hours of infection control training and lack of understanding of infection control procedures (Siegel et al, 2007).

Patient education bulletin boards provided by the IPC practitioner can include information on hospital-specific topics such as hand hygiene, MDROs, SSIs, urinary tract infections, or ventilator-associated pneumonias. Education information could also be related to public health and prevention topics such as community-acquired MDROs, influenza, respiratory syncytial virus, sexually transmitted diseases, and tuberculosis, to name a few. The IPC practitioner as an educator has a potentially enormous effect on the quality of patient care and the safety of the OR and SPD staff.

The IPC practitioner is among the most consulted professionals in the health care setting. The IPC practice covers many different topics and disciplines, requiring partnerships like few other professions. Frequent cooperation takes place between the IPC practitioner and the following: microbiology laboratory, infectious disease physicians, epidemiologists, primary care physicians, surgeons, community and public health professionals, occupational health professionals, pharmacists, facility management, veterinarians, industrial hygiene, housekeeping staff, OR and SPD staff, and IPC representatives and staff from all patient care areas.

The IPC practitioner is both a patient and staff advocate. Working with the all health care staff members to improve compliance with hand hygiene, educating staff about compliance with standard and transmission-based precautions, and educating the housekeeping staff regarding appropriate cleaning standards for patient care areas are all activities of patient and staff advocacy.

STANDARD AND TRANSMISSION-BASED PRECAUTIONS

Standard Precautions

The most recent release of standard precautions by the CDC in 2007 evolved from the universal precautions mandated by OSHA. Standard precautions combine universal precautions and body substance isolation and are based on the principle that all blood, body fluids, secretions, excretions except sweat, nonintact skin, and mucous membranes may contain transmissible infectious agents (Siegel et al, 2007). Standard precautions include a combination of infection prevention and control measures such as hand hygiene (HH); use of gloves, gowns, masks, eye protection, or face shield, depending on the anticipated exposure; safe injection practices; respiratory hygiene and cough etiquette; and use of masks for insertion of catheters or injection of material into spinal or epidural spaces via lumbar puncture procedures (Siegel et al, 2007). Standard precautions should be used for all patients regardless of whether an infectious illness is confirmed or unconfirmed and based upon the anticipated level of exposure (AORN, 2009).

Hand Hygiene

HH has been demonstrated to be one of the most important activities to prevent the spread of infection in the health care setting (Siegel et al, 2007). HH is important because it minimizes the risk for transmitting infection to and between patients, as well as staff. A complete HH program not only minimizes risk, but also offers convenient HH options designed to maximize staff compliance (AORN, 2009). Most HH programs offer a selection of traditional or antiseptic hand soap, an alcohol-based hand sanitizer, a surgical hand antiseptic, and hand lotion. Selection of the appropriate HH agent is situationally dependent and must be approved by the hospital's infection control committee. A staff member's awareness of a patient illness when choosing the appropriate method of HH is imperative. For example, when a staff member is caring for a patient with a spore-forming illness (e.g., *Clostridium difficile* or *Bacillus anthracis*), alcohol-based hand sanitizers are ineffective and a hand wash must be performed. A hand wash should also be performed when hands are visibly soiled. HH should be performed at the beginning and end of a work shift, before and after patient contact and after removing gloves, before and after eating, before and after entering the restroom, anytime there has been a possibility of contact with blood or potentially infectious materials, and anytime when hands are or may have been soiled. In addition, the maintenance of health skin integrity with the frequent application of skin-moisturizing lotions is very important to minimize the portal of entry for infectious disease.

BOX 24-1 Safe Donning of Personal Protective Equipment (PPE)

GOWN
- Fully cover torso from neck to knees, arms to end of wrist, and wrap around the back
- Fasten in back at neck and waist

MASK OR RESPIRATOR
- Secure ties or elastic band at middle of head and neck
- Fit flexible band to nose bridge
- Fit snug to face and below chin
- Fit-check respirator

GOGGLES/FACE SHIELD
- Put on face and adjust to fit

GLOVES
- Use non-sterile for isolation
- Select according to hand size
- Extend to cover wrist of isolation gown

SAFE WORK PRACTICES
- Keep hands away from face
- Work from clean to dirty
- Limit surfaces touched
- Change when torn or heavily contaminated
- Perform hand hygiene

From Siegel JD et al: *Guideline for isolation precautions: preventing transmission of infectious agents in healthcare settings*, June 2007, Centers for Disease Control and Prevention, available at http://www.cdc.gov/ncidod/dhqp/pdf/guidelines/Isolation2007.pdf. Accessed August 29, 2009.

Personal Protective Equipment

Personal protective equipment (PPE) refers to a variety of barriers and equipment used alone or in combination to protect mucous membranes, the airway, skin, and clothing from contact with infectious agents (Friedman and Petersen, 2004; Siegel et al, 2007). PPE includes gloves, masks, goggles, face shields, glasses, and gowns. PPE is intended to prevent the spread of microorganisms from patient to caregiver and from caregiver to patient by creating a barrier between the patient and caregiver and between caregiver, patient, and an infectious organism (Boxes 24-1 and 24-2) (Friedman and Petersen, 2004).

Gloves are indicated when it is anticipated that contact with blood or bodily fluids will occur. There are different types of gloves, and gloves are made of many different materials (Friedman and Petersen, 2004). The type of glove used should be based on the specific activity, allergy of the wearer, and personal preference (Friedman and Petersen, 2004). The use of sterile surgical gloves during surgical and invasive procedures protects not only the patient, but also the staff member from the risk for infection. The practice of double gloving for surgical procedures should always be standard practice in the surgical setting for various patient and staff safety reasons. First, the imperviousness of sterile surgical gloves may not be completely intact. The U.S. Food and Drug Administration (FDA) accepts a failure rate of 2.5% for new unused sterile gloves in quality control tests (Berguer and Heller, 2005). Although 2.5% may be a very small and acceptable number according to the FDA, the potential risk to patients and staff is too high not to double glove

BOX 24-2 Safe Removal of Personal Protective Equipment (PPE)

Remove PPE at doorway before leaving patient room or in anteroom.

GLOVES

- Outside of gloves are contaminated!
- Grasp outside of glove with opposite gloved hand; peel off
- Hold removed glove in gloved hand
- Slide fingers of ungloved hand under remaining glove at wrist

GOGGLES/FACE SHIELD

- Outside of goggles or face shield are contaminated!
- To remove, handle by "clean" head band or ear pieces
- Place in designated receptacle for reprocessing or in waste container

GOWN

- Gown front and sleeves are contaminated!
- Unfasten neck, then waist ties
- Remove gown using a peeling motion; pull gown from each shoulder toward the same hand
- Gown will turn inside out
- Hold removed gown away from body, roll into a bundle and discard into waste or linen receptacle

MASK OR RESPIRATOR

- Front of mask/respirator is contaminated—DO NOT TOUCH!
- Grasp ONLY bottom then top ties/elastics and remove
- Discard in waste container

HAND HYGIENE

- Perform hand hygiene immediately after removing all PPE!

From Siegel JD et al: *Guideline for isolation precautions: preventing transmission of infectious agents in healthcare settings*, June 2007, Centers for Disease Control and Prevention, available at http://www.cdc.gov/ncidod/dhqp/pdf/guidelines/Isolation2007.pdf. Accessed August 29, 2009.

and minimize risk. Secondly, double gloving can reduce the risk for exposure to patient blood by as much as 87% when the outer glove is punctured (Berguer and Heller, 2005). Furthermore, the volume of blood on a suture needle is reduced 95% when passed through two glove layers (Berguer and Heller, 2005).

Masks, goggles, face shields, and glasses also constitute PPE. These protect the mucous membranes of the nose, mouth, and eyes during procedures and activities that generate splashes, splatters, sprays, or aerosols of blood or other potentially infectious materials (AORN, 2009). The choice of eye wear protection—whether it is goggles, a face shield, or glasses—is based upon the staff member's perceived level of anticipated exposure and personal preferences. In the OR and SPD setting the potential level of exposure is high; therefore eye protection should be worn consistently in these high-risk environments.

Impervious gowns and aprons must be used to protect the skin and clothing during activities that generate splashes, splatters, sprays, or aerosols of blood or other potentially infectious materials. Scrub attire, laboratory jackets, and warm-up jackets are not considered adequate for PPE because they are not impervious. Grossly soiled scrub attire and laboratory and warm-up jackets should be changed as soon as feasible (OSHA, 2008).

Sharps Injury Prevention

Sharps injury prevention in the OR and SPD setting is of immense importance. The occurrence of sharps injuries in the OR remains too high despite measures to mitigate the risk for injury. Standard procedures to diminish the occupational hazard of handling sharps in the OR include engineered safety devices and establishing hands-free passing of sharps at the surgical field. Engineered safety devices used in the OR include needleless hubs on intravenous lines, safety devices on hypodermic needles to negate the need to recap a needle, safety guards on scalpels, and encouraging the use of blunt suturing needles. The availability and variety of these engineered safety devices have increased drastically since OSHA's bloodborne pathogens regulation (2008) took effect.

Implementing work practice controls such as hands-free passing of sharps and prohibiting recapping of needles with a two-handed technique can greatly reduce the number of sharps injuries in the OR (Berguer and Heller, 2005). According to the National Surveillance System for Health Care Workers, the OR has the second-highest rate of sharps injury at 27% of the injuries overall (CDC, 2008). AORN (2009) recommends perioperative-specific sharps injury risk reduction strategies (Box 24-3).

If a bloodborne pathogen exposure occurs, the site should be washed with soap and water and mucous membranes should be flushed copiously with water (Friedman and Petersen, 2004). There is no evidence of benefit for using antiseptics or disinfectants or for squeezing the puncture site to minimize or prevent infection (APIC, 2005). The use of bleach or other caustic agents should be avoided (APIC, 2005). Although the

BOX 24-3 Perioperative-Specific Sharps Injury Risk Reduction Strategies

- Adopt and incorporate safe habits into daily work activities when preparing and using sharps devices
- Focus attention on the intent of the action when working with sharp items, minimize rushing and distractions while applying safety techniques during critical moments
- During preparation for operative or other invasive procedures:
  - Inspect the surgical field for adequate lighting and space to perform the procedure
  - Organize the work area so that the sharps are always pointed away from staff members
  - Establish a separate area to place a reusable sharp for safe handling during the procedure
  - Use standardized sterile field set-ups
  - Include the identification of the neutral zone in the preoperative briefing
- During the operative or other invasive procedure:
  - Wear two pairs of gloves
  - Monitor gloves for punctures
  - Encourage the use of blunt suture needles
  - Use neutral or hands-free technique for passing sharp items whenever possible or practical, instead of passing hand to hand
  - Give verbal notifications when passing a sharp device
  - Keep visual contact with the procedure site and the sharp device
  - Take steps to control the location of the sharp device
  - Be aware of other staff members in the area when handling a sharp device
  - Contain used sharps on the sterile field in a designated, disposable, puncture-resistant needle container, and replace it as necessary
  - Check to be sure the disposable, puncture-resistant needle container is securely closed before handing it off the sterile field
  - Load suture needles using the suture packet to assist in mounting the suture needle in the needle holder, and use the appropriate instrument to adjust and unload the needle
  - Remove the needle from the suture before tying, or use "controlled release" sutures that allow the needle to be removed with a straight pull on the needle holder
  - Activate the safety feature of a safety engineered device immediately after use according to manufacturers' instructions
- Keep hands away from the surgical site when sharp items are in use
  - Use one-handed or blunt instrument–assisted suturing techniques to avoid finger contact with the suture needle or tissue being sutured
  - Provide a barrier between the hands and the needle after use
  - Use gloves and an instrument to pick up sharp items (i.e., suture needles, hypodermic needles, scalpel blades) that have fallen on the floor
- During post procedure clean up:
  - Inspect the surgical set-up used during the procedure for sharps
  - Transport reusable sharps in a closed, secure container to the designated cleanup area
  - Inspect the sharps container for overfilling before discarding disposable sharps in it
  - Make sure the sharps container is large enough to accommodate the entire device
  - Avoid bringing hands close to the opening of a sharps container
  - Do not place hands or fingers into a container to dispose of a device
  - Keep hands behind the sharp tip when disposing

Modified from Association of periOperative Registered Nurses: *Perioperative standards and recommended practices*, Denver, 2009, The Association.

aforementioned statements from the Association for Professionals in Infection Control and Epidemiology (APIC) appears rational, other institutions' guidance for specific disease exposures may contradict APIC's. The postexposure protocols of the occupational health program should be presented annually to staff to ensure that staff understand the process.

The most recent version of standard precautions includes new elements that enhance patient and staff safety. The new requirements include safe injection practices, respiratory hygiene and cough etiquette, and special lumbar puncture procedures (Siegel et al, 2007).

The safe injection practices include the use of a sterile, single-use, disposable needle and syringe for each injection given and prevention of contamination of injection equipment and medication (Siegel et al, 2007). Whenever possible, use of single-dose vials is preferred over multiple-dose vials, especially when medications will be administered to multiple patients (Siegel et al, 2007). The inclusion of safe injection practices in the 2007 standard precautions emphasizes the importance of maintaining very basic IPC practices. Performing safe injection practices protects the patient and staff members. Not using a sterile, single-use, disposable needle and syringe not only is potentially a catastrophic event for the patient, but also places the individual staff member at risk for an injury from a contaminated needle.

Respiratory Concerns

The respiratory hygiene and cough etiquette elements include educating staff members, patients, and visitors about respiratory hygiene and cough etiquette. Post signs with instructions to patients and accompanying family members or friends about when and how to use respiratory hygiene and cough etiquette. Education includes the following information: (1) employ source control measures such as using a surgical mask to cover a cough, when tolerated, or, when the mask is not tolerated, covering coughs with a tissue and promptly disposing of the used tissue; (2) perform hand hygiene immediately after contact with respiratory secretions; and (3) maintain spatial separation of ideally more than 3 feet from individuals with respiratory infections (Siegel et al, 2007). Using respiratory hygiene and cough etiquette can assist in preventing the spread of infection in the OR setting by minimizing the spread of droplet secretions among our waiting patients, visitors, and staff within the preoperative setting (Siegel et al, 2007).

Special lumbar puncture procedures include wearing a face mask to limit the dispersal of oropharyngeal droplets when placing a catheter or injecting material into the spinal or epidural space (Siegel et al, 2007). Wearing a mask when injecting into the spinal or epidural spaces can also potentially protect the staff member from any spray from a needle pop-off during the process of the injection.

Transmission-Based Precautions

The three categories of transmission-based precautions are contact precautions, droplet precautions, and airborne precautions. Transmission-based precautions are used when the routes of transmission are not completely interrupted using standard precautions alone (Siegel et al, 2007). Transmission-based precautions in the perioperative setting should essentially be the same as in any other setting with a few very specific exceptions.

When transmission-based precautions are indicated, all efforts must be made to educate the patient and family regarding the rationale for the precautions and to counteract possible adverse effects. Education and explanations of the precautions may prevent negative patient feelings such as anxiety, depression, mood disturbances, and perceptions of stigma and reduced contact with clinical staff. Educational engagement of the patient also may help improve acceptance and compliance by the patient (Siegel et al, 2007).

Contact Precautions

Contact precautions are intended to prevent transmission of infectious agents that are spread by direct or indirect contact with the patient or the patient's environment (Siegel et al, 2007). The intent of contact precautions is to put a barrier between the patient with a contact precaution illness and an uninfected person to prevent transmission. Wear gloves for contact with the patient and for contact with any environmental item(s) touched by the patient. Wear fluid-resistant gowns when entering the room if clothing will come in contact with the patient or if working close to the patient (Siegel et al, 2007). Before leaving the room the staff member removes all PPE and conducts HH. Post a sign on all doors to notify and inform staff that contact precautions are in use (Figure 24-2, *A*). Infectious agents for which contact precautions are indicated are found in Appendix B and include methicillin-resistant *Staphylococcus aureus* (MRSA), vancomycin-resistant enterococci (VRE), *Acinetobacter baumannii*, noroviruses and other intestinal tract pathogens, and respiratory syncytial virus and other respiratory tract pathogens.

Contact precautions are by far the most common form of transmission-based precaution used in the OR. MDROs, for example, continue to be a challenge to manage in the OR and in today's health care environment. However, by implementing contact precautions the impact can be greatly minimized. In the OR the first step in minimizing the negative effect of MDROs begins with staff awareness, understanding, and practicing of meticulous hand hygiene. In addition, ensure that OR staff are properly trained and knowledgeable about when and how to implement contact precautions. OR staff must proactively communicate the patient's medical history to the unit of disposition to ensure continuity of care for the patient. Providing the unit of disposition timely notification that the patient will require contact precautions is a professional courtesy that should be adhered to. The OR staff should also provide the same professional courtesy communication to the SPD staff about the use of contact precautions during the specific procedure.

Droplet Precautions

Droplet precautions are intended to prevent transmission of pathogens that are spread through respiratory or mucous membrane contact with large-droplet respiratory secretions. Pathogens requiring droplet precautions do not remain infectious over long distances because the large droplets settle quickly, usually within 3 feet of the

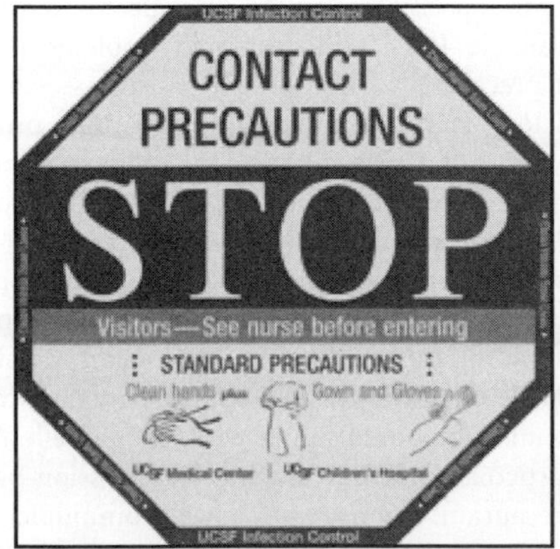

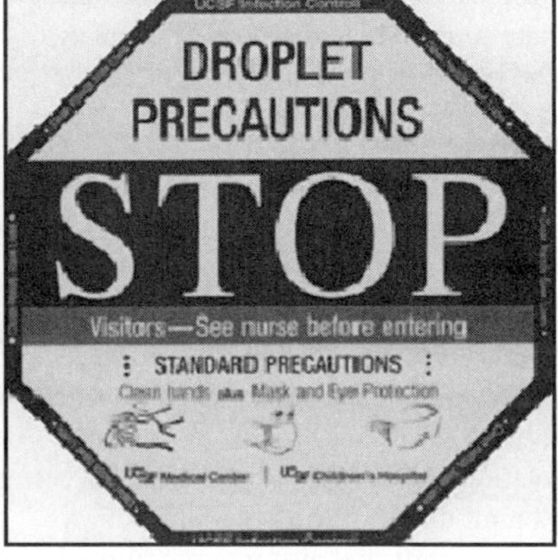

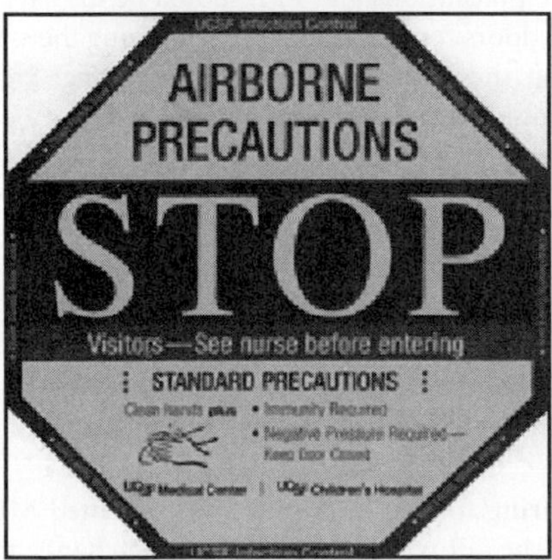

FIGURE 24-2 Transmission-based precaution signs. **A**, Contact precautions. **B**, Droplet precautions. **C**, Airborne precautions. (From University of California at San Francisco Children's Hospital: *Infection control: standard and transmission-based precautions.*)

ill patient, and therefore do not require special air handling and ventilation. Droplet precautions simply require the wearing of a surgical mask for contact or activity within 3 feet of the patient or reservoir. A sign should be posted on all doors to notify and inform the staff that droplet precautions are in use (see Figure 24-2, *B*). Infectious agents for which droplet precautions are indicated are found in Appendix B and commonly include *Bordetella pertussis*, influenza virus, adenovirus, rhinovirus, *Neisseria meningitides*, and group A streptococcus (Siegel et al, 2007).

Management of a patient infected with an illness requiring droplet precautions intuitively seems easy to manage in the OR setting. The perioperative staff must continue wearing of the surgical mask, especially before induction of general anesthesia and after extubation of the airway device. After extubation of the airway device a patient's airway may be irritated, potentially leading to an increase in coughing and dispersal of infectious droplets. Ideally it is best for the patient to wear a mask as soon as tolerated to minimize dispersal of infectious droplets. A simple oxygen mask would be appropriate to minimize dispersal of droplets. Following the need for oxygen the patient can be transitioned to a simple surgical face mask.

Airborne Precautions

Airborne precautions prevent transmission of infectious agents that remain infectious over long distances when suspended in the air (Siegel et al, 2007). To effectively implement airborne precautions it is necessary to use an airborne infection isolation room (AIIR) (Siegel et al, 2007). Post a sign on all doors of the isolation room to notify and inform staff that airborne precautions are in use (see Figure 24-2, *C*). For an isolation room to qualify as an AIIR it must meet the following criteria: (1) it is capable of maintaining negative pressure, (2) it is capable of 12 or more air exchanges per hour, (3) air should be either exhausted directly to the outside or recirculated only after high-efficiency particulate air (HEPA) filtration, and (4) the room is fitted with self closing doors to assist with the maintenance of proper airflow (APIC, 2005). Infectious agents for which airborne precautions are found in Appendix B and commonly include *Mycobacterium tuberculosis*, rubella virus (measles), and varicella-zoster virus (chickenpox) (Siegel et al, 2007).

One of the most common illnesses requiring airborne precautions is tuberculosis, or *M. tuberculosis*. When possible, the best practice is to postpone surgery on the tuberculosis-positive patient until the patient is determined to be noninfectious (CDC, 2005). When surgery is urgent, efforts should be made to minimize staff and patient exposure. Using an OR that meets the above AIIR criteria is optimal. If an AIIR-compliant OR is unavailable, portable HEPA filters and ultraviolet germicidal irradiation can be used to improve the air quality (CDC, 2005). Anesthesia and surgical staff members should wear at least a National Institute for Occupational Safety and Health–approved N95 respirator. A bacterial filter of 0.3 μm should also be placed on the endotracheal tube to reduce the risk for contaminating the ventilator or anesthesia equipment and to prevent discharging tubercle bacilli into the ambient air when operating (CDC, 2005).

Perioperative staff members must be aware of and knowledgeable about transmission-based precautions and the procedures for implementing the specific precaution. Organized and readily available PPE facilitates rapid implementation of precautions based on the patient assessment, history, and communications with other professional staff. It also enhances the ability to respond to a CBRNE (***C***hemical, ***B***iological, ***R***adiologic, ***N***uclear, and ***E***xplosive) event. Stocked rolling carts are a convenient way to organize supplies and can be positioned outside the OR entrances, providing the appropriate PPE to staff members before entering the OR. Both the surgical communication board and schedule should reflect the particular patient's specific transmission-based precaution. Appropriate signage communicating the precautions and PPE should be displayed on all doors for the specific OR notifying the staff to don the required PPE before entering. Signage should also be placed on the patient's bed or gurney (Gruendeman and Mangum, 2001).

SPECIFIC ILLNESS CONSIDERATIONS IN THE OPERATING ROOM

Multidrug-Resistant Organism Implications

Caring for patients with a documented MDRO in the OR will result in little or no change in the care they or other patients receive. Caring for patients with MDROs does, however, require significant planning and preparedness. Educating the OR staff regarding care improvements to mitigate spread of the MDRO is imperative. These improvements include improved compliance with hand hygiene, use of contact precautions until the patient's cultures are negative for the target MDRO, enhanced environmental cleaning, active surveillance cultures, and improvements in communication about patients with MDROs within and between health care facilities (Siegel et al, 2006). These improvements or enhancements of basic care are imperative to diminish the threat of MDRO outbreaks. Staff commitment to improving compliance with hand hygiene and implementing the appropriate transmission-based precaution is essential and begins many times with the perioperative nurse. An example of enhanced environmental cleaning may include terminally cleaning the OR following every patient that has an MDRO. Some facilities actively culture all patients to screen them for MDROs or concern that the patient may have an MDRO before any surgery. Enhancement of communication regarding a patient with an MDRO within and between facilities is very important. The importance of this is emphasized by The Joint Commission (2009) making communication between organizations regarding a patient's infectious status an element of performance in the 2009 standards. Just as important and often overlooked is communication between professionals within the organization.

Decolonization Regimens for MRSA-Colonized Staff

A MRSA-colonized staff member has been shown to have a limited role in transmission (Siegel et al, 2006). A MRSA-colonized staff member has an increased potential to transmit if the following are present: chronic sinusitis, upper respiratory infection, or dermatitis (Siegel et al, 2006). Staff that are colonized with MRSA but are asymptomatic and have not been linked epidemiologically to transmission do not require decolonization. If a staff member is linked epidemiologically as a source of transmission to patients, consideration of a decolonization regimen is indicated (Siegel et al, 2006). Colonization with MRSA in health care workers, who are generally healthy young adults, may be successfully eradicated with a combination of various antibiotics (Simor et al, 2007). Because of the fear of antibiotic resistance, a consultation with a microbiologist before administration may be prudent to ascertain any resistance (Siegel et al, 2006).

BIOTERRORISM AND EMERGING INFECTIONS

Medical facilities have broad disaster management plans to assist with bioterrorism events, but the OR and the SPD must also be prepared to manage emerging infections and illnesses associated with bioterrorism in our specific environments (AORN, 2009). OR and SPD leadership not only should be present for facility disaster management discussions, but also should work in partnership to develop section and department plans to ensure fluid operations in the possibility of such an event. Written plans must be developed, reviewed, refined, and rehearsed to ensure staff knowledge, compliance, and comfort with policies. In addition, incorporation of disaster preparedness plans into competency-based orientations of OR, SPD, and environmental services can assist with staff knowledge and comfort. The development and inclusion of quick references such as a table for signs, symptoms, appropriate precautions, and treatments may assist staff members in the care of patients with a known or suspected bioterrorism agent (Table 24-1). Collaborating with infection prevention and control professionals within the organization to develop and request educational materials and in-service programs is encouraged to ensure the safety of the patients and staff. The CDC has identified anthrax *(B. anthracis)* and smallpox (variola major) as the two most likely biological weapons (Rothrock, 2007). Other infectious illnesses associated with bioterrorism are pneumonic plague *(Yersinia pestis)*, tularemia *(Francisella tularensis)*, and botulism toxin *(Clostridium botulinum)* (Perry, 2006).

Anthrax is caused by a gram-positive, spore-forming bacterial rod (Rothrock, 2007). Anthrax spores are very hearty and can survive for many decades in the soil (Rothrock, 2007). Anthrax infection can occur in three forms: inhalation, cutaneous, and gastrointestinal (APIC, 2005). Anthrax is a lethal illness and, if effectively aerosolized, could have catastrophic effects on the recipient population. The World Health

Text continued on page 326

TABLE 24-1 Bioterrorism Quick Reference Guide

	BACTERIAL AGENTS								VIRUSES				BIOLOGICAL TOXINS			
	Anthrax	*Brucellosis*	*Cholera*	*Glanders (rarely seen)*	*Bubonic Plague*	*Pneumonic Plague*	*Tularemia*	*Q Fever*	*Smallpox*	*Venez Equine Encephalitis*	*Viral Encephalitis*	*Viral Hemor Fever*	*Botulism*	*Ricin*	*T-2 Mycotoxins*	*Staph Enterotoxin B*
ISOLATION PRECAUTION																
Standard precautions for all aspects of patient care	X	X	X	X	X	X	X	X	X	X	X	X	X	X	X	**X**
Contact precautions		X			X				X			X				
Airborne precautions				X					X			X*				
Use of **N95** mask by **all** individuals entering the room that have not had recent immunization (5 yrs)									X							
Droplet precautions						X				X						
Hand hygiene with alcohol-based product or antimicrobial		X	X						X			X				
PATIENT PLACEMENT																
No restrictions	X						X						X	X	X	X
Cohort "like" patients when private room unavailable			X		X	X		X			X					
Private room		X	X	X	X	X			X	X		X				

Negative pressure									X							
Door closed at all times				X					X							
PATIENT TRANSPORT																
No restrictions	X						X	X			X		X	X	X	X
Limit movement to essential medical purposes only		X	X	X	X	X			X	X		X				
Place mask on patient to minimize dispersal of droplets				X		X			X	X						
CLEANING, DISINFECTION OF EQUIPMENT																
Routine terminal cleaning of room with hospital-approved disinfectant upon discharge			X	X			X	X	X	X	X		X	X	X	X
Disinfect surfaces with bleach/water sol. (10% sol.)	X	X			X	X						X				
Dedicated equipment disinfected before leaving room		X							X			X				
Linen management as with all other patients	X	X	X	X	X	X	X	X	X	X	X	X	X	X	X	X
RMW handled per hospital policy	X	X	X	X	X	X	X	X	X	X	X	X	X	X	X	X
DISCHARGE MANAGEMENT																
No special discharge instruction necessary	X		X	X			X	X		X	X		X	X	X	X
Home care providers need to be taught principles of standard precautions	X	X			X	X						X				
Not discharged from hospital until determined no longer infectious						X			X			X				
Patient usually not discharged until 72 hours of antibiotics completed						X										

Continued

TABLE 24-1 Bioterrorism Quick Reference Guide—cont'd

	BACTERIAL AGENTS								VIRUSES				BIOLOGICAL TOXINS			
	Anthrax	*Brucellosis*	*Cholera*	*Glanders (rarely seen)*	*Bubonic Plague*	*Pneumonic Plague*	*Tularemia*	*Q Fever*	*Smallpox*	*Venez Equine Encephalitis*	*Viral Encephalitis*	*Viral Hemor Fever*	*Botulism*	*Ricin*	*T-2 Mycotoxins*	*Staph Enterotoxin B*
POSTMORTEM CARE																
Follow principles of standard precautions	X	X	X	X	X	X	X	X	X	X	X	X	X	X	X	X
Droplet precautions						X										
Airborne precautions									X							
Use of **N95** mask by **all** individuals entering the room									X							
Negative pressure									X							
Contact precautions									X			X				
Routine terminal cleaning of room with hospital-approved disinfectant upon autopsy/transport		X	X	X			X	X	X	X	X		X	X	X	X
Disinfect surfaces with bleach/water sol. (10% sol.)	X				X	X						X				

STANDARD PRECAUTIONS—Standard precautions prevent direct contact with all body fluids (including blood), secretions, excretions, nonintact skin (including rashes), and mucous membranes. Standard precautions routinely practiced by health care providers include hand hygiene, gloves when contact with above, mask/eye protection/face shield while performing procedures that cause splash/spray, and gowns to protect skin and clothing during procedures.

SIGNS AND SYMPTOMS																
Cardiovascular																
Chest pain	X			X			X	X							X	X
Cyanosis						X										
Edema												X				
Hypotension												X				
Respiratory																
Cough	X						X	X						X	X	X
Dyspnea	X					X							X		X	
Pulmonary edema														X		
Shortness of breath														X		X
Stridor	X					X										
Musculoskeletal																
Arthralgia/myalgia		X	X	X				X		X		X		X	X	X
Backache									X							
Cervical adenopathy				X		X										
Paralysis													X			
Rigors				X					X	X						
Weakness		X	X									X	X	X	X	
Hemodynamic																
Bleeding												X		X		
Chills		X				X	X									X
Diaphoresis	X															
Fatigue	X	X														

Continued

TABLE 24-1 Bioterrorism Quick Reference Guide—cont'd

	BACTERIAL AGENTS								VIRUSES				BIOLOGICAL TOXINS			
	Anthrax	*Brucellosis*	*Cholera*	*Glanders (rarely seen)*	*Bubonic Plague*	*Pneumonic Plague*	*Tularemia*	*Q Fever*	*Smallpox*	*Venez Equine Encephalitis*	*Viral Encephalitis*	*Viral Hemor Fever*	*Botulism*	*Ricin*	*T-2 Mycotoxins*	*Staph Enterotoxin B*
Fever	X	X		X	X	X	X	X	X	X		X		X		X
Hemoptysis						X									X	
Septicemia					X	X	X									
Shock												X			X	X
Sweating		X		X												
Toxemia						X										
Dermatologic																
Petechiae												X				
Flushed face and chest												X			X	
Rash (macular/papular eruptions)	X			X					X							
Skin pain, pruritus, redness, necrosis														X	X	
Gastrointestinal																
Diarrhea	X		X					X		X		X		X	X	X
Intestinal cramping	X		X					X				X				
Weight loss							X	X								

Nausea leading to vomiting			X						X	X		X		X	X	X
Neurologic																
Ataxia															X	
Depression and mental status changes		X						X								
Dizziness													X			
Headache		X	X	X		X	X	X	X	X		X				X
Other Miscellaneous																
Lymph node tenderness					X	X										
Malaise	X				X		X		X	X		X				
Nasal discharge															X	
Photophobia										X						
Ptosis													X			
Splenomegaly				X												
Sore throat						X				X					X	
Red eyes												X				
Death Occurs in																
24–36 hours	X													X		
Fatal without treatment			X	X											X	
INCUBATION																
< 1 day							X		X	X				X	X	X
2–3 days			X			X							X			
1–6 days	X									X						

Continued

TABLE 24-1 Bioterrorism Quick Reference Guide—cont'd

	BACTERIAL AGENTS								VIRUSES				BIOLOGICAL TOXINS			
	Anthrax	*Brucellosis*	*Cholera*	*Glanders (rarely seen)*	*Bubonic Plague*	*Pneumonic Plague*	*Tularemia*	*Q Fever*	*Smallpox*	*Venez Equine Encephalitis*	*Viral Encephalitis*	*Viral Hemor Fever*	*Botulism*	*Ricin*	*T-2 Mycotoxins*	*Staph Enterotoxin B*
2–10 days					X		X									
2–21 days												X				
7–14 days				X				X	X							
1–2 months		X														
TREATMENT OPTIONS																
Medications																
Bactrim		X		X												
Carbapenem					X											
Ceftazidime				X												
Ciprofloxacin	X		X	X	X	X	X									
Doxycycline	X	X	X	X	X	X	X	X								
Erythromycin			X													

Gentamicin		X		X	X	X	X									
Ofloxacin		X														
Penicillin	X															
Ribavirin												X				
Rifampin		X		X												
Streptomycin		X			X	X	X									
Tetracycline			X		X	X	X	X								
Vaccine available	X		X		X	X	X	X	X	X		X	X			
Fluid replacement management			X													X
Supportive care										X		X	X	X		X
Tracheostomy													X			

Hemor, Hemorrhagic; *RMW*, regulated medical waste; *sol*, solution; *Staph*, Staphlococcal; Venez, Venezuelan.

* Use N-95 or greater mask when aerosol-producing procedures are performed.

From Thomas Winthrop, Walter Reed Army Medical Center: *Infection control user manual,* revised 2005, Infection Control Service.

Organization (WHO) estimated that 50 kg of aerosolized anthrax dispersed in ideal conditions over a city of 500,000 people would kill nearly half (Perry, 2006). Although anthrax is difficult to treat, transmission of anthrax is easily preventable with standard precautions. Person-to-person transmission is unlikely, although direct contact with draining skin lesions caused by cutaneous anthrax may result in infection (APIC, 2005). Early recognition and treatment with antibiotics is imperative for survival (Rothrock, 2007). Environmental cleaning following a procedure on a patient with anthrax should be conducted with a sporicidal agent.

Smallpox is caused by the variola major virus (Rothrock, 2007). Smallpox is a highly communicable disease transmitted by inhalation of droplets and aerosols, as well as direct and indirect contact (Rothrock, 2007). Patients are considered infectious beginning the day the first lesions appear and remain infectious until all scabs have fallen off (APIC, 2005). Recommendations for care of the surgical patient with smallpox include the following: (1) all staff should use an N95 mask; (2) all nonessential equipment and supplies should be removed from the OR; (3) institute strict airborne and contact precautions; (4) the room is restricted to minimal, essential personnel only; (5) all waste, PPE, and unopened supplies are considered regulated medical waste; and (6) instrumentation should be marked "smallpox" to communicate to the SPD staff that the instrumentation is contaminated with smallpox contagions (Rothrock, 2007).

Plague is caused by the bacterium *Y. pestis*, a gram-negative coccobacillus (Perry, 2006). The three forms of plague are bubonic, septicemic, and pneumonic (APIC, 2005). Bubonic and septicemic plagues are transmitted by the bites of infected fleas (Perry, 2006). Pneumonic plague occurs after direct inhalation of aerosolized organism, often in the form of droplets or as a biological weapon (Perry, 2006). Bubonic and septicemic plagues require only standard precautions (APIC, 2005). Pneumonic plague requires isolation and droplet precautions (APIC, 2005). Standard environmental cleaning is appropriate with no special procedures required (APIC, 2005).

Tularemia is a zoonotic disease caused by the small aerobic, gram-negative coccobacillus *F. tularensis* bacterium (APIC, 2005). Tularemia is highly communicable from rabbits, hares, muskrats, their ticks, flies, and mosquitoes, but human-to-human transmission is rare (Otaiza and Pessoa Da Silva, 2008). Infection can also occur with exposure to contaminated water, soil, or vegetation (Rothrock, 2007). Tularemia requires standard precautions and no special environmental cleaning.

Emerging infections that are currently having an effect on the OR and will most likely continue to have an effect in the future are the coronaviruses, influenza virus, and prion-based diseases such as Creutzfeldt–Jakob disease (CJD).

The coronavirus is associated with SARS. Surgery for a patient with SARS should be postponed until the patient is not considered to be infectious. However, patient condition may prohibit postponing surgery (AORN, 2009). If the patient requires an urgent surgical intervention, the procedure should be scheduled at the end of the day or at a time that best minimizes other patient and staff exposure (AORN, 2009). The patient is transported directly to the OR, bypassing the holding area (OSHA, 2007). Implementation of contact and airborne precautions is imperative. Environmental services personnel should also understand and comply with the indicated transmission-based precautions during the OR terminal cleaning.

The influenza virus is spread primarily through large-droplet transmission; therefore implementation of droplet precautions and contact precautions with added eye protection is appropriate (AORN, 2009). When patients with confirmed or suspected influenza are transported, they should wear a mask or cover their coughs and sneezes with tissues. Surgery for a patient with influenza would be limited to the very rare emergency.

CJD is a neurologically degenerative disease caused by a group of protein particles called prions (APIC, 2005). CJD and other diseases such as kuru and Gerstmann-Sträussler-Scheinker (GSS) syndrome are categorized as transmissible spongiform encephalopathies (TSEs) (APIC, 2005). The risk for transmission of TSEs is associated with direct contact with infectious tissues. Highly infectious tissues include brain, dura mater, spinal cord, and eyes (APIC, 2005). Lower-risk tissues include cerebral spinal fluid, liver, lymph nodes, kidney, tonsil, and spleen (APIC, 2005). Current diagnostic tests must include a sample of brain tissue to confirm CJD; therefore proper precautions must be taken to minimize exposure to infectious tissue during the procedure to harvest diagnostic tissue (APIC, 2005). Current postexposure protocols (PEPs) for a needlestick injury from a patient with confirmed or suspected TSE include gently bleeding the site; gently washing the site, avoiding scrubbing, with warm soapy water; drying; and covering with dressing (British Department of Health, 2007). The WHO (1999) PEP recommends for maximum safety exposing the injury for 1 minute to a 1:10 dilution of bleach solution. Immediate PEP for an eye exposure includes a copious flush with normal saline or tap water (WHO, 1999).

STERILIZATION AND QUALITY ASSURANCE

Increased emphasis on quality assurance and process improvement initiatives is imperative to maintaining a high-quality work environment. The importance of developing and maintaining a continuous quality improvement culture within the SPD is a crucial part of patient and staff safety. The mantra "If it's not clean, it's not sterile" should be part of the vernacular of not only SPD staff, but all health care workers. Whether it is a surgical instrument or a wheelchair that is being cleaned, it should be cleaned of soil before being sterilized or disinfected (Freeman et al, 2009). When cleaning and disinfecting surgical instruments, how does a staff member know if and when the instruments are free of infectious agents and therefore rendered safe to handle? Quality assurance checks validate the effectiveness of cleaning and decontamination processes, ensuring the safety of patients and the staff.

The perioperative nurse's role as a patient advocate includes ensuring that the instruments used to perform surgery are indeed clean and therefore sterile. There is a level of trust between the perioperative staff members and their SPD colleagues, because the perioperative nurse obviously cannot perform all required processes and quality assurance tests for every instrument set used in surgery. The expectation is that the processes required to return the sterile instrument set to the OR for surgery were refined and conducted using the highest standard of care. The highest standard of care includes quality assurance testing and repeat demonstrations of positive process performances. Although the expectation is that the instrument set is sterile, it does not release the perioperative nursing staff from ensuring that all instruments are clean and functioning properly. Any sterile instruments with blood or bioburden are not acceptable and should be immediately removed from the surgical field. As a patient advocate, the perioperative staff member is responsible for removing the set and getting a clean and sterile replacement. The SPD staff must be notified so that a prompt review of the cleaning and decontamination processes and procedures can be conducted. If a set is found to be contaminated after or during use, an incident report should be provided to the IPC service, as well as hospital risk management.

It is important (1) to define the entire cleaning and decontamination process, (2) to discuss validation and verification of the cleaning and decontamination processes, mitigating the risk for inadequately decontaminated instruments, and (3) to discuss proper PPE to be used during cleaning and decontamination.

In reference to instruments that will be further processed for sterilization, the definition of cleaning is the removal of all visible and nonvisible soil and any foreign material from any medical devices being processed (Bird et al, 2007). The definition of decontamination is the use of physical or chemical means to remove, inactivate, or destroy all pathogenic organisms on a surface or item to the point where they are no longer capable of transmitting infectious particles and the surface or item is rendered safe for handling, use, or disposal (Association for the Advancement of Medical Instrumentation [AAMI], 2006). Cleaning and decontamination may be manual or mechanical depending on the type of surgical instruments and the manufacturer's written instructions for processing the instrument for sterilization (AAMI, 2006). Again, sterilization of any instrument cannot take place without effective cleaning and decontamination.

Devices that are commonly cleaned manually are microsurgical instruments, lensed or fiberoptic instruments, flexible endoscopes, and air-powered drills (AAMI, 2006). Manual cleaning and decontamination that is completed following a step-by-step validated procedure is an effective, cost-efficient method of cleaning and decontaminating surgical instruments.

Mechanical or automated cleaning methods include the following: ultrasonic, washer-sanitizers, washer-pasteurizers, washer-decontaminators, transesophageal echocardiogram probe cleaners, automatic endoscopic reprocessors, and washer-sterilizers. Mechanical or automated cleaning is beneficial because of the validated, consistent performance devoid of individual performance variation (AAMI, 2006).

Ideally the process of cleaning and decontamination begins at the point of use. Sterile water should be used to wipe down the instruments throughout the surgical procedure, preventing the drying and coagulating of blood and other bioburden on the instruments. The use of saline for point-of-use cleaning should not be encouraged because of the corrosive effect it has on the instrument finish. Removing gross contamination immediately at the point of use minimizes bioburden, the formation of biofilms, and adherence of blood and proteinaceous materials to the instrument surfaces. To ensure staff safety, contaminated surgical instruments should be checked and double-checked to ensure that no disposable sharps are present and that reprocessable sharps are segregated and contained. Before leaving the OR the contaminated instruments should be moistened either by spraying or soaking with an enzymatic detergent or water (Bird et al, 2007). This prevents any further coagulation of blood or bioburden remaining on the instruments.

Transportation of the contaminated instruments to the SPD requires precautions to prevent transmission of infectious disease to patients or staff. Instruments should be contained either in a completely enclosed case cart or, if an enclosed case cart is not used, in a leakproof bin for transport (Bird et al, 2007). Transportation carts and equipment used to transport contaminated surgical instruments to the SPD should be clearly marked as biohazardous (Bird et al, 2007). For example, a traditional, enclosable metal case cart can be marked with a magnetic biohazard sign. Leakproof, sealable containers can be purchased with the biohazard warning present on the container (Bird et al, 2007). Special care and caution must be used if transport from the OR to the SPD requires passage through patient-accessible corridors. A cart carrying contaminated instruments always yields the right of way to patients and patient transports.

When the cart reaches the receiving, cleaning, and decontamination area of the SPD, the cleaning and decontamination process continues with a manual cleaning and decontamination of the instruments. During this process it is of the utmost importance to use proper PPE, which includes a face mask and shield, gloves, and a gown or apron. Cleaning and decontamination of the instruments is then conducted according to the manufacturer's validated guidelines.

A manual cleaning and decontamination typically is conducted by wiping, brushing, and flushing and using mechanical aids such as water, detergents, and enzymes to remove foreign debris (Bird et al, 2007). Ideally a three-sink method is used to manually clean and decontaminate. The first sink consists of water and detergent solution, the second sink is plain tap water, and the third sink is distilled water to help prevent spotting and to prevent the redeposit of minerals, microbes, and pyrogens (Bird et al, 2007). The final rinse in the cleaning and decontamination process should be with distilled water. All brushes and other cleaning implements used for manual cleaning and decontamination should be disinfected and sterilized daily (AAMI, 2006).

The cleaning and decontamination process can continue further with mechanical decontamination or be completed with manual decontamination depending on the instrument manufacturer's validated instructions and the SPD policy. The instruments will ideally be processed further through a mechanical process such as a quality assurance–tested ultrasonic cleaner or an automated washer.

Following the cleaning and decontamination processes the instruments should be inspected for visible soil. Failure to effectively clean and decontaminate instruments will result in the ineffective penetration of the sterilant (AAMI, 2006). A magnification device or a chemical blood indicator can be used to verify effective cleaning and decontamination. Once the instruments are inspected, they are allowed to dry before proceeding to the preparation, assembly, and packing area.

Historically SPDs have focused primarily on validating the sterilization process, but not on the cleaning and decontamination processes. Each step in the decontamination process should be validated to ensure that the processes are both effective and efficient. Maximizing efforts to ensure that instruments are clean in turn maximizes the efforts to ensure sterility and therefore maximizes patient safety. Consequently, by ensuring that our cleaning and decontamination processes are effective, we maximize patient safety by ensuring sterile instruments, and we make them safer for our SPD staff during the preparation and packing processes.

Quality assurance testing and controls for cleaning and decontamination areas include water quality testing, ultrasonic testing to validate effective cavitation, artificial soil devices, temperature-monitoring devices, and blood and protein detection kits.

Water quality testing is important for many reasons. Water quality can influence and hinder the effectiveness of enzymatic and detergent cleaners. The ability to demonstrate an effective cleaning process begins with demonstrating water quality. Most enzymatic and detergent manufacturers recommend an optimal pH and hardness for their product (AAMI, 2006). Water testing as it relates to the SPD includes pH levels, hardness, temperature, and purity (Bird et al, 2007). The pH level is a measure of alkalinity or acidity (Bird et al, 2007). The pH level and hardness of water are important because they can influence the effectiveness of enzyme and detergent cleaners; at extreme pH and hardness levels cleaners can be completely inactivated or degraded (Bird et al, 2007).

Quality assurance testing and controls of the ultrasonic machine include ensuring that the machine is being operated and maintained according to the manufacturer's recommendations, as well as temperature and cavitation testing. An excellent way to ensure that any piece of equipment is operated properly is to include the operating instructions as part of the competency-based orientation. Another method is to have posters displayed at the machinery point of use to assist and provide a quick, easy reference for the SPD staff. An ultrasonic machine works by converting ultrahigh-frequency sound waves into mechanical vibrations, which create microscopic bubbles that attach to an instrument's surface and burst inward, or cavitate (AAMI, 2006). The cavitation of the bubbles attached to the instrument's surface results in a vacuum action that pulls soil and debris off the instrument (AAMI, 2006). Before the ultrasonic machine is used, a process called degassing must take place (Bird et al, 2007). Degassing removes excess air or gas in the fluid to maximize the ultrasonic energy that causes cavitations to occur (Bird et al, 2007). Degassing begins with the complete filling of the reservoir. The machine is then turned on for approximately 5 to 10 minutes to complete the degassing process (Bird et al, 2007). Various tests for effective cavitation processes are commercially available, or a homemade verification device may be adequate. One commercially available cavitation test changes color when sufficient ultrasonic energy or cavitations are occurring within the fluid in the test. Other simple tests for effective cavitation include the aluminum foil and glass slide tests (Cole-Parmer, n.d.).

Temperature checks of the ultrasonic fluid should also occur to ensure an ideal temperature range of 80° F (26.6° C) to 109° F (42.7° C) and no greater than 140° F (60° C) (Bird et al, 2007). Temperature checks are an important quality assurance check for the ultrasonic cleaner because temperatures greater than 140° F (60° C) can coagulate protein residue on the instruments, making it very difficult to remove (Bird et al, 2007). Ultrasonic fluid should be changed when visibly soiled or at least daily (AAMI, 2006). The ultrasonic chamber should be cleaned according to the manufacturer's instructions and between changing of the fluid.

Quality assurance testing and controls for mechanical decontamination processes generally include artificial soil devices, temperature monitoring devices, and blood and protein detection kits. Artificial soil devices are used to demonstrate the effectiveness of various washer-disinfectors (AAMI, 2006). Some manufacturers' products mimic human blood coagulation on an instrument's surface and also provide a penetration challenge that mimics hinges and other difficult-to-reach areas for the washer-disinfector. Although these tests are a great indicator of the washer-decontaminator performance and effectiveness, further evidence of and redundancy in the processes' effectiveness is good. Spot checks with blood and protein detection kits should also be conducted at scheduled intervals to further validate the washer-decontaminator processes. Temperature-monitoring devices are also a critical quality assurance test for the washer-decontaminator. Verification of cycle-dependent and temperature-sensitive enzymatics and disinfectants is imperative for an effective washer-decontaminator quality assurance test.

Detailed record keeping and incorporating these quality assurance tests and controls for cleaning and decontamination into a continuous quality improvement program are ideal. The maintenance of cleaning and decontamination records and results should be as important as maintaining the records and results of sterilizer quality assurance tests. Quality assurance results should be shared with IPC professionals and patient safety representatives from your facility.

STAFF TRAINING

Fostering the relationship between housekeeping staff and the OR, SPD, and IPC leadership is essential to an effective infection prevention plan. Negotiate with housekeeping management to ensure continuity of housekeeping staff working in the OR and SPD areas, which will allow adequate time for appropriate initial training. Collaborate with the OR, the SPD, the IPC service, and housekeeping management to develop the initial training program for the housekeeping staff to ensure that expectations are met and that the best practices are being employed.

Develop and implement a competency-based orientation (CBO) for the OR and SPD housekeeping staff. Collaborate to develop the CBO with input from all the stakeholders, including the OR, the SPD, the IPC service, and housekeeping management and staff. During the initial orientation brief of OR and SPD housekeeping staff, extensively review the CBO and answer any questions even before the orientation process begins. Provide copies of the CBO to the housekeeping staff to minimize surprise expectations during the formal orientation process. In addition, if the housekeeping staff members feel they need some further training on a specific section of the CBO, they can ask their supervisor for that training.

Initial briefings and CBO completions will start the housekeeping staff on the right foot; however, to ensure their continued success and the quality of their services, they must have a continuing education program. The IPC service is instrumental in ensuring an effective continued education program. Some examples and essential components of a continuing education program include infection prevention principles, terminal cleaning techniques following transmission-based precautions, hand hygiene techniques, cleaning product efficacy and application review, a review of facility environmental cleaning policies, and disposal of regulated medical waste.

Finally, recognizing the housekeeping staff for their part in preventing infection for both our patients and staff members is essential to maintaining a top-quality housekeeping staff. Recognition comes in many forms, but it could be as simple as a certificate of appreciation or nomination for employee of the month for a job well done. Acknowledging their commitment and effort, and that they are members of the team will increase retention of good housekeeping staff; in addition, the other housekeepers will become aware that the OR and SPD are desirable places to work.

MAINTAINING A SAFE, CLEAN WORK ENVIRONMENT

Following proper environmental parameters and proper cleaning procedures in the OR and the SPD is one of the most effective ways to minimize exposure to infectious disease. Maintaining these parameters is complex and takes the coordinated efforts of many professionals, including OR and SPD staff, facility and HVAC personnel, industrial hygiene personnel, and environmental services/housekeeping staff. Recommended air handling, humidity, and temperatures in the OR and SPD are environmental considerations that minimize conditions favorable for microbial growth (Sehulster et al, 2004). These parameters should be monitored daily and recorded as a quality assurance control.

Ensuring that proper environmental cleaning procedures are followed is also very challenging. This is accomplished with the assistance of quality personnel, effective training programs, and effective supervision. Fundamental to correctly implementing these procedures is a thorough orientation process with a competency-based orientation for environmental services staff. Maintaining a clean OR and SPD environment protects our patients and staff members.

Occupational Screening and Exposure Prevention

The infection prevention and control aspect of an occupational health screening of employees includes preemployment medical evaluations, education regarding facility infection prevention and control policies and practices, and immunization policies and procedures (APIC, 2005).

Preemployment and periodic medical evaluations and screenings ensure that a worker will not pose a risk for infection to patients or other staff members (APIC, 2005). Incorporated into the screenings are opportunities for educating and reviewing with staff the topics of bloodborne pathogens, proper use of personal protective equipment, and safety practices and procedures for reporting occupational exposures and communicable diseases (Friedman and Petersen, 2004).

Medical evaluations and screenings also determine the staff member's occupational risk and subsequent need for additional protective devices such as a respirator (Friedman and Petersen, 2004). Occupational health policies should be explicit and address personnel with infections and nonintact skin in the workplace (AORN, 2009). Personnel should refrain from working in the OR, SPD, or other high-risk environments until such infections or healing of nonintact skin is resolved (AORN, 2009).

During the occupational health screening process appropriate immunizations such as the hepatitis B vaccine; measles, mumps, rubella (MMR) live vaccine; influenza vaccine; and the varicella zoster live vaccine should be provided or offered (Friedman and Petersen, 2004). All staff members working in the OR and SPD work areas must receive the hepatitis B vaccination (OSHA, 2007). The vaccination is a requirement unless medically contraindicated (AORN, 2009). The hepatitis B virus can remain infectious for a week or longer on environmental surfaces (AORN, 2009). Mandatory hepatitis B vaccination has been an overwhelming success in health care workers, with occurrence of hepatitis B declining by 93% from 12,000 cases in 1985 to 800 cases a decade later (Friedman and Petersen, 2004).

A culture of prevention is superior to a culture of treatment. Engineered safety devices designed to mitigate risk on the surgical field are mandated by OSHA but now seem so practical as to be common sense. Common medically engineered safety devices such as hypodermic needles, intravenous catheters, and scalpels have been refined to greatly enhance function compared with when they were first introduced. Sharps with engineered controls must be used when deemed acceptable (AORN, 2009). There are still bastions of resistance to these engineered medical safety devices within the surgical community, but they are fading and the devices are slowly becoming ubiquitous within the operative settings.

Unfortunately, even with engineered controls on many of the sharps used in the OR, injuries continue to occur (Berguer and Heller, 2005). Given this fact, it is imperative for staff members to understand the policies and procedures following a sharps injury. Techniques such as using a neutral zone or hands-free technique for passing sharps can have a major effect on these injuries (AORN, 2009).

CONCLUSION

This chapter provides some insight into a wide variety of topics related to infectious disease exposure in the OR, SPD, and IPC nursing practices. Through teamwork, collaboration, and recognition in these specialty nursing areas the development of effective and innovative approaches to preventing infectious disease exposure will greatly benefit the nursing profession. We have touched briefly on the evolution and development of infectious disease prevention and control and discussed the infectious disease process and mitigating strategies. Future challenges for the IPC, OR, and SPD areas include MDROs, emerging diseases, and bioterrorism agents. Initiatives that can improve the quality of service the OR, SPD, and IPC areas provide include SPD decontamination quality assurance initiatives, fostering the development of environmental cleaning services, and occupational health screening and preventive services.

REFERENCES

Association for Professionals in Infection Control and Epidemiology: *Text of infection control and epidemiology, vols I-II, Essential elements*, Washington, DC, 2005, The Association.

Association for the Advancement of Medical Instrumentation: *Comprehensive guide to steam sterilization and sterility assurance in health care facilities*, publication no. ST 79 Annapolis Junction, Md, 2006, The Association.

Association of periOperative Registered Nurses: *Perioperative standards and recommended practices*, Denver, 2009, The Association.

Bellis M: *Louis Pasteur Dec. 27, 1822-Sept. 28, 1895*, 2009, available at http://inventors.about.com/library/inventors/blpasteur.htm. Accessed April 26, 2009.

Berguer R, Heller PJ: Strategies for preventing sharps injuries in the operating room, *Surg Clin North Am* 85:1299–1305, 2005.

Bird TB, et al: In Lind N, Ninemeier JD, editors: *International Association of Healthcare Central Service Material Management: Central services technical manual*, ed 7, Chicago, 2007, The Association.

British Department of Health, Advisory Committee on Dangerous Pathogens, TSE working group, Transmissible Spongiform Encephalopathy Agents: *Safe working and the prevention of infection—infection control of CJD and related disorders in the healthcare setting*, 2007, available from http://www.advisorybodies.doh.gov.uk/acdp/tseguidance/tseguidancepart4-30mar07.pdf. Accessed May 13, 2009.

Centers for Disease Control and Prevention: Guidelines for preventing the transmission of *Mycobacterium tuberculosis* in health-care settings, *MMWR* 54(RR-17):1–121, 2005.

Centers for Disease Control and Prevention, National Surveillance System for Health Care Workers: *Workbook for designing, implementing, and evaluating a sharps injury prevention program*, 2008, available at http://www.cdc.gov/sharpssafety/pdf/sharpsworkbook_2008.pdf. Accessed May 17, 2009.

Cole-Parmer Technical Library: *Ultrasonic cleaner frequently asked questions*. n.d. http://www.coleparmer.com/techinfo/techinfo.asp?htmlfile=ultrasoniccleaner_faq.htm Accessed May 14, 2009.

Freeman SS, et al: An evidence-based process for evaluating infection control policies, *AORN J* 89:489–507, 2009.

Friedman C, Petersen KH: *Infection control in ambulatory care*, Sudbury, Mass, 2004, Jones & Bartlett.

Gruendeman BJ, Mangum SS: *Infection prevention in surgical settings*, Philadelphia, 2001, Saunders.

Miller JT, et al: *History of infection control and its contributions to the development and success of brain tumor operations*, Augusta, Ga, 2005, Department of Neurosurgery, Medical College of Georgia, available at http://www.medscape.com/viewarticle/503947. Accessed April 26, 2009.

Occupational Safety and Health Administration: *Pandemic influenza preparedness and response guidance for healthcare workers and healthcare employers*, Washington, DC, 2007, U.S. Department of Labor.

Occupational Safety and Health Administration: *Bloodborne pathogens*, Standard number 1910.1030, 2008, available at http://www.osha.gov/pls/oshaweb/owadisp.show_document?p_table=STANDARDS&p_id=10051. Accessed September 6, 2009.

Otaiza F, Pessoa Da Silva C: Infection prevention and control. In Heymann DL, editor: *Control of communicable diseases manual*, ed 19, Washington, DC, 2008, American Public Health Association.

Perry WB: Biological weapons: an introduction for surgeons, *Surg Clin North Am* 86:649–663, 2006.

Phillips NF: *Berry and Kohn's operating room technique*, ed 10, St. Louis, 2004, Mosby.

Rothrock JC: *Alexander's care of the patient in surgery*, ed 13, St. Louis, 2007, Mosby.

Sehulster LM, et al: *Guidelines for environmental infection control in healthcare facilities, recommendations from CDC and the Healthcare Infection Control Practices Advisory Committee*, Chicago, 2004, American Society for Healthcare Engineering/American Hospital Association, available at http://www.cdc.gov/ncidod/dhqp/pdf/guidelines/Enviro_guide_03.pdf. Accessed August 29, 2009.

Siegel JD, et al: *Management of multidrug-resistant organisms in healthcare settings*, 2006, Centers for Disease Control and Prevention, available at http://www.cdc.gov/ncidod/dhqp/pdf/ar/mdroguideline2006.pdf. Accessed August 29, 2009.

Siegel JD, et al: *Guideline for isolation precautions: preventing transmission of infectious agents in healthcare settings*, 2007, Centers for Disease Control and Prevention, available at http://www.cdc.gov/ncidod/dhqp/pdf/guidelines/Isolation2007.pdf. Accessed August 29, 2009.

Simor AE, et al: Randomized controlled trial of chlorhexidine gluconate for washing, intranasal mupirocin, and rifampin and doxycycline versus no treatment for the eradication of methicillin-resistant *Staphylococcus aureus* colonization, *Clin Infect Dis* 44:178–185, 2007.

The Joint Commission: *Standards for ambulatory care*, Oakbrook Terrace, Ill, 2009, Joint Commission Resources.

World Health Organization: *Communicable disease surveillance and control, infection control guidelines for transmissible spongiform encephalopathies*, 1999, available from http://www.who.int/entity/csr/resources/publications/bse/whocdscsraph2003.pdf. Accessed May 13, 2009.

DEALING WITH DISRUPTIVE BEHAVIOR IN THE PERIOPERATIVE SETTING

Beverly A. Kirchner, BSN, RN, CNOR, CASC

DEFINING DISRUPTIVE BEHAVIOR

Any action that causes one to feel less than safe is known as disruptive behavior. There are four types of disruptive behavior seen in the workplace. The most common type of disruptive behavior is verbal. Christmas (2007) defined verbal abuse as communication delivered via a behavior, tone, or words that were meant to make an individual feel attacked or humiliated. The words delivered are meant to demean, isolate, belittle, threaten, or accuse a person of an action that is not founded in truth or facts. Psychologic abuse involves aggressive behavior that overtaxes a person's ability to cope. A bully is one who uses psychologically abusive behavior to control the victim. Bullying is a purposeful exertion of power or intimidation that is physically or emotionally threatening to the victim (Kolanko et al, 2006). In the workforce we are able to identify two types of bullying. Direct bullying includes overt acts of verbal or physical aggression. Indirect bullying involves the use of passive-aggressive behavior or social isolation to intimidate the target. Physical abuse inflicts harm intentionally on another individual. Sexual abuse is accomplished when a person is forced into physical contact that has the sole purpose of humiliating the victim. Disruptive behavior can cross lines of authority and job hierarchy. An example of crossing lines of authority is when a surgeon bullies a certified registered nurse anesthetist (CRNA) and the anesthesiologist gets involved and retaliation occurs (Figure 25-1). The cycle of disruptive behavior is born and will spread quickly throughout the department if not stopped (Figure 25-2). Defining disruptive behavior is the first step toward stopping the behavior in the workplace. The following examples provide insight into what a nurse may experience as a direct result of disruptive behavior and bullying:

- I changed my perception of the entire institution where it happened as a result of the incident.
- I considered the incident to be a major factor in deciding whether or not to leave the institution and work somewhere else entirely.
- My supervisors were unsupportive of me during or after the incident.
- I felt as though I had to give in to the attacker's demands to avoid disciplinary action from my supervisors.
- I felt as though my professional decisions were being monitored and being called into question after the incident.
- I felt others made subtle "behind the back" negative comments about the incident after it occurred.
- I felt management made me give in and compromise to maintain my status as a satisfactory employee.
- I believe patient care was affected by the incident in a way that could have resulted, or actually did result, in an error or a compromise of patient safety.

Bullying Origins

According to Namie and Namie (2003) 81% of the bullies in the workplace are managers. This is a frightening number in our workplace that can destroy a culture of safety. Every nurse must ask, "What can we do in our workplace to eliminate the bully?" First we have to understand the person and the motivation that causes an individual to define his or her worth by destroying someone else. Where do we first see a bully? The answer is easy; we were first introduced to the bully in school. We noticed the behavior on the playground and in the lunchroom more than in the classroom. Women are far more likely to be bullies than men. The reason is that girls are presumably more likely to get away with passive-aggressive behavior, social isolation of others, and gossip. Young boys tend to

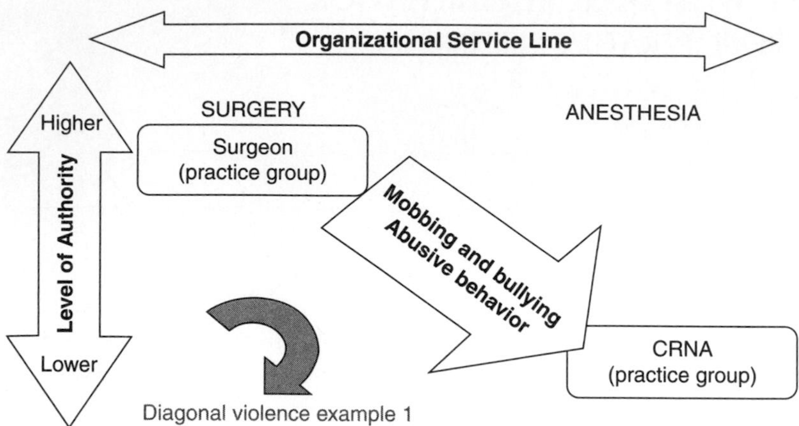

FIGURE 25-1 Disruptive behavior crossing lines of authority between surgery and anesthesia. (From Beverly Kirchner, RN, BSN, CNOR, CASC; Jeanie Zelanko, RN, BSN, MSN, PhD; Richard Gilder, RN, BSN, MS.)

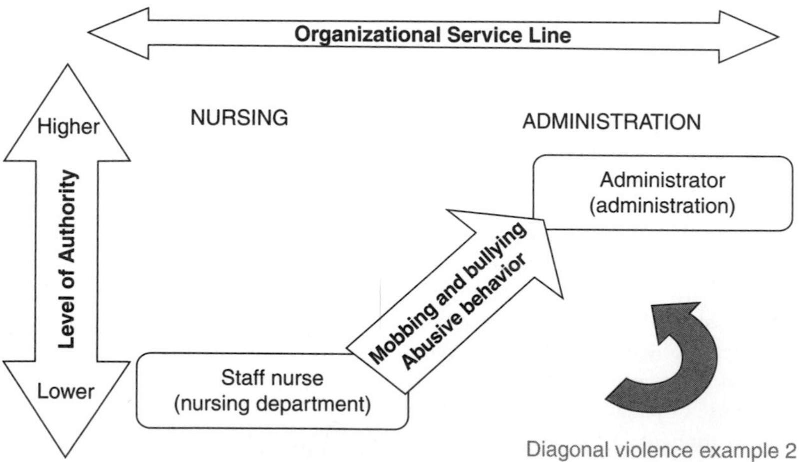

FIGURE 25-2 Disruptive behavior crossing lines of authority between nursing and administration. (From Beverly Kirchner, RN, BSN, CNOR, CASC; Jeanie Zelanko, RN, BSN, MSN, PhD; Richard Gilder, RN, BSN, MS.)

be overt and aggressive in behavior when angry or wanting to control a situation. In contrast, young girls resort to note passing, gossip, and avoidance to isolate another girl who was targeted by the bully. Boys—being overt—get into trouble, whereas girls—passing notes and being passive-aggressive—are not disciplined as often and thus the behavior becomes acceptable.

Bullies in the Workplace

In our workplace we now see this person as an individual who puts self above anyone else to control another human being. The bully seeks to control the targeted victim through the use of humiliation and the withholding of information and resources. If the workplace bully is left unchecked, the results can be an environment that is hostile, and everyone will suffer. An ignored workplace bully can put the whole organization at risk for employee trauma and/or possible litigation. Bullies at work are malicious individuals that can be considered to be endangering the health of the bully's intended victim. The bully will repeat the behavior of attacking an individual over and over again. The bully's target will often eventually leave the organization.

BOX 25-1 Survey Questions to Assess Effects of Bullying

EXAMPLES OF OPEN-ENDED QUESTIONS

1. During the last 6 months of working here, have you changed your perception of this entire institution because of bullying or mobbing (fellow employees and/or supervisors "ganging up" on you)?
2. Do you consider the mobbing-bullying incident you just described above to be a major factor in deciding whether or not to leave the institution and work somewhere else entirely?
   If yes to this question, please describe, in your opinion, the factors that changed your mind about staying here and trying to make things work out.
3. If you answered yes to any of the previous questions, in your opinion, were your supervisors unsupportive of you during or after the mobbing or bullying incident?
   If yes to this question, please describe the details (who, what, when, where, how, and why), in your opinion, about your supervisors being unsupportive of you during or after the bullying or mobbing took place.
4. During the last 6 months of working here, have you ever felt as though you had to give in to the demands made upon you by those doing the mobbing or bullying to avoid disciplinary action from your supervisors?
   If you answered yes to this question, please describe the details (who, what, when, where, how, and why), in your opinion, about being subjected to the "sham peer review" as an aspect of being bullied or mobbed.

The bully will seek another victim after the target has left the organization. Bullies cannot survive without victims, and victims want nothing to do with bullies. A bully has low self-esteem and uses the target to feel better about his or her behavior. Workplace bullies usually have a lifelong history of disrespecting the needs of others. Namie and Namie (2003) claim that bullies are inadequate, defective, and poorly developed people that destroy others' self-esteem to feel good about themselves.

Targets are the bully's victims. Targets are vulnerable people who often make self-effacing statements, are private, and use several forms of self-denial for protection. In other words, some targets feel after a while that they deserve the abuse. The target makes statements like "If only I had …" Targets perceive themselves as victims. Targets find it hard to work with bullies. The target is brought into the relationship involuntarily, whereas the bully controls when to attack, when to hold back, and whom to perform in front of for the best results. The bully's goal is to control the target completely. Weapons that the bully uses may vary from gossip to sabotage. Targets do suffer emotional damage at the hands of a bully. Targets often have problems with sleep and become fatigued. The fatigued health care worker/victim then places the patient at risk, because fatigue has been identified as one of the leading causes of medical errors in health care. When targets are being intimidated by the bully, they will not speak up, thus leaving the most vulnerable person in the perioperative environment—the patient—at risk. Targets are not the only ones who suffer in this type of work environment. The other staff members will suffer if they witness the behavior. The more the behavior is repeated, the greater the damage the work environment will suffer.

CORE ISSUES OF DISRUPTIVE BEHAVIOR

Survey Preparation and Distribution

Every health care facility has to examine the work environment to identify the core issues. The first step toward identifying core issues is to prepare and distribute surveys to physicians and employees (Box 25-1). The survey needs to be designed to explore specific concerns regarding the work environment. Successful data collection depends on ensuring the respondents' confidentiality. Several concerns that need to be addressed in the survey design include ensuring that the respondents cannot be identified by their description of specific events or handwriting. Using an outside company is one way of providing this guarantee. A facility may be able to work with the information technology department and devise a plan for respondents to answer and feel safe using internal resources. No matter how the plan is designed and implemented, a baseline must be obtained to determine the work environment's core issues according to the members who work in the environment.

Analyzing Responses

The second step in the process involves analysis of the responses received in the survey. It is important to analyze the data and identify key responses to questions, as well as examples of incidents the respondents describe. During the analysis phase the core issues will become apparent and guide the next steps: providing a safe work environment (Box 25-2).

Strategic Goals

Once the core issues have been identified, develop a strategy to address each issue. The strategy should be simple because the real goal is to develop tools to prevent disruptive behavior and to describe the behavior that is expected in the workplace. The strategic plan should address the risk factors for disruptive behavior found in the workplace environment. The first strategic goal should address the position the facility takes concerning a safe work environment. The second strategic goal should be the development of a "zero tolerance" policy. The third strategic goal should address communication in the workplace, including what, how, and to whom to communicate when the behavior displayed does not meet the core values of the work environment. The fourth strategic goal is to train leaders in how to assess and respond to an incident so there will be minimum negative effects of disruptive behavior on the work environment. The fifth strategic goal is to train the team in how to identify, report, and reduce disruptive behavior in the workplace. The sixth strategic goal is to assess the plan on a regular basis to ensure that the plan is meeting the objective of a safe work environment.

Developing a position statement or a "fit format" will address the first strategic goal. A position statement describes the behavior expected to be displayed in the workplace. A fit format describes the behavior employees are expected to display at work and how employees will be continuously evaluated on this behavior (Box 25-3). A sample fit format is seen in Figure 25-3.

BOX 25-2 Sample Core Issues

- Communication is inappropriate between service X and service Y. The staff in each service line is laying blame on the other team.
- Communication between anesthesiologist A and the nurses is abusive.
- Employees call in frequently when they are scheduled to work with B.
- Employees working in service Z are displaying symptoms of depression.
- The staff working in service W cannot locate a vital instrument when the charge nurse is off (potential sabotage).

BOX 25-3 Fit Format Process

1. All new employees will receive a fit format evaluation on the thirtieth day of employment.
2. The employee fits the organization if he or she scores 4.2 or greater. The employee may fit the organization if he or she scores 3.5 to 4.2. The employee will be put on probation for 30 days if his or her score is below 4.2. The supervisor will discuss with the employee in detail the action needed to fit the organization. If the employee's score is below 3.5, you must terminate his or her employment on the thirtieth day when completing the fit format review with the employee.
3. You will review the employee on probation exactly 30 days after the original evaluation. If the employee does not reach the goal of 4.2 or greater, the employee will be terminated at this time.
4. The fit format can be used at any time to discuss how an employee is fitting with the organization. An employee's behavior can change throughout his or her employment with the organization for many reasons. If the employee does not fit the behavior expected, use this tool to identify the problem and the expectation you have of the employee.

From Beverly Kirchner, RN, BSN, CNOR, CASC; Jeanie Zelanko, RN, BSN, MSN, PhD; Richard Gilder, RN, BSN, MS.

Developing a zero tolerance policy is the simple part of the strategic goal, whereas enforcing it is the tough part. A zero tolerance policy should contain the following elements: (1) definitions of acceptable behavior, (2) responsibilities of each team member, (3) how someone who reports poor behavior will be protected, (4) how an investigation will be conducted in the facility, and (5) consequences of the behavior. The zero tolerance procedure will outline in detail what

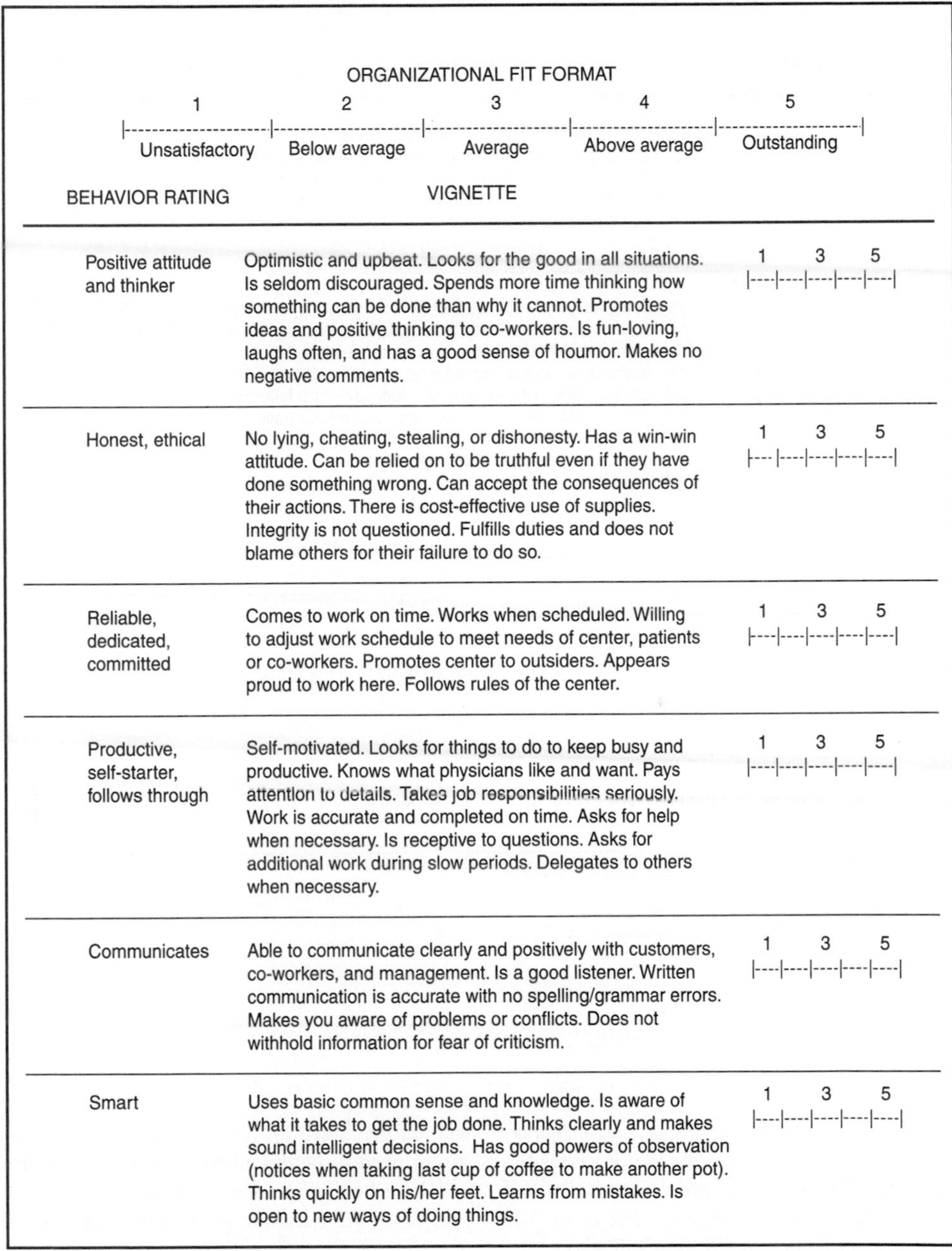

ORGANIZATIONAL FIT FORMAT

1	2	3	4	5
Unsatisfactory	Below average	Average	Above average	Outstanding

BEHAVIOR RATING	VIGNETTE	
Positive attitude and thinker	Optimistic and upbeat. Looks for the good in all situations. Is seldom discouraged. Spends more time thinking how something can be done than why it cannot. Promotes ideas and positive thinking to co-workers. Is fun-loving, laughs often, and has a good sense of houmor. Makes no negative comments.	1 3 5
Honest, ethical	No lying, cheating, stealing, or dishonesty. Has a win-win attitude. Can be relied on to be truthful even if they have done something wrong. Can accept the consequences of their actions. There is cost-effective use of supplies. Integrity is not questioned. Fulfills duties and does not blame others for their failure to do so.	1 3 5
Reliable, dedicated, committed	Comes to work on time. Works when scheduled. Willing to adjust work schedule to meet needs of center, patients or co-workers. Promotes center to outsiders. Appears proud to work here. Follows rules of the center.	1 3 5
Productive, self-starter, follows through	Self-motivated. Looks for things to do to keep busy and productive. Knows what physicians like and want. Pays attention to details. Takes job responsibilities seriously. Work is accurate and completed on time. Asks for help when necessary. Is receptive to questions. Asks for additional work during slow periods. Delegates to others when necessary.	1 3 5
Communicates	Able to communicate clearly and positively with customers, co-workers, and management. Is a good listener. Written communication is accurate with no spelling/grammar errors. Makes you aware of problems or conflicts. Does not withhold information for fear of criticism.	1 3 5
Smart	Uses basic common sense and knowledge. Is aware of what it takes to get the job done. Thinks clearly and makes sound intelligent decisions. Has good powers of observation (notices when taking last cup of coffee to make another pot). Thinks quickly on his/her feet. Learns from mistakes. Is open to new ways of doing things.	1 3 5

FIGURE 25-3 Sample fit format process tool. (From Beverly Kirchner, RN, BSN, CNOR, CASC; Jeanie Zelanko, RN, BSN, MSN, PhD; Richard Gilder, RN, BSN, MS.)

Continued

Organizational Fit Format Form, Page 2

1	2	3	4	5
Unsatisfactory	Below average	Average	Above average	Outstanding

BEHAVIOR RATING	VIGNETTE	
Team player, supportive	Knows that no one alone can win the game. Helpful and willing to assist others (including the other centers). Willing to learn other staff members' job responsibilities to be more helpful. Promotes center and teamwork. Willing to go the extra mile. Respectful, appreciative of what we have and how we got it. Demonstrates empathy and caring.	1 3 5 |----|----|----|----|----|
Professional	Always treats everyone with respect. Thinks before speaking and keeps private conversations to a minimum, especially in patient care areas. Treats everyone as a "customer"—patients, physicians, and co-workers. Sets and maintains high standards. Constantly evaluates successes and failures and identifies how to improve. Observes what others have done better and emulates them. Keeps up with the changes in health care. Seeks educational opportunities.	1 3 5 |----|----|----|----|----|

Comments: ______________________________

I understand what was reviewed with me today concerning my fit in the organization.

Signature ____________ Date ____________

I have reviewed with the employee how he/she fits in the organization.

Signature ____________ Date ____________

SCORE: ____________

RE-EVALUATE ____________

Figure 25-3—cont'd

a person should do to report disruptive behavior. The procedure will describe the processes the facility has put in place to protect the individual reporting the disruptive behavior. The procedure will also describe how the facility will resolve the reported disruptive behavior and the methods of communication to be used for both the victim and the abuser. The consequences that the facility will enforce based on the findings of the investigation need to be described in detail. The policy will describe the type of education the facility will provide to the team and how often the team will receive education on reporting and handling disruptive behavior.

The third strategic goal the facility needs to address involves describing appropriate communication within the workplace. To effectively eliminate disruptive behavior, the facility must teach the team how to communicate appropriately. Communication education should include how to appropriately communicate verbally, nonverbally, and in writing. E-mail and text messaging should also be addressed. Gossip needs to be addressed under communication. Gossip is a very destructive form of communication; because of this, every facility needs to address gossip as a separate issue. The facility needs to have an ongoing education schedule addressing communication. The Joint Commission (2007) has reported that the number one cause of a sentinel event is poor communication or lack of communication. If perioperative team members learn to communicate appropriately, this will eliminate a significant portion of disruptive behavior (Box 25-4).

Training leaders is the fourth strategic goal in eliminating disruptive behavior. Leaders need tools to prevent the disruptive behavior, to manage the problem quickly to reduce the severity of the results of the behavior on another individual or group of individuals, and to manage the results of a severe act of disruptive behavior. All levels of team members should take active roles and be responsible for eliminating disruptive behavior, but the ultimate responsibility belongs to the leaders of the facility. The facility should provide ongoing formal training for its leaders.

Training every member of the team in how to prevent disruptive behavior and how to report the act is the fifth strategic goal. Like leaders, team members should receive ongoing training that is reinforced frequently. Prevention is the proactive way to eliminate the results of disruptive behavior in the work environment.

WORK MODEL FOR DISRUPTIVE BEHAVIOR

Prevention of disruptive behavior is the primary goal of any facility. A facility must set goals that support the facility leader's ability to manage disruptive behavior. Facilities should look at disruptive behavior the way nurses look at patient care and use a process similar to the nursing process to prevent or manage the results of disruptive behavior. Then leaders will have a chance to prevent—and if not prevent then address—disruptive behavior quickly to minimize the damage. Leaders must define personnel guidelines for addressing disruptive behavior. The leadership team must be proactive in preventing disruptive behavior by identifying behaviors in team members that display potential for disruptive behavior. Addressing the behaviors before an incident occurs is essential in prevention. Leaders cannot prevent the behavior alone. All team members need to participate in the prevention of the disruptive behavior by identifying and eliminating behaviors that instigate and support the spread of disruptive behavior and by knowing and following the no tolerance policy.

Secondary prevention of disruptive behavior involves the treatment and management of the problem after it occurs. In secondary prevention the facility's plan for managing disruptive behavior is activated when the incident is reported. A critical incident debriefing should occur, following the protocols defined in the policy for debriefing. Once the incident debriefing is completed and the investigation has taken place, the facility must follow through with instigator discipline as outlined by the facility's policy. The team's role in secondary prevention is to be responsible and report incidents when they occur. The team needs to actively participate in the debriefing when appropriate. The debriefing should be kept confidential to protect the integrity of the environment and promote a safe environment for reporting incidents. The process for dealing with disruptive behavior should be completed as described in the no tolerance plan and policy.

When a facility has to invoke tertiary prevention, the incident is one that can leave devastating effects on a team member, members, or an innocent victim such as a patient. When a severe incident occurs, such as psychologic abuse that has devastated an individual or individuals, the leader must act quickly to limit the effects. The leader will need to provide personnel necessary to support the victims, which may include the following: psychologist, nurse practitioner trained in dealing with victims of abuse, psychiatrist, social worker, clergy, attorney, human resource representative, and potentially law enforcement. These personnel not only help the victim, but also assess the need to reform the perpetrator's coping skills. The facility should have tertiary prevention goals that include required participation in education programs that address disruptive behavior, providing an environment that encourages reporting of ongoing stress

BOX 25-4 Sample Code of Conduct

PURPOSE: To define the expected behavior of all employees in the facility.

POLICY STATEMENT

A. Ethical Conduct

Each employee has an obligation to act in an ethical manner in dealings with Facility, with coemployees, with patients, and with any third party. In this regard each employee is required to be honest and forthright and to not take any action or make statements or engage in any conduct that is unethical or improper or that could create the appearance of impropriety. In addition, each employee shall not engage in any conduct, take any actions, or make statements that negatively reflect upon Facility and/or in any way harm or potentially cause harm to Facility's image, reputation, or good will. It is expected that all staff of Facility will maintain the highest level of job performance and professional decorum. Each member of the staff is expected to support the mission, goals, business interest, and reputation of the organization.

B. Antiharassment

Facility is committed to providing a work environment that is free of discrimination and unlawful harassment. Actions, words, jokes, or comments based on an individual's sex, race, national origin, age, religion, disability, or any other legally protected characteristic will not be tolerated. As an example, sexual harassment (both overt and subtle) is a form of employee misconduct that is demeaning to another person, undermines the integrity of the employment relationship, and is strictly prohibited.

Sexual harassment is defined as unwelcome sexual advances, requests for sexual favors, and other verbal or physical conduct of a sexual nature when (1) submission to such conduct is made, either explicitly or implicitly, as a term or condition of an individual's employment, (2) submission to or rejection of such conduct by an individual is used as the basis for employment decisions affecting such individual, or (3) such conduct has the purpose or effect of unreasonably interfering with an individual's work performance or creating an intimidating, hostile, or offensive work environment. Sexual harassment could include, among other things, displaying sexually suggestive material in the workplace, unwelcome advances, requests for sexual favors, or any other offensive words or actions of a sexual nature.

Sexual harassment is unlawful, it violates Facility's policy, and it will not be permitted. No officer, manager, supervisor, or employee has the authority to require another employee to submit to sexual harassment, to condition retention of an employee's job or benefits on submission, or in any way to make submission to such conduct a term or condition of employment.

C. Patient Privacy and Confidentiality

Each employee of Facility is required to comply with the Facility Patient Privacy Compliance Program. That program provides, among other things, that all patient information is strictly confidential and can be shared only with those who have a "need to know" in the due course of business and operations, and only in a secure area. The "need to know" is defined as the need for information that is necessary for a person to perform his or her specific job responsibilities adequately. The forwarding, transmittal, downloading, or other reproduction or transmission of protected health information for purposes unrelated to the treatment of a patient, obtaining payment for medical services, or the operations of Facility, or that is not authorized by the employee's supervisor, is prohibited.

Any information concerning the business of Facility, its patients, suppliers, subcontractors, dealers, employees, or personnel associated with the Facility is confidential and restricted. You may not reveal any such information except under the direction of your supervisor or with their approval. If you are not sure about whether particular information is subject to this confidentiality duty, refer inquiries to your supervisor or the Chief Compliance Officer.

D. Attendance

You must notify your supervisor, as far as possible in advance of your scheduled workday, whenever you will be late or absent, to state the reason for such lateness or absence, and to advise when you expect to return to work. If your supervisor is not available when you call, you must call administration. If you are physically unable to make a personal call, you must have someone else call for you. A written medical excuse may be requested at the discretion of Facility. Following these steps does not excuse the absence. No absence is automatically considered to be "excused" as such. Chronic, habitual, or excessive absenteeism or lateness, as judged by Facility in its discretion, may result in disciplinary

BOX 25-4 Sample Code of Conduct—cont'd

action, up to and including termination, in circumstances including but not limited to the following:

- Frequent short-term absences and/or lateness in violation of Facility rules
- Absence from work for three (3) consecutive scheduled workdays without notifying Facility during the absence of an illness or accident preventing you from working (as evidenced by written certification of a medical doctor if requested by Facility) or other satisfactory reason for such absence, as determined by Facility
- Failure to return to work within two (2) consecutive scheduled workdays after being released for duty by a doctor, unless specifically requested not to do so by your supervisor, or after being notified of recall from layoff status by Facility
- Subject to applicable law and our policy on family and medical leave and policies regarding accommodations (as applicable), absence from work for any reason, including but not limited to illness, on- or off-the-job injury, layoff, or leave of absence, for a period in excess of three (3) consecutive months since your last day worked for Facility, or for a period exceeding the length of your continuous service with Facility, whichever is shorter

E. Keep Facility Up-To-Date

Up-to-date, personal information is necessary for a number of reasons, including ensuring the administration of your employee benefits. It is your responsibility to notify Facility promptly of any change in your address, telephone number, marital status, number of dependents, beneficiary designation, or anything else that would affect your employee benefits or our ability to contact you quickly.

F. Remember Courtesy

Facility views service to its patients and business family as one of its most important responsibilities. You are expected to help Facility carry out this policy by extending every courtesy and all assistance necessary, not only to your fellow employees, but also to any patients, callers, or business visitors to the Facility. If someone asks for assistance that you are unable to give, refer him or her to your supervisor.

G. Be Aware of Your Personal Appearance

Individual appearances are an important aspect of Facility's overall image, and each employee has a responsibility to be properly dressed at all times. Your common sense should lead you to practice good personal hygiene and to wear clean and neat clothing. Consult with your supervisor for the specific guidelines regarding personal appearance in your work area.

H. Respect Our Policies on E-mail, Computers, and Other Communications Equipment

All electronic and telephonic communication systems, computers, and other business equipment and communications, including Facility-provided phone mail, e-mail, Internet access, fax machines, and similar business devices, are the sole property of Facility. Any information transmitted by, received from, or stored in such equipment is also the property of Facility. Employees do not have any expectation of privacy in any of the above devices, systems, communications, and transmissions or in their desks or workspaces. Employees should use these systems only for legitimate business purposes to advance the business interests of Facility and not for their own personal use. These systems must not be used to transmit or download solicitations or offensive, vulgar, or otherwise disruptive messages or materials, including, but not limited to, those that contravene Facility's policies regarding equal employment opportunity and antiharassment. All messages and materials transmitted by, retrieved from, or stored within the business systems of Facility shall be regarded as nonpersonal, business communications. Facility reserves the right to monitor and intercept electronic or telephonic communications in the ordinary course of business and may monitor or download computers or software, in accordance with applicable law. Employees should not use passwords or retrieve any stored communications or files without prior authorization. Passwords are "on loan" to employees and, at all times, remain the property of Facility. Employees found to have violated these policies shall be subject to disciplinary action, up to and including termination of employment.

This is not a complete copy of a code of conduct but an example of how to start one for your facility.
From Beverly Kirchner, RN, BSN, CNOR, CASC; Jeanie Zelanko, RN, BSN, MSN, PhD; Richard Gilder, RN, BSN, MS.

symptoms to leaders, and monitoring of compliance to the policies and procedures addressing disruptive behavior.

CONCLUSION

Disruptive behavior is a problem that can be identified in every facility in the country. The cost of this behavior to our health care system according to Hutton (2006) is estimated to be $4.2 billion a year. Preventing the behavior is crucial to creating a safe work environment and safe patient care. Leaders have to be the driver of the strategic plan and goals for prevention of the disruptive behavior. The team plays a significant role in the prevention of disruptive behavior in the facility. If the team participates in the education and follows policy on reporting disruptive behavior, the leaders will be able to eliminate or at least decrease the effects of disruptive behavior in the facility. A safe work environment is essential to a team that is providing care to others. It takes everyone participating in the prevention of disruptive behavior to make a difference. Breaking the cycle of disruptive behavior in a facility is the goal.

REFERENCES

Christmas K: Workplace abuse: finding solutions, *Nurse Econ* 25(6):365–376, 2007.

Hutton SA: Workplace incivility: state of science, *J Nurs Adm* 36(1):22–27, 2006.

Kolanko KM, et al: Academic dishonesty, bullying, incivility, and violence: difficult challenges facing nurse educators, *Nurs Educ Perspect* 27(1):34–43, 2006.

Namie G, Namie R: *The bully at work: what you can do to stop the hurt and reclaim your dignity on the job*, Naperville, Ill, 2003, Sourcebooks, Inc.

The Joint Commission: *Improving America's hospitals: The Joint Commission's annual report on quality and safety*, 2007, available at http://www.jointcommissionreport.org/pdf/JC_2007_Annual_Report.pdf. Accessed September 1, 2009.

SAFETY IN THE PERIOPERATIVE SETTING

Vendor Support

Chapter 26

Peggy Camp, MSN, BSN, RN

Managing patient safety in the perioperative setting continues to be a major challenge. Managers of surgical services departments develop and implement multiple equipment-related and safe practices policies and procedures to minimize safety risk for the staff and surgical patients. In addition, managers must develop and implement policies that balance the need for industry representatives (vendors) in the operating room (OR) and other high-risk procedural areas within a facility (e.g., cardiac catheterization laboratory, endoscopy unit, interventional radiology departments). It is an accepted practice to allow vendors in various procedural areas, including the OR. This is especially important when the physicians and staff are unfamiliar with a specific supply item or piece of equipment (ECRI, 2007).

As professional caregivers, the perioperative staff and physicians have a responsibility to ensure that patient safety is maintained at all times regardless of the setting. Patient safety continues to be an area that regulatory agencies, government agencies, and professional associations closely track and research in an effort to identify practices that can be implemented to minimize untoward patient outcomes. "Healthcare is one of the last, complex high-technology industries to adopt a systematic approach to safety and typically relies on the resolve and vigilance of individual clinicians to avoid bad outcomes for the patient" (Webster, 2005). There is no question that vendors provide the perioperative team with education and information that is necessary in these times with rapidly changing and sophisticated technology (ECRI, 2007). At the same time, the importance of controlling access to the OR is essential for maintaining a safe patient environment. It is not acceptable for vendors to be present in perioperative areas without a designated purpose. Facilities should implement controls and guidelines for vendor access, and it is important for every perioperative team member to be aware of policies governing access.

As facilities look to ensure safety in the OR related to vendor access, there are several key considerations. Every vendor must be qualified to support the equipment or supply the vendor represents. The vendor should be trained in general hospital policies and protocols such as Health Insurance Portability and Accountability Act of 1996 (HIPAA) regulations, fire safety, and aseptic practice principles. The vendor should be a reputable individual who demonstrates awareness of and follows all facility policies regarding introduction of new products. Another issue is the surgeon's request for vendor presence in the OR. Although difficult to determine, consider if there are known financial relationships between the physician and vendor. Staff comfort level with the vendor in the room is another important aspect. Are there documented policies that identify vendor access in the OR? Consider the possibility of an increased risk for infection when outside individuals are allowed access to the OR. A defined policy on patient consent to having a vendor in the OR during a procedure is necessary.

These issues need to be addressed by every facility with vendors in the OR and will be covered in detail in this chapter.

VENDOR QUALIFICATIONS

Product Knowledge and Expertise

Facility policies and procedures should identify the process to determine vendor qualifications to support the supply or equipment the vendor represents. The majority of large, nationally known vendors will have formalized education and training programs for their sales representatives. However, there is a growing number of small companies that do not have resources to provide extended training for their field representatives. In addition, many equipment or supply manufacturers contract with local companies or individuals to support their products in the clinical setting. An example of this would be a small implant company (e.g., bone, tissue, spine, trauma) that hires individuals to cover its products and that has limited resources to train those individuals on the products they are promoting.

Over the past decade the verification of vendor knowledge, skill, and expertise has been embraced in varying degrees with inconsistent requirements and expectations. Currently there are no regulatory agencies such as The Joint Commission (2009) that require facilities to implement organized systems. However, The Joint Commission (2009) expects implementation of standards that "are relevant to any individual that enters a health care organization who directly impacts the quality and safety of patient care." These standards include the following: Standard EC.02.01.01, which states that to protect patient safety, accredited health care organizations need to be aware of who is entering their organization and what these individuals are doing in their organization; Standard RI.01.01.01, which states that accredited health care organizations need to take steps to ensure that patient rights are respected; and Standard IC.02.01.01, which states that accredited health care organizations need to take steps to ensure that infection control precautions are followed.

Given the rising concerns about patient safety and liability, many facilities are implementing clearly identified processes to control vendor access. Many facility policies and procedures require a formal request by the surgeon and/or staff before allowing a vendor into the OR. Vendor access to sell or promote products in public areas such as staff and physician lounges may not be permitted in some facilities. Many facilities have implemented a policy that if a vendor does not have a scheduled appointment, the vendor will not be permitted in any clinical area, including the OR. The unfortunate reality is that health care professionals are inundated with new technology every day. It is unreasonable and unrealistic to expect that the surgeon and perioperative team will have the knowledge, skills, and understanding to use every piece of equipment, supply, or implant in a manner that is safe and optimizes patient outcomes.

Most facilities have implemented processes requiring new product evaluation by a thorough detailed analysis before being allowed into the OR. The analysis includes U.S. Food and Drug Administration (FDA) approval for the procedure that the product is being used in, comparison with similar products already available, cost and reimbursement for the new product(s), and end-user education and support. Even with these type of controls in place, facilities may be held liable for all nonemployed individuals that participate directly or indirectly in surgical procedures. In a highly publicized case in New York, a sales representative was in the OR during a laparoscopic procedure. The patient died during the procedure, and the facility was cited on several counts, including an allegation that the sales representative operated the equipment during the procedure (Murphy, 2001).

Most state laws dictate that only licensed physicians can perform surgery; although physicians may use assistants, vendors do not (generally) have the proper training to be legally recognized assistants (Pennsylvania Patient Safety Authority [PSA], 2006). This presents questions about the level of involvement and facility/surgeon liability in procedures where implants are used. Specifically in spine, orthopedic, trauma, and plastic surgery, the vendor is generally in the OR in the role of advising and collaborating with the surgeon on the proper implant size and placement. The continued growth of technology and advancements in the implant arena makes it difficult, if not impossible, for the surgeon to be knowledgeable about every system and implant that could be used—this fact further complicates the situation.

There are also safety, liability, and ethical concerns if the vendor is denied access. Is the patient placed at a greater risk than if the vendor is allowed to be present? Hospitals have documented that vendors in the OR can be a distraction that may contribute to adverse patient outcomes. In one case the patient was undergoing bilateral knee replacement surgery. The vendor handed the surgeon the wrong knee implant, and it was placed in the patient (Maryland Department of Health and Mental Hygiene, 2007). In another case a warning light came on during a gynecologic procedure. The vendor turned off the alarm, and the patient had a bowel burn requiring emergency surgery a few days later (*Smart v Johnson and Johnson et al*, 1998). Although these may be isolated incidents, they support the need for advance review and approval of all new products. Allowing vendors in the OR and limiting access both have pros and cons. Although new product review and approval are not going to eliminate risk and untoward outcomes, the process will help to minimize some of the patient safety risks and concerns.

Policies and procedures for vendor representatives in the OR must be well-defined and include the following:

1. Defined oversight for all vendor access
2. Policies and procedures requiring documentation of appropriate training and education on the product the vendor is representing and promoting
3. Policies and procedures to ensure appropriate training and education on internal processes (e.g., aseptic technique, fire safety, electrical safety, HIPAA, and infection control)
4. Policies and procedures requiring documented evidence that the vendor has been provided with a copy of the expectations for presence and performance at the facility

Personal and Professional Competencies

Health care providers and facilities have the responsibility to ensure that nonemployed individuals are competent to support a safe patient environment while in the facility. To accomplish this, vendors must meet specific criteria before being given access into the facility. Vendors must be able to validate that they are trustworthy, honest, have integrity, and are professional in addition to having clinical competencies. For facilities that have formal credentialing processes in place, this information is generally included in the application process. The first step should be to obtain a background check, which can be done by the credentialing agency or the facility or obtained from the vendor parent company. Another initial verification should be that the parent company meets federal regulations (e.g., Office of Inspector General [OIG], U.S. General Services Administration [GSA] Exclusion check). Screening vendors for criminal or malpractice violations is critical, given that they are in close proximity to patients, and failing to produce evidence of a solid personal and professional history should be a cause for concern. Many facilities do not approve vendor access if the vendor and/or parent company fails to pass these requirements.

Once the vendor and parent company have satisfied the background and OIG/GSA requirements, they can move forward to verify credentials for the individual's clinical competencies. Unfortunately, facilities can ask for verification of the vendor training and education, but it is up to each company to develop vendor training programs because there are no universally accepted training methods. There remain great variations in the programs. For example, some companies have training programs that are several weeks long, whereas others are only a few days. It is expected that all vendors must have the ability to support the product and equipment and adhere to policies and procedures of the complex OR environment. Many companies hire nurses and scrub technicians to support their sales force; it is important to verify that the "clinical company resource" individuals are also required to meet the same criteria as the sales representatives. Again, it is not safe to assume that an individual is competent just because the individual has practiced as a clinician in the past. For this reason, the OR director, manager, or designee should complete a formal or informal assessment of the vendor or clinical support person's ability to perform while in the OR. In addition to the initial assessment, the facility may request information that includes the following:

1. A letter of competence from other institutions where the vendor is credentialed.
2. Documentation of training that is specific to the product or equipment in the following areas:
   a. The medical system, device, or procedure for which approval is sought, which should

include evidence of initial participation in a mentorship program supervised by an experienced vendor or company trainer and evidence that the individual has provided services or technical support on at least (X) occasions in the past (X) months for the product being represented

b. Working in the OR or other procedural setting, which includes the following:
   (1) Evidence of completion of an OR protocols course
   (2) Training in the Universal Protocol (i.e., time-out and verification of correct patient identity, correct side and site, agreement on the procedure to be done, correct patient position, and availability of correct implants and any special equipment [including any brought by the vendor] or special requirements)
   (3) Training in aseptic principles and techniques, including any cleaning or sterilization requirements for any device or equipment brought by the vendor, including any requirements related to disposal, storage, or reprocessing of single-use devices
   (4) Proper surgical attire
   (5) Fire prevention related to heat sources
   (6) Knowledge of sterile fields and traffic patterns
c. Standard infection control practices and bloodborne pathogens, which may include use of personal protection equipment, standard precautions, and hand hygiene procedures
d. Fire, electrical, and other safety protocols as applicable to the clinical area where vendor services are performed
e. Patient rights, specifically confidentiality and HIPAA compliance requirements
f. Human subject experimentation if the vendor will be providing services in conjunction with a product that is experimental or "off-label" as defined by the FDA
g. Patient safety, including applicable Joint Commission National Patient Safety Goals, and procedures for reporting concerns about patient safety or quality of care
h. Emergency response protocol

3. Evidence of current licensure, certification, or registration as required by law or regulation to practice as a professional in the performance of providing services, or when required by facility policy.
4. Evidence (documentation) of applicable health screening and vaccinations, including immunity/vaccination for tuberculosis and hepatitis B.
5. Signed agreement by the vendor that the individual will not participate in the delivery of services when symptoms of any contagious disease or illness exist and/or when the person is taking any medications for transmissible diseases.
6. Vendor agreement to follow standard for sales calls (e.g., making an appointment, securing an identification badge).
7. Vendor follow-up to complete department-specific orientation with OR director, manager, or designee.
8. Vendor agreement to maintain professional behaviors and refrain from any behaviors that create conflict or disruption.
9. Vendor agreement to limit personal business while in the clinical setting.
10. Vendor agreement to provide proof of professional services errors and omissions insurance coverage (to be determined on an individual facility basis).
11. Vendors are generally required to sign a facility confidentiality agreement and/or a business associate agreement (ECRI, 2007). These agreements often include adherence to FDA regulations involving the promotion of products or equipment for off-label use. They may also include some statement related to the Medicare and Medicaid Patient Protection Act of 1987, which prohibits accepting gifts or incentives for promoting products or services.

Although having the above documentation does not ensure the competence and subsequent safe practice of the vendor, it ensures with some level of confidence that the facility has an organized process to validate vendor competence to the best of its ability. This information needs to be organized and placed in a secure area, but it needs to be accessible as needed or requested by the department director, manager, or designee. Finally, there needs to be an ongoing process or requirement that these competencies be reviewed at least every 2 years or as dictated by facility policy.

GENERAL HOSPITAL POLICIES, PROTOCOLS, AND PROCEDURES

Facilities should follow regulatory, state, and federal recommendations as well as the recommendations of professional associations. Both the Association of periOperative Registered Nurses (AORN) and the American College of Surgeons (ACS) have published statements or recommendations for health care industry representatives in the OR (ACS, 2005; AORN, 2006). These recommendations provide a framework for facilities to create internal policies and procedures governing the requirements for vendor education and training in internal practices. In addition to creating the policies and procedures, facilities need to have a well-organized plan that defines the process for collecting and storing the information. The information should be readily accessible to staff, managers, and administration. As more and more facilities and health care systems move to outsourcing vendor credentialing, the company or agency contracted for this service must ensure that the information collected is consistent with a facility's internal policy and procedures. It is critical that the facility or health care system work closely with credentialing services to communicate the required education and training. Most of the credentialing companies have approved online courses covering the topics of aseptic techniques, fire and electrical safety, and infection control.

One of the areas that is often overlooked in internal policy is outlining nonemployee activities when in the OR. This is a facility-specific policy and procedure and may include restrictions on touching the patient, participating directly in a procedure, serving as an assistant in the procedure, opening sterile supplies (e.g., implants, sutures, gowns, gloves), troubleshooting equipment that is specific to the vendor, and performing tasks designated as staff responsibilities. Staff should understand that it is an expectation to not make requests of the vendors to perform identified restricted activities. In cases in which the vendor is not compliant with the policy and procedures of the facility, a policy should outline the appropriate action that will be taken. The action plan is facility specific and may include a verbal warning with a written plan for performance improvement and/or subsequent suspension of privileges in cases of noncompliance with facility policy. Repeated failure to correct behaviors can result in the vendor being permanently banned from the facility. Creating a safe patient environment requires that all employed and nonemployed individuals not only have proper training and skills, but also are compliant with written policies and procedures.

NEW-PRODUCT PROTOCOLS

In an effort to provide a safe patient environment, more and more facilities are putting processes in place to control the flow of new supplies and equipment. Many facilities require that a formal request be submitted, analyzed, and approved before new equipment is brought into the OR. Some facilities have a policy that they will not pay for a product that has not been preapproved. This position primarily affects products and equipment that are being requested on an elective as opposed to an emergent basis. Although having a new product approved before being used creates additional work for staff, it is a key foundation for ensuring that the patient's safety is considered at all times. The analysis can reveal that the product is not FDA approved for the procedure it has been requested for. It can also show that there is no need for the new product because there are comparable products currently available. It can help the facility to predetermine the financial effect of the new product, including the initial and ongoing cost and the facility's ability to get reimbursed for the product. It also will show if there is education and/or training required before bringing the new product into the OR. It is not unusual for requests for new products to be denied for safety and financial reasons. Although the primary concern is maintaining a safe patient environment, health care providers also have an obligation to be good stewards of the funds entrusted to them.

Other factors that need to be considered when creating new-product protocols include documentation of the vendor's competence in demonstrating use of the new product, arranging the schedule for when the new product will be used and with whom, and arranging space to accommodate the new supply or equipment. For any new equipment there needs to be sufficient time for the equipment to be brought into the facility and checked by biomedical engineering for functionality, safety, and FDA approval before use.

This information needs to be forwarded to the perioperative services director so that there is documentation in the event of product failure or adverse patient outcomes. Evaluation forms need to be created to validate that the product worked as expected. Finally, there needs to be a process to notify and gain patient consent when new supply/implant/technology is being used.

FDA Approval

It is important to note that FDA oversight and approval of medical devices is intended to protect the patient, the caregiver, and the facility. Medical device companies have incentives to bring products to market that are safe, will be embraced by health care providers, and will improve patient outcomes. There have been reports of companies that provide limited information to the FDA to avoid having their request for approval of a new product denied. In a landmark case an infant died after having a pacemaker implanted. The device was new on the market, and the size was compatible with that needed for an infant or small child. When it approved the device, the FDA was unaware that the manufacturer planned to market the device for infants and had failed to advise the FDA that the leads used with the device had not been tested on infants or children (Gregory, 2009). The health care community has come to rely on FDA approvals as a guiding light when using new products. This should cause organizations to carefully review every new product request, especially if it is considered to be a lifesaving device and is new to market. In addition, requests to use FDA-approved products off label should be carefully reviewed before approval. Off-label use of critical and noncritical products should be evaluated based on clinical needs and potential limitation and benefits, and patients must be advised in advance that they will be receiving a product that does not have FDA approval.

Surgeon Requests

In the past surgeon requests for new products (equipment and supplies) have been unregulated; most facilities did not question such requests. This is changing, however, as the flow of new technology continues to escalate and the requests to trial new products and technology continue to grow as well. In the past it was not unusual for a vendor to show up in the OR at the request of a surgeon. This practice creates a potential liability for the facility, staff, and the surgeon related to lack of specific knowledge of the product.

When there is a request for a new supply or equipment, the staff should first verify the request. Unless there is an urgent or emergent need, administration and staff need to educate surgeons and anesthesiologists and communicate the process for obtaining approval to use new products. As health care providers become more cognizant of the potential safety concerns with bringing new supplies and equipment into the OR, hospital administration is taking a firmer stand on adherence to new-product protocols.

When a surgeon or an anesthesiologist requests a non-FDA-approved product or an off-label application, this request needs to be forwarded to the medical staff overseeing the service and to risk management. Most facilities have processes in place to approve trials of non–FDA-approved equipment and/or off-label use, but these situations need to be approved by the facility's internal review board well in advance of the product's being brought into the facility. As the patient's advocate, the facility is responsible for ensuring that patient safety and well-being take priority over vendor, physician, and staff requests for new products. When new companies present requests to trial their products, some facilities are requiring a letter of sponsorship from the requesting physician (ECRI, 2007).

PHYSICIAN AND VENDOR RELATIONSHIPS RELATIVE TO MEDICAL SUPPLIES AND EQUIPMENT

Physician and vendor relationships in regard to promotion of products or equipment have recently come under intense investigation at the federal, state, and local level. In the past some vendors have offered physicians financial incentives to both use and promote their products. This practice creates not only a conflict of interest for both the physician and the vendor, but also ethical and risk issues for the physician, the vendor, and the facility. In addition, it may pose safety concerns for patients and staff. When physicians have financial incentives to use one product over another, they are unable to make fair, objective decisions regarding the product. The American Academy of Orthopaedic Surgeons (AAOS) (2007) issued a standard that required surgeons to disclose to patients any financial relationship with vendors and, when conflicts of interest were in question, that required the surgeon to support decisions that favored the patient's best interests. As concerns about physician conflicts of interest have grown, a number of health care facilities and systems have adopted rigid protocols to ensure that they control physician-vendor relationships in an effort to guarantee that the patients' best interests and safety are the driving forces behind decisions about new technology and products used in the OR.

STAFF AND VENDOR RELATIONSHIPS

At some facilities, OR staff may find themselves in a difficult position when new products are brought into the OR. A vendor may arrive just before the case is ready to start per surgeon request for a product trial. The staff may not have been informed in advance that the vendor would be there and that there would be a new and unknown product being trialed.

The initiation of any procedure is a stressful and demanding time. The staff are extremely busy ensuring that the routine supplies and equipment are ready and available and that the patient is being cared for in the best possible manner. Having a vendor show up unannounced and with an unknown product at the beginning of a case is an example of unnecessary, unacceptable intrusion for the staff and the patient. The staff often feel caught in a situation in which they have little, if any, control. Historically staff have been conditioned not to challenge physician requests—often creating a lose-lose situation when a new product is presented for use without prior knowledge. The vendor may also feel caught in the middle because the surgeon has requested a trial of the product. As efforts to control the flow of new products into the OR grow and expand, it is critical to ensure that there are developed policy and procedures defining the expectations and process that are expected of the vendor and the surgeon in this situation to safeguard the patient. In addition, the facility administration must be knowledgeable and supportive of the policies to fully enforce them. Health care providers are becoming increasingly aware of the risks to themselves and to patients if they do not adhere to policy and procedures for new-product evaluation.

Another consideration needs to be taken into account related to staff-vendor relationships. There are vendors who present in the OR who are knowledgeable, professional, and truly "add value" to the physician, staff, and the patient by being there. At the same time there are vendors who are marginal relative to the safety of their product and the value brought to the case. If there is ever any question of vendor performance, representation, value, or patient safety concern, the situation should be brought to the attention of the facility director and/or senior administration. The facility's administrators should never permit marginal vendors inside the ORs when there are concerns that patient safety and/or outcomes have the potential to be compromised.

INFECTION CONTROL CONSIDERATIONS

Controlling hospital-acquired conditions, including postoperative wound infections, continues to be a high priority for health care organizations. Regulatory agencies and payers are creating report cards for individual facilities on several key complications, including postoperative wound infections, and health care organizations are closely tracking their rates. As health care organizations seek to put protocols in place to address the control of these infections, we should ask ourselves a number of questions: (1) Is there an increased risk when nonessential employed and nonemployed individuals (including vendors and service providers) are present in the OR? (2) Is there documented evidence that postoperative wound infections occur more frequently in cases in which there are more individuals in the room? (3) Can the rates be linked through facility data to a specific case or team? (4) Do ORs need to create additional controls for access before and during operative procedures for nonessential personnel to minimize the risks for postoperative wound infections? (5) Is there valid evidence that vendors in the OR increase the risk for postoperative infections? Although these are valid concerns, there is limited evidence-based research that can quantify and validate that vendors specifically contribute to an increased incidence of postoperative wound infections. However, it is a well-documented fact that increased traffic and personnel in the OR are a contributing factor for the incidence of postoperative wound infections. This supports limiting access to anyone considered nonessential. All vendors in a procedure must have a specific purpose (e.g., to support the trial of a new product). In addition, vendors seeking access need to be compliant with facility policies regarding immunization and not being present when they have active symptoms of an infectious disease.

PATIENT CONSENT

A critical consideration in allowing vendor access to the OR and trialing new products is gaining the consent of the patient. Health care providers and physicians have an obligation to inform the patient that a vendor will be in the room during the patient's procedure. An increasing number of facilities have incorporated this information as part of their consent documents, but many have not. Facilities need to be clear that allowing a vendor in the OR without obtaining the patient's consent could be argued as an invasion of the patient's privacy. Further, if the vendor is permitted to touch the patient, this could be argued as a battery on the patient.

In the past, patient consent has not been a requirement outlined in facility policy, and in many cases there has not been a requirement to document the vendor presence in the OR as part of the operative record. It is important to note that the patient is well informed and expects to be informed when additional individuals (including vendors) are allowed access to the OR during the patient's procedure. It is the responsibility of the surgeon to advise the patient that there will be a vendor in the room during the procedure and to obtain the patient's consent. Most patients are open to this and accept the physician's recommendations. Should staff become aware that the patient has not been informed or has not consented to the vendor being allowed access to the OR for the patient's procedure, they have an obligation to notify the surgeon, vendor, and administration that vendor access has been denied because there has not been patient agreement to this condition. If consent is in place, the staff should follow facility policy on documentation. The vendor should be recorded on the intraoperative record. This serves as a protection to the staff, physician, and facility should a claim arise in the future.

MANAGING VENDORS IN THE OPERATING ROOM

Facilities have a responsibility to establish expectations for vendors when they are in the facility. It is critical that the expectations are communicated to vendors when they initially are credentialed or approved by a facility. It is important for vendors to understand that cross selling other vendor products or speaking in negative terms about other vendors or their products will not be tolerated. Vendors will be required to follow the facility procedure when accessing the facility, and vendors without badges will be denied access to clinical areas. Vendors are not allowed to promote products that are not approved when in the procedure area and are not allowed to promote any and all products that are not currently on contract. As noted earlier, they may not be permitted in physician or staff lounges unless they have a preapproved appointment according to policy and procedure. Vendors are expected to respect the privacy of patients, other staff, and any other information that they have access to while in the facility (e.g., competitors and/or competitor products). Vendors are expected to follow the requests of staff and management, including leaving a procedural area when requested. Vendors are not allowed to "cruise" the OR for the purpose of promoting products. In a situation in which a vendor asks to take photographs during a procedure, the facility policy on the taking of photographs must be followed (PSA, 2006). In addition, there must be consent from both the patient and the facility to do so.

PROS AND CONS OF VENDORS IN THE OPERATING ROOM

There is no doubt that the majority of vendors "add value" to the staff, physicians, and ultimately the patient and the facility in general. Today's ORs are complex, high-intensity environments that are continually confronted with new products and technology. Physicians and staff do not have the time to learn about all of the new products and technology and thus rely on the vendors to provide this information and support. Without the vendor's help, there is a potential risk for the patient, the staff, and the physician. Courses in technology are generally not part of the curriculum for either physicians or nurses. Most of their education is "hands on" once they are in the practice area. Although the majority of new products used in the OR are fairly routine and do not require in-depth education and support, the growing number of highly technical systems and equipment can be overwhelming for even the most experienced perioperative team. The team in the OR relies on the vendor to help support the growing number of implants for orthopedics, spine, plastic, and general surgery, to name a few. Medical device companies are continually adding improvements or upgrades to existing equipment such as electrosurgical generators, laparoscopic operating systems, and lasers, which adds to the need for vendor education and support. Facilities can sometimes rely on internal resources such as biomedical engineering to assist in the education process, but even they may not be current on the new technologies that are being brought into the facility. It is obvious that the health care community at large has a need for education on new technology, and at this time the vendor appears to be the one best qualified to provide it.

On the other hand, ORs need to be more cautious and selective about the products they allow into their department. Not every new supply or piece of equipment needs to be considered—many of the new products being presented are similar to those already being used and in many cases may not offer any clinical or outcome improvements. Responsibility for being selective about which new products will be approved for evaluation rests with the management team and product evaluation team in the OR. Evaluating new equipment generally means that the vendors will have access to the OR. The addition of nonhospital personnel in an already complex, high-stress area can create disruption, causing the staff to direct their attention to something other than the patient. This results in potential risk and liability.

Each facility needs to weigh all of the pros and cons as they receive requests to trial new products. The OR staff, physicians, and administration need to be proactive in establishing an organized, controlled process for new-product introduction and vendors in their OR. Once the policy is established, it should be adhered to and closely monitored. Policy is only as good as its enforcement, and, in cases where there is a policy and it is not followed, the facility is placed at even more risk.

CONCLUSION

It is fair to expect that ORs and health care providers in general are cognizant of the need for having formal policies and procedures governing vendor access and the introduction of new products within their facilities. Vendor access should be considered a privilege and not a right. In addition, OR leaders need to continue to educate and support staff to report any and all situations in which the patient's safety or privacy is placed at risk directly or indirectly by a vendor. The health care community has been entrusted by the public to make their safety the priority. The OR staff and management need to work on developing more collaborative relationships with our physician partners and vendors through education and communication. The facility's managers and senior administration are the driving force in establishing policies, procedures, and protocols that ensure patient safety is maintained at the highest levels, not only in the hospital, but also across the full continuum of care.

REFERENCES

American Academy of Orthopaedic Surgeons: *Standards of professionalism: orthopaedist-industry conflicts of interest*, 2007, available at http://www3.aaos.org/member/profcomp/SOPConflictsIndustry.pdf. Accessed October 11, 2009.

American Colleges of Surgeons: *Statement on healthcare industry representatives in the operating room*, revised September 2005, available at http://www.facs.org/fellows_info/statements/st-33.html. Accessed October 6, 2009.

Association of periOperative Registered Nurses: Guidance statement: the role of the health care industry representative in the perioperative setting, *AORN J* 83(4):930–934, 2006.

Brennan TA: Health industry practices that create conflicts of interest: a policy proposal for academic medical centers, *JAMA* 295(4):429–433, 2006.

ECRI Institute: Sales representatives and other outsiders in the OR, *Operating Room Risk Management* (2):1–14, 2007.

Gregory K: Wanted: common sense reforms at FDA, *Mass Device (MD)*, available at http://www.massdevice.com/blogs/karin-gregory/wanted-common-sense-reforms-fda. Accessed October 11, 2009

Maryland Department of Health and Mental Hygiene; Office of Health Care Quality: An unnecessary distraction: vendors in the operating room, *Clinical Alert* 4(3):1–2, 2007.

Murphy EK: The presence of sales representative in the OR, *AORN J* 73(4):822–824, 2001.

Pennsylvania Patient Safety Authority: Healthcare industry representatives: maximizing benefits and reducing risks, *Pa Patient Saf Advis* 3(1):13–19, 2006.

Smart v Johnson and Johnson et al, No. 120272/98 (NY Sup Ct 1998).

The Joint Commission: *Frequently asked questions, healthcare industry/vendor representatives,* 2009, available at http://www.jointcommission.org/AccreditationPrograms/LongTermCare/Standards/09_FAQs/HR/hc_industry_vendor_representatives.htm. Accessed October 11, 2009.

Webster CS: The iatrogenic-harm cost equation and new technology, *Anaesthesia* 60:843–846, 2005 (invited editorial).

USING HUMAN FACTORS TO BALANCE YOUR OPERATING ROOM

Chasity Burrows Walters, MSN, RN • Aileen Killen, PhD, RN • Jill Garrett, RN, CPHQ

Health care is an inherently risky business, and with that risk errors are inevitable. Medical errors represent a public health issue that has been increasingly well recognized since the sentinel Institute of Medicine report (Kohn et al, 2000) was published a decade ago. Since then, the demands on health care to redesign processes to ensure a safer system have been increasing. Despite the efforts of health care leaders, policy makers, and public health advocates, however, the number of errors continues to rise (HealthGrades Inc., 2006). As one of the most complex work environments in health care (Christian et al, 2006), the operating room (OR) is a common site for adverse events (Leape, 1994). It involves teams of highly trained professionals interacting with advanced technology in high-risk situations, and the nature of such work places these teams at risk for errors. The largest numbers of errors result from treatment provided in the OR (Gawande et al, 2003; Brennan et al, 2004). The causes of these errors are variable and include technical errors (Gawande et al, 2003; Rogers et al, 2006) and communication deficiencies (Sexton et al, 2000; Christian et al, 2006; Rogers et al, 2006).

Although surgical safety has long been an area of concern (Wachter, 2008), why do these errors persist? Safety in the OR historically has been viewed as a matter of individual human factors. Although health care continued to perpetuate a culture of blame and shame, other industries successfully adopted a systems approach to errors. This approach has left the health care industry lagging behind other high-reliability industries, such as aviation, when it comes to designing safer systems. Shifting focus from the notion of errors resulting from human failure to errors as a consequence of the underlying systemic inefficiencies requires a change in thinking, and it is gaining momentum. This change is imperative to create and sustain health care environments conducive to patient safety. However, it requires an understanding of work systems not traditionally taught to the nurses, surgeons, or allied health providers who are so well intentioned about the pursuit of safety. This chapter provides an introduction to concepts used in a systems approach followed by strategies that can be implemented to cultivate a safer OR.

THE OPERATING ROOM AS A MICROSYSTEM

A work system is essentially any environment in which work is performed. In the OR, for example, the work system can be described as a microsystem in which small, interdependent groups of people work as a team to provide patient care. The microsystem typically consists of 5 to 15 people, including the surgeon, assistants, anesthesia providers, scrub person, circulating nurse, unlicensed assistive personnel (e.g., nursing assistants, equipment technicians, housekeeping personnel), perfusionists, monitoring technicians, and possibly others. The large number of participants gets further complicated by hierarchical issues within the system and the multiple handoffs that take place during a typical case. Although each member of the microsystem has a specific role, one member cannot function effectively without the support of others. Finally, this group needs to perform in routine situations and highly specialized or crisis situations. These factors describe some issues that occur daily in the OR that are not generally considered in their entirety in attempts to create a safe environment.

Viewing the OR as a microsystem provides a basis for understanding the complexity of systems, and this shifting of approach may allow for a significant decrease in errors (Weigmann et al, 2007). From the systems perspective, errors are viewed as a consequence of a system breakdown rather than being caused by an individual working in the system. This thinking is fundamental to the field of human factors, which has been used in other complex industries to balance the components of work (Yourstone and Smith, 2002).

HUMAN FACTORS

Human factors is an umbrella term that refers to the interaction of humans on and by the system in which humans work. Historically the term *human factors* has been used in the United States, and the term *ergonomics* has been used in Europe. Much of the current literature uses the terms interchangeably. The Human Factors and Ergonomics Society (n.d.) defines the terms as "concerned with the understanding of interactions among humans and other elements of a system, and the profession that applies theory, principles, data, and other methods to design in order to optimize human well-being and overall system performance." Human factors science offers a way to understand the interactions among the elements of the work system, as opposed to addressing the elements individually. It takes into account human strengths and limitations with the goal of offering solutions that limit the dependence of the work system on less-reliable human characteristics (i.e., memory) and places greater emphasis on systems processes (e.g., standardization).

In their study of work systems, Smith and Sainfort (1989) developed the Balance Theory to conceptualize the interaction of five human factors components within the system: the individual, tasks, tools and technologies, the environment, and organizational factors (Figure 27-1). These components work together to create a "stress load" that challenges an individual's biological, psychologic, and behavioral resources (Carayon and Smith, 2000). These five components should be considered equally when designing a product, process, or system to achieve effective, efficient, and safe results. This chapter presents those human factor components as they relate to the OR and discusses how balancing all five factors within a work system can improve patient safety.

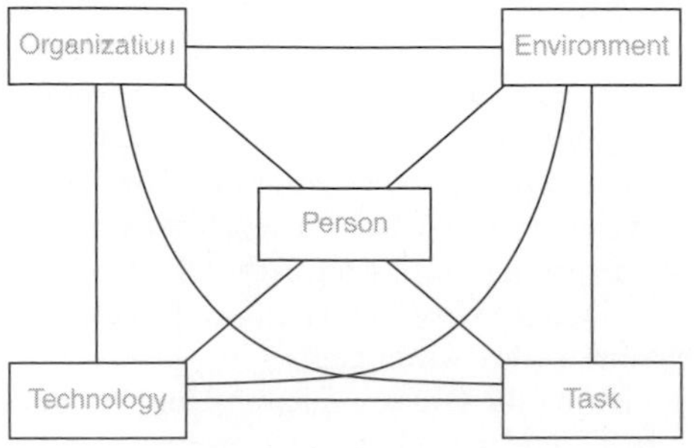

FIGURE 27-1 Smith and Sainfort work system model. (From Smith MJ, Sainfort PC: A balance theory of job design for stress reduction, *Int J Ind Ergon* 4:67–79, 1989.)

BALANCE THEORY

Individual

The characteristics of an individual in the work system include everything the perioperative nurse "brings" to work, including individual characteristics such as past experience, abilities, physical and emotional health, motivation, and professional aspirations. Many of these characteristics are not static. Fatigue, for example, has been implicated in errors in disasters such as the *Exxon Valdez* oil spill, Chernobyl nuclear disaster, and Three Mile Island situation (Mitler et al, 1988). Adverse surgical outcomes have been linked to fatigue (Gaba and Howard, 2002), and, although little is known specifically about the impact of fatigue on the practice of OR nursing, it presents some unique challenges.

Fatigue

In addition to working a full-time schedule, perioperative nurses often need to take call. Balancing work and personal obligations becomes more difficult, which can force nurses to work without adequate sleep. Lack of sleep impairs one's ability to deliver safe care. Research has shown that after 17 hours without sleep, performance is equivalent to having a blood alcohol level of 0.05% (Page et al, 2009); it further degrades to 0.10% after 24 hours without sleep (Rosekind et al, 1997). Recognizing fatigue as an important factor in the OR, the Association of periOperative Registered Nurses (AORN) has issued a position statement based on an extensive review of the literature outlining recommendations for safe on-call practices (AORN, 2008).

Experience Level

Another individual characteristic that demands consideration in the designing of a safe OR is the experience level. Like other specialty nurses, perioperative nurses bring varying degrees of knowledge, skills, and experience to the OR. The gap between available experienced perioperative nurses and the needs of ORs around the country has required creative hiring and training practices by perioperative leaders. New graduate nurses and experienced nurses from other specialties are choosing perioperative nursing for their career paths. Compounded by the aging surgical patient population and the complexity of modern surgical interventions, orientation and ongoing skill development are crucial to balance the work environment. Addressing this issue, AORN published a position statement, "Orientation of the Registered Professional Nurse to the Perioperative Setting" (AORN, 2005), which provides suggested timelines for orientation of novice and experienced perioperative nurses. These guidelines provide justification for perioperative leaders as they request resources of time, staff, and money. The fallout of this phenomenon is complex; the need for ongoing preceptorship programs can burden the experienced staff who are adding this additional responsibility to their full workload. Training and development only go so far to facilitate transition to perioperative nursing. Novice perioperative nurses who have expertise in other clinical areas of practice also may require special support as they move from being "expert" nurses in one specialty to "novice" perioperative nurses.

Although this section focuses on individual human factors, including fatigue and experience, several other characteristics can be managed by targeting elements within the work system. Human factor limitations and error reduction strategies can be implemented to compensate for them. Some of those factors include the following:

- Humans have a limited short-term memory capacity, so use checklists to reduce reliance on memory.
- Sensory overload in the OR requires staff to be constantly alert to everything around them. Limiting the availability of choices, such as by using unit dose medication whenever possible, can decrease the likelihood of a medication error.
- Cognitive tunnel vision can occur related to stress in high-intensity situations. Using forcing functions whenever possible, such as automatic shut-off valves on warming devices, can mitigate this risk.

Task

According to the Balance Theory, the tasks of the work system affect and are impacted by the individual, technology, and the environment (Carayon and Smith, 2000). The tasks required in the OR must be considered to achieve a balanced work system, necessitating attention to concepts such as the appropriate use of skills, workload, and work pressures.

The ability to identify and prioritize the enormous number of individual tasks required of a perioperative nurse is a skill that evolves along the novice-to-expert continuum. Time pressures, combined with high-level multitasking, are routine. Nurses face significant competition for attention during routine and critical points in a surgical procedure (Christian et al, 2006). The workload in the OR varies and is affected by the need to retrieve additional resources, such as supplies and equipment, and the need to perform safety-related activities, such as "count" and handoff. The requirements of these tasks are physical and cognitive. Standardization and simplification should be the mantra for developing error reduction strategies for the task component of a balanced work system. As part of the "Safe Surgery Saves Lives" campaign, the World Health Organization (WHO) (2008) developed the WHO Surgical Safety Checklist, which can be used to remind the surgical team of key tasks to be performed in the preoperative, intraoperative, and immediate postoperative phases of care (World Alliance for Patient Safety, 2008).

Situational awareness, a concept borrowed from high-reliability organizations (Weick and Sutcliffe, 2001), allows members of the team to have an accurate understanding of "what's going on" and "what is likely to happen next." It allows the entire team to be on the same page. Institutions across the country are identifying ways to increase situational awareness in their ORs. Memorial Health System in Colorado Springs, Colorado, identified briefings as the first step in creating situational awareness. The elements of briefing were determined by the Unit Practice Council and were designed into the current "count board," which offers the appropriate visual cue when in the OR scrubbed and standing at the table (Figure 27-2). Electronic documentation of a physician-led briefing was later added to facilitate the collection of metrics for this process improvement (Figure 27-3).

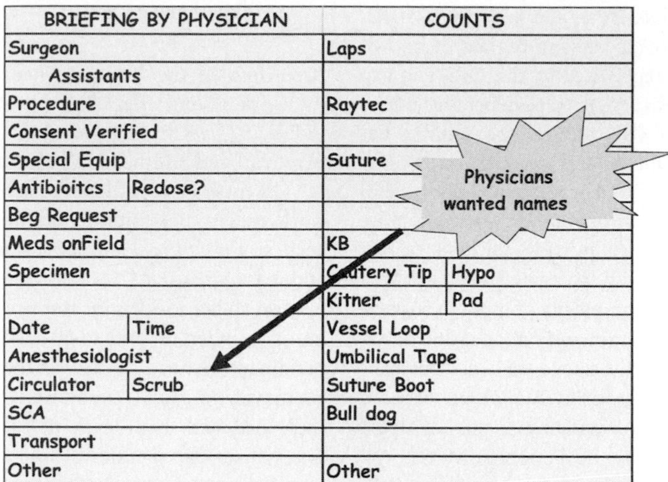

BRIEFING BY PHYSICIAN		COUNTS	
Surgeon		Laps	
Assistants			
Procedure		Raytec	
Consent Verified			
Special Equip		Suture	
Antibioitcs	Redose?		
Beg Request			
Meds onField		KB	
Specimen		Cautery Tip	Hypo
		Kitner	Pad
Date	Time	Vessel Loop	
Anesthesiologist		Umbilical Tape	
Circulator	Scrub	Suture Boot	
SCA		Bull dog	
Transport			
Other		Other	

FIGURE 27-2 Memorial Hospital count board. (From Walters, et al: Using human factors to "balance" your operating room, *Perioper Nurs Clin* 3(4):277–285, 2008.)

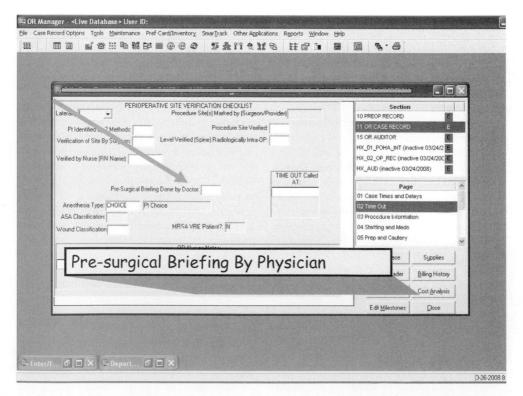

FIGURE 27-3 Memorial Hospital electronic documentation. (From Walters, et al: Using human factors to "balance" your operating room, *Perioper Nurs Clin* 3(4):277–285, 2008.)

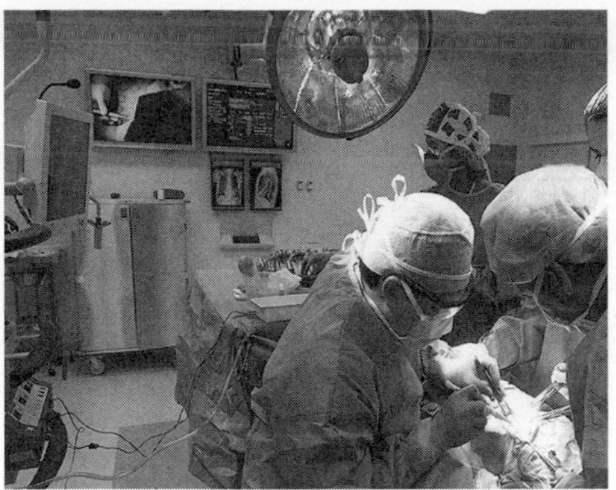

FIGURE 27-4 Wall of knowledge. (From Walters, et al: Using human factors to "balance" your operating room, *Perioper Nurs Clin* 3(4):277–285, 2008.)

Likewise, during the design and construction of their OR platform, Memorial Sloan Kettering Cancer Center in New York developed the concept of the "wall of knowledge" (Figure 27-4). One component of the wall of knowledge is the "OR dashboard," which displays continuous real-time data to all members of the surgical team regarding patient information, the progress of the case, and team members.

In addition to these strategies involving task management and awareness, other error reduction strategies can be implemented to simplify tasks and processes:

- Support the most appropriate use of skills by considering the redistribution of work to ancillary personnel.
- Use checklists and automated reminders when possible to remind staff of critical activities. Multitasking can lead to errors.
- Decrease number of choices by using prepacked custom procedure packs.
- Decrease number of steps necessary to complete a task. Design a pass-through cabinet to obtain supplies from central core to OR (which has the added value of decreasing the number of staff coming into and out of the room).
- Reduce reliance on memory and experience by using up-to-date preference cards.

Technology

The modern OR is a technologically sophisticated work environment. Battles and Keyes (2002) described the relationship between technology and patient safety as a "two-edged sword." Technology can assist perioperative nurses by automating repetitive, time-consuming, and error-prone tasks, yet it may provide distractions and competition for attention. The addition of new technology can burden individuals who need to acquire new skills or who may be concerned about changes to their job functions as a result of adoption of new technology. The two-edged sword of new technologies (Battles and Keyes, 2002) can be told in a "tale of two communication devices." When a new OR communication system was being designed at Memorial Sloan Kettering Cancer Center, a hands-free phone was selected for the nurses' documentation station. The phone plugged into a USB port on the computer. A surgeon picked up the phone at the end of the case to call a patient's family, and the phone number was entered in the nurses' documentation fields because the computer could not tell the difference between the phone and the keyboard! On the other hand, a hands-free wireless communication system (Vocera Communications) was implemented and was hugely successful in facilitating communication between anesthesia and nursing staff and nursing staff and support personnel.

Seeking technologic solutions is often thought to provide a simple answer to complex problems. A wise colleague once said, "Never automate a broken system." Perioperative managers need to be mindful of the use of technology to "balance" the work system. Kukla et al (1992) suggested that safety concerns for automated systems should be addressed by a design that is easy to use and provides a better way for staff to do their work (or at least as good as current methods). Before implementation of any automated system, a detailed analysis of the current work flow should be undertaken. The Institute for Healthcare Improvement is an excellent resource when getting started with the documentation of work flow.

In this technologic era, new tools are created daily that are intended to improve care in the OR. Error reduction strategies using some of these newer technologies are as follows:

- Advances are plentiful in the field of electronic documentation. This not only benefits the patient by timely and institution-wide availability of information, but also allows data retrieval for clinical and administrative report cards.

- Limit repetitive tasks when possible. Radiofrequency identification technology, for example, is an emerging technology that offers new solutions for time-consuming tasks, such as sponge and instrument counts.
- Investigate bar code technology for use with implants, medications, and supplies to facilitate documentation and tracking.

Environment

Human factors science requires that the physical environment be considered in balancing the work system. Interaction among all components of the work system involves the environment, yet in health care, space constraints, outdated work areas, and inefficient planning can overcome any efforts to balance the system. With the increase in outpatient surgeries, technology, and concern regarding the conservation of resources, the physical environment is demanding attention. This presents an invaluable opportunity to bring human factor concepts to the OR.

One of the challenges in OR design and construction is to provide an efficient and safe environment for patients and staff. Standardization is the mainstay of error reduction strategies and should be considered in the design of the environment. During the design phase of a new 21-suite OR platform, Memorial Sloan Kettering Cancer Center developed principles to guide the design (Figure 27-5). These principles were based on expert consultation and experience of the design team and were agreed upon by the executive committee. One of these guiding principles, "Promote familiarly and utility in room design though 95% similarity," addressed this notion of standardization. Just as agreeing on a process may make deviations from the norm more likely to be noted (Wachter, 2008), agreeing on a design of the OR may lead to surgical staff working more efficiently when stakes are high.

Vigilance refers to a person's state of alertness and is particularly critical in risky conditions, such as in the OR. Promoting vigilance can be accomplished with the design of a nurses' workstation with full line of sight to the surgical field. At Memorial Sloan Kettering Cancer Center the optimal height of the workstation was determined to be "transactional" height (42 inches) so that a nurse can sit or stand while accomplishing tasks. The controls for operating room lights, surgical equipment, and audiovisual integration were all designed to be within easy reach of nurses (Figure 27-6). Sometimes consideration of human factors, including the details of the environment, requires thinking out of the box. The openness to an "asymmetrical" orientation to the OR table, in which the OR table and light fixtures are not in the geographic center of the room, maximizes areas for sterile setup and circulation. Regardless of the design, it is critical to get input from staff who work in the space. To the extent that it is financially and physically feasible, building a realistic mock-up of the space to "play" in is an invaluable way to assess design plans.

Although the ideas presented for addressing the environment as a component of the system are resource intensive, other strategies to consider might include the following:

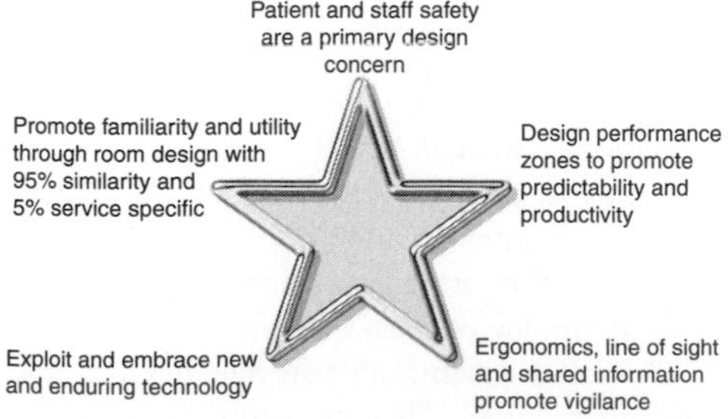

FIGURE 27-5 Memorial Sloan Kettering Cancer Center operating room design principles. (From Walters, et al: Using human factors to "balance" your operating room, *Perioper Nurs Clin* 3(4):277–285, 2008.)

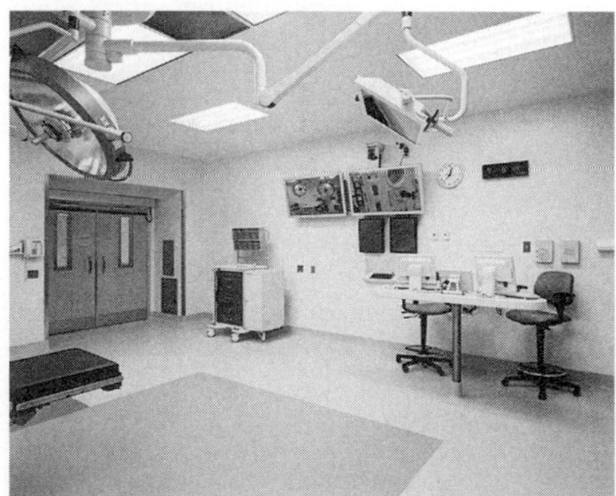

FIGURE 27-6 Operating room workstation. (From Walters, et al: Using human factors to "balance" your operating room, *Perioper Nurs Clin* 3(4):277–285, 2008.)

- Lighting is important in the work environment. Multiple-zone fluorescent lights are useful for maximum control for maximally and minimally invasive procedures. Green lights can be considered for visualization by circulating staff and anesthesia during minimally invasive procedures.
- Temperature of the environment can affect the work balance. Design space outside the walls of the OR for electronic equipment. This approach allows for technical support from outside the procedure area, decreases the heat produced in the OR, and frees up valuable space around the patient.
- Planning flooring can save problems later. Consider hardness and cleanability, and test several surfaces in a mock setup if possible.
- Decrease number of steps necessary for staff when working in an environment. This goal can be accomplished by examining the work flow to identify locations for refuse, sharps, and laundry containers.

Organization

The organizational context has implications for the work produced by the individual. To promote safety in the OR, emphasis on the importance of a safety culture throughout the organization is paramount. The value of a safety culture must be driven by senior leadership and diffuse to frontline staff. Programs that identify and involve patient safety champions or stars are useful in disseminating information to and from frontline staff. Cultivating this environment takes time, but several initiatives can facilitate the change.

Reporting Concerns

The strongest predictor of a safety culture on the unit level is agreement with the statement "I am encouraged by my colleagues to report any patient safety concerns I may have" (Perspectives on Safety, n.d.). Emphasis on reporting mechanisms can provide a rewarding start to building an organization conducive to patient safety. Although nurses traditionally have been the reporters of error (Lawton and Parker, 2002), responsibility should extend to include anyone involved in patient care. The reporting of errors should be simple, and well-designed computer-based programs are available to encourage reporting. For example, when Memorial Sloan Kettering Cancer Center instituted a computer-based reporting system, the reporting of actual events doubled. The organization also moved from reporting only incidents to reporting near misses, which was driven by use of a systems perspective.

Because near misses occur more often than errors, emphasis on near misses allows for the collection of more data, enabling organizations to most effectively identify weaknesses in the system that could lead to patient harm if not addressed. Reading groups, which consist of frontline and patient safety staff, review aggregate data for themes and process improvement opportunities that ultimately can serve the system in decreasing the number of "work-arounds." Work-arounds are first-order problem solving (Edmonson, 2004) and remove the immediate obstacle to getting work done but do nothing to change the probability of the event reoccurring. Whatever the mechanism of reporting chosen, feedback and nonpunitive discussions are critical in the development of trust in the system.

As in other industries, levels of teamwork in the OR correlate with the frequency of surgical errors (Catchpole et al, 2008). Industries such as aviation have moved toward a culture that affords questioning by the crew and recognizes human limitations (Sexton et al, 2000). When attitudes toward teamwork and communication were examined among OR staff, however, nurses reported low levels of teamwork, whereas surgeons were in support of a hierarchy that functions to suppress the questioning of others' behavior or decisions (Sexton et al, 2000). Explicit opportunities for nurses and other staff must be made to encourage communication about concerns and specific patient issues. At Memorial Health System in Colorado Springs, 260 perioperative staff and physicians participated in 4 hours of focused human factor training. Before the training, the safety attitudes questionnaire (Sexton et al, 2006) was completed by more than 100 perioperative staff and physicians. This survey was repeated after the training and 1 year later after voluntary briefings had begun. The graph in Figure 27-7 represents five areas of significant improvement in regard to the perception of safety in the OR.

In addition to increasing reporting and facilitating teamwork, which are commitment-intensive strategies, organizations can cultivate a safer environment through the following means:

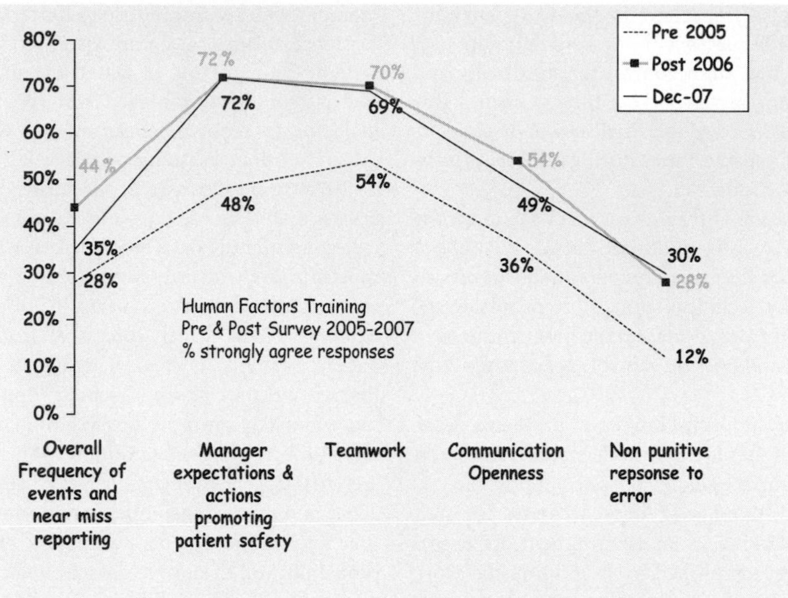

FIGURE 27-7 Safety attitudes survey results. (From Walters, et al: Using human factors to "balance" your operating room, *Perioper Nurs Clin* 3(4):277–285, 2008.)

- Review policies pertaining to work schedules, corrective action, whistle blowing, and cultural competence with the human resources department.
- Shifting focus from the individual to the system gets to the real issues in the OR and fosters job security through fairness.
- Consider institutional hiring practices. Balancing the work system may be made easier through careful selection of personnel. Southwest Airlines has a reputation for its "Hire for attitude, train for skill" philosophy (Carbonara, 1996).
- Provide opportunities for professional development, such as a clinical ladder program and promotional opportunities. Participation in institutional committees and performance improvement projects not only increases perspective but also builds confidence and contentment with work.

DIRECTIONS FOR FUTURE RESEARCH

The use of systems models, such as the Balance Theory, has not been readily tested within the context of health care systems. Although the use of strategies adopted in other systems can offer a unique and helpful approach, those lessons can take the health care system only so far. The Balance Theory provides a framework for thought in the design of a safer OR; however, research is needed to explore the fit of the components to the OR system. Research designs that support testing the relationships between the elements as they pertain to the OR are necessary in the strategic development of interventions. This testing of relationships facilitates evidence-based efforts to build a safer OR, which in time can be further tested to delineate the components that are predictors of a safe OR work system.

CONCLUSION

This chapter uses the Balance Theory to describe characteristics of the OR work system from a human factors perspective. Although examples have been provided within the context of each component, it is worth mentioning that there is considerable overlap among the components. The key is to use the model as a framework to guide thinking in a systems direction, offering new and different insights into the design of a safer work system in the OR.

Although there are several ways to conceptualize work in the OR, the Balance Theory offers an advantage in that no one particular aspect is highlighted. Instead, it examines the system as a whole to evaluate which potentially positive elements can be highlighted to balance potentially negative aspects (Carayon and Smith, 2000). This is especially helpful because it can be manipulated to serve particular work systems to best allocate resources. For example, if limited resources are available to address the technology component, more emphasis can be applied to the task component, thus balancing the model as a whole.

REFERENCES

Battles JB, Keyes MA: Technology and patient safety: a two-edged sword, *Biomed Instrum Technol* 36(2):84–88, 2002.

Brennan TA, et al: Incidence of adverse events and negligence in hospitalized patients: results of the Harvard medical practice study I, 1991, *Qual Saf Health Care* 13(2):145–151, 2004.

Carayon P, Smith MJ: Work organization and ergonomics, *Appl Ergon* 31:649–662, 2000.

Carbonara P: *Hire for attitude, train for skill*, 1996, available at http://www.starttogether.org/docs/hiring.pdf. Accessed July 9, 2008.

Catchpole K, et al: Teamwork and error in the operating room: analysis of skills and roles, *Ann Surg* 247:699–706, 2008.

Christian CK, et al: A prospective study of patient safety in the operating room, *Surgery* 139:159–173, 2006.

Edmonson AC: Learning from failure in health care: frequent opportunities, pervasive barriers, *Qual Saf Health Care* 13(Suppl 2):ii3–ii9, 2004.

Gaba DM, Howard SK: Patient safety: fatigue among clinicians and the safety of patients, *N Engl J Med* 347:1249–1255, 2002.

Gawande AA, et al: Analysis of errors reported by surgeons at three teaching hospitals, *Surgery* 133:614–621, 2003.

HealthGrades, Inc.: *Third annual patient safety in American hospitals study*, April 2006, available at http://www.healthgrades.com/media/dms/pdf/patientsafetyinamericanhospitalsstudy2006.pdf. Accessed June 18, 2008.

Human Factors and Ergonomic Society: n.d., available at http://www.hfes.org/WEB/AboutHFES/about.html. Accessed June 11, 2008.

Institute for Healthcare Improvement: n.d., available at http://www.ihi.org/IHI/Topics/Improvement/ImprovementMethods/Tools/Flowchart.htm. Accessed on June 19, 2008.

Kohn LT, et al: *To err is human: building a safer health system*, Washington, DC, 2000, National Academy Press.

Kukla CD, et al: Designing effective systems: a tool approach. In Adler P, Winogard T, editors: *Usability: turning technology into tools*, New York, 1992, Oxford University Press.

Lawton R, Parker D: Barriers to incident reporting in a healthcare system, *Qual Saf Health Care* 11:15–18, 2002.

Leape L: Error in medicine, *JAMA* 242:1851–1857, 1994.

Page A, et al: *Keeping patients safe: transforming the work environment of nurses*, Washington, DC, 2009, National Academies Press, available at http://www.nap.edu/openbook/0309090679/html/1.html. Accessed December 2, 2009.

Perspectives on safety: in conversation with Bryan Sexton: n.d., available at http://www.webmm.ahrq.gov/perspective.aspx?perspectiveID=34. Accessed June 14, 2008.

Rogers SO Jr, et al. Analysis of surgical errors in closed malpractice claims at 4 liability insurers, *Surgery* 140:25–33, 2006.

Rosekind M, et al: Managing fatigue in operational settings. II. An integrated approach, *Hosp Top* 75:31–35, 1997.

Sexton JB, et al: Error, stress, and teamwork in medicine and aviation: cross sectional surveys, *BMJ* 320(7237):745–749, 2000.

Sexton JB, et al: The safety attitudes questionnaire: psychometric properties, benchmarking data, and emerging research, *BMC Health Serv Res* 6:44, 2006.

Smith MJ, Sainfort PC: A balance theory of job design for stress reduction, *Int J Ind Ergon* 4:67–79, 1989.

Weick KE, Sutcliffe KM: *Managing the unexpected*, San Francisco, 2001, Jossey-Bass.

Weigmann DA, et al: Disruptions in surgical flow and their relationship to surgical errors: an exploratory investigation, *Surgery* 142:658–665, 2007.

World Alliance for Patient Safety: *World Health Organizaton (WHO) surgical safety checklist*, Geneva, Switzerland, 2008, WHO, available at http://www.who.int/patientsafety/safesurgery/ss_checklist/en/index.html. Accessed December 2, 2009.

World Health Organization: *Safe surgery saves lives*, 2008 available at http://www.who.int/patientsafety/safesurgery/en/. Accessed June 17, 2008.

Yourstone SA, Smith HL: Managing system errors and failures in health care organizations: suggestions for practice and research, *Health Care Manage Rev* 27:50–61, 2002.

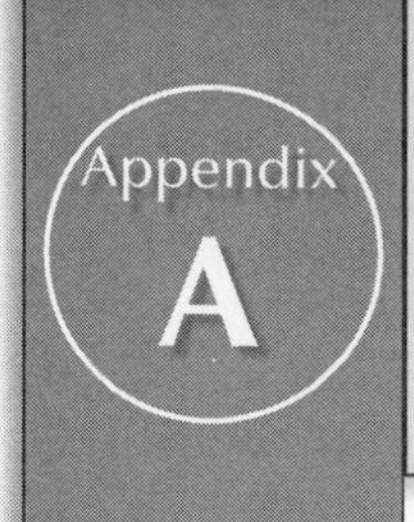

SAMPLE SURGICAL COUNT POLICY AND PROCEDURE PERIOPERATIVE PATIENT CARE SERVICES POLICY AND PROCEDURE

SUBJECT: Counts, Surgical: Sponge, Sharps, and Instruments

SCOPE: Perioperative Patient Care Services

PURPOSE

To prevent the unintentional retention of a foreign body (e.g., sponge, sharp, or instrument) when the patient leaves the operating room (OR).

RESPONSIBILITY

All members of the surgical team (e.g., registered nurse, surgical technologist, and surgeon).

POLICY

1. A sponge, sharps, and designated miscellaneous item count is performed for all procedures.

Designated miscellaneous items include, but are not limited to, the following:

Antifogging solution and sponge	Penrose drain
Bulldog clamps	Rubber shods
Cautery scratch pads	Safety pins
Cautery tips	Stapler reloads
Fogarty inserts	Suture booties
Hemoclip cartridges	Throat packs
Knitter dissector	Vaginal packs
Laparotomy sponge rings	Vessel loops
Linen shod	

Also include in the count any other small item(s) (e.g., adapters or wing nuts) that have the potential for being retained in the surgical wound.

Exceptions for required counts are the following:

- When procuring cadaveric donor organs, perform an initial and final count.
- In extreme emergencies when the time required to conduct a surgical count may jeopardize the patient's life, all counts are aborted. An occurrence report will be completed, and an x-ray film of the surgical wound will be taken before the patient leaves the OR.
- Instrument counts may be omitted for orthopedic and other procedures when fluoroscopy is used to scan the cavity for retained items before beginning the closure of the cavity. The surgeon of record will document in the immediate postoperative note that no inadvertent retained foreign bodies were noted on fluoroscopic evaluation of the surgical cavity or area.

2. All instruments, sponges, sharps, and designated miscellaneous items are counted when the following body cavities are entered:
   - Abdominal
   - Mediastinal
   - Pelvic
   - Retroperitoneal
   - Thoracic

This includes endoscopic minimally invasive surgery involving those cavities for which an instrument count is indicated when the possibility exists of an "open" procedure or the depth or location of the wound is such that an instrument could be left in the patient.

3. Incorrect counts necessitate that the surgeon explore the wound while a search for items on and off the sterile field is conducted by nursing.
   a. An x-ray film of the surgical site must be taken and read as negative for retained foreign body before the drapes are removed and before the instrument table is broken down.
   b. An x-ray film is not warranted for missing needles that are less than or equal to 17 mm; studies have demonstrated that suture needles 17 mm and smaller may not be detectable on x-ray examination.
   c. All incorrect or unresolved counts necessitate an occurrence report.
4. Radiopaque towels will be used on all open chest and abdominal procedures (i.e., intracavity procedures) and included in the surgical count using the counting process as described for sponges.

PROCEDURES

General Procedures for Counting

1. Counts will be performed in the same sequence each time.
   a. The count begins at the surgical site and the immediate surrounding areas, proceeds to the Mayo stand, back table, and finally to items that have been discarded from the field.
2. Perform all counts audibly, and have them reviewed concurrently by the registered nurse (RN) circulator and scrub person.
3. Remove any package containing an incorrect number of sponges from the field; bag, label, and isolate them from the rest of the sponges in the room.
4. On multiple procedures, which require separate table setups, perform a separate count for each operative site and record separately on the count sheet and/or whiteboard.
5. Whenever possible, only x-ray-detectable items will be used during a counted operative procedure.
6. Dressing sponges (i.e., non–x-ray-detectable sponges) will not be placed on the sterile field until the final sponge count is completed.
7. Disassembled, cut, or broken instruments, needles, or other items (e.g., red rubber catheters) must be accounted for in their entirety, including all parts of the instrument(s) or item disassembled.
   a. Verify that all pieces of disassembled or broken item(s) or instrument(s) are part of the count and tracked on the count sheet and/or whiteboard during the procedure.
8. Do not remove ANY countable items, linen, or trash (e.g., waste containers) from the room until ALL counts are completed and/or resolved.
9. Items not visible after draping and/or items placed within a cavity (e.g., throat pack) are noted on the count sheet and/or whiteboard (e.g., four towel clips).
10. Perform subsequent counts at the following times:
    a. When additional sponges, sharps, or other countable items are added to the sterile field.
    b. As wound closure begins.
    c. Upon permanent relief of the scrub person a full surgical count (i.e., instruments, sponges, sharps, and designated miscellaneous items) is performed.
    d. At skin closure or end of procedure.
    e. When requested by the scrub person, circulator, and/or surgeon.
    f. Before closure of a cavity within a cavity (e.g., closure of the uterus) an instrument count is not required.
    g. Upon permanent relief of the circulator, instrument counts are not required.
11. Empty suture packs will remain accessible to the scrub person and will not be discarded until the final count is resolved or the search for a missing needle has stopped.
    a. Empty suture packs may be used as an immediate reference but may not be used to resolve the needle count.
    b. Do not discard empty suture packs inside the garbage bag on the field. It is below the sterile field, and it is an occupational risk to retrieve items after discarding.
12. If the count is interrupted, the count for those items must be restarted.
13. The circulating RN is responsible for notifying the surgeon of the outcome of all counts whether correct or incorrect.
    a. If a count is incorrect, the steps under incorrect counts are followed.

Additional Count Procedures

The following specific count procedures will be performed in addition to the general procedures for counting as outlined earlier in this document.

1. Sponges
   a. Remove packaging band before counting packs of sponges.
   b. Separate sponges when counting.
   c. Count sponges in units of 5 or 10, according to packaging.
   d. Radiopaque towels will be counted in units of 4.
   e. Remove from the operative field packages of sponges that contain more or less than expected packaged number.
   f. Maintain knowledge of location of sponges on the sterile field.
   g. Record running total of all sponges on the count sheet and/or whiteboard throughout the procedure.
   h. Discard used sponges in plastic-lined kick bucket.

i. Fully open discarded sponges to properly visualize them.
j. Count discarded sponges before bagging.
k. Place counted sponges in clear plastic bag in groups of 5 or 10 as they accumulate.

2. Radiopaque towels will be counted using the process outlined above for sponges in multiples of 4 on all open intracavity procedures of the chest and/or abdomen.
3. Sharps
   a. Count suture needles according to the number indicated on the package.
   b. Verify the number of suture needles with the circulating nurse when the package is opened.
   c. Place used needles, blades, and hypodermic needles on a needle pad or counter.
   d. Maintain knowledge of location of sharps on the sterile field.
   e. Hand needles to the surgeon on an exchange basis when possible.
   f. Account for all pieces of broken sharps.
   g. Record total number of knife blades and hypodermic needles as separate counts from the total number of suture needles.
   h. Record a running total of all needles on the count sheet and/or whiteboard throughout the procedure.
   i. In the event a needle less than or equal to 17 mm is missing, a radiologic film of the operative site is not indicated, yet an occurrence report is warranted.
4. Instruments
   a. Maintain knowledge of location of instruments on and off the field.
   b. Isolate and account for all pieces of broken instruments.
   c. Any instruments not visible (e.g., towel clips) during the closing count are recorded on the count sheet and/or whiteboard and verbally counted, as well as visualized, at the end of the case when the drapes are removed and the instruments are retrieved.
5. Incorrect Counts
   a. Notify the surgeon of incorrect count, and recount.
   b. Search for lost items on and off the sterile field (e.g., field, floor, trash, and laundry).
   c. Notify charge nurse so extra assistance may be provided.
   d. In the event of an incorrect recount, the surgeon will explore the surgical wound.
   e. If the count has not been resolved, immediately request a plain radiographic film of the surgical site while the patient remains in the OR.
      (1) In the event a needle less than or equal to 17 mm is missing, a radiologic film of the operative site is not indicated, yet an occurrence report is warranted.
   f. The patient must remain in the OR under anesthesia until the surgeon or radiologist has read the film and confirmed the findings to the surgical team.
      (1) The operative surgeon will include the findings of the film in the immediate postoperative note.
   g. Complete an occurrence report.
   h. Document the respective count as incorrect on the operative record.
6. Packing

   If counted sponges are intentionally used for postoperative packing (e.g., abdomen, chest) and the patient leaves the OR with this packing in place, perform the following:
   a. Document the number, location, and type of packing (e.g., sponges) on the operative record in the nursing notes.
   b. Complete an occurrence report noting location, type, and number of items packed into the surgical wound.
   c. Document the count on the operative record as correct, given that all sponges are accounted for as documented in 6a and 6b above.
7. Removal of Packing

   In the event the patient returns to the OR for packing removal-closure, perform the following:
   a. Number and type of packing (e.g., retained sponges) removed are documented on the operative record as part of the procedure or in the nurses' notes.
   b. Circulating nurse is responsible for confirming the number, location, and type of packing against the documentation when it was placed as described in 6a and 6b above.
   c. If the number, type, and location of the packing removed are the same as the number, type, and location of the packing placed, the count is considered correct. If the number removed differs from the number packed, then the count is considered incorrect and the process for an incorrect count is followed.

d. Complete an occurrence report describing the number, type, and location of packing removed.

DOCUMENTATION

1. Documentation of counts on the perioperative record includes the type of count performed, names of the personnel completing the count, and the results of the final count.
2. In the event any counted item is removed from the room (e.g., dropped needle, put in needle box or sharps container, clamp), it will be subtracted from the count worksheet and/or whiteboard.

STATEMENT OF COLLABORATION

Perioperative Nursing, Surgery, Labor and Delivery, Patient Safety/Risk Management, Department of Radiology.

REFERENCES

Association of periOperative Registered Nurses: *Perioperative nursing data set*, ed 2, Denver, 2002, The Association.

Association of periOperative Registered Nurses: Recommended practices for sponge, sharp and instrument counts. In Association of periOperative Registered Nurses: *Perioperative standards and recommended practices*, Denver, 2008, The Association.

Association of periOperative Registered Nurses: *AORN position statement on orientation of the registered professional nurse to the perioperative setting*, April 2005, available at: http://www.aorn.org/PracticeResources/AORNPositionStatements/Position_OrientationOfTheRegisteredProfessionalNur/. Accessed December 21, 2009.

Association of periOperative Registered Nurses: *AORN position statement on safe work/on-call practices*, March 2008, available at: http://www.aorn.org/PracticeResources/AORNPositionStatements/Position_SafeWorkOnCallPractices/. Accessed December 21, 2009.

Egorova NN, et al: Managing the prevention of retained surgical instruments: what is the value of counting? *Ann Surg* 247(1):13–18, 2008.

Gawande A, et al: Risk factors for retained instruments and sponges after surgery, *N Engl J Med* 348(3):228–235, 2003.

King CA: To count or not to count: a surgical misadventure, *Perioper Nurs Clin* 3(4):395–400, 2008.

Macilquham MD, et al: Identifying lost surgical needles using radiographic techniques, *AORN J* 78(1):73–78, 2003.

Milter, et al: Catastrophes, sleep, and public policy: consensus report, *Sleep* 11(1):100–109, 1988.

Patterson P: How ORs decide when to count instruments, *OR Manager* 16(4):1–14, 2000.

Ponrartana S, et al: Accuracy of plain abdominal radiographs in the detection of retained surgical needles in the peritoneal cavity, *Ann Surg* 247(1):8–12, 2008.

Rothrock JC: *Alexander's care of the patient in surgery*, ed 12, Philadelphia, 2003, Mosby.

Wachter RM: *Understanding patient safety*, New York, 2008,McGraw Hill.

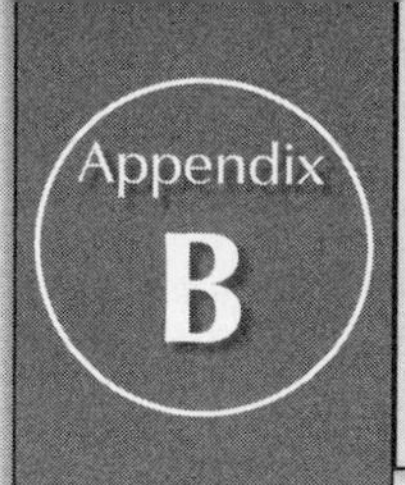

2007 GUIDELINE FOR ISOLATION PRECAUTIONS: PREVENTING TRANSMISSION OF INFECTIOUS AGENTS IN HEALTH CARE SETTINGS

The mode(s) and risk for transmission for each specific disease agent included in Appendix B were reviewed. Principal sources consulted for the development of disease-specific recommendations for Appendix B included infectious disease manuals and textbooks (Mandell et al, 2000; COID, 2003; Heymann, 2005). The published literature was searched for evidence of person-to-person transmission in health care and non–health care settings with a focus on reported outbreaks that would assist in developing recommendations for all settings where health care is delivered. Criteria used to assign transmission-based precautions categories follow:

A transmission-based precautions category was assigned if there was strong evidence for person-to-person transmission via droplet, contact, or airborne routes in health care or non–health care settings and/or if patient factors (e.g., diapered infants, diarrhea, draining wounds) increased the risk for transmission.

Transmission-based precautions category assignments reflect the predominant mode(s) of transmission.

If there was no evidence for person-to-person transmission by droplet, contact, or airborne routes, standard precautions were assigned.

If there was a low risk for person-to-person transmission and no evidence of health care–associated transmission, standard precautions were assigned.

Standard precautions were assigned for blood-borne pathogens (e.g., hepatitis B and C viruses, human immunodeficiency virus) as per Centers for Disease Control and Prevention (CDC) (1988) recommendations for universal precautions issued in 1988. Subsequent experience has confirmed the efficacy of standard precautions to prevent exposure to infected blood and body fluid (CDC, 2001b; Occupationally acquired human immunodeficiency virus [HIV] infection, 2003; CDC, 2005d).

Additional information relevant to use of precautions was added in the comments column to assist the caregiver in decision making. Citations were added as needed to support a change in or provide additional evidence for recommendations for a specific disease and for new infectious agents (e.g., SARS-CoV, avian influenza) that have been added to Appendix B.

REFERENCES

Abulrahi HA, et al: *Plasmodium falciparum* malaria transmitted in hospital through heparin locks, *Lancet* 349(9044):23–25, 1997.

Al-Saigul AM, et al: Nosocomial malaria from contamination of a multidose heparin container with blood, *Infect Control Hosp Epidemiol* 21(5):329–330, 2000.

Ammari LK, et al: Secondary measles vaccine failure in healthcare workers exposed to infected patients, *Infect Control Hosp Epidemiol* 814(2):81–86, 1993.

Arvin A, Whitley R: Herpes simplex virus infections. In Remington JS, Klein JO, editors: *Infectious diseases of the fetus and newborn infant*, ed 5, Philadelphia, 2001, Saunders.

Barker J, et al: Effects of cleaning and disinfection in reducing the spread of norovirus contamination via environmental surfaces, *J Hosp Infect* 58(1):42–49, 2004.

Behrman A, et al: A cluster of primary varicella cases among healthcare workers with false-positive varicella zoster virus titers, *Infect Control Hosp Epidemiol* 24(3):202–206, 2003.

Beyt BE Jr, Waltman SR: Cryptococcal endophthalmitis after corneal transplantation, *N Engl J Med* 298(15):825–826, 1978.

Bolyard EA, et al: Guideline for infection control in healthcare personnel, 1998, Hospital Infection Control Practices Advisory Committee, *Infect Control Hosp Epidemiol* 19(6):407–463, 1998.

Book LS, et al: Clustering of necrotizing enterocolitis: interruption by infection-control measures, *N Engl J Med* 297(18):984–986, 1977.

Borio L, et al: Hemorrhagic fever viruses as biological weapons: medical and public health management, *JAMA* 287(18):2391–2405, 2002.

Brooks S, et al: Reduction in vancomycin-resistant *Enterococcus* and *Clostridium difficile* infections following change to tympanic thermometers, *Infect Control Hosp Epidemiol* 19(5):333–336, 1998.

APPENDIX B Type and Duration of Precautions Recommended for Selected Infections and Conditions

Infection/Condition	PRECAUTIONS Type*	Duration†	Comments
Abscess			
Draining, major	C	DI	Use no dressing or containment of drainage until drainage stops or can be contained by dressing.
Draining, minor or limited	S		Dressing covers and contains drainage.
Acquired human immunodeficiency syndrome (HIV)	S		Provide postexposure chemoprophylaxis for some blood exposures (CDC, 2005d).
Actinomycosis	S		Not transmitted from person to person
Adenovirus infection (see agent-specific guidance under gastroenteritis, conjunctivitis, pneumonia)			
Amebiasis	S		Person-to-person transmission is rare. Transmission in settings for the mentally challenged and in a family group has been reported (Vreden et al, 2000). Use care when handling diapered infants and mentally challenged persons (Thacker et al, 1981).
Anthrax	S		Infected patients do not generally pose a transmission risk.
Cutaneous	S		Transmission through nonintact skin contact with draining lesions is possible, therefore use contact precautions if there is a large amount of uncontained drainage. Hand washing with soap and water is preferable to use of waterless alcohol-based antiseptics because alcohol does not have sporicidal activity (Weber et al, 2003).
Pulmonary	S		Not transmitted from person to person
Environmental: aerosolizable spore-containing powder or other substance		DE	Until decontamination of environment is complete (Inglesby et al, 2002). Wear respirator (N95 mask or PAPRs), protective clothing; decontaminate persons with powder on them (http://www.cdc.gov/mmwr/preview/mmwrhtml/mm5135a3.htm) **Hand hygiene**: Hand washing for 30–60 seconds with soap and water or 2% chlorhexidine gluconate after spore contact (alcohol hand rubs inactive against spores) (Weber et al, 2003) **Postexposure prophylaxis following environmental exposure**: 60days of antimicrobials (either doxycycline, ciprofloxacin, or levofloxacin) and postexposure vaccine under IND
Antibiotic-associated colitis (see *Clostridium difficile*)			

Continued

APPENDIX B Type and Duration of Precautions Recommended for Selected Infections and Conditions—cont'd

Infection/Condition	PRECAUTIONS Type*	Duration†	Comments
Arthropod-borne viral encephalitides (eastern, western, Venezuelan equine encephalomyelitis; St. Louis, California encephalitis; West Nile virus) and viral fevers (dengue, yellow fever, Colorado tick fever)	S		Not transmitted from person to person except rarely by transfusion, and for West Nile virus by organ transplant, breast milk or transplacentally (Sampathkumar, 2003; CDC, 2005e). Install screens in windows and doors in endemic areas. Use DEET-containing mosquito repellants and clothing to cover extremities.
Ascariasis	S		Not transmitted from person to person
Aspergillosis	S		Use contact precautions and airborne precautions if there is massive soft tissue infection with copious drainage and repeated irrigations are required (Pegues et al, 2002).
Avian influenza (see influenza, avian)			
Babesiosis	S		Not transmitted from person to person except rarely by transfusion
Blastomycosis, North American, cutaneous, or pulmonary	S		Not transmitted from person to person
Botulism	S		Not transmitted from person to person
Bronchiolitis (see respiratory infections in infants and young children)	C	DI	Use mask according to standard precautions.
Brucellosis (undulant, Malta, Mediterranean fever)	S		Not transmitted from person to person except rarely via banked spermatozoa and sexual contact (Vandercam et al, 1990; Ruben et al, 1991). Provide antimicrobial prophylaxis following laboratory exposure (Robichaud et al, 2004).
Campylobacter gastroenteritis (see gastroenteritis)			
Candidiasis, all forms, including mucocutaneous	S		
Cat-scratch fever (benign inoculation lymphoreticulosis)	S		Not transmitted from person to person
Cellulitis	S		

Chancroid (soft chancre) *(Haemophilus ducreyi)*	S		Transmitted sexually from person to person
Chickenpox (see varicella)			
Chlamydia trachomatis			
Conjunctivitis	S		
Genital (lymphogranuloma venereum)	S		
Pneumonia (infants ≤3 mo of age)	S		
Chlamydia pneumoniae	S		Outbreaks in institutionalized populations have been reported, rarely (Ekman et al, 1993; Troy et al, 1997).
Cholera (see gastroenteritis)			
Closed-cavity infection			
Open drain in place; limited or minor drainage	S		Use contact precautions if there is copious uncontained drainage.
No drain or closed drainage system in place	S		
Clostridium			
C. botulinum	S		Not transmitted from person to person
C. difficile (see gastroenteritis, *C. difficile*)	C	DI	
C. perfringens			
Food poisoning	S		Not transmitted from person to person
Gas gangrene	S		Transmission from person to person is rare; one outbreak in a surgical setting has been reported (Eickhoff, 1962). Use contact precautions if wound drainage is extensive.
Coccidioidomycosis (valley fever)			
Draining lesions	S		Not transmitted from person to person except under extraordinary circumstances because the infectious arthroconidial form of *Coccidioides immitis* is not produced in humans (Kohn et al, 1992).
Pneumonia	S		Not transmitted from person to person except under extraordinary circumstances (e.g., inhalation of aerosolized tissue-phase endospores during necropsy, transplantation of infected lung) because the infectious arthroconidial form of *C. immitis* is not produced in humans (Kohn et al, 1992; Wright et al, 2003).

Continued

APPENDIX B Type and Duration of Precautions Recommended for Selected Infections and Conditions—cont'd

Infection/Condition	PRECAUTIONS Type*	Duration†	Comments
Colorado tick fever	S		Not transmitted from person to person
Congenital rubella	C	Until 1 yr of age	Use standard precautions if nasopharyngeal and urine cultures are repeatedly negative after 3 mo of age.
Conjunctivitis			
Acute bacterial	S		
Chlamydial	S		
Gonococcal	S		
Acute viral (acute hemorrhagic)	C	DI	Adenovirus is most common; enterovirus 70 (Maitreyi et al, 1999) and Coxsackie virus A24 (CDC, 2004) are also associated with community outbreaks. It is highly contagious; outbreaks in eye clinics, pediatric and neonatal settings, and institutional settings have been reported. Eye clinics should follow standard precautions when handling patients with conjunctivitis. Routine use of infection control measures in the handling of instruments and equipment will prevent the occurrence of outbreaks in this and other settings (Warren et al, 1989; Buffington et al, 1993; Jernigan et al, 1993; Montessori et al, 1998; Chaberny et al, 2003; Faden et al, 2005).
Coronavirus associated with SARS (SARS-CoV) (see severe acute respiratory syndrome)			
Coxsackie virus disease (see enteroviral infection)			
Creutzfeldt-Jakob disease (CJD, vCJD)	S		Use disposable instruments or special sterilization/disinfection for surfaces and objects contaminated with neural tissue if CJD or vCJD is suspected and has not been ruled out. No special burial procedures (http://www.cdc.gov/ncidod/dvrd/cjd/qa_cjd_infection_control.htm)
Crimean-Congo fever (see viral hemorrhagic fever)	S		
Croup (see respiratory infections in infants and young children)			
Cryptococcosis	S		Not transmitted from person to person, except rarely via tissue and corneal transplant (Beyt and Waltman, 1978; Wang et al, 2005)

Cryptosporidiosis (see gastroenteritis)			
Cysticercosis	S		Not transmitted from person to person
Cytomegalovirus infection, including in neonates and immunosuppressed patients	S		No additional precautions for pregnant HCWs
Decubitus ulcer (see pressure ulcer)			
Dengue fever	S		Not transmitted from person to person
Diarrhea, acute-infective etiology suspected (see gastroenteritis)			
Diphtheria			
Cutaneous	C	CN	Until two cultures taken 24 hr apart are negative
Pharyngeal	D	CN	Until two cultures taken 24 hr apart are negative
Ebola virus (see viral hemorrhagic fevers)			
Echinococcosis (hydatidosis)	S		Not transmitted from person to person
Echovirus (see enteroviral infections)			
Encephalitis or encephalomyelitis (see specific etiologic agents)			
Endometritis (endomyometritis)	S		
Enterobiasis (pinworm disease, oxyuriasis)	S		
Enterococcus species (see multidrug-resistant organisms if epidemiologically significant or vancomycin resistant)			
Enterocolitis, *C. difficile* (see gastroenteritis, *C. difficile*)			
Enteroviral infections (i.e., group A and B Coxsackie viruses and echoviruses) (excludes poliovirus)	S		Use contact precautions for diapered or incontinent children for duration of illness and to control institutional outbreaks.
Epiglottitis, due to *Haemophilus influenzae* type b	D	U 24 hr	See specific disease agents for epiglottitis due to other causes.

Continued

APPENDIX B Type and Duration of Precautions Recommended for Selected Infections and Conditions—cont'd

Infection/Condition	PRECAUTIONS Type*	Duration†	Comments
Epstein-Barr virus infection, including infectious mononucleosis	S		
Erythema infectiosum (also see parvovirus B19)			
Escherichia coli gastroenteritis (see gastroenteritis)			
Food poisoning			
Botulism	S		Not transmitted from person to person
C. perfringens or *Clostridium welchii*	S		Not transmitted from person to person
Staphylococcal	S		Not transmitted from person to person
Furunculosis, staphylococcal	S		Use contact precautions if drainage is not controlled. Follow institutional policies if MRSA.
Infants and young children	C	DI	
Gangrene (gas gangrene)	S		Not transmitted from person to person
Gastroenteritis	S		Use contact precautions for diapered or incontinent persons for the duration of illness or to control institutional outbreaks of gastroenteritis caused by all of the agents below.
Adenovirus	S		Use contact precautions for diapered or incontinent persons for the duration of illness or to control institutional outbreaks.
Campylobacter species	S		Use contact precautions for diapered or incontinent persons for the duration of illness or to control institutional outbreaks.
Cholera *(Vibrio cholerae)*	S		Use contact precautions for diapered or incontinent persons for the duration of illness or to control institutional outbreaks.
C. difficile	C	DI	Discontinue antibiotics if appropriate. Do not share electronic thermometers (Brooks et al, 1998; Jernigan et al, 1998); ensure consistent environmental cleaning and disinfection. Hypochlorite solutions may be required for cleaning if transmission continues (Wilcox et al, 2003). Hand washing with soap and water is preferred because of the absence of sporicidal activity of alcohol in waterless antiseptic hand rubs (Weber et al, 2003).
Cryptosporidium species	S		Use contact precautions for diapered or incontinent persons for the duration of illness or to control institutional outbreaks.

E. coli			
Enteropathogenic O157:H7 and other Shiga toxin–producing strains	S		Use contact precautions for diapered or incontinent persons for the duration of illness or to control institutional outbreaks.
Other species	S		Use contact precautions for diapered or incontinent persons for the duration of illness or to control institutional outbreaks.
Giardia lamblia	S		Use contact precautions for diapered or incontinent persons for the duration of illness or to control institutional outbreaks.
Noroviruses	S		Use contact precautions for diapered or incontinent persons for the duration of illness or to control institutional outbreaks. Persons who clean areas heavily contaminated with feces or vomitus may benefit from wearing masks because virus can be aerosolized from these body substances (Sawyer et al, 1988; Cheesbrough et al, 2000; Marks et al, 2003); ensure consistent environmental cleaning and disinfection with focus on restrooms even when apparently unsoiled (CDC, 2001a; Widdowson et al, 2005). Hypochlorite solutions may be required when there is continued transmission (Doultree et al, 1999; Barker et al, 2004; Inactivation of caliciviruses, 2004). Alcohol is less active, but there is no evidence that alcohol antiseptic hand rubs are not effective for hand decontamination (Gehrke et al, 2004). Cohorting of affected patients to separate airspaces and toilet facilities may help interrupt transmission during outbreaks.
Rotavirus	C	DI	Ensure consistent environmental cleaning and disinfection and frequent removal of soiled diapers. Prolonged shedding may occur in both immunocompetent and immunocompromised children and older adults (Wood et al, 1988; Mori et al, 2002).
Salmonella species (including *S. typhi*)	S		Use contact precautions for diapered or incontinent persons for the duration of illness or to control institutional outbreaks.
Shigella species (bacillary dysentery)	S		Use contact precautions for diapered or incontinent persons for the duration of illness or to control institutional outbreaks.
Vibrio parahaemolyticus	S		Use contact precautions for diapered or incontinent persons for the duration of illness or to control institutional outbreaks.
Viral (if not covered elsewhere)	S		Use contact precautions for diapered or incontinent persons for the duration of illness or to control institutional outbreaks.
Yersinia enterocolitica	S		Use contact precautions for diapered or incontinent persons for the duration of illness or to control institutional outbreaks.

Continued

APPENDIX B Type and Duration of Precautions Recommended for Selected Infections and Conditions—cont'd

Infection/Condition	PRECAUTIONS Type*	Duration†	Comments
German measles (see rubella; see congenital rubella)			
Giardiasis (see gastroenteritis)			
Gonococcal ophthalmia neonatorum (gonorrheal ophthalmia, acute conjunctivitis of newborn)	S		
Gonorrhea	S		
Granuloma inguinale (donovanosis, granuloma venereum)	S		
Guillain-Barré syndrome	S		Not an infectious condition
Haemophilus influenzae (see disease-specific recommendations)			
Hand, foot, and mouth disease (see enteroviral infection)			
Hansen disease (see leprosy)			
Hantavirus pulmonary syndrome	S		Not transmitted from person to person
Helicobacter pylori	S		
Hepatitis, viral			
Type A	S		Provide hepatitis A vaccine post exposure as recommended (CDC, 1999b).
Diapered or incontinent patients	C		Maintain contact precautions in infants and children <3 yr of age for duration of hospitalization; for children 3–14 yr of age for 2 weeks after onset of symptoms; >14 yr of age for 1 week after onset of symptoms (Carl et al, 1982; Rosenblum et al, 1991; COID, 2003).
Type B—HBsAg positive; acute or chronic	S		See specific recommendations for care of patients in hemodialysis centers (CDC, 2001b).

Type C and other unspecified non-A, non-B	S		See specific recommendations for care of patients in hemodialysis centers (CDC, 2001b).
Type D (seen only with hepatitis B)	S		
Type E	S		Use contact precautions for diapered or incontinent individuals for the duration of illness. (Robson et al, 1992).
Type G	S		
Herpangina (see enteroviral infection)			
Herpes simplex (*Herpesvirus hominis*)			
Encephalitis	S		
Mucocutaneous, disseminated or primary, severe	C	Until lesions dry and crusted	
Mucocutaneous, recurrent (skin, oral, genital)	S		
Neonatal	C	Until lesions dry and crusted	Also use for asymptomatic, exposed infants delivered vaginally or by C-section and if mother has active infection and membranes have been ruptured for more than 4 to 6 hr until infant surface cultures obtained at 24–36 hr of age are negative after 48-hr incubation (Arvin and Whitley, 2001; Enright and Prober, 2002).
Herpes zoster (varicella zoster) (shingles)			
Disseminated disease in any patient Localized disease in immuno-compromised patient until disseminated infection ruled out	A,C	DI	Susceptible HCWs should not enter room if immune caregivers are available; there is no recommendation for protection of immune HCWs; there is no recommendation for type of protection (i.e., surgical mask or respirator) for susceptible HCWs.
Localized in patient with intact immune system with lesions that can be contained/covered	S	DI	Susceptible HCWs should not provide direct patient care when other immune caregivers are available.
Histoplasmosis	S		Not transmitted from person to person
Hookworm	S		

Continued

APPENDIX B Type and Duration of Precautions Recommended for Selected Infections and Conditions—cont'd

Infection/Condition	PRECAUTIONS Type*	Duration†	Comments
Human immunodeficiency virus (HIV)	S		Provide postexposure chemoprophylaxis for some blood exposures (CDC, 2005d).
Human metapneumovirus	C	DI	HAI has been reported (Esper et al, 2003), but route of transmission has not been established (Mejias et al, 2004). It is assumed to have contact transmission as for RSV because the viruses are closely related and have similar clinical manifestations and epidemiology. Wear masks according to standard precautions.
Impetigo	C	U 24 hr	
Infectious mononucleosis	S		
Influenza			
Human (seasonal influenza)	D	5 days except DI in immuno-compromised persons	Place in single-patient room when available or cohort; avoid placement with high-risk patients; mask patient when transported out of room; provide chemoprophylaxis/vaccine to control/prevent outbreaks (CDC, 2005b). Use gown and gloves according to standard precautions; this may be especially important in pediatric settings. Duration of precautions for immunocompromised patients cannot be defined; prolonged duration of viral shedding (i.e., for several weeks) has been observed; implications for transmission are unknown (Weinstock et al, 2003).
Avian (e.g., H5N1, H7, H9 strains)			See http://www.cdc.gov/flu/avian/professional/infect-control.htm for current avian influenza guidance.
Pandemic influenza (also a human influenza virus)	D	5 days from onset of symptoms	See http://www.pandemicflu.gov for current pandemic influenza guidance.
Kawasaki syndrome	S		Not an infectious condition
Lassa fever (see viral hemorrhagic fevers)			
Legionnaires' disease	S		Not transmitted from person to person
Leprosy	S		
Leptospirosis	S		Not transmitted from person to person
Lice			See http://www.cdc.gov/ncidod/dpd/parasites/lice/default.htm.

Head (pediculosis)	C	U 4 hr	
Body	S		Transmitted person to person through infested clothing; wear gown and gloves when removing clothing; bag and wash clothes according to CDC guidance above.
Pubic	S		Transmitted person to person through sexual contact
Listeriosis (*Listeria monocytogenes*)	S		Person-to-person transmission is rare; cross-transmission in neonatal settings has been reported (Farber et al, 1991; Schuchat et al, 1991; Pejaver et al, 1993; Colodner et al, 2003).
Lyme disease	S		Not transmitted from person to person
Lymphocytic choriomeningitis	S		Not transmitted from person to person
Lymphogranuloma venereum	S		
Malaria	S		Not transmitted from person to person except rarely through transfusion and through a failure to follow standard precautions during patient care (Abulrahi et al, 1997; Al-Saigul et al, 2000; Piro et al, 2001; Jain et al, 2005). Install screens in windows and doors in endemic areas. Use DEET-containing mosquito repellants and clothing to cover extremities.
Marburg virus disease (see viral hemorrhagic fevers)			
Measles (rubeola)	A	4 days after onset of rash; DI in immune compromised	Susceptible HCWs should not enter room if immune care providers are available; there is no recommendation for face protection for immune HCW; there is no recommendation for type of face protection for susceptible HCWs (i.e., mask or respirator) (Ammari et al, 1993; Behrman et al, 2003). For exposed susceptibles, provide postexposure vaccine within 72 hr or immune globulin within 6 days when available (Ruuskanen et al, 1978; Bolyard et al, 1998; CDC, 1998). Place exposed susceptible patients on airborne precautions, and exclude susceptible health care personnel from duty from day 5 after first exposure to day 21 after last exposure, regardless of postexposure vaccine (Bolyard et al, 1998).
Melioidosis, all forms	S		Not transmitted from person to person
Meningitis			
Aseptic (nonbacterial or viral; also see enteroviral infections)	S		Contact precautions for infants and young children
Bacterial, gram-negative enteric, in neonates	S		
Fungal	S		

Continued

APPENDIX B Type and Duration of Precautions Recommended for Selected Infections and Conditions—cont'd

Infection/Condition	PRECAUTIONS Type*	Duration†	Comments
H. influenzae, type b known or suspected	D	U 24 hr	
L. monocytogenes (see listeriosis)	S		
Neisseria meningitidis (meningococcal) known or suspected	D	U 24 hr	See meningococcal disease.
Streptococcus pneumoniae	S		
Mycobacterium tuberculosis	S		Concurrent, active pulmonary disease or draining cutaneous lesions may necessitate addition of contact and/or airborne precautions. For children, use airborne precautions until active tuberculosis is ruled out in visiting family members (see tuberculosis) (Munoz et al, 2002).
Other diagnosed bacterial	S		
Meningococcal disease: sepsis, pneumonia, meningitis	D	U 24 hr	Provide postexposure chemoprophylaxis for household contacts, HCWs exposed to respiratory secretions; provide postexposure vaccine only to control outbreaks (Bolyard et al, 1998; CDC, 2000).
Molluscum contagiosum	S		
Monkeypox	A,C	A—Until monkeypox confirmed and smallpox excluded C—Until lesions crusted	See http://www.cdc.gov/ncidod/monkeypox for most current recommendations. Transmission in hospital settings is unlikely (Fleischauer et al, 2005). Preexposure and postexposure smallpox vaccine is recommended for exposed HCWs.
Mucormycosis	S		
Multidrug-resistant organisms (MDROs), infection or colonization (e.g., MRSA, VRE, VISA/VRSA, ESBLs, resistant *S. pneumoniae*)	S/C		MDROs judged by the infection control program, based on local, state, regional, or national recommendations, to be of clinical and epidemiologic significance. Contact precautions recommended in settings with evidence of ongoing transmission, acute care settings with increased risk for transmission, or wounds that cannot be contained by dressings. See recommendations for management options in *Management of Multidrug-Resistant Organisms in Healthcare Settings* (2006). Contact state health department for guidance regarding new or emerging MDROs.

Mumps (infectious parotitis)	D	U 9 days	After onset of swelling; susceptible HCWs should not provide care if immune caregivers are available. NOTE: Recent assessment of outbreaks in healthy 18- to 24-year-olds has indicated that salivary viral shedding occurred early in the course of illness and that 5 days of isolation after onset of parotitis may be appropriate in community settings; however, the implications for health care personnel and high-risk patient populations remain to be clarified.
Mycobacteria, nontuberculosis (atypical)			Not transmitted person to person
Pulmonary	S		
Wound	S		
Mycoplasma pneumonia	D	DI	
Necrotizing enterocolitis	S		Use contact precautions when cases are clustered temporally (Book et al, 1977; Rotbart and Levin, 1983; Rotbart et al, 1983; Gerber et al, 1985).
Nocardiosis, draining lesions or other presentations	S		Not transmitted person to person
Norovirus (see gastroenteritis)			
Norwalk agent gastroenteritis (see gastroenteritis)			
Orf	S		
Parainfluenza virus infection, respiratory in infants and young children	C	DI	Viral shedding may be prolonged in immunosuppressed patients (Elizaga et al, 2001; Nichols et al, 2001). Reliability of antigen testing to determine when to remove patients with prolonged hospitalizations from contact precautions is uncertain.
Parvovirus B19 (erythema infectiosum)	D		Maintain precautions for duration of hospitalization when chronic disease occurs in an immunocompromised patient. For patients with transient aplastic crisis or red-cell crisis, maintain precautions for 7 days. Duration of precautions for immunosuppressed patients with persistently positive PCR has not been defined, but transmission has occurred (Lui et al, 2001).
Pediculosis (lice)	C	U 24 hr after treatment	

Continued

APPENDIX B Type and Duration of Precautions Recommended for Selected Infections and Conditions—cont'd

Infection/Condition	PRECAUTIONS Type*	Duration†	Comments
Pertussis (whooping cough)	D	U 5 days	Placement in single-patient room is preferred. Cohorting is an option. Provide postexposure chemoprophylaxis for household contacts and HCWs with prolonged exposure to respiratory secretions (CDC, 2005c). Recommendations for Tdap vaccine in adults are under development.
Pinworm infection (enterobiasis)	S		
Plague (*Yersinia pestis*)			
Bubonic	S		
Pneumonic	D	U 48 hr	Provide antimicrobial prophylaxis for exposed HCW (Kool, 2005).
Pneumonia			
Adenovirus	D, C	DI	Outbreaks in pediatric and institutional settings have been reported (Singh-Naz et al, 1993; Sanchez et al, 1997; Uemura et al, 2000; Hatherill et al, 2004). In immunocompromised hosts, extend duration of droplet and contact precautions due to prolonged shedding of virus (van Tol et al, 2005).
Bacterial not listed elsewhere (including gram-negative bacterial)	S		
Burkholderia cepacia patients with CF, including respiratory tract colonization	C	Unknown	Avoid exposure to other persons with CF; private room is preferred. Criteria for droplet and contact precautions have not been established. See CF Foundation guideline (Saiman and Siegel, 2003).
B. cepacia patients without CF (see multidrug-resistant organisms)			
Chlamydia	S		
Fungal	S		
H. influenzae, type b			
Adults	S		
Infants and children	D	U 24 hr	
Legionella spp.	S		
Meningococcal	D	U 24 hr	See meningococcal disease.

Multidrug-resistant bacteria (see multidrug-resistant organisms)			
Mycoplasma (primary atypical pneumonia)	D	DI	
Pneumococcal pneumonia	S		Use droplet precautions if there is evidence of transmission within a patient care unit or facility (Nuorti et al, 1998; Gleich et al, 2000; Carter et al, 2005; Fry et al, 2005).
Pneumocystis jiroveci (Pneumocystis carinii)	S		Avoid placement in the same room with an immunocompromised patient.
Staphylococcus aureus	S		For MRSA, see MDROs.
Streptococcus, group A			
Adults	D	U 24 hr	See streptococcal disease (group A streptococcus) below. Use contact precautions if skin lesions are present.
Infants and young children	D	U 24 hr	Use contact precautions if skin lesions are present.
Varicella zoster (see varicella zoster)			
Viral			
Adults	S		
Infants and young children (see respiratory infectious disease, acute, or specific viral agent)			
Poliomyelitis	C	DI	
Pressure ulcer (decubitus ulcer, pressure sore) infected			
Major	C	DI	If no dressing or containment of drainage, use until drainage stops or can be contained by dressing.
Minor or limited	S		Use if dressing covers and contains drainage.
Prion disease (see Creutzfeldt-Jakob disease)			
Psittacosis (ornithosis) *(Chlamydia psittaci)*	S		Not transmitted from person to person
Q fever	S		

Continued

APPENDIX B Type and Duration of Precautions Recommended for Selected Infections and Conditions—cont'd

Infection/Condition	PRECAUTIONS Type*	Duration†	Comments
Rabies	S		Person-to-person transmission is rare; transmission via corneal, tissue, and organ transplants has been reported (Houff et al, 1979; Srinivasan et al, 2005). If patient has bitten another individual or saliva has contaminated an open wound or mucous membrane, wash exposed area thoroughly and administer postexposure prophylaxis (CDC, 1999a).
Rat-bite fever (*Streptobacillus moniliformis* disease, *Spirillum minus* disease)	S		Not transmitted from person to person
Relapsing fever	S		Not transmitted from person to person
Resistant bacterial infection or colonization (see multidrug-resistant organisms)			
Respiratory infectious disease, acute (if not covered elsewhere)			
Adults	S		
Infants and young children	C	DI	
Respiratory syncytial virus infection, in infants, young children and immunocompromised adults	C	DI	Wear mask according to standard precautions (LeClair et al, 1987; Madge et al, 1992; Hall, 2000). In immunocompromised patients, extend the duration of contact precautions due to prolonged shedding (Hall et al, 1986). Reliability of antigen testing to determine when to remove patients with prolonged hospitalizations from contact precautions is uncertain.
Reye syndrome	S		Not an infectious condition
Rheumatic fever	S		Not an infectious condition
Rhinovirus	D	DI	Droplet is most important route of transmission (Dick et al, 1987; Hayden, 2004). Outbreaks have occurred in NICUs and LTCFs (Valenti et al, 1982; Chidekel et al, 1997; Louie et al, 2005). Add contact precautions if copious moist secretions and close contact are likely to occur (e.g., young infants) (COID, 2003; Musher, 2003).
Rickettsial fevers, tick-borne (Rocky Mountain spotted fever, tick-borne typhus fever)	S		Not transmitted from person to person except through transfusion, rarely

Rickettsialpox (vesicular rickettsiosis)	S		Not transmitted from person to person
Ringworm (dermatophytosis, dermatomycosis, tinea)	S		Rarely, outbreaks have occurred in health care settings (e.g., NICU [Drusin et al, 2000], rehabilitation hospital [Lewis and Lewis, 1997]). Use contact precautions for outbreak.
Ritter's disease (staphylococcal scalded skin syndrome)	C	DI	See staphylococcal disease, scalded skin syndrome below.
Rocky Mountain spotted fever	S		Not transmitted from person to person except through transfusion, rarely
Roseola infantum (exanthem subitum; caused by HHV-6)	S		
Rotavirus infection (see gastroenteritis)			
Rubella (German measles) (also see congenital rubella)	D	U 7 days after onset of rash	Susceptible HCWs should not enter room if immune caregivers are available. There is no recommendation for wearing face protection (e.g., a surgical mask) if immune. Pregnant women who are not immune should not care for these patients (Fliegel and Weinstein, 1982; Bolyard et al, 1998). Administer vaccine to nonpregnant susceptible individuals within 3 days of exposure. Place exposed susceptible patients on droplet precautions; exclude susceptible health care personnel from duty from day 5 after first exposure to day 21 after last exposure, regardless of postexposure vaccine.
Rubeola (see measles)			
Salmonellosis (see gastroenteritis)			
Scabies	C	U 24	
Scalded skin syndrome, staphylococcal	C	DI	See staphylococcal disease, scalded skin syndrome below.
Schistosomiasis (bilharziasis)	S		
Severe acute respiratory syndrome (SARS)	A, D, C	DI plus 10 days after resolution of fever, provided respiratory symptoms are absent or improving	Airborne precautions are preferred; use D if AIIR is unavailable. Use N95 or higher respiratory protection; use surgical mask if N95 is unavailable; use eye protection (goggles, face shield). Aerosol-generating procedures and "supershedders" have highest risk for transmission via small droplet nuclei and large droplets (Scales et al, 2003; Fowler et al, 2004; Loeb et al, 2004). Provide vigilant environmental disinfection (see http://www.cdc.gov/ncidod/sars).

Continued

APPENDIX B Type and Duration of Precautions Recommended for Selected Infections and Conditions—cont'd

Infection/Condition	PRECAUTIONS Type*	Duration†	Comments
Shigellosis (see gastroenteritis)			
Smallpox (variola; see vaccinia for management of vaccinated persons)	A, C	DI	Use precautions until all scabs have crusted and separated (3–4 weeks). Nonvaccinated HCWs should not provide care when immune HCWs are available; use N95 or higher respiratory protection for susceptible and successfully vaccinated individuals; postexposure vaccine provided within 4 days of exposure is protective (Dixon, 1948; Gelfand and Posch, 1971; Fenner et al, 1988; CDC, 2001c; Fulginiti et al, 2003).
Spirillum minor disease (rat-bite fever)	S		Not transmitted from person to person
Sporotrichosis	S		
Staphylococcal disease (*S. aureus*)			
Skin, wound, or burn			
Major	C	DI	No dressing or dressing does not contain drainage adequately
Minor or limited	S		Dressing covers and contains drainage adequately
Enterocolitis	S		Use contact precautions for diapered or incontinent children for duration of illness.
Multidrug-resistant (see multidrug-resistant organisms)			
Pneumonia	S		
Scalded skin syndrome	C	DI	Consider health care personnel as potential source of nursery, NICU outbreak (Saiman et al, 1998).
Toxic shock syndrome	S		
Streptobacillus moniliformis disease (rat-bite fever)	S		Not transmitted from person to person
Streptococcal disease (group A streptococcus)			
Skin, wound, or burn			
Major	C, D	U 24 hr	No dressing or dressing does not contain drainage adequately

Minor or limited	S		Dressing covers and contains drainage adequately
Endometritis (puerperal sepsis)	S		
Pharyngitis in infants and young children	D	U 24 hr	
Pneumonia	D	U 24 hr	
Scarlet fever in infants and young children	D	U 24 hr	
Serious invasive disease	D	U 24 hr	Outbreaks of serious invasive disease have occurred secondary to transmission among patients and health care personnel (Schwartz et al, 1992; Ramage et al, 1996; Kakis et al, 2002; O'Brien et al, 2002; Greene et al, 2005). Use contact precautions for draining wound as above; follow recommendation for antimicrobial prophylaxis in selected conditions (CDC, 2002).
Streptococcal disease (group B streptococcus), neonatal	S		
Streptococcal disease (not group A or B) unless covered elsewhere	S		
Multidrug-resistant (see multidrug-resistant organisms)			
Strongyloidiasis	S		
Syphilis			
Latent (tertiary) and seropositivity without lesions	S		
Skin and mucous membrane, including congenital, primary, secondary	S		
Tapeworm disease			
Hymenolepis nana	S		Not transmitted from person to person
Taenia solium (pork)	S		
Other	S		

Continued

APPENDIX B Type and Duration of Precautions Recommended for Selected Infections and Conditions—cont'd

Infection/Condition	PRECAUTIONS Type*	Duration†	Comments
Tetanus	S		Not transmitted from person to person
Tinea (e.g., dermatophytosis, dermatomycosis, ringworm)	S		Rare episodes of person-to-person transmission
Toxic shock syndrome (staphylococcal disease, streptococcal disease)	S		Use droplet precautions for the first 24 hours after implementation of antibiotic therapy if group A streptococcus is a likely cause.
Toxoplasmosis	S		Transmission from person to person is rare; vertical transmission from mother to child, transmission through organs and blood transfusion rare
Trachoma, acute	S		
Transmissible spongiform encephalopathy (see Creutzfeldt-Jakob disease [CJD, vCJD])			
Trench mouth (Vincent angina)	S		
Trichinosis	S		
Trichomoniasis	S		
Trichuriasis (whipworm disease)	S		
Tuberculosis *(M. tuberculosis)*			
Extrapulmonary, draining lesion	A, C		Discontinue precautions only when patient is improving clinically and drainage has ceased or there are three consecutive negative cultures of continued drainage (Hutton et al, 1990; Frampton, 1992). Examine for evidence of active pulmonary tuberculosis.
Extrapulmonary, no draining lesion, meningitis	S		Examine for evidence of pulmonary tuberculosis. For infants and children, use airborne precautions until active pulmonary tuberculosis in visiting family members is ruled out (Munoz et al, 2002).
Pulmonary or laryngeal disease, confirmed	A		Discontinue precautions only when patient on effective therapy is improving clinically and has three consecutive sputum smears negative for acid-fast bacilli collected on separate days (http://www.cdc.gov/mmwr/preview/mmwrhtml/rr5417a1.htm?s_cid=rr5417a1_e) (CDC, 2005a).

Pulmonary or laryngeal disease, suspected	A		Discontinue precautions only when the likelihood of infectious tuberculosis disease is deemed negligible and either (1) there is another diagnosis that explains the clinical syndrome or (2) the results of three sputum smears for AFB are negative. Each of the three sputum specimens should be collected 8–24 hr apart, and at least one should be an early morning specimen.
Skin-test positive with no evidence of current active disease	S		
Tularemia			
Draining lesion	S		Not transmitted from person to person
Pulmonary	S		Not transmitted from person to person
Typhoid *(Salmonella typhi)* fever (see gastroenteritis)			
Typhus			
Rickettsia prowazekii (epidemic or louse-borne typhus)	S		Transmitted from person to person through close personal or clothing contact
Rickettsia typhi	S		Not transmitted from person to person
Urinary tract infection (including pyelonephritis), with or without urinary catheter	S		
Vaccinia (vaccination site, adverse events following vaccination)*			Only vaccinated HCWs have contact with active vaccination sites and care for persons with adverse vaccinia events; if unvaccinated, only HCWs without contraindications to vaccine may provide care.
Vaccination site care (including autoinoculated areas)	S		Vaccination recommended for vaccinators; for newly vaccinated HCWs: use semipermeable dressing over gauze until scab separates, with dressing change as fluid accumulates, ~3–5 days; use gloves, hand hygiene for dressing change; vaccinated HCW or HCW without contraindication to vaccine provides care for dressing changes (http://www.bt.cdc.gov/agent/smallpox/; Wharton et al, 2003; Talbot et al, 2004).
Eczema vaccinatum	C	Until lesions dry and crusted, scabs separated	For contact with virus-containing lesions and exudative material
Fetal vaccinia	C		
Generalized vaccinia	C		
Progressive vaccinia	C		

Continued

APPENDIX B Type and Duration of Precautions Recommended for Selected Infections and Conditions—cont'd

Infection/Condition	PRECAUTIONS Type*	Duration†	Comments
Postvaccinia encephalitis	S		
Blepharitis or conjunctivitis	S/C		Use contact precautions if there is copious drainage.
Iritis or keratitis	S		
Vaccinia-associated erythema multiforme (Stevens-Johnson syndrome)	S		Not an infectious condition
Secondary bacterial infection (e.g., *S. aureus*, group A beta hemolytic streptococcus	S/C		Follow organism-specific (strep, staph most frequent) recommendations, and consider magnitude of drainage.
Varicella zoster	A, C	Until lesions dry and crusted	Susceptible HCWs should not enter room if immune caregivers are available; there is no recommendation for face protection of immune HCWs; there is no recommendation for type of protection (i.e., surgical mask or respirator) for susceptible HCWs. In immunocompromised host with varicella pneumonia, prolong duration of precautions for duration of illness. Postexposure prophylaxis: provide postexposure vaccine as soon as possible but within 120hr; for susceptible exposed persons for whom vaccine is contraindicated (immunocompromised persons, pregnant women, newborns whose mother's varicella onset is ≥5days before delivery or within 48hr after delivery), provide VZIG, when available, within 96hr; if unavailable, use IVIG. Use airborne precautions for exposed susceptible persons, and exclude exposed susceptible HCWs beginning 8 days after first exposure until 21 days after last exposure or 28 days if received VZIG, regardless of postexposure vaccination (Watson et al, 2000).
Variola (see smallpox)			
Vibrio parahaemolyticus (see gastroenteritis)			
Vincent angina (trench mouth)	S		
Viral hemorrhagic fevers due to Lassa, Ebola, Marburg, Crimean-Congo fever viruses	S, D, C	DI	Single-patient room is preferred. Emphasize (1) use of sharps safety devices and safe work practices; (2) hand hygiene; (3) barrier protection against blood and body fluids upon entry into room (single gloves and fluid-resistant or impermeable gown, face/eye protection with masks, goggles or face shields); and (4) appropriate waste handling. Use N95 or higher respirators when performing aerosol-generating procedures. Largest viral load is in final stages of illness when hemorrhage may occur; additional PPE, including double gloves, leg and shoe coverings, may be used, especially in resource-limited settings where options for cleaning and laundry are limited. Notify public health officials immediately if Ebola is suspected (http://www.bt.cdc.gov/agent/vhf; CDC, 1995; Borio et al, 2002; CDC, 2003).

Viral respiratory diseases (not covered elsewhere)			
Adults	S		
Infants and young children (see respiratory infectious disease, acute)			
Whooping cough (see pertussis)			
Wound infections			
Major	C	DI	No dressing or dressing does not contain drainage adequately
Minor or limited	S		Dressing covers and contains drainage adequately.
Yersinia enterocolitica gastroenteritis (see gastroenteritis)			
Zoster (varicella zoster) (see herpes zoster)			
Zygomycosis (phycomycosis, mucormycosis)	S		Not transmitted person to person

AFB, Acid-fast bacilli; *AIIR*, airborne infection isolation room; *CF*, cystic fibrosis; *DEET*, diethyltoluamide; *ESBL*, extended-spectrum beta-lactamase; *HAI*, health care–associated infection; *HCW*, health care worker; *HHV-6*, human herpesvirus-6; *IND*, investigational new drug; *IVIG*, intravenous immunoglobulin; *LTCF*, long-term care facility; *MRSA*, methicillin-resistant *Staphylococcus aureus; NICU*, neonatal intensive care unit; *PAPR*, powered air-purifying respirator; *PPE*, personal protective equipment; *RSV*, respiratory syncytial virus; *SARS*, severe acquired respiratory syndrome; *SARS-CoV*, SARS-associated coronavirus; *Tdap*, diphtheria and reduced tetanus toxoids and acellular pertussis vaccine; *vCJD*, variant Creutzfeldt-Jakob disease; VISA, vancomycin-intermediate *Staphylococcus aureus; VRE*, vancomycin-resistant enterococci; *VRSA*, vancomycin-resistant *Staphylococcus aureus; VZIG*, varicella-zoster immune globulin.

* Type of precautions: *A*, Airborne precautions; *C*, contact; *D*, droplet; *S*, standard; when A, C, and D are specified, also use S.

† Duration of precautions: *CN*, Until off antimicrobial treatment and culture negative; *DI*, duration of illness (with wound lesions, *DI* means until wounds stop draining); *DE*, until environment is completely decontaminated; *U*, until time specified in hours (hr) after initiation of effective therapy; *Unknown*: criteria for establishing eradication of pathogen has not been determined.

Modified from Siegel JD et al: *2007 Guideline for isolation precautions: preventing transmission of infectious agents in healthcare settings*, available at http://www.cdc.gov/ncidod/dhqp/pdf/guidelines/Isolation2007.pdf.

Buffington J, et al: Epidemic keratoconjunctivitis in a chronic care facility: risk factors and measures for control, *J Am Geriatr Soc* 41(11):1177–1181, 1993.

Carl M, et al: Excretion of hepatitis A virus in the stools of hospitalized hepatitis patients, *J Med Virol* 9(2):125–129, 1982.

Carter RJ, et al: Failure to control an outbreak of multidrug-resistant *Streptococcus pneumoniae* in a long-term-care facility: emergence and ongoing transmission of a fluoroquinolone resistant strain, *Infect Control Hosp Epidemiol* 26(3):248–255, 2005.

Centers for Disease Control and Prevention (CDC): Update: universal precautions for prevention of transmission of human immunodeficiency virus, hepatitis B virus, and other bloodborne pathogens in health-care settings, *MMWR Morb Mortal Wkly Rep* 37(24):377–382, 1988.

Centers for Disease Control and Prevention (CDC): Recommendations for preventing the spread of vancomycin resistance: recommendations of the Hospital Infection Control Practices Advisory Committee (HICPAC), *MMWR Recomm Rep* 44(RR-12):1–13, 1995.

Centers for Disease Control and Prevention (CDC): Measles, mumps, and rubella—vaccine use and strategies for elimination of measles, rubella, and congenital rubella syndrome and control of mumps: recommendations of the Advisory Committee on Immunization Practices (ACIP), *MMWR Recomm Rep* 47(RR-8):1–57, 1998.

Centers for Disease Control and Prevention (CDC): Human rabies prevention—United States, 1999 Recommendations of the Advisory Committee on Immunization Practices (ACIP), *MMWR Recomm Rep* 48(RR-1):1–21, 1999a.

Centers for Disease Control and Prevention (CDC): Prevention of hepatitis A through active or passive immunization: recommendations of the Advisory Committee on Immunization Practices (ACIP), *MMWR Recomm Rep* 48(RR-12):1–37, 1999b.

Centers for Disease Control and Prevention (CDC): Guidelines for preventing opportunistic infections among hematopoietic stem cell transplant recipients: recommendations of CDC, the Infectious Disease Society of America, and the American Society of Blood and Marrow Transplantation, *MMWR Morb Mortal Wkly Rep* 49(RR-10):1–125, 2000.

Centers for Disease Control and Prevention (CDC): "Norwalk-like viruses": public health consequences and outbreak management, *MMWR Morb Mortal Wkly Rep* 50(RR-09): 1–18, 2001a (June).

Centers for Disease Control and Prevention (CDC): Updated U.S. Public Health Service guidelines for the management of occupational exposures to HBV, HCV, and HIV, *MMWR Recomm Rep* 50(RR-11):1–52, 2001b.

Centers for Disease Control and Prevention (CDC): Vaccinia (smallpox) vaccine: recommendations of the Advisory Committee on Immunization Practices (ACIP), 2001, *MMWR Recomm Rep* 50(RR-10):1–25, 2001c quiz CE1–7.

Centers for Disease Control and Prevention (CDC): Prevention of invasive group A streptococcal disease among household contacts of case patients and among postpartum and postsurgical patients: recommendations from the Centers for Disease Control and Prevention, *Clin Infect Dis* 35(8): 950–959, 2002.

Centers for Disease Control and Prevention (CDC): *Emergency preparedness and response*, 2003, available at www.bt.cdc.gov.

Centers for Disease Control and Prevention (CDC): Acute hemorrhagic conjunctivitis outbreak caused by coxsackievirus A24—Puerto Rico, 2003, *MMWR Morb Mortal Wkly Rep* 53(28):632–634, 2004.

Centers for Disease Control and Prevention (CDC): Guidelines for preventing the transmission of *Mycobacterium tuberculosis* in health-care settings, 2005, *MMWR Recomm Rep* 54(17):1–141, 2005a.

Centers for Disease Control and Prevention (CDC): Prevention and control of influenza: recommendations of the Advisory Committee on Immunization Practices (ACIP), *MMWR Recomm Rep* 54(RR-8):1–40, 2005b.

Centers for Disease Control and Prevention (CDC): Recommended antimicrobial agents for the treatment and postexposure prophylaxis of pertussis: 2005 CDC guidelines, *MMWR Recomm Rep* 54(RR-14):1–16, 2005c.

Centers for Disease Control and Prevention (CDC): Updated U.S. Public Health Service guidelines for the management of occupational exposures to HIV and recommendations for postexposure prophylaxis, *MMWR Recomm Rep* 54(RR-9):1–17, 2005d.

Centers for Disease Control and Prevention (CDC): West Nile virus infections in organ transplant recipients—New York and Pennsylvania, August-September, 2005, *MMWR Morb Mortal Wkly Rep* 54(40):1021–1023, 2005e.

Chaberny IE, et al: An outbreak of epidemic keratoconjunctivitis in a pediatric unit due to adenovirus type 8, *Infect Control Hosp Epidemiol* 24(7):514–519, 2003.

Cheesbrough JS, et al: Widespread environmental contamination with Norwalk-like viruses (NLV) detected in a prolonged hotel outbreak of gastroenteritis, *Epidemiol Infect* 125(1):93–98, 2000.

Chidekel AS, et al: Rhinovirus infection associated with serious lower respiratory illness in patients with bronchopulmonary dysplasia, *Pediatr Infect Dis J* 16(1):43–47, 1997.

Colodner R, et al: *Listeria monocytogenes* cross-contamination in a nursery, *Am J Infect Control* 31(5):322–324, 2003.

Committee on Infectious Diseases (COID): 2003 Report of the Committee on Infectious Diseases. In Red Book, Elk Grove Village, Ill, 2003, American Academy of Pediatrics.

Dick EC, et al: Aerosol transmission of rhinovirus colds, *J Infect Dis* 156(3):442–448, 1987.

Dixon CW: Smallpox in Tripolitania, 1946: an epidemiological and clinical study of 500 cases, including trials of penicillin treatment, *J Hyg (Lond)* 46:351–377, 1948.

Doultree JC, et al: Inactivation of feline calicivirus, a Norwalk virus surrogate, *J Hosp Infect* 41(1):51–57, 1999.

Drusin LM, et al: Nosocomial ringworm in a neonatal intensive care unit: a nurse and her cat, *Infect Control Hosp Epidemiol* 21(9):605–607, 2000.

Eickhoff TC: An outbreak of surgical wound infections due to *Clostridium perfringens*, *Surg Gynecol Obstet* 114:102–108, 1962.

Ekman MR, et al: An epidemic of infections due to *Chlamydia pneumoniae* in military conscripts, *Clin Infect Dis* 17(3): 420–425, 1993.

Elizaga J, et al: Parainfluenza virus 3 infection after stem cell transplant: relevance to outcome of rapid diagnosis and ribavirin treatment, *Clin Infect Dis* 32(3):413–418, 2001.

Enright AM, Prober CG: Neonatal herpes infection: diagnosis, treatment and prevention, *Semin Neonatol* 7(4):283–291, 2002.

Esper F, et al: Human metapneumovirus infection in the United States: clinical manifestations associated with a newly emerging respiratory infection in children, *Pediatrics* 111(6 Pt 1):1407–1410, 2003.

Faden H, et al: Outbreak of adenovirus type 30 in a neonatal intensive care unit, *J Pediatr* 146(4):523–527, 2005.

Farber JM, et al: Neonatal listeriosis due to cross-infection confirmed by isoenzyme typing and DNA fingerprinting, *J Infect Dis* 163(4):927–928, 1991.

Fenner F, et al: The epidemiology of smallpox. In *Smallpox and its eradication*, Geneva, Switzerland, 1988, World Health Organization.

Fleischauer AT, et al: Evaluation of human-to-human transmission of monkeypox from infected patients to health care workers, *Clin Infect Dis* 40(5):689–694, 2005.

Fliegel PE, Weinstein WM: Rubella outbreak in a prenatal clinic: management and prevention, *Am J Infect Control* 10(1): 29–33, 1982.

Fowler RA, et al: Transmission of severe acute respiratory syndrome during intubation and mechanical ventilation, *Am J Respir Crit Care Med* 169(11):1198–1202, 2004.

Frampton MW: An outbreak of tuberculosis among hospital personnel caring for a patient with a skin ulcer, *Ann Intern Med* 117(4):312–313, 1992.

Fry AM, et al: Persistence of fluoroquinolone-resistant, multidrug-resistant *Streptococcus pneumoniae* in a long-term-care facility: efforts to reduce intrafacility transmission, *Infect Control Hosp Epidemiol* 26(3):239–247, 2005.

Fulginiti VA, et al: Smallpox vaccination: a review. I. Background, vaccination technique, normal vaccination and revaccination, and expected normal reactions, *Clin Infect Dis* 37(2):241–250, 2003.

Gehrke C, et al: Inactivation of feline calicivirus, a surrogate of norovirus (formerly Norwalk-like viruses), by different types of alcohol in vitro and in vivo, *J Hosp Infect* 56(1): 49–55, 2004.

Gelfand HM, Posch J: The recent outbreak of smallpox in Meschede, West Germany, *Am J Epidemiol* 93(4):234–237, 1971.

Gerber AR, et al: Increased risk of illness among nursery staff caring for neonates with necrotizing enterocolitis, *Pediatr Infect Dis* 4(3):246–249, 1985.

Gleich S, et al: *Streptococcus pneumoniae* serotype 4 outbreaks in a home for the aged: report and review of recent outbreaks, *Infect Control Hosp Epidemiol* 21:711, 2000.

Greene CM, et al: Cluster of deaths from group A streptococcus in a long-term care facility—Georgia, 2001, *Am J Infect Control* 33(2):108–113, 2005.

Hall CB: Nosocomial respiratory syncytial virus infections: the "Cold War" has not ended, *Clin Infect Dis* 31(2):590–596, 2000.

Hall CB, et al: Respiratory syncytial viral infection in children with compromised immune function, *N Engl J Med* 315(2):77–81, 1986.

Hatherill M, et al: Evolution of an adenovirus outbreak in a multidisciplinary children's hospital, *J Paediatr Child Health* 40(8):449–454, 2004.

Hayden FG: Rhinovirus and the lower respiratory tract, *Rev Med Virol* 14(1):17–31, 2004.

Heymann DL, editor: *Control of communicable diseases manual*, ed 18, Washington, DC, 2005, American Public Health Association.

Houff SA, et al: Human-to-human transmission of rabies virus by corneal transplant, *N Engl J Med* 300(11):603–604, 1979.

Hutton MD, et al: Nosocomial transmission of tuberculosis associated with a draining abscess, *J Infect Dis* 161(2): 286–295, 1990.

Inactivation of caliciviruses, *Appl Environ Microbiol* 70(8): 4538–4543, 2004.

Inglesby TV, et al: Anthrax as a biological weapon, 2002: updated recommendations for management, *JAMA* 287(17): 2236–2252, 2002.

Jain SK, et al: Nosocomial malaria and saline flush, *Emerg Infect Dis* 11(7):1097–1099, 2005.

Jernigan JA, et al: Adenovirus type 8 epidemic keratoconjunctivitis in an eye clinic: risk factors and control, *J Infect Dis* 167(6):1307–1313, 1993.

Jernigan JA, et al: A randomized crossover study of disposable thermometers for prevention of *Clostridium difficile* and other nosocomial infections, *Infect Control Hosp Epidemiol* 19(7):494–499, 1998.

Kakis A, et al: An outbreak of group A streptococcal infection among health care workers, *Clin Infect Dis* 35(11): 1353–1359, 2002.

Kohn GJ, et al: Acquisition of coccidioidomycosis at necropsy by inhalation of coccidioidal endospore, *Diagn Microbiol Infect Dis* 15(6):527–530, 1992.

Kool JL: Risk of person-to-person transmission of pneumonic plague, *Clin Infect Dis* 40(8):1166–1172, 2005.

LeClair JM, et al: Prevention of nosocomial respiratory syncytial virus infections through compliance with glove and gown isolation precautions, *N Engl J Med* 317(6):329–334, 1987.

Lewis SM, Lewis BG: Nosocomial transmission of *Trichophyton tonsurans* tinea corporis in a rehabilitation hospital, *Infect Control Hosp Epidemiol* 18(5):322–325, 1997.

Loeb M, et al: SARS among critical care nurses, Toronto, *Emerg Infect Dis* 10(2):251–255, 2004.

Louie JK, et al: Rhinovirus outbreak in a long term care facility for elderly persons associated with unusually high mortality, *Clin Infect Dis* 41(2):262–265, 2005.

Lui SL, et al: Nosocomial outbreak of parvovirus B19 infection in a renal transplant unit, *Transplantation* 71(1):59–64, 2001.

Madge P, et al: Prospective controlled study of four infection-control procedures to prevent nosocomial infection with respiratory syncytial virus, *Lancet* 340(8827):1079–1083, 1992.

Maitreyi RS, et al: Acute hemorrhagic conjunctivitis due to enterovirus 70 in India, *Emerg Infect Dis* 5(2):267–269, 1999.

Management of multidrug-resistant organisms in healthcare settings, 2006, 2006, CDC, available at www.cdc.gov/ncidod/dhqp/pdf/ar/mdroguideline2006.pdf. Accessed 2007.

Mandell GL, et al: *Mandell, Douglas and Bennett's principles and practice of infectious diseases*, ed 5, Philadelphia, 2000, Churchill Livingstone.

Marks PJ, et al: A school outbreak of Norwalk-like virus: evidence for airborne transmission, *Epidemiol Infect* 131(1):727–736, 2003.

Mejias A, et al: Human metapneumovirus: a not so new virus, *Pediatr Infect Dis J* 23(1):1–7, 2004; quiz 8–10.

Montessori V, et al: Epidemic keratoconjunctivitis outbreak at a tertiary referral eye care clinic, *Am J Infect Control* 26(4): 399–405, 1998.

Mori I, et al: Prolonged shedding of rotavirus in a geriatric inpatient, *J Med Virol* 67(4):613–615, 2002.

Munoz FM, et al: Tuberculosis among adult visitors of children with suspected tuberculosis and employees at a children's hospital, *Infect Control Hosp Epidemiol* 23(10):568–572, 2002.

Musher DM: How contagious are common respiratory tract infections?, *N Engl J Med* 348(13):1256–1266, 2003.

Nichols WG, et al: Parainfluenza virus infections after hematopoietic stem cell transplantation: risk factors, response to antiviral therapy, and effect on transplant outcome, *Blood* 98(3):573–578, 2001.

Nuorti JP, et al: An outbreak of multidrug resistant pneumococcal pneumonia and bacteremia among unvaccinated nursing home residents, *N Engl J Med* 338(26):1861–1868, 1998.

O'Brien KL, et al: Epidemiology of invasive group A streptococcus disease in the United States, 1995–1999, *Clin Infect Dis* 35(3):268–276, 2002.

Occupationally acquired human immunodeficiency virus (HIV) infection: national case surveillance data during 20 years of the HIV epidemic in the United States, *Infect Control Hosp Epidemiol* 24(2):86–96, 2003.

Pegues DA, et al: Cluster of cases of invasive aspergillosis in a transplant intensive care unit: evidence of person-to-person airborne transmission, *Clin Infect Dis* 34(3):412–416, 2002.

Pejaver RK, et al: Neonatal cross-infection with *Listeria monocytogenes*, *J Infect* 26(3):301–303, 1993.

Piro S, et al: Hospital-acquired malaria transmitted by contaminated gloves, *J Hosp Infect* 47(2):156–158, 2001.

Ramage L, et al: An outbreak of fatal nosocomial infections due to group A streptococcus on a medical ward, *Infect Control Hosp Epidemiol* 17(7):429–431, 1996.

Robichaud S, et al: Prevention of laboratory-acquired brucellosis, *Clin Infect Dis* 38(12):e119–e122, 2004.

Robson SC, et al: Hospital outbreak of hepatitis E, *Lancet* 339(8806):1424–1425, 1992.

Rosenblum LS, et al: Hepatitis A outbreak in a neonatal intensive care unit: risk factors for transmission and evidence of prolonged viral excretion among preterm infants, *J Infect Dis* 164(3):476–482, 1991.

Rotbart HA, Levin MJ: How contagious is necrotizing enterocolitis?, *Pediatr Infect Dis* 2(5):406–413, 1983.

Rotbart HA, et al: An outbreak of rotavirus-associated neonatal necrotizing enterocolitis, *J Pediatr* 103(3):454–459, 1983.

Ruben B, et al: Person-to-person transmission of *Brucella melitensis*, *Lancet* 337(8732):14–15, 1991.

Ruuskanen O, et al: Measles vaccination after exposure to natural measles, *J Pediatr* 93(1):43–46, 1978.

Saiman L, Siegel J: Infection control recommendations for patients with cystic fibrosis: microbiology, important pathogens, and infection control practices to prevent patient-to-patient transmission, *Infect Control Hosp Epidemiol* 24(5 Suppl):S6–S52, 2003.

Saiman L, et al: Molecular epidemiology of staphylococcal scalded skin syndrome in premature infants, *Pediatr Infect Dis J* 17(4):329–334, 1998.

Sampathkumar P: West Nile virus: epidemiology, clinical presentation, diagnosis, and prevention, *Mayo Clin Proc* 78(9):1137–1143, 2003; quiz 1144.

Sanchez MP, et al: Outbreak of adenovirus 35 pneumonia among adult residents and staff of a chronic care psychiatric facility, *J Infect Dis* 176(3):760–763, 1997.

Sawyer LA, et al: 25- to 30-nm virus particle associated with a hospital outbreak of acute gastroenteritis with evidence for airborne transmission, *Am J Epidemiol* 127(6):1261–1271, 1988.

Scales D, et al: Illness in intensive-care staff after brief exposure to severe acute respiratory syndrome, *Emerg Infect Dis* 9(10):1205–1210, 2003.

Schuchat A, et al: Outbreak of neonatal listeriosis associated with mineral oil, *Pediatr Infect Dis J* 10(3):183–189, 1991.

Schwartz B, et al: Clusters of invasive group A streptococcal infections in family, hospital, and nursing home settings, *Clin Infect Dis* 15(2):277–284, 1992.

Singh-Naz N, et al: Nosocomial adenovirus infection: molecular epidemiology of an outbreak, *Pediatr Infect Dis J* 12(11): 922–925, 1993.

Srinivasan A, et al: Transmission of rabies virus from an organ donor to four transplant recipients, *N Engl J Med* 352(11):1103–1111, 2005.

Talbot TR, et al: Risk of vaccinia transfer to the hands of vaccinated persons after smallpox immunization, *Clin Infect Dis* 38(4):536–541, 2004.

Thacker SB, et al: Parasitic disease control in a residential facility for the mentally retarded: failure of selected isolation procedures, *Am J Public Health* 71(3):303–305, 1981.

Troy CJ, et al: *Chlamydia pneumoniae* as a new source of infectious outbreaks in nursing homes, *JAMA* 277(15):1214–1218, 1997.

Uemura T, et al: A recent outbreak of adenovirus type 7 infection in a chronic inpatient facility for the severely handicapped, *Infect Control Hosp Epidemiol* 21(9):559–560, 2000.

Valenti WM, et al: Concurrent outbreaks of rhinovirus and respiratory syncytial virus in an intensive care nursery: epidemiology and associated risk factors, *J Pediatr* 100(5):722–726, 1982.

van Tol MJ, et al: Adenovirus infection in children after allogeneic stem cell transplantation: diagnosis, treatment and immunity, *Bone Marrow Transplant* 35(Suppl 1):S73–S76, 2005.

Vandercam B, et al: Isolation of *Brucella melitensis* from human sperm, *Eur J Clin Microbiol Infect Dis* 9(4):303–304, 1990.

Vreden SG, et al: Outbreak of amebiasis in a family in The Netherlands, *Clin Infect Dis* 31(4):1101–1104, 2000.

Wang CY, et al: Nosocomial transmission of cryptococcosis, *N Engl J Med* 352(12):1271–1272, 2005.

Warren D, et al: A large outbreak of epidemic keratoconjunctivitis: problems in controlling nosocomial spread, *J Infect Dis* 160(6):938–943, 1989.

Watson B, et al: Postexposure effectiveness of varicella vaccine, *Pediatrics* 105(1 Pt 1):84–88, 2000.

Weber DJ, et al: Efficacy of selected hand hygiene agents used to remove *Bacillus atrophaeus* (a surrogate of *Bacillus anthracis*) from contaminated hands, *JAMA* 289(10): 1274–1277, 2003.

Weinstock DM, et al: Prolonged shedding of multidrug-resistant influenza A virus in an immunocompromised patient, *N Engl J Med* 348(9):867–868, 2003.

Wharton M, et al: Recommendations for using smallpox vaccine in a pre-event vaccination program: supplemental recommendations of the Advisory Committee on Immunization Practices (ACIP) and the Healthcare Infection Control Practices Advisory Committee (HICPAC), *MMWR Recomm Rep* 52(RR-7):1–16, 2003.

Widdowson MA, et al: Probable transmission of norovirus on an airplane, *JAMA* 293(15):1859–1860, 2005.

Wilcox MH, et al: Comparison of the effect of detergent versus hypochlorite cleaning on environmental contamination and incidence of *Clostridium difficile* infection, *J Hosp Infect* 54(2):109–114, 2003.

Wood DJ, et al: Chronic enteric virus infection in two T-cell immunodeficient children, *J Med Virol* 24(4):435–444, 1988.

Wright PW, et al: Donor-related coccidioidomycosis in organ transplant recipients, *Clin Infect Dis* 37(9):1265–1269, 2003.

INDEX

Note: Page numbers followed by *b* indicates boxes; *f* indicates figures; *t* indicates tables.